Clinical Dentistry Daily Reference Guide

Clinical Dentistry Daily Reference Guide

William A. Jacobson, DMD, MPH

General Dentist
One Community Health
Sacramento, CA, USA

Assistant Clinical Professor
Preventive and Restorative Dental Sciences
University of California, San Francisco (UCSF) School of Dentistry
San Francisco, CA, USA

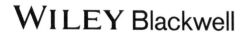
WILEY Blackwell

Registered Office
John Wiley & Sons, Inc., 111 River Street, Hoboken, NJ 07030, USA

Editorial Office
111 River Street, Hoboken, NJ 07030, USA

For details of our global editorial offices, customer services, and more information about Wiley products visit us at www.wiley.com.

Wiley also publishes its books in a variety of electronic formats and by print-on-demand. Some content that appears in standard print versions of this book may not be available in other formats.

Library of Congress Cataloging-in-Publication Data applied for

PB ISBN: 9781119690719

Cover Design: Wiley
Cover Image: © William A. Jacobson, DMD, MPH

Set in 9.5/12.5pt STIXTwoText by Straive, Pondicherry

SKY10084002_090624

Brief Contents

Contents

About the Author

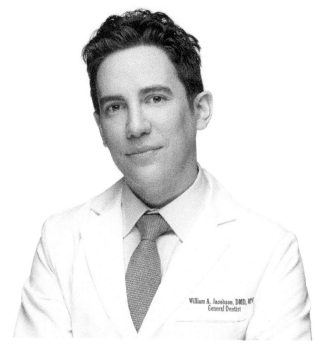

Courtesy: Kevin Fiscus Photography

Dr. William Jacobson is a general dentist and an educator. He completed his Bachelor of Arts in Fine Arts at University of San Francisco. Dr. Jacobson received a Doctor of Dental Medicine, Master of Public Health, and various awards of recognition at Case Western Reserve University. To further his training, he completed a General Practice Residency at University of Southern California where he treated medically compromised patients at LAC+USC Medical Center and at the Los Angeles Veterans Affairs. Since completing residency, Dr. Jacobson has been practicing general dentistry at community clinics treating the underserved. He is an Assistant Clinical Professor at University of California, San Francisco School of Dentistry. Dr. Jacobson is also a consultant for the curriculum committee at California Northstate University, College of Dental Medicine.

Dr. Jacobson is a member of the American Dental Association, California Dental Association, and the Sacramento District Dental Society. He is a native Spanish speaker and in his free time enjoys painting.

To contact the author, email CDDRGauthor@gmail.com

Preface

Why I Wrote this Book?

Picture the following scenario. Monday morning you arrive to work:

8 a.m. You need to figure out how to calculate the dosage for amoxicillin in liquid form for a 40-pound child.

9 a.m. A teenager shows up with an avulsed tooth from a skateboard accident and you need to review the dental trauma guidelines before treating the patient.

10 a.m. A patient is requesting nitrous oxide sedation for a filling and you need to quickly review all the indications, contraindications, and steps for administering nitrous, since it has been over a year since you last did this.

11 a.m. A patient comes in for an extraction and reports a history of radiation and chemotherapy and you are unsure if any treatment modifications are necessary.

11 a.m. You are double booked with a patient whose cast metal partial denture just broke and you are not sure what the dental lab needs from you. Just the broken partial? An opposing impression? A bite? A pick-up impression?

The scenarios are endless and it can be overwhelming having to scramble through various sources, from consulting other providers to websites to phone apps to books, to find critical information in a timely manner in order to provide our patients with the safest and best possible care.

The philosopher Plato said, "necessity is the mother of invention," and for me as a practicing dentist and educator, a book like this is indispensable. For this reason, I made it my goal to write this book to make our lives easier as dentists.

The Journey from Conception to a Published Book

In dental school we entered clinic full time in third year. To cope with the fears that came along with treating human patients (non-manikin) for the first time, I made it my mantra to "learn from every patient encounter," regardless of the procedure. Every night I would go home and write in my journal. These "daily lessons" included reflecting on the clinical experiences of the day, along with researching answers to questions my patients would ask or I would ask myself. Later I learned that this is referred to as self-directed learning. The "daily lesson" journal entries continued through my General Practice Residency, working at community clinics, and teaching dental students. While teaching dental students at UCSF I came to realize that these students could benefit from my "daily lessons" journal entries that are mostly collecting dust on a bookshelf.

Someone told me "if you have dreams chase them." Writing this book was one of my dreams and I was determined to realize it, but how? One day I sat on my sofa staring at my bookshelf of dental books. I homed in on the names of the various publishing companies and decided to pitch my idea to them with a formal book proposal. I was ecstatic to hear that John Wiley & Sons, Inc. was intrigued and believed in my vision.

Writing a book is an arduous process. Many challenges were faced, including how to create a book that is both concise and comprehensive, how to write to an audience ranging from dental students to seasoned dentists, how to make time to write a book while teaching dental students and working at a community clinic, and finding dental and medical professionals willing to offer their time to review my chapters.

The manuscript writing process involved clinical information from many sources. I consolidated my "daily lessons" notes from dental school, general practice residency and practicing dentistry, and teaching dental students. Contributions also came from continuing education courses, textbooks, and journal articles. I added my clinical photos, made illustrations, created tables, and obtained permissions to reprint clinical guidelines and figures from various sources. Lastly I consulted with general dentists, dental specialists, lab technicians, pharmacists, pediatricians, academicians, and dental assistants.

To my Readers

Thank you for your support! Whether you are a dental student, a dental resident, a new graduate, a seasoned dentist, a dental educator, or other dental professional, I hope this book provides you with the tools you need to offer the safest, ethical, and best dentistry you can for your patients.

If you have questions or suggestions contact me at CDDRGauthor@gmail.com

Acknowledgments

Thank you John Wiley & Sons, Inc. for believing in my vision and for giving me this opportunity to create a book designed to help dental professionals navigate dentistry which ultimately helps patients. A special thank you to Erica, Tanya, Ranjit, Hari, Susan, and Angela at Wiley.

To the following reviewers, thank you for your time, encouragement, and input:

- Richard Green, DDS, MSEd, FACD, FIDC
- Mark Mehrali, DDS
- Dawn Stock, DDS
- Jim Grisdale, DDS, Dip. Prosth, Dip. Perio., MRCD(C)
- Craig Noblett, DDS, MS
- Rich Hirschinger, DDS, MBA
- Mark Horton, DMD, MSD
- Craig Alpha, DDS
- Carl Choi, DDS, MD
- Justin Shek, DDS
- Joy Vongspanich Dray, PharmD, BCACP, AAHIVP
- Tamara Todd, MD FAAP
- The Certified Dental Technicians at Laguna Dental Arts in Elk Grove, California especially Chris, Su, Layne, Mark and Carrie
- Andrea Francillette, RDA

Special thanks to:

- Merissa Ferrar DDS, CCA
- Maria Theresa Hernandez, RDA

Thank you to my students that inspire me, and to my patients who are my greatest teachers. Thank you to my friends, family, and colleagues for your encouragement, especially:

- Mom, gracias por todo que me has dado, tu amor, pacencia, y tiempo.
- Dad, for your wisdom, for helping me keep things in perspective, and for never making me feel like a loser.
- John, my brother, for being a visionary and for assuring me during the days of my pre-dental science courses that the other students in my classes did not have higher IQs than me but that success comes by working hard.
- Larissa, my big sister, for always brightening my day no matter how gray.
- My best friend Catherine for being my boulder, my confidant, and my muse.
- And to Pamela Caviness, my previous Dental Director and now friend, for telling me "Don't doubt yourself for a second" before embarking on this project.

List of Abbreviations

AAE	American Association of Endodontists
AAO	American Association of Orthodontists
AAOS	American Academy of Orthopedic Surgeons
AAP	American Academy of Pediatrics; American Academy of Periodontology
AAPD	American Academy of Pediatric Dentistry
AAT	animal-assisted therapy
AB	antibiotics
ADA	American Dental Association
AED	automated external defibrillator
AIDS	acquired immunodeficiency syndrome
ALT	alanine aminotransferase
AMA	Against Medical Advice (form)
Appt	appointment
aPTT	activated partial thromboplastin time
ART	antiretroviral therapy
AST	aspartate aminotransferase
ASAP	as soon as possible
B	buccal
BLS	Basic Life Support
BMI	body mass index
BOP	bleeding on probing
BP	blood pressure
bpm	beats per minute
BRONJ	bisphosphonate-related osteonecrosis of the jaw
BW	bitewing (radiograph)
CABG	coronary artery bypass graft
CAL	clinical attachment level
CAMBRA	Caries Management by Risk Assessment
CAR	conservative adhesive restoration
CBC	complete blood count
CBCT	cone beam computed tomography
CC	chief complaint
CDC	Centers for Disease Control and Prevention
CDT	Current Dental Terminology
CEJ	cementoenamel junction

Chp	chapter
COE	comprehensive oral evaluation
COMT	catechol-O-methyltransferase
COPD	chronic obstructive pulmonary disease
CPAP	continuous positive airway pressure
CPR	cardiopulmonary resuscitation
CR	centric relation
CVA	cerebrovascular accident
D	distal
DEA	Drug Enforcement Administration
DM	diabetes mellitus
DOB	date of birth
DP	distal palatal
DVT	deep vein thrombosis
EDTA	ethylenediaminetetraacetic acid
e.g.	for example
EMS	emergency medical services
EOE	extraoral exam
ER	emergency room
F	facial
FDA	Food and Drug Administration
FMX	full-mouth examination
FPD	fixed partial denture
GERD	gastroesophageal reflux disease
GI	glass ionomer
HBSS	Hanks' balanced salt solution
HCR	high caries risk
HIPAA	Health Insurance Portability and Accountability Act
HIV	human immunodeficiency virus
HOCL	height of contour line
HPV	human papillomavirus
HTN	hypertension
HVE	high volume evacuator
IANB	inferior alveolar nerve block
i.e.	that is
INR	international normalized ratio
IOE	intraoral exam
IRT	interim therapeutic restorations
IV	intravenous
L	lingual
LED	light-emitting diode
LSTR	lesion sterilization/tissue repair
M	mesial
MAOI	monoamine oxidase inhibitor
MI	myocardial infarction
MICP	maximum intercuspation
Misc	miscellaneous

MME	morphine milligram equivalents
MP	mesial palatal
MR	marginal ridge
MRD	maximum recommended dose
MRONJ	medication-related osteonecrosis of the jaw
MRSA	methicillin-resistant *Staphylococcus aureus*
MS	multiple sclerosis
MTA	mineral trioxide aggregate
NIDCR	National Institute for Dental and Craniofacial Research
NPI	National Provider Identifier
NSAID	nonsteroidal anti-inflammatory drug
NV	next visit
O	occlusal
OCS	oral cancer screening
OHI	Oral Hygiene Index
OMFS	oral and maxillofacial surgeon
ORN	osteoradionecrosis
OTC	over the counter
PA	periapical (radiograph)
PARL	periapical radiolucency
PCP	primary care physician
PD	probing depth
PDL	periodontal ligament
PDMP	Prescription Drug Monitoring Program
PECS	picture exchange communication system
PFM	porcelain fused to metal
PIP	pressure-indicating paste
POE	periodic oral evaluation
PPS	posterior palatal seal
prophy	prophylaxis
PRR	preventive resin restoration
Pt	patient
Pt's	patient's
Pts	patients
Pts'	patients'
PT	prothrombin time
PTSD	post-traumatic stress disorder
PVS	polyvinyl siloxane
QTH	quartz–tungsten–halogen
RA	rheumatoid arthritis
RCT	root canal treatment
RIND	reversible ischemic neurologic deficit
RMGI	resin-modified glass ionomer
RPD	removable partial denture
rpm	revolutions per minute
RX	prescription
SADE	sensory-adapted dental environments

SDF	silver diamine fluoride
SLOB	same lingual opposite buccal (rule)
SM	space maintainer
SRP	scaling and root planing
SSRI	selective serotonin reuptake inhibitor
TB	tuberculosis
TIA	transient ischemic attack
TMD	temporomandibular joint disorder
TMJ	temporomandibular joint
USS	ultrasonic scaler
VDO	vertical dimension of occlusion
VDR	vertical dimension at rest
VPS	vinyl polysiloxane
vs.	versus
WBC	white blood cell (count)
WHO	World Health Organization
WL	working length
WNL	within normal limits
WOR	wax occlusal rims
WW	wrought wire

How to Read this Book

This book is not intended to be read cover to cover like a novel. How you choose to read this book is up to you. You may want to:

- Review Procedural Steps the night before a procedure.
- Consult Troubleshooting and Clinical Tips for a specific topic.
- Quickly reference information such as the Dental Trauma Guidelines or Health History Treatment Modifications.
- Understand the relevance of a topic and test your knowledge by reading Real-Life Clinical Questions.

When applicable, each chapter follows the same framework:

- Chapter Outline
- Real-Life Clinical Questions
- Relevance
- Clinical and Radiographic Exam
- Treatment Planning
- Referrals
- Informed Consent
- Procedural Steps
- Alternative Steps
- Lab Prescriptions
- Postoperative Instructions
- Pearls: Troubleshooting and Tips
- Real-Life Clinical Questions Answered

1

Health History Treatment Modifications

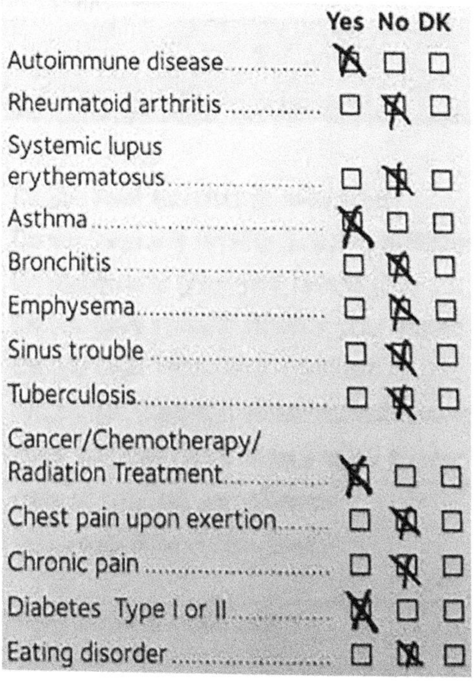

Figure 1.1 A sample health history form filled out by a patient. DK, Don't know.

Chapter Outline

- Real-Life Clinical Questions
- Relevance
- Treatment Planning
- ADA Health History Form
- General Guidelines
- Demographic Data
- Dental Information
- Medical History

Clinical Dentistry Daily Reference Guide, First Edition. William A. Jacobson.
© 2022 John Wiley & Sons, Inc. Published 2022 by John Wiley & Sons, Inc.

- Alphabetized Conditions with Treatment Modifications
- Medications
- Lab Values
  - Miscellaneous Terms
- ASA Physical Status Classification System
- Medical Consultations
  - Sample Form
- Charting Template
- Clinical Pearls
  - Troubleshooting
  - Tips
- Real-Life Clinical Questions Answered
- References

Real-Life Clinical Questions

Dental Student's Comment

- "My patient has asthma and is here for a filling."

Dental Assistants' Questions

- "Doc, how often do we have the patient fill out the health history form?"
- "Doctor, the pulse is really high, is that OK?"
- "If I take his temperature, what temperature is considered a fever?"

Patient's Daughter's Comment

- "She [the patient] is my mother and I will translate for her."

Patients' Comments

- "Yeah I take medications, but you don't need to know which ones I'm taking, you're just working on my teeth."
- "I stopped my blood thinner medication a few days before this appointment."
- "I took about 10 aspirin the last two days before today's extraction appointment."
- "My INR is always 2 so I'll be fine."
- "I have a newborn!"
- "I have HIV but I'm undetectable."
- "I had radiation to my head."
- "I had a heart attack last week but don't worry about it, I'm fine just pull the tooth."
- "I feel fine so I'm not going to the emergency room because of my blood pressure."

Patients' Questions

- "I'm pregnant. Is it safe to get dental treatment?"
- "I'm just here for my denture, so why do you need to take my blood pressure?"
- "I was diagnosed with cancer and I need a dental clearance signed."

Relevance

While you are not expected to be a physician, as a dentist you are expected to understand the patient's health history well enough to know:

- if any **treatment modifications** are necessary
- when to obtain a **medical consultation** and what to ask
- when to **refer** the patient to another provider for consultation and/or treatment.

Treatment Planning

Obtaining and updating patients' health histories is critical and occurs at various treatment planning phases. See Table 1.1

Table 1.1 Treatment planning phases related to health history.

Treatment phase	Description (may or may not apply)
Emergency phase	Urgent treatment of pain, infection, trauma, and/or esthetic emergency (provide a health history form and medical consultation as necessary)
Data gathering phase	Medical history: medical consultation as necessary
Stabilization phase (to control disease)	At every appointment ask if any changes to health history (document)
Definitive phase	At every appointment ask if any changes to health history (document)
Maintenance phase	New health history form every two years (document date) [1]

ADA Health History Form

See figure 1.2

General Guidelines

- Follow up with any questions marked "Yes" or "DK" (i.e. "Don't Know). See Figure 1.1.
- Do not allow the patient to leave any response unanswered.
- Do not allow the patient to mark one long line through all the "No" answers.
- Make sure the patient signs and dates.
- Do not provide any dental treatment to the patient until you review the entire health history form.

Demographic Data

Name: Ask "How would you like to be addressed?" Some patients are offended if they are not addressed as Mr., Mrs., Miss, Dr., etc.

   Pronouns: It's important to respect and affirm a patient's identity. If unsure which pronoun to use, ask "What pronouns would you like me to use when I refer to you?" (e.g. she/her/hers, he/him/his, they/them/theirs).

   Address: If the patient is homeless, when writing a prescription write "general delivery" [2]. However controlled substances requires an address. Ask for a form of identification and discuss with the pharmacist.

Health History Form

Email: _____ Today's Date: _____

As required by law, our office adheres to written policies and procedures to protect the privacy of information about you that we create, receive or maintain. Your answers are for our records only and will be kept confidential subject to applicable laws. Please note that you will be asked some questions about your responses to this questionnaire and there may be additional questions concerning your health. This information is vital to allow us to provide appropriate care for you. This office does not use this information to discriminate.

Name: _____ *Last* _____ *First* _____ *Middle*

Home Phone: *Include area code* ( )
Business/Cell Phone: *Include area code* ( )

Address: _____ *Mailing address*

City: _____ State: ____ Zip: ____

Occupation: _____

Height: ____ Weight: ____ Date of Birth: ____ Sex: M F

SS# or Patient ID: _____ Emergency Contact: _____

Relationship: _____ Home Phone: *Include area code* ( ) Cell Phone: *Include area code* ( )

If you are completing this form for another person, what is your relationship to that person?

Your Name _____ *Relationship* _____

Do you have any of the following diseases or problems: (*Check DK if you Don't Know the answer to the the question*)

	Yes	No	DK
Active Tuberculosis	☐	☐	☐
Persistent cough greater than a 3 week duration	☐	☐	☐
Cough that produces blood	☐	☐	☐
Been exposed to anyone with tuberculosis	☐	☐	☐

If you answer yes to any of the 4 items above, please stop and return this form to the receptionist.

Dental Information *For the following questions, please mark (X) your responses to the following questions.*

	Yes	No	DK
Do your gums bleed when you brush or floss?	☐	☐	☐
Are your teeth sensitive to cold, hot, sweets or pressure?	☐	☐	☐
Is your mouth dry?	☐	☐	☐
Have you had any periodontal (gum) treatments?	☐	☐	☐
Have you ever had orthodontic (braces) treatment?	☐	☐	☐
Have you had any problems associated with previous dental treatment?	☐	☐	☐
Is your home water supply fluoridated?	☐	☐	☐
Do you drink bottled or filtered water?	☐	☐	☐

If yes, how often? *Circle one:* DAILY / WEEKLY / OCCASIONALLY

	Yes	No	DK
Are you currently experiencing dental pain or discomfort?	☐	☐	☐

	Yes	No	DK
Do you have earaches or neck pains?	☐	☐	☐
Do you have any clicking, popping or discomfort in the jaw?	☐	☐	☐
Do you brux or grind your teeth?	☐	☐	☐
Do you have sores or ulcers in your mouth?	☐	☐	☐
Do you wear dentures or partials?	☐	☐	☐
Do you participate in active recreational activities?	☐	☐	☐
Have you ever had a serious injury to your head or mouth?	☐	☐	☐

Date of your last dental exam:
What was done at that time?

Date of last dental x-rays:

What is the reason for your dental visit today?

How do you feel about your smile?

Medical Information *Please mark (X) your response to indicate if you have or have not had any of the following diseases or problems.*

	Yes	No	DK
Are you now under the care of a physician?	☐	☐	☐

Physician Name: _____ Phone: *Include area code* ( )

Address/City/State/Zip:

	Yes	No	DK
Are you in good health?	☐	☐	☐
Has there been any change in your general health within the past year?	☐	☐	☐

If yes, what condition is being treated?

Date of last physical exam:

	Yes	No	DK
Have you had a serious illness, operation or been hospitalized in the past 5 years?	☐	☐	☐

If yes, what was the illness or problem?

	Yes	No	DK
Are you taking or have you recently taken any prescription or over the counter medicine(s)?	☐	☐	☐

If so, please list all, including vitamins, natural or herbal preparations and/or dietary supplements:

_____
_____
_____
_____
_____

Figure 1.2 ADA Health History Form. *Source:* Copyright © 2012 American Dental Asssociation. All rights reserved. Reprinted with permission.

Medical Information *Please mark (X) your response to indicate if you have or have not had any of the following diseases or problems.*

(Check DK if you Don't Know the answer to the question)

	Yes	No	DK
Do you wear contact lenses?	☐	☐	☐

Joint Replacement. Have you had an orthopedic total joint (hip, knee, elbow, finger) replacement? ☐ ☐ ☐

Date: _____ If yes, have you had any complications? _____

Are you taking or scheduled to begin taking an antiresorptive agent (like Fosamax®, Actonel®, Atelvia, Boniva®, Reclast, Prolia) for osteoporosis or Paget's disease? ☐ ☐ ☐

Since 2001, were you treated or are you presently scheduled to begin treatment with an antiresorptive agent (like Aredia®, Zometa®, XGEVA) for bone pain, hypercalcemia or skeletal complications resulting from Paget's disease, multiple myeloma or metastatic cancer? ☐ ☐ ☐

Date Treatment began: _____

Allergies. Are you allergic to or have you had a reaction to: To all **yes** responses, specify type of reaction.

	Yes	No	DK
Local anesthetics _____	☐	☐	☐
Aspirin _____	☐	☐	☐
Penicillin or other antibiotics _____	☐	☐	☐
Barbiturates, sedatives, or sleeping pills _____	☐	☐	☐
Sulfa drugs _____	☐	☐	☐
Codeine or other narcotics _____	☐	☐	☐

	Yes	No	DK
Do you use controlled substances (drugs)?	☐	☐	☐
Do you use tobacco (smoking, snuff, chew, bidis)?	☐	☐	☐

If so, how interested are you in stopping?
Circle one: VERY / SOMEWHAT / NOT INTERESTED

	Yes	No	DK
Do you drink alcoholic beverages?	☐	☐	☐

If yes, how much alcohol did you drink in the last 24 hours? _____
If yes, how much do you typically drink i n a week? _____

WOMEN ONLY Are you:

	Yes	No	DK
Pregnant?	☐	☐	☐
Number of weeks: _____			
Taking birth control pills or hormonal replacement?	☐	☐	☐
Nursing?	☐	☐	☐

	Yes	No	DK
Metals _____	☐	☐	☐
Latex (rubber) _____	☐	☐	☐
Iodine _____	☐	☐	☐
Hay fever/seasonal _____	☐	☐	☐
Animals _____	☐	☐	☐
Food _____	☐	☐	☐
Other _____	☐	☐	☐

Please mark (X) your response to indicate if you have or have not had any of the following diseases or problems.

	Yes	No	DK
Artificial (prosthetic) heart valve	☐	☐	☐
Previous infective endocarditis	☐	☐	☐
Damaged valves in transplanted heart	☐	☐	☐
Congenital heart disease (CHD)			
Unrepaired, cyanotic CHD	☐	☐	☐
Repaired (completely) in last 6 months	☐	☐	☐
Repaired CHD with residual defects	☐	☐	☐

Except for the conditions listed above, antibiotic prophylaxis is no longer recommended for any other form of CHD.

	Yes	No	DK
Cardiovascular disease	☐	☐	☐
Angina	☐	☐	☐
Arteriosclerosis	☐	☐	☐
Congestive heart failure	☐	☐	☐
Damaged heart valves	☐	☐	☐
Heart attack	☐	☐	☐
Heart murmur	☐	☐	☐
Low blood pressure	☐	☐	☐
High blood pressure	☐	☐	☐
Other congenital heart defects	☐	☐	☐

	Yes	No	DK
Mitral valve prolapse	☐	☐	☐
Pacemaker	☐	☐	☐
Rheumatic fever	☐	☐	☐
Rheumatic heart disease	☐	☐	☐
Abnormal bleeding	☐	☐	☐
Anemia	☐	☐	☐
Blood transfusion	☐	☐	☐
If yes, date: _____			
Hemophilia	☐	☐	☐
AIDS or HIV infection	☐	☐	☐
Arthritis	☐	☐	☐

	Yes	No	DK
Autoimmune disease	☐	☐	☐
Rheumatoid arthritis	☐	☐	☐
Systemic lupus erythematosus	☐	☐	☐
Asthma	☐	☐	☐
Bronchitis	☐	☐	☐
Emphysema	☐	☐	☐
Sinus trouble	☐	☐	☐
Tuberculosis	☐	☐	☐
Cancer/Chemotherapy/ Radiation Treatment	☐	☐	☐
Chest pain upon exertion	☐	☐	☐
Chronic pain	☐	☐	☐
Diabetes Type I or II	☐	☐	☐
Eating disorder	☐	☐	☐
Malnutrition	☐	☐	☐
Gastrointestinal disease	☐	☐	☐
G.E. Reflux/persistent heartburn	☐	☐	☐
Ulcers	☐	☐	☐
Thyroid problems	☐	☐	☐
Stroke	☐	☐	☐

	Yes	No	DK
Glaucoma	☐	☐	☐
Hepatitis, jaundice or liver disease	☐	☐	☐
Epilepsy	☐	☐	☐
Fainting spells or seizures	☐	☐	☐
Neurological disorders	☐	☐	☐
If yes, specify: _____			
Sleep disorder	☐	☐	☐
Do you snore?	☐	☐	☐
Mental health disorders	☐	☐	☐
Specify: _____			
Recurrent infections	☐	☐	☐
Type of infection: _____			
Kidney problems	☐	☐	☐
Night sweats	☐	☐	☐
Osteoporosis	☐	☐	☐
Persistent swollen glands in neck	☐	☐	☐
Severe headaches/ migraines	☐	☐	☐
Severe or rapid weight loss	☐	☐	☐
Sexually transmitted disease	☐	☐	☐
Excessive urination	☐	☐	☐

Has a physician or previous dentist recommended that you take antibiotics prior to your dental treatment? ☐ ☐ ☐
Name of physician or dentist making recommendation:

Phone: *Include area code*
( )

Do you have any disease, condition, or problem not listed above that you think I should know about? ☐ ☐ ☐
Please explain:

NOTE: Both doctor and patient are encouraged to discuss any and all relevant patient health issues prior to treatment.
I certify that I have read and understand the above and that the information given on this form is accurate. I understand the importance of a truthful health history and that my dentist and his/her staff will rely on this information for treating me. I acknowledge that my questions, if any, about inquiries set forth above have been answered to my satisfaction. I will not hold my dentist, or any other member of his/her staff, responsible for any action they take or do not take because of errors or omissions that I may have made in the completion of this form.

Signature of Patient/Legal Guardian: _____ Date: _____

Signature of Dentist: _____ Date: _____

FOR COMPLETION BY DENTIST

Comments: _____

Figure 1.2 (Continued)

Occupation: Helps you learn about the patient and build good rapport. Also provides insight to their educational level and how to best communicate with the patient.

Height and weight: Weight is especially important with children for determining maximum dosage of local anesthetic and medications. See Chapter 16.

Date of birth: If the patient is a minor, an adult legal caretaker must complete the health history form, sign treatment plans, sign consent forms, and accompany the patient.

If you are completing this form for another person, what is your relationship to that person? Is this a parent, sibling, other relative, court appointed conservator or legal guardian? Can the patient understand? Is an interpreter needed? Avoid family/friends interpreting due to bias, patient confidentiality, barriers to patient understanding, and ability to communicate medical/dental terms [3]. Use a professional medical interpreter.

Tuberculosis screening: See *Tuberculosis* (all subsequent cross-references to topics in section Alphabetized Conditions with Treatment Modifications are italicized).

Dental Information

Do your gums bleed when you brush or floss? Likely indicates gingivitis or periodontal disease. See Chapter 6.

Are your teeth sensitive to cold, hot, sweets or pressure? Possible recession, decay, pulpal or periapical disease. See Chapter 10.

Is your mouth dry? Risk for gum disease, caries, or sore spots from removable appliances. Determine cause. See Chapter 5.

Have you had any periodontal (gum) treatment? Useful to know if there is a history of periodontal disease and if any previous surgical/nonsurgical periodontal treatment. Currently seeing a periodontist? See Chapter 6.

Have you ever had orthodontic (braces) treatment? Ask if the patient wears a retainer. Be aware that if the patient has a retainer it may not fit after treatment (e.g. crowns). Orthodontic treatment can reveal the reason for missing teeth (e.g. premolars). If the patient is interested in braces, the orthodontist should require a "clearance" from the general dentist indicating no active dental disease (i.e. caries/periodontitis). If you are unsure about the patient's periodontal condition, do not give "clearance" and refer to a periodontist. Emphasize oral hygiene and a lifelong commitment to wearing a retainer.

Have you ever had any problems associated with previous dental treatment? Find out what type of problems. Trouble becoming anesthetized? Extractions where teeth were not successfully removed? Complications with bleeding? This is valuable information to be aware of when offering similar treatment. If the patient speaks poorly of their previous dentist, the patient could do the same thing next time about you. Don't take sides, be objective with what you see today both clinically and radiographically. Simply present the facts and contact previous dentists with any questions.

Is your home water supply fluoridated? Helps determine caries risk and knowledge level/views on fluoride. See Chapters 5 and 16.

Do you drink bottled or filtered water? Helps determine caries risk (inadequate fluoride and may be acidic). See Chapters 5 and 16.

Are you currently experiencing dental pain or discomfort? See Chapter 10.

Do you have earaches/neck pain? May be related to impacted third molar, pulpal and/or periapical disease (Chapter 8), dry socket (Chapter 9), or temporomandibular joint disorder (TMD) (Chapter 15).

Do you have any clicking, popping, or discomfort in the jaw? Related to TMD. See Chapter 15.

Do you brux or grind? Related to TMD. See Chapter 15.

Do you have sores or ulcers in your mouth? Could be related to their systemic health (Chapter 1), oral cancer (Chapter 2), to removable appliances (Chapters 12 and 13), or may require medication (Chapter 16).

Do you wear dentures or partials? See Chapters 12 and 13.

Do you participate in active recreational activities? Sports? See Chapter 15.

Have you ever had a serious injury to your head and mouth? Dental trauma? See Chapter 10. Prevention of future trauma, see Chapter 15.

Date of your last dental exam? Useful to know if the patient is overdue and the reason. Even if patient is seen by a dentist frequently, complete a thorough exam without bias (may find undiagnosed gum disease, caries, and other pathology).

What was done at that time? Helpful to know if the patient was mid-treatment, or believed all the necessary work was completed.

Find out the reason for changing offices. Did the patient move? Was the patient unhappy with the previous provider or treatment and if so why? Was the office switch related to finances?

Date of last dental X-ray? Recent? See Chapter 3.

What is the reason for your dental visit today? This is the patient's chief complaint (CC)! Listen more than you speak and ask open-ended questions. Be sure to address all the patient's CCs in the initial exam appointment.

How do you feel about your smile? Relates to the CC. Important to understand what the patient may be unhappy with esthetically so that treatment alternatives can be offered.

Medical History

Physician name/phone number/address: Provides contact information for a medical consultation. If the patient is not under the care of a physician, determine if you can treat the patient safely. If there are any red flags in the health history (or other signs and symptoms), recommend obtaining assistance from a medical provider. You are ultimately liable for whatever treatment you provide even if you consulted with a medical provider.

Has a physician or previous dentist recommended taking antibiotics prior to your dental treatment? Some patients mark "Yes" because they've been prescribed antibiotics without understanding that this question refers to prophylactic premedication with antibiotics before every dental visit. This needs to be clarified. Some patients require antibiotic premedication. See *Heart conditions*, *Joint replacement*, *Diabetes mellitus*, *HIV*, and *Splenectomy* in the following section.

Alphabetized Conditions with Treatment Modifications

A

Abnormal bleeding
In general
1) Determine the cause: bleeding disorder, medications, liver disease, alcoholism, kidney disease, or other.
2) Consult a physician or hematologist to determine if laboratory investigation is necessary and if any treatment modifications are needed for the proposed treatment plan. See section Lab Values.

3) Avoid nonsteroidal anti-inflammatory drugs (NSAIDs). Instead prescribe acetaminophen with or without codeine [4].

4) Use local hemostatic agents [4] with procedures that may cause bleeding.

5) If this is an urgent appointment and you are unable to consult beforehand, provide the least invasive treatment possible (e.g. referring to an oral maxillofacial surgeon, prescribing analgesics, pulpectomy with careful rubber dam clamp placement to reduce tissue damage, or antibiotics if indicated).

Specific disorders

Bleeding disorder: If suspected (by exam, history, or relatives), refer to a physician for a consultation prior to treatment.

Thrombocytopenia: Consult a hematologist to obtain a platelet count to determine if replacement therapy is needed before surgery. Obtain a white blood cell (WBC) count to determine if an antibiotic premed is indicated for a low WBC. See *Alcoholism, Hemophilia, Hepatitis, Kidney problems, Liver disease, von Willebrand disease.*

Medications: Obtain a complete list. Do not allow the patient to stop taking any medications without consulting a physician. See section Medications.

Adrenal issues: Goal is to avoid adrenal crisis, which is a rare and potentially lethal complication that requires prompt medical attention. A medical consultation is recommended to determine type, stability, postoperative analgesic plan, and whether a physician must prescribe supplemental corticosteroids for dental surgery, infection, trauma, and postoperative pain. There is a higher risk of adrenal crisis in primary adrenal insufficiency. Signs are nonspecific and sudden and can lead to hypovolemic shock and cardiovascular failure (tachycardia, hypotension, sweating, confusion, fever, etc.) [5]. There are several types including:

Primary adrenal insufficiency (Addison's disease): May require supplemental corticosteroids for dental surgery, stress reduction (nitrous or sedatives), long-acting local anesthetic, and blood pressure (BP) measurement every five minutes to monitor for hypotension [4].

Secondary adrenal insufficiency: Majority do not require supplemental corticosteroids, but may cause delayed healing and susceptibility to infection [4].

Hyperadrenalism (usually Cushing's syndrome): Avoid NSAIDs, monitor BP throughout appointment, and follow up due to delayed wound healing. The patient may have osteoporosis, diabetes mellitus (DM), hypertension, and peptic ulcer disease. See *Osteoporosis, Diabetes, Hypertension, Ulcers.*

Steroids: For patients on long-term steroids (months to years) consult a physician for possible supplemental steroids for dental surgery, infection, trauma, and postoperative pain.

Acquired immunodeficiency syndrome (AIDS): See *HIV and AIDS.*

Alcoholism: Determine amount of alcohol being consumed. If alcohol is on the breath, do not allow patient to consent to treatment. Report to police if the patient is under the influence, departs the office and gets into their car and drives as you could be liable. A higher dosage of local anesthetic may be required. Avoid alcohol-containing mouth rinses (Listerine, Peridex) and narcotics/sedatives due to a risk of relapse. Postpone elective care. Consult physician/clinical pharmacist when prescribing medications regarding dosage. If suspicious oral lesions are present, refer for biopsy due to higher risk for oral and pharyngeal cancer (see Chapter 2). Bleeding of the gingiva and with oral surgery is also common due to vitamin K deficiency, thrombocytopenia, or cirrhosis (alcoholic liver disease). If there is a history of alcoholic liver disease or alcohol abuse, obtain labs. Main concerns are bleeding tendencies, unpredictable drug metabolism, and risk for spread of infection. For surgery obtain the following: complete blood count (CBC) with differential, aspartate aminotransferase (AST), alanine aminotransferase (ALT), platelet count, thrombin time, activated partial thromboplastin time (aPTT), and international normalized ratio (INR) [4]. See section Lab Values. Good idea to obtain labs if an acute alcoholic seems jaundice, emaciated, etc.

Allergies: Determine if there is a true allergy or simply an adverse drug reaction. Document the reaction (e.g. anaphylactic shock) *and* how it was managed.

Local anesthetic: Always believe the patient and investigate further. Ask the patient to describe the reaction and how it was managed (medical intervention may point to true allergy), what position they were in at the time of reaction (syncope more common if not supine), whether treatment continued after the episode (minor/nonallergic), whether emergency medical provision was required (more severe), which anesthetic was given and how much (overdose), whether the anesthetic contained a vasoconstrictor or preservative (bisulfite allergy), and whether they were taking other medications at the time (drug–drug interaction). Possibly call the previous dentist or locate dental records. If still concerned, refer the patient for allergy testing and provide a list of all anesthetics used in your office.

Epinephrine: No human has a true allergy to epinephrine; however, patients may have palpitations or be sweaty or nervous due to anxiety or sensitivity to dose amount [6].

Antibiotics: If allergic to penicillin/amoxicillin recommend azithromycin or clindamycin. See Chapter 16.

Sulfa drugs (sulfonamide antibiotics): No cross-allergenicity between sulfites and "sulfa" antibiotics [6].

Bisulfites/sodium bisulfite/sulfite: Preservative in local anesthetics containing vasoconstrictors (epinephrine or levonordefrin) used to prolong the shelf-life [6]. If allergic or sensitive to these additives, use plain anesthetic instead.

Narcotics: True allergy to narcotics is not common. Some patients indicate that they have an allergy when in fact it is an adverse effect (gastrointestinal issues are the most common), or if in recovery to avoid being prescribed narcotics. See *Controlled substances* and Chapter 16.

Metals: Nickel may be a constituent of porcelain fused to metal (PFM) base metal crowns/bridges; 4.5% of the population is sensitive to nickel [7]. It is possible to request nickel-free base metal from the lab. If the patient has a silver allergy avoid silver diamine fluoride [8]. Use caution with removable partial denture (RPD) framework metals (contact lab technician for types of metals) and cast posts and cores.

Latex: Use the non-latex versions of gloves, rubber dams, and BP cuffs/stethoscope. The rubber stopper inside local anesthetic cartridges is latex free [6].

Iodine: Avoid 10% povidone iodine for scaling and root planing [9].

Lactose: Caution with milk-based proteins in prescription toothpaste.

Anemia: Determine which form and its severity, and if there is any management of it (this may require a medical consultation). If severe, only treat for emergencies. There are various oral manifestations.

Aplastic anemia: Medical consult prior to invasive treatment due to low platelet count and need for antibiotic premedication.

Iron-deficiency anemia: No treatment modifications, unless rare cases of low WBC and platelets.

Pernicious anemia: No treatment modifications.

Sickle cell trait: No risk unless severe hypoxia, infection or dehydration.

Sickle cell anemia: Antibiotic premedication with penicillin for surgical procedures to prevent wound infection or osteomyelitis (must consult physician to discuss premed and if blood transfusion indicated). For nonsurgical treatment avoid local anesthetics with epinephrine. For surgical treatment use a maximum of two cartridges of local anesthetic with epinephrine. Avoid dehydration when infection is present or postoperatively. If infection is present, treat aggressively with heat, incision and drainage, antibiotics, and procedure. Safe to use acetaminophen with or without codeine. Recommend aggressive preventive care [4].

Angina: See *Heart conditions*.

Anorexia: Patient may have xerostomia, atrophic mucosa, or enlarged parotid glands [4]. Dry mouth increases the risk of caries and periodontal disease [10]. Refer to physician for evaluation; note that there is a 20% mortality rate from cardiac arrest and suicide [4]. Be prepared for cardiopulmonary resuscitation (CPR). Patient may also be bulimic (see *Bulimia*). If patient is a minor, the parent/guardian must be informed; refer patient to physician for evaluation/treatment [4]. High caries risk. See Chapter 5.

Anxiety: Inquire about previous negative dental experiences and any of the patient's concerns. The patient may require numerous trips to the restroom, and recommend that they go before the appointment. Inform the patient when to expect discomfort and inform when things are going well. Patient may require oral sedation (Chapter 16) or nitrous (Chapter 18). Some oral diseases have psychological components, such as TMD, myofascial pain, aphthous ulcers, lichen planus, and geographic tongue [4]. Consider silver diamine fluoride (see Chapter 5).

Arteriosclerosis: Determine if the patient is taking any blood thinners or has a history of angina, heart attack, stroke, or heart surgeries (need for antibiotic premedication?). For patients with coronary atherosclerosis or ischemic heart disease, limit anesthetic with vasoconstrictor to two cartridges and show caution with NSAIDs [4].

Arthritis: The patient may have problems with manual dexterity for oral hygiene (recommend electric toothbrush and floss aids or possible help from a caregiver). Ensure the patient is in a comfortable position (pillow/towel) and make shorter appointments (temporomandibular joint involvement).

> **Rheumatoid arthritis (RA)**: Determine if the patient also has a prosthetic (see *Joint replacement*). For invasive treatment, the medications patients take for RA may be immunosuppressive, increasing infection risk. Obtain CBC.
>
> **Osteoarthritis**: Similar to RA.
>
> **Fibromyalgia**: Similar to RA.
>
> **Systemic lupus erythematosus (lupus)**: Determine the extent of systemic involvement (heart, kidneys, etc.) with a medical consult. Obtain CBC with differential (25% of these patients have thrombocytopenia, i.e. low platelets causing abnormal bleeding). If leukopenia (low WBC) is present and patient is taking corticosteroids or cytotoxic medications, consider antibiotic premedication for invasive treatment. If the patient is taking corticosteroids consult their primary care physician (PCP). The patient may require supplemental corticosteroids if surgery is anticipated or patient exhibits extreme anxiety. Provide palliative treatment of oral lesions [4].

Artificial (prosthetic) heart valve: See *Heart conditions*.

Asthma: The goal is to prevent an asthma attack during the dental appointment. Determine severity of previous asthma attacks (trips to ER?), frequency, how attacks are managed, and triggers (to avoid). If severe/unstable, consult the physician and postpone nonurgent dental treatment. Avoid prescribing NSAIDs (can trigger attacks) and narcotics (respiratory depression). Recommend the patient brings their inhaler to appointments and to use prophylactically in moderate to severe cases. Be prepared to manage the asthma attack. For oral conditions (dry mouth, gingivitis, caries, oral candidiasis) recommend using a "spacer" and rinsing with water after every use of inhaler [4]. If rinsing is not carried out, fungal infection of the mouth can develop.

Autism: Inquire about seizures (>30%) (see *Epilepsy*). Plan a desensitization appointment for the patient to become familiar with the dental setting. Recommend they bring a comfort item. Reduce sensory input, avoid interruptions, limit staff, and attempt to keep the same conditions (staff/operation/time) for all visits. Ensure all visits are kept short and to the point. Keep instruments out of sight, using a "tell, show, do" approach. About 25% have bruxism (see Chapter 15). Electric toothbrushes may be too stimulating. Refer for sedation or general anesthesia if complex surgical/

restorative needs [11]. Consider silver diamine fluoride to keep procedures shorter and less invasive (see Chapter 5).

Autoimmune disease: Refer to specific disease.

B

Bariatric surgery: Exercise caution in prescribing *all* medications, and consult with physician/pharmacist. Do not prescribe NSAIDs (risk of stomach ulcers); for any other medication you may have to change dosage and form (crush pills or take medication in liquid form) [12]. These patients are at higher risk for caries, periodontal disease, tooth wear, tooth hypersensitivity, and tooth erosion (frequent gastroesophageal reflux and vomiting) [13]. Treat as high risk for caries/periodontitis. With vomiting, recommend baking soda mouth rinse as soon as possible after vomiting [4] (two teaspoons of baking soda in 8 ounces [226 ml] of water, made fresh). Patient should wait 40 minutes before brushing their teeth after vomiting to reduce enamel abrasion; dentist should consider fabricating upper/lower mouthguards for harm reduction. Inquire about the patient's diet, duration of eating/drinking, and frequency (due to small stomach capacity) as it relates to oral pH, caries and periodontitis risk. Before bariatric surgery discuss with the patient these oral risks and prepare a preventative plan. See Chapter 5.

Bed bugs: Inform the patient and refer to a medical provider. Be sure to replace plastic chair covers. Inspect any furniture patient was in contact with. May have to contact an exterminator.

Bell's palsy: Can cause xerostomia, food accumulation on the affected side (see Chapter 5), and angular cheilitis [14].

Bipolar 1 and 2: Same treatment modifications as depression (see *Depression*).

Birth control pills: If prescribing antibiotics, inform the patient that antibiotics can potentially reduce the effectiveness of oral contraceptives, and discuss with the patient's physician additional nonhormonal means of contraception [4]. If extracting teeth, these patients are twice as likely to develop dry socket [15].

Bleeding conditions: See *Abnormal bleeding*.

Blood transfusion: Discover the reason for the blood transfusion, such as trauma, surgery, or a bleeding disorder.

Bronchitis: See *Chronic obstructive pulmonary disease*.

Bulimia: Tooth erosion occurs mostly on maxillary lingual and occlusal tooth surfaces. Enlarged parotid glands may be present. Recommend that patient performs baking soda mouth rinse (two teaspoons of baking soda in 8 ounces [226 ml] of water made fresh) after vomiting [4], avoids rinsing with tap water, and waits 40 minutes before brushing teeth. Consider fabricating upper/lower mouthguards for patient to wear when vomiting, 1.1% neutral fluoride gel trays, and a 0.5% fluoride daily rinse [16]. Treat tooth sensitivity (e.g. desensitizing medicaments, desensitizing toothpaste, avoid whitening toothpaste). Avoid prophy polish (use fluoride toothpaste instead) and complex restoratives until stable; restorations may fail if relapse. Use composite (minimally invasive) instead of crown if possible. Recommend nutritional counseling (may be high-carbohydrate/carbonated diet). Dry mouth increases risk of caries and periodontal disease [10]. If patient is a minor the parent must be informed, and refer patient to physician for evaluation/treatment [4]. High caries risk (see Chapter 5).

C

Cancer/chemotherapy/radiation treatment: Determine the type and status of cancer, and the status and timing of treatment. Various oral manifestations are associated (See Table 1.2).

Table 1.2 Cancer treatment type and dental modifications before, during, and after.

Treatment type	Before	During	After
Chemotherapy	Medical consult with oncologist prior to treatment: • WBC (<2000/μl) or neutrophils (<500/μl)? • Need for antibiotic premed and antibiotic during healing for first week if invasive treatment[a]? • Platelets <50000/μl: need for transfusion if invasive treatment? Extract teeth with questionable/poor long-term prognosis (deep decay, pockets 6+) a minimum of three weeks prior to radiation or one week prior to chemotherapy. Treat any active dental disease, eliminate any potential future dental disease, smooth any sharp edges, verify well-fitting prothesis, RCT (minimum one week prior) if restorable and good compliance, prophy, SRP especially purulent pockets for excellent periodontal health Provide an aggressive oral hygiene/preventative plan (CHLX, custom fluoride trays, prescription-strength F toothpaste, topical F, nutritional counseling). Maintain excellent oral hygiene	Only emergency treatment with medical consult Medical consult with oncologist prior to treatment: • WBC (<2000/μl) or neutrophils (<500/μl)? • Need for antibiotic premed and antibiotic during healing for first week if invasive treatment? • Platelets <50000/μl: need for transfusion if invasive treatment? Best treated 17–20 days after chemotherapy Provide an aggressive oral hygiene/preventative plan (CHLX, custom fluoride trays, prescription-strength F toothpaste, topical F, nutritional counseling). Maintain excellent oral hygiene Antibiotics may be indicated if a central venous catheter is placed. Consult with treating oncologist [17]	Medical consult with oncologist prior to treatment: • In remission, cured, metastasized, in palliative care? • Please send current CBC with WBC and platelets to check if lab values are within normal range • Do you recommend antibiotic premed for procedures that may cause bleeding? • Was the patient on any IV/oral bisphosphonate or other IV/oral drugs (e.g. antiresorptive or antiangiogenic medications) that may lead to necrosis of jaw with oral surgery or trauma? Provide an aggressive oral hygiene/preventative plan (CHLX, custom fluoride trays, prescription-strength F toothpaste, topical F, nutritional counseling). Maintain excellent oral hygiene

| Radiation to the head and neck (this does not include radioactive iodine for thyroid conditions/cancers) | Warn the patient of future risks of oral infections, caries, BRONJ, MRONJ, ORN | Only emergency treatment with medical consult

Radiation: daily stretching exercises for trismus

Treat oral conditions (ex/ mucositis, fungal infections, xerostomia)

Provide an aggressive oral hygiene/preventative plan (CHLX, custom fluoride trays, prescription-strength F toothpaste, nutritional counseling). Maintain excellent oral hygiene

Refer extractions to oral surgeon

Endo preferred over extractions (RCT + coronectomy vs. extraction) | Medical consult with the oncologist or the radiation oncologist prior to treatment:

• Where was the port (location) of the radiation? Was the radiation beam collimated? If the radiation beam was directly through the surgical area, more concern about healing potential of the bone vs. if beam was further away
• Could ask if total dose over 60 Gy
• Risk of ORN with the following treatment plan?

Minimized vasoconstrictor usage with local anesthetic

Avoid wearing dentures for first six months after radiation therapy

Endo preferred over extractions (RCT + coronectomy vs. extraction). If dose >60 Gy (or 6000 cGy) do not extract, do RCT/restore or if not restorable RCT/coronectomy

Provide an aggressive oral hygiene/preventative plan (CHLX, custom fluoride trays, prescription-strength F toothpaste, topical F, nutritional counseling, frequent recalls every 3–4 months). Maintain excellent oral hygiene

Treat caries early

Signs/symptoms of ORNJ refer to oral surgeon |

(*Continued*)

Table 1.2 (Continued)

Treatment type	Before	During	After
IV or oral bisphosphonates (and Denosumab)	Extract teeth with questionable/poor long-term prognosis (deep decay, pockets 6+), treat any active dental disease and eliminate any potential future dental disease, smooth any sharp edges, verify well-fitting prothesis, RCT if restorable and good compliance, prophy, SRP especially purulent pockets for excellent periodontal health Ideally, extraction followed by a 3-week postoperative appointment prior to IV bisphosphonates Warn the patient of MRONJ/BRONJ, and educate about the signs/symptoms and report if any appear Maintain excellent oral hygiene	Obtain a medical consult In general, routine dental care can be provided (fillings, SRP, RCT) Refer any extractions to an OMFS	Obtain medical consult Inform patient of risk of BRONJ with dentistry Treat oral disease early, nonsurgical approaches preferred, refer any extractions to an OMFS Oral surgery: discuss alternative to extraction (RCT/coronectomy allowing roots to exfoliate) [18] Risk of MRONJ is higher with IV bisphosphonates (1–10%) vs. oral bisphosphonates (0.001–0.01%) [19] Signs/symptoms of MRONJ refer to OMFS

BRONJ, bisphosphonate-related osteonecrosis of the jaw; CHLX, chlorhexidine; MRONJ, medication-related osteonecrosis of the jaw; OMFS, oral and maxillofacial surgeon; ORN, osteoradionecrosis; prophy, prophylaxis; RCT, root canal treatment; SRP, scaling and root planing.

[a] Invasive treatment is any treatment that is going to induce an inflammatory response to heal.

Source: Little et al. [4].

Cardiovascular disease: See *Heart conditions, Stroke, Rheumatic heart disease, Deep vein thrombosis, Pulmonary embolism*.

Celiac disease: Various oral manifestations such as enamel defects, dry mouth. Treat recurrent aphthous ulcers palliatively, encourage prevention (avoid gluten), possible association with corticosteroids [20, 21]. The FDA (U.S. Food and Drug Administration) encourages but does not require drug manufacturers to label drugs products as gluten-free. Gluten is rarely contained in any dental product (even when not labeled gluten-free) and may not contain enough gluten to even meet the definition of gluten-containing [20].

Cerebral palsy: Displays a range of intellectual disability, and may require referral to special needs clinic/hospital for general anesthesia. Ask if seizure history (30–50% have seizures) [22] (see *Epilepsy*). Consider mouth props for exam/treatment/for caregiver providing home hygiene. If feeding tube is in place, position patient upright to prevent aspiration [20]. Consider silver diamine fluoride (see Chapter 5).

Cerebrovascular accident: See *Stroke*.

Chest pain upon exertion: See *Angina*.

Chronic pain: Determine the location of pain and history (e.g. back pain from a car accident). Is the patient taking narcotics? Consult pain management doctor for managing acute dental pain. Patient is usually on a "pain contract" and can only have a certain amount of opioids per month. Beware acetaminophen overdose if the patient is taking an acetaminophen/opioid combination. See *Controlled substances* and Chapter 16.

Crohn's disease: See *Gastrointestinal disease*.

Clostridium difficile: See *Pseudomembranous colitis*.

Cold: Similar symptoms to flu, may be indistinguishable [23]. See *Flu*.

Congenital heart diseases: See *Heart conditions*.

Congestive heart failure: See *Heart conditions*.

Contraceptives: See *Birth control pills*.

Controlled substances: Is the patient able to consent to treatment?

> **Cocaine**: Absolute contraindication to use of vasoconstrictor (e.g. epinephrine in local anesthetic), which within 24 hours can be fatal (e.g. dysrhythmias, myocardial infarction [MI], cardiac arrest). Postpone treatment [6]. Ask the patient if any use within last 24 hours.

> **IV drug usage**: Recommend patient be tested for human immunodeficiency virus (HIV)/hepatitis B and C [4]. Also recommend patient talks to PCP about pre-exposure prophylaxis for prevention of HIV.

> **Narcotics**: Complex when prescribing analgesics (see Chapter 16). Oral findings include xerostomia, severe caries, occlusal wear (see Chapter 5). Patient may be taking opioids for chronic pain, or taking opioids (buprenorphine, suboxone, and methadone) to reduce the "cravings," or be actively seeking opioids due to addiction or to sell illegally. See Chapter 16.

> **Marijuana**: Oral manifestations include xerostomia, gingivitis, periodontal disease, and high caries risk (see Chapters 5 and 6). Avoid epinephrine if within 24 hours of usage; be vigilant for gingival hyperplasia, tongue carcinoma [24, 25]. Faulty logic in thinking marijuana is risk-free because it is "natural."

> **Methamphetamines**: Oral manifestations include xerostomia, and "meth mouth" (black rotting teeth, typically buccal smooth surfaces and anterior interproximal). Avoid vasoconstrictors in local anesthetic, and consider occlusal guard (due to bruxism/occlusal wear).

Consult physician when prescribing analgesics, caution with nitrous sedation [24]. Inform your patients meth leads to rampant tooth decay and if meth is continued any dental treatment will fail. Provide patients with the free confidential national helpline (1800-662-HELP) which has trained counselors to provide referral to local treatment facilities, support groups, and community-based organizations [64]. Use an aggressive approach for caries management such as fluoride varnish applications every 3 months, SDF, glass ionomers, prescribe fluoride toothpaste and chrlorhedixine rinse, provide oral hygiene instructions and nutritional counseling.

Vaping (electronic cigarettes, electronic nicotine delivery systems): Scientists do not know the long-term health effects. Various health risks involved including addiction (nicotine), exposure to toxins, aerosols with cancer-causing agents, development of lung disease, and fires/explosions causing injuries. FDA has not approved these as aids to quitting smoking [26–28]. Discourage use and document.

Chronic obstructive pulmonary disease (includes **Bronchitis** and **Emphysema**): Obtain a medical consult if severe (e.g. shortness of breath at rest), undiagnosed, or uncertain. Use pulse oximetry during treatment especially if the patient is showing signs of distress. If oxygen saturation <95% provide supplemental oxygen at a rate of 2–3 l/min; this is essential if oxygen saturation <91%. Treat semi-supine/upright. If rubber dam or bilateral palatal or mandibular blocks are used, provide oxygen to prevent the sensation of airway constriction. Avoid narcotics (respiratory depression). Nitrous oxide sedation (and general anesthesia) is contraindicated; instead use low-dose oral diazepam [4]. Ask the patient "Do you have a home oxygen tank?" Ask about history of tobacco (periodontitis/oral cancer risk).

D

Damaged heart valves: See *Heart conditions*.

Deaf or hearing impaired: Ask the patient their preferred form of communication. Decide how best to communicate between the patient and dental office (e.g. scheduling) [29]. Not all deaf people can read lips, and there are limitations (only one-third of what's spoken is understood). Don't assume everbody speaks English, and there are limits to communication in writing. For lengthy conversations, the Americans with Disabilities Act requires dentists to provide the patient with a free interpreter. Avoid family/friends interpreting due to bias, patient confidentiality, barriers to understanding, and communicating medical/dental terms [3]. Patient may prefer to adjust or turn off hearing aids when using instruments (auditory discomfort) [30].

Deep vein thrombosis (DVT): Check medication list. Patient is likely on anticoagulants such as warfarin [31]. See section Medications.

Defibrillator: See *Pacemaker and implantable cardioverter-defibrillators*.

Dementia: May be caused by Alzheimer's disease. Determine if the patient's cognitive abilities allow consent to treatment. Consent, both written and verbal/implied, is needed from the legal guardian, not from an unauthorized family member/caregiver. Written consent must come from the legal guardian. Communication should be verbal (short words and sentences, with repetition) and nonverbal. Emphasize preventative treatment and frequent recalls (every three months). In advanced stages the patient may be hostile, uncooperative, and require sedation. The patient may lack interest and/or ability for self-care. Instruct the caregiver about proper oral hygiene (see Chapter 5). Patient may be prone to candidiasis, periodontal diseases, and caries, and medications may cause xerostomia. May be taking antipsychotics (see section Medications).

Depression: During depressive stage oral hygiene neglect increases risk of caries and periodontitis, and medications may cause xerostomia (see Chapters 5 and 6). Limit epinephrine to two cartridges if patient taking tricyclic antidepressants (hypertension reaction), monoamine oxidase inhibitors (hypertensive reaction), and antipsychotic drugs (hypotensive reaction). Be cautious when prescribing narcotics due to respiratory depression. Medication side effects include thrombocytopenia (lower platelets), leukopenia (low WBC), and hypotension (check vitals), and avoid NSAIDs if taking lithium [4].

Diabetes mellitus (types 1, 2, and gestational): Antibiotic premedication not indicated with insulin pumps [4]. Manage acute oral infections aggressively by incision and drainage, warm intraoral rinses, antibiotics, and treatment (pulpectomy or extraction). Consult physician to determine if patient requires insulin or increased dosage of insulin [4]. Many oral manifestations exist with DM, including xerostomia, bacterial, viral and fungal infections, caries, periodontal disease, and burning mouth syndrome [4]. The rate of periodontitis progression is "slow" if patient is normoglycemic, "moderate" if HbA1c <7.0%, and "rapid" if HbA1c >7.0% [32]. If DM is poorly controlled and invasive treatment is planned, the patient is at higher risk of infection from blood entering the circulation and of delayed wound healing. The goal is to determine the patient's level of knowledge/participation in their condition and any signs that it is not well controlled, in order to determine if medical consultation, laboratory investigation and treatment modifications are necessary (Table 1.3).

Table 1.3   Questions to ask diabetics, rationale, and treatment modifications.

Ask	Rationale	Treatment modification
Last visit with physician?	Being monitored regularly by physician? Should be every 3 months	If >3 months, obtain a medical consultation/lab results (A1c, blood glucose)
HbA1c or "A1c" level?	Patient should know. If not, medical consult to obtain results	• If patient does not know A1c, obtain a medical consult and lab results (A1c and blood glucose) and limit treatment to palliative care • If A1c <6.5%, no treatment modifications • If A1c 7–9%, possible antibiotics for invasive procedures (prophy, SRP, extractions) • If A1c >10%, obtain a medical consult, avoid elective treatment, and consider antibiotics for invasive procedures (prophy, SRP, extractions). Schedule one-week postoperative visit for extractions to verify healing, or as needed. Consider referring to oral surgeon • If uncontrolled, avoid elective treatments (e.g. implants) until well controlled. Still recommend treatment of dental disease. Delaying treatment could worsen the dental disease and DM status

(Continued)

Table 1.3 (Continued)

Ask	Rationale	Treatment modification
Fasting blood glucose level (or glucometer reading)? How often do you test it?	Determine if the patient takes morning fingerstick, and is aware of normal values	• If patient does not know blood glucose but knows A1c, refer to previous entry for A1c • If patient does not know blood glucose or A1c, obtain a medical consult/labs (A1c, blood glucose) • If <70 mg/dl, provide sugar in office. Consider referring to oral surgeon • If 80–120 mg/dl, no treatment modifications • If 120–180 mg/dl, possible antibiotic for invasive procedures (prophy, SRP, extractions) • If >200 mg/dl, obtain medical consult, avoid elective treatment, and consider antibiotic for invasive procedures (prophy, SRP, extractions) • Consider referring to OMFS. If you extract, schedule one-week postoperative visit for extractions to verify healing, or as needed • Knowing the HbA1c is useful; however the patient may not know or it could be out of date (>3 months old). Same-day fingerstick blood sugar is more useful to know. Provide fingerstick blood sugar reading the day of treatment if the patient did not check it themselves • Delay treatment if blood sugar is very high (≥300 mg/dl) as there is risk of acute cardiac issues if the patient goes into diabetic ketoacidosis
Taking medications regularly?	Determines level of compliance. If not, higher risk	Obtain a medical consult/labs (A1c, blood glucose)
Previous hospitalizations?	May indicate poorly controlled	If concerned, obtain medical consult/labs (A1c, blood glucose)
Frequent hunger, thirst, urination, weight loss, paresthesia, vision problems?	Signs of poorly controlled (or undiagnosed)	Obtain medical consult/labs (A1c, blood glucose)
Had a meal and took insulin prior to appointment?	Risk of hypoglycemia in dental chair	If patient skipped meal and took insulin, high risk of hypoglycemic event. Be prepared to handle emergency
How do you feel today? Any hunger or weakness?	Risk of hypoglycemia in dental chair	Be prepared to handle emergency. Tell patient to inform dentist/staff if any symptoms of hypoglycemia

Dialysis/hemodialysis: See *Kidney problems.*

Down syndrome: Talk to the parent/caregiver to determine the patient's intellectual and functional abilities. There are many oral manifestations, including early onset of severe periodontitis. Various comorbidities exist, so determine presence of any cardiac conditions and need for antibiotic premed. If the patient has a feeding tube there is risk of aspiration, so position upright with good water control. Consider daily chlorhexidine (brush if patient unable to rinse and expectorate) [30, 33] Similar treatment modifications as autism (see *Autism*). Introduce yourself to the patient, speak at the patient's eye level, don't use baby talk, and don't ignore the patient.

E

Eating disorder: Which disorder(s)? See *Anorexia* or *Bulimia*.

Emphysema: See *Chronic obstructive pulmonary disease.*

Endocarditis/previous infective endocarditis: See *Heart conditions.*

Epilepsy/seizures: The goal is to prevent a seizure during the dental appointment. Schedule appointments within hours of the patient taking anticonvulsant medication. Have patient warn you if they sense an aura. Determine severity (past trips to ER?), frequency, typical seizure duration, how managed, and any triggers (to avoid). Be prepared to manage the seizure. If poorly controlled obtain a medical consult. Medications for epilepsy/seizures can cause gingival overgrowth. Prevent and decrease the severity with meticulous oral hygiene. The patient may require gingivectomy. Fixed prosthodontics preferred over removable to avoid dislodgement. All metal preferred over porcelain. Avoid NSAIDs/aspirin if taking valproic acid [4]. May want to recommend a mouthguard for patient to prevent tooth trauma if able to sense aura ahead of time. See Chapter 15.

Excessive urination: Helps screen a patient for diabetes [4] or prostate issues. Refer to physician.

F

Fainting spells or seizures: See *Syncope* or *Seizures.*

Flu: If the patient has a flu or fever postpone any elective dental treatment [34] (see *Vitals*) until at least 24 hours after the fever is gone [35, 36]. Make sure the patient allows their toothbrush to air dry and replacement not necessary unless immunocompromised [37]. The Centers for Disease Control and Prevention (CDC) recommends yearly flu vaccine for everyone to protect against influenza and its complications [35, 36].

G

Gastric bypass: See *Bariatric surgery.*

Gastric sleeve: See *Bariatric surgery.*

Gastrointestinal disease: Find out which disease (see *Gastroesophageal reflux disease, Pseudomembranous colitis, Ulcers*). If inflammatory bowel disease (ulcerative colitis or Crohn's disease), 20% develop oral manifestations including aphthous-like lesions (use topical steroids). Oral manifestations resolve when the disease is controlled. Offer flexible scheduling with dental appointments. CBC if taking sulfasalazine (may have thrombocytopenia). Avoid NSAIDs [4].

Gastroesophageal reflux disease (GERD)/heartburn: The patient is at risk for Barrett's esophagus, which is a risk factor for esophageal cancer [38]. Patient with history of reflux/enamel erosion should be referred to a physician [4] if untreated. May require treatment for tooth sensitivity and prescription fluoride toothpaste. Oral manifestations include tooth wear, loss of enamel (erosion), and loss of vertical dimension. Recommend mouthguards for known periods of reflux.

Glaucoma: No specific treatment modifications. However, anyone with visual impairment may need additional personalized oral hygiene instructions/assistance. See *Vision impaired* and Chapter 5.

Gout: Ensure the patient is comfortable in the dental chair, and consider shorter appointments [4]. Rarely affects the head and neck but consider gout in differential diagnosis when TMD is present [39]. Refer to oral and maxillofacial surgeon (OMFS) or orofacial pain specialist, and physician.
Graves' disease: See *Thyroid problems.*

H

Hemophilia: Caution! Excessive bleeding even with minor trauma. Avoid dental treatment until medical consult with the hematologist to determine severity of condition, whether replacement therapy (e.g. factor VIII) is needed to prevent uncontrollable bleeding before/after treatment, labs (prothrombin time [PT], aPTT, thrombin time, platelet count), and if hospitalization is needed for dental treatment. Avoid NSAIDs and block anesthetic injections, use topical hemostatic agents, and follow up 24–48 hours after invasive treatment. If urgent treatment, consider endodontic therapy instead of extraction to minimize bleeding risk [4].
Hearing impaired: See *Deaf.*
Heart attack: See *Heart conditions.*
Heartburn: See *Gastroesophageal reflux disease.*
Heart conditions: For all the following conditions, determine if antibiotic premed is indicated (See Table 1.4) and if patient is taking blood thinners. Limit to a maximum of two cartridges of local anesthetic with epinephrine. May have to avoid epinephrine if taking digoxin. Reduce stress/anxiety/pain (sedatives, nitrous, analgesics). In conditions requiring antibiotic premedication, emphasize that optimal oral health and hygiene are important for reducing chance of bacteremia from daily exposure [4]. See Chapters 5 and 16.

> **Angina:** Determine if stable or unstable. For patients with stable angina, the patient is at intermediate cardiac risk, so limit to two cartridges with epinephrine, have nitroglycerin and oxygen available, and be prepared to perform CPR and activate emergency medical services (EMS). For patients with unstable angina, the patient is at major cardiac risk, so obtain medical consult, postpone elective care, and treat only for dental emergencies (bleeding, infection, pain) best done in a hospital setting [4]. Antibiotic premed not indicated.

Table 1.4 Indications for antibiotic prophylaxis for the prevention of infective endocarditis (when a dental visit involves the manipulation of gingival tissue or the periapical region of teeth or perforation of oral mucosa[a].

Prosthetic cardiac valves, including transcatheter-implanted prostheses and homografts

Prosthetic material used for cardiac valve repairs, such as annuloplasty rings and chords

History of infective endocarditis

Cardiac transplant with valve regurgitation due to a structurally abnormal valve

The following congenital heart diseases:

- Unrepaired cyanotic congenital heart disease, including palliative shunts and conduits
- Any repaired congenital heart defects with residual shunts or valvular regurgitation at the site of or adjacent to the site of a prosthetic patch or a prosthetic device

[a] If the antibiotic premed dose is accidently missed, it can be administered up to two hours after the procedure. If back-to-back appointments, it still warrants repeat doses. If the patient is already taking an antibiotic, select one from a different class [17].
Source: Based on American Dental Association [17].

Artificial heart valve: Antibiotic premed indicated. Includes transcatheter-implanted prosthesis, homografts, and prosthetic material used for cardiac valve repair, such as annuloplasty ring and chords [17].

Coronary artery bypass graft: Antibiotic premed not indicated [4].

Cardiac arrhythmia: If taking digoxin avoid epinephrine. May have pacemaker (see *Pacemaker*). Antibiotic premed not indicated.

Congenital heart disease/defect: Antibiotic premed indicated for "unrepaired cyanotic congenital heart disease, including palliative shunts and conduits," "any repaired congenital heart defect with residual shunts or valvular regurgitation at the site of or adjacent to the site of a prosthetic patch or a prosthetic device," or repaired (completely) in last six months [17].

Congestive heart failure: Recommend medical consult. If asymptomatic, any dental treatment may be carried out. Avoid NSAIDs. If taking digoxin, avoid epinephrine. Supine position may not be tolerable. Antibiotic premed not indicated. If symptomatic, urgent care only (infection/bleeding/pain). If poorly controlled, monitor BP throughout procedure for significant increase/decrease. Be prepared for cardiac arrest, call EMS, and institute BLS [4].

Coronary artery disease/stent/balloon angioplasty: Antibiotic premed not indicated [4].

Damaged valves in transplanted heart (with valve regurgitation due to structurally abnormal valve): Antibiotic premed indicated [17].

Endocarditis/previous infective endocarditis: Antibiotic premed indicated (Table 1.4) [17]. See Chapter 16.

Heart attack/MI: Antibiotic premed not indicated. Determine date of heart attack and document. If <30 days ago, avoid elective treatment, obtain a medical consult, and best treat in hospital setting as the patient has a major cardiac risk. Consider prophylactic nitroglycerin before the procedure and administer oxygen. Be prepared for medical emergency (nitroglycerin, oxygen, BLS, EMS). If >30 days, the patient is at lower risk [4]. Avoid use of ibuprofen in presence of recent MI, increased risk for MI, or stroke (instead use naproxen for less than seven days) [40].

Heart murmur: Antibiotic premed no longer indicated [4].

Mitral valve prolapse: Antibiotic premed no longer indicated [4].

Pacemaker and implantable cardioverter-defibrillators: Antibiotic premed not indicated. See *Pacemaker*.

Quadruple bypass: Antibiotic premed not indicated for bypass. See *Coronary artery bypass graft*.

Heart murmur: See *Heart conditions*.

Herpes: See *Sexually transmitted diseases*.

High blood pressure: See *Hypertension*.

HIV and AIDS: Always use standard precautions [4]. The transmission risk is low from patient to dentist, so-called "rule of 3's" (hepatitis B 30%, hepatitis C 3%, HIV 0.3%) [4]. If needlestick exposure occurs, consult PCP immediately for evaluation to determine if post-exposure prophylaxis needs to be started along with HIV testing [4]. Many possible interactions with antiretroviral therapy (ART), so check before prescribing/recommending over the counter (OTC) medications. Many oral manifestations, such as oral candidiasis, hairy leukoplakia, specific forms of periodontal disease, and Kaposi sarcoma. Consider obtaining a medical consultation to determine the drugs a patient is taking, lab results, drug interactions for any dental prescriptions, and presence of other illnesses. May require follow-up medical consult based on laboratory values. Lab results should be obtained within one year (See Table 1.5).

Table 1.5   HIV/AIDS tests and treatment modifications.

Lab test to order	Test	Quantity	Treatment modifications
HIV-1 RNA	HIV-1 RNA ("viral load")	<20 copies/ml is considered "undetectable"	If viral load is undetectable and CD4 count is not low, then no treatment modifications necessary. If detectable, the higher the copies of virus per milliliter of blood, the higher the risk for the practitioner. Higher amount related to susceptibility to opportunistic infections and rate of disease progression [4]
Lymphocyte subset panel	Absolute CD4+ ("T cells," "CD4 count")	>600 cells/μl	No increased risk of opportunistic infections [18]
		200–400 cells/μl	Appearance of opportunistic infections [18]
		<200 cells/μl	AIDS diagnosis, high risk of life-threatening AIDS-defining infections [18]. No elective treatment. Medical consult to determine if antibiotic premed recommended
CBC with differential	WBC	If <2000 cells (or <2000/μl)	Medical consult for antibiotic premed [4]
	Absolute neutrophils	If <500 cells/μl	Medical consult for antibiotic premed [4]
	Platelets	If <50000/μl	Medical consult, may require platelet transfusion or hospital setting for treatment

Sources: Based on Little et al. [4] and Newland et al. [18].

Hypertension (HTN): Only a physician can diagnose HTN, although the dentist can inform the patient of high BP readings. Determine if the patient is compliant with taking medications and if any taken the day of the appointment. Avoid long-term (more than two weeks) NSAIDs, which can interfere with the effectiveness of HTN medication. Primary concern with dental treatment is a sudden rise in BP due to stress/anxiety, injection of vasoconstrictor (epinephrine), which can lead to a stroke or heart attack. If BP <180/110 mmHg, use a maximum of two cartridges of local anesthetic with epinephrine. If anxious, recommend sedative (consult physician as patient may need dosage reduced due to medication interaction) or nitrous. Defer dental treatment if BP >180/110 mmHg. Anticipate possible medical emergencies including angina, stroke, arrhythmia, and heart attack [4] (Table 1.6).

Discuss with the patient that BP readings are taken at every dental visit. Some patients may have undiagnosed HTN, while others have been diagnosed but are poorly controlled. HTN is often referred to as a "silent killer" as there can be no symptoms but can cause severe damage to the heart, brain, and other organs. High BP readings affect dental treatment.

Document in chart: BP readings, patient denies symptoms (with list of symptoms), referral to physician, patient warned of consequences including heart attack and stroke. If patient refuses to go to ER, get them to sign an AMA form. Have a protocol in place in dental office for the dental team. Do not schedule next visit until BP under control.

Antihypertensive medications may take several weeks until BP under control [41]. In medical consult provide date of dental visit and the high BP readings.

Table 1.6 Blood pressure readings protocol.

Range (mmHg)	Determine if symptomatic	Protocol
Systolic ≤120 or Diastolic ≤80		Any dental treatment [4]
Systolic 121–159 or Diastolic 81–99		Any dental treatment. Encourage patient to see physician [4]
Systolic 160–179 or Diastolic 100–109 [4]		Any dental treatment. Refer to physician for medical consult within one month. Periodic monitoring of BP during dental treatment [4]. Some dentists may choose to defer treatment until medical consult
Systolic ≥180 or Diastolic ≥110 and Asymptomatic [4]	Do you have a headache, dizziness, vision changes, shortness of breath, difficulty speaking, chest pain, numbness, weakness, or radiating pain? (Document)	*Asymptomatic*: Repeat BP reading in five minutes. If same or higher, postpone dental procedure. If urgent dental treatment consult with physician. Refer to physician promptly within one week [4]
Systolic ≥180 or Diastolic ≥110 and Symptomatic [4]		*Symptomatic*: Repeat BP reading in five minutes. If same or higher, postpone dental procedure. Call EMS for patient to go to the ER [4]. If patient refuses, have the patient sign an Against Medical Advice (AMA) form

Source: Little et al. [4].

Hypotension: Be prepared to manage orthostatic hypotension and syncope. If the BP drops below 100/60 mmHg seek medical attention [4].

Hepatitis, jaundice, or liver disease: Main concerns involve bleeding and drug metabolism. Various oral manifestations.

Liver cirrhosis: Most severe form of liver disease, due to alcohol or chronic infection. See *Alcoholism*.

Liver disease: Medical consult to determine type of liver disease, liver function status, laboratory findings if surgery is planned (PT, INR, platelet count), drug selection and dosage for medications that may be prescribed [4]. Labratory tests related to liver disease include PT, aPTT, INR, platelet count, liver function tests (AST, ALT, alkaline phosphatase and bilirubin). See section Lab Values.

Hepatitis (strains A, B, C, D, E): Use standard precautions.

Active hepatitis: consult physician, emergency treatment only, minimize aerosols, PT and bleeding time prior to surgery (may require platelet transfusion and/or fresh frozen plasma), and avoid drugs metabolized in liver.

History of hepatitis: consult physician for status. Hepatitis B/C: consult physician for liver function status. Minimize use of drugs metabolized by liver. Before dental surgery obtain PT and platelet count. Use a maximum of three cartridges of lidocaine; articaine is safe to use. Caution with NSAIDs and acetaminophen (no significant changes in the short term, but in the long term all medications are a risk, especially acetaminophen). Medical consult to determine liver function status, laboratory findings if surgery is planned (PT, INR, platelet count), drug selection and dosage for medications that may be prescribed [4].

Jaundice: If signs or symptoms of hepatitis/cirrhosis are present, defer dental treatment and refer to a physician immediately [4].

J

Jaundice: See *Hepatitis*.

Joint replacement: Total joint replacement includes shoulders, hips, and knees. This does not refer to nonmobile hardware including plates, pins, and screws (Figure 1.3). According to the ADA,

Management of patients with prosthetic joints undergoing dental procedures

Clinical Recommendation:

In general, for patients with prosthetic joint implants, prophylactic antibiotics are *not* recommended prior to dental procedures to prevent prosthetic joint infection.

For patients with a history of complications associated with their joint replacement surgery who are undergoing dental procedures that include gingival manipulation or mucosal incision, prophylactic antibiotics should only be considered after consultation with the patient and orthopedic surgeon.* To assess a patient's medical status, a complete health history is always recommended when making final decisions regarding the need for antibiotic prophylaxis.

Clinical Reasoning for the Recommendation:

- There is evidence that dental procedures are not associated with prosthetic joint implant infections.
- There is evidence that antibiotics provided before oral care do not prevent prosthetic joint implant infections.
- There are potential harms of antibiotics including risk for anaphylaxis, antibiotic resistance, and opportunistic infections like *Clostridium difficile*.
- The benefits of antibiotic prophylaxis may not exceed the harms for most patients.
- The individual patient's circumstances and preferences should be considered when deciding whether to prescribe prophylactic antibiotics prior to dental procedures.

ADA. **Center for Evidence-Based Dentistry**™

*In cases where antibiotics are deemed necessary, it is most appropriate that the orthopedic surgeon recommend the appropriate antibiotic regimen and when reasonable write the prescription.
Sollecito T, Abt E, Lockhart P, et al. The use of prophylactic antibiotics prior to dental procedures in patients with prosthetic joints: Evidence-based clinical practice guideline for dental practitioners — a report of the American Dental Association Council on Scientific Affairs. JADA. 2015;146(1):11-16.

Figure 1.3 Management of patients with prosthetic joints undergoing dental procedures.
Source: Copyright © 2012 American Dental Association. All rights reserved. Reprinted with permission.

in general, for patients with prosthetic joint implants, prophylactic antibiotics are not recommended prior to dental procedures to prevent prosthetic joint infection. [If] a history of complication associated with their joint replacement surgery, prophylaxis antibiotics should only be considered after consultation with the patient and the orthopedic surgeon.

If necessary it is "most appropriate that the orthopedic surgeon recommend the appropriate antibiotic regimen and when reasonable write the prescription" [42]. For dosage, see Chapter 16.

Determine when the surgery took place (date) and the history of any complications. Use the American Academy of Orthopedic Surgeons (AAOS) tool. If unsure, discuss the patient's planned procedure with their orthopedic surgeon. You can provide a copy of the ADA chairside guidelines (See Figure 1.3). Also ask the surgeon about how long they recommended that antibiotics be prescribed (for a specific period after surgery or for life). If you do not agree with patient's need for an antibiotic premed, have the patient's orthopedic surgeon write the prescription with refills.

The AAOS tool "Appropriate use criteria: management of patients with orthopedic implants undergoing dental procedures (2016)" is available at https://aaos.webauthor.com/go/auc/terms.cfm?auc_id=224995&actionxm=Terms. Simply answer the questions and a recommendation is provided (yes or no to antibiotic premed). Questions include type of dental procedure, immuno-compromised status, diabetic glycemic control, history of joint infection, and years since joint replacement [43].

K

Kidney problems/kidney disease: Determine stage. If stage 3 or greater, obtain a medical consultation to determine status, and input for drug selection/dosage; if dental surgery is planned, obtain labs (platelet count, PT, aPTT). Local anesthetics can be used safely. Avoid NSAIDs. Monitor BP throughout appointment. Emphasize meticulous oral hygiene to avoid infections [4].

Dialysis/hemodialysis: Do not take BP on the arm with the arteriovenous shunt. Consult the nephrologist regarding labs, concerns about postoperative bleeding, drug selection/dosage, and need for corticosteroids. If surgery is planned, obtain aPTT and platelet count to determine the bleeding risk. Provide treatment the day after hemodialysis (patient fatigued and bleeding risk same day), or at least six hours after dialysis. Use additional hemostatic agents. Avoid drugs metabolized in the kidneys. Antibiotic premedication for incision and drainage [4]. Recommend surgery be done on the off day from dialysis. If surgery is directly after dialysis, the patient is anticoagulated with heparin. Do not perform surgery immediately before dialysis as there may be prolonged bleeding once dialysis starts.

L

Lice: Spread most commonly from hair-to-hair contact, which is unlikely in the dental office [44]. Be sure to replace plastic chair covers that the patient's head was resting on. Inform the patient and refer to a medical provider.

Liver cirrhosis: See *Hepatitis*.

Liver disease: See *Hepatitis*.

Low blood pressure: See *Hypotension* and *Vitals*.

Lupus: See *Arthritis*.

M

Malnutrition: Evaluate for oral signs of vitamin deficiencies including angular cheilitis, glossitis, gingival bleeding, periodontal disease, poorly mineralized bone, and erythema of oral mucosa. May be due to malabsorption syndromes, anorexia (see *Anorexia*), or alcoholism (see *Alcoholism*) [45]. Refer to a physician and a registered dietician. Emphasize the importance of nutrition when recovering from dental surgery: increased nourishment improves healing rate and lowers risk of infection, and improves the ability of tissue to withstand dentures. Recommend high-calorie high-protein foods and multivitamin before surgery [46]. See Chapter 9.

Mental health disorders: Specify type. See *Anxiety*, *Bipolar 1 and 2*, *Depression*, *Post-traumatic stress disorder*, and *Schizophrenia*.

Metastatic cancer: See *Cancer.*

Mitral valve prolapse: See *Heart conditions.*

Mononucleosis/infectious mononucleosis: If symptomatic, including fever or tonsillar exudate or malaise, refer to a physician. Similar precautions as flu; however, delay routine dental care until four weeks after recovery [23]. See *Flu.*

Methicillin-resistant *Staphylococcus aureus* (MRSA)/any *Staphylococcus* infection: Use standard precautions including good hand hygiene. Patient should cover any scrapes/wounds until healed. If symptoms are present, refer to physician promptly [47].

Multiple myeloma: See *Cancer.*

Myocardial infarction: See *Heart conditions.*

N

Narcotics: See *Controlled substances* and Chapter 16.

Neurological disorders: Specify type. See *Dementia* (Alzheimer's), *Epilepsy*, and *Stroke.*

Multiple sclerosis (MS): Optimal treatment is during remission. In advanced disease, may require a caregiver to transport patient to the dental chair and assist with oral hygiene. Schedule morning appointments due to afternoon fatigue. Consult a physician if the patient is taking corticosteroids requiring increased dose for dental surgery. MS patients are more likely to have trigeminal neuralgia [4].

Parkinson's disease: Determine ability to maintain oral hygiene due to muscle rigidity and tremors; patient may require assistance. Consider frequent recall visits. Schedule appointment within first three hours of medications. If movements are severe patient may require sedation. Prone to imbalance/falls, so use caution when patient is getting in and out of dental chair. If patient is on catechol-*O*-methyltransferase (COMT) inhibitors, limit to two cartridges of local anesthetic with epinephrine. One-quarter develop dementia [4]. See *Dementia.*

Hydrocephalus: Cerebrospinal fluid shunt is not an indication for antibiotic premedication [4].

Night sweats: Refer patient to physician.

Nursing: The main concern is drug safety for the baby. If prescribing any medications, check if nursing/breastfeeding is safe (Table 1.7). X-rays/radiation: no risk to lactation. Review the Oral Hygiene Index (OHI) for babies. See Chapter 5.

Table 1.7 Drugs and nursing safety.

Drug type	Nursing safe	Nursing caution/avoid
Injectable local anesthetics	Lidocaine, prilocaine, bupivacaine, mepivacaine	Articaine
Topical local anesthetics	Lidocaine, lidocaine + prilocaine	Benzocaine and tetracaine
Sedatives	Nitrous, lorazepam, and oxazepam	Other benzodiazepines
Analgesics	Acetaminophen, ibuprofen	Narcotics (can cause drowsiness, CNS depression, and death)
Antibiotics	Penicillin (VK, G), amoxicillin, amoxicillin + clavulanic acid, clindamycin, nystatin, acyclovir, valacyclovir, chlorhexidine	Other antibiotics
OTC medication	Use lowest possible dose for shortest possible time	Extra-strength [48]

O

Organ transplant: See *Transplant*.

Osteoarthritis: See *Arthritis*.

Osteopenia/osteoporosis: Patient may be on bisphosphonates. See section Medications and *Cancer/chemotherapy/radiation treatment*.

Other congenital heart defects: See *Heart conditions*.

P

Pacemaker and implantable cardioverter-defibrillators: Contraindications to ultrasonic devices include cardiac pacemakers, especially those placed before the mid 1980s due to possible electromagnetic interferences [9]. Many electronic dental devices exist, including ultrasonic scaler, apex locator, electronic pulp test, electrosurgery instruments, curing lights, gutta percha devices, ultrasonic cleaning systems, curing light, osseointegration tools, and electric toothbrushes. Evidence is conflicting. Consult with patient's cardiologist to determine if ultrasonic or electronic devices may be used safely. "It may reduce the risk to avoid waving device or its cords over the patient's pectoral region and turn off the equipment when not in use" [49]. The pacemakers made in the USA since around 2010 are shielded. Consult with the physician and ask if the pacemaker is shielded.

Paget's disease: Patient may be taking bisphosphonates. See section Medications and *Cancer/chemotherapy/radiation treatment*. Cotton wool appearance on X-ray, with hypercementosis/ankylosed teeth. Expanding jaw leads to dentures becoming tighter, with need for replacement and formation of diastemas [45].

Persistent swollen glands in neck: Likely due to an infection. Treat if a dental infection (antibiotics may be indicated); if not odontogenic refer the patient to their physician.

Post-traumatic stress disorder (PTSD): May report atypical facial pain, glossodynia, TMD, and bruxism. During the depressive stage there is neglect of oral hygiene, increasing the risk of caries and periodontal disease. See *Anxiety* and Chapters 5 and 6 [4]. Inquire about alcohol/drug usage (see *Alcoholism* and *Controlled substances*). Consider silver diamine fluoride (see Chapter 5).

Pregnancy

Goal: To prevent and manage dental disease. Delaying treatment may result in more complex problems.

For prescriptions and dental materials, check if pregnancy-safe. See Chapter 16.

Ask about trimester, changes in BP, oral changes, previous miscarriages, name and address of obstetrician/gynecologist.

If pregnant woman is healthy, consultation is not needed. If comorbid conditions are present or it is a high-risk pregnancy, obtain medical consult with obstetrician/gynecologist.

Medical consultation: Ask if any contraindications or restrictions to the proposed treatment plan, list potential local anesthetics/medications to be prescribed, ask expected delivery date, any specific treatment recommendations, any medical complications as a result of pregnancy (e.g. DM, HTN).

Miscellaneous: Patient may have tooth mobility of upper incisors that resolved postpartum. All women experience pregnancy gingivitis (peaks at eight months) that resolves postpartum, so plaque control important. Pyogenic granuloma/pregnancy tumor.

The ADA and American College of Obstetricians and Gynecologists recommend that dentists "reassure patients that the prevention, diagnosis, and treatment of oral conditions, including dental X-rays (wish shielding of the abdomen and thyroid) and local anesthesia (lidocaine with or without epinephrine), are safe during pregnancy" [50].

Four bitewings (0.005 milligray [mGy]) and a panoramic X-ray (0.01 mGy) constitute one-third the radiation of a full-mouth X-ray (0.035 mGy). The risk-free fetal radiation dose is <50 mGy. Provide appropriate treatment and have a justification for your decision. If the patient is in pain and is refusing radiography, do not treat the patient without an X-ray. The standard of care does not allow you to provide treatment without proper diagnostic information (Table 1.8).

Table 1.8   Pregnancy and dental treatment.

Pregnancy trimester	Safe	Avoid/caution	Miscellaneous
Unknown pregnancy status			Defer treatment, refer to physician for pregnancy test
1, 2, 3	Lidocaine (maximum eight cartridges), acetaminophen, chlorhexidine, diphenhydramine, nystatin (topical), penicillin, amoxicillin, augmentin, clindamycin, fluoride (water and toothpaste). Removal and placement of amalgam/composite with rubber dam (minimize inhalation)	Benzocaine, nitrous, sedatives, ibuprofen (in third trimester), narcotics	Emphasize OHI. Educate the patient that the "tooth for every pregnancy" is a myth, calcium in stable crystalline form [4]. Limit sugary foods/drinks which lead to decay. If vomiting, immediately swish with baking soda and water and avoid brushing for 40 minutes
1	OHI, prophy/SRP, emergency treatment	Elective treatment, routine radiographs	
2	OHI, prophy/SRP, elective dental treatment	Routine radiographs	
3	OHI, prophy/SRP, control of oral disease, elective treatment (except second half of third trimester)	Minimize radiographs. Appointments >30 minutes (pressure on bladder and risk of supine hypotensive syndrome) [48]	

Sources: Based on Little et al. [4] and Skouteris [48].

Pseudomembranous colitis/*Clostridium difficile/C. diff*: Only prescribe antibiotics judiciously when indicated and warn patient of signs of *C. diff*. Some antibiotics associated with *C. diff* include clindamycin, ampicillin, and cephalosporins. High risk if patient is taking antibiotics, aged 65 or older, has a weakened immune system, previous *C. diff*, and is in hospital or nursing home [51]. *C. diff* signs and symptoms can occur within 4–10 days of antibiotics but can also occur up to eight weeks later [4].

Concerned about catching *C. diff* from a patient? The organisms are found in the feces of a carrier and onward transmission depends on he or she not washing their hands after going to the bathroom. If the carrier touches you, or a surface which you contact, then when you go to eat the *C. diff* spores reach the intestines and are activated. If you are healthy and have not received antibiotics recently, you may not get sick [52]. *C. diff* has not been reported after clindamycin usage as an antibiotic premed. Postpone elective treatment until patient is stable. Patient may have oral fungal infections with use of antibiotics for treating C. diff [4]. Wear gloves and disposable gown. For antibiotics, see Chapter 16.

Pulmonary embolism: Ask about medications; patient is likely on anticoagulants such as warfarin [31]. See section Medications.

Pulmonary hypertension: A type of hypertension (see *Hypertension*). Ask about medications; patient is likely on anticoagulants such as warfarin [31]. See section Medications.

R

Radiation treatment: See *Cancer/chemotherapy/radiation treatment*.

Recreational drugs: See *Controlled substances*.

Recurrent infections: Specify type.

Rheumatoid arthritis: See *Arthritis*.

Rheumatic fever: Can damage heart valves, but not listed as an indication for antibiotic premedication [17].

Rheumatic heart disease: Antibiotic premed not indicated. See Chapter 16 [17].

S

Scabies: Use standard precautions, since contagious by skin-to-skin contact. If patient has crusted scabies they are highly contagious via skin-to-skin contact or via contaminated items such as furniture. Avoid handshaking [53]. Refer patient to physician. If history of scabies, verify if treatment was successful.

Schizophrenia: Consult physician regarding patient's status, medications, and ability to consent. Inquire about patient's ability to perform home hygiene; may have to teach family member [4]. Additional treatment modifications same as depression (see *Depression*). Consider silver diamine fluoride (see Chapter 5).

Seizures: See *Epilepsy*.

Severe headaches/migraines: May be the source of nonodontogenic pain (see Chapter 10). May be related to TMD (see Chapter 15).

Severe or rapid weight loss: Determine cause. May be related to anorexia, DM, HIV/AIDs, tuberculosis, or malignancy [4] (see *Anorexia, Diabetes mellitus, HIV and AIDS*, and *Tuberculosis*). The opposite, weight gain, is also associated with diabetes.

Sexually transmitted diseases: Determine which disease and current status. Practice standard precautions. Various oral manifestations exist. Obtain medical consultation if undiagnosed or uncertain [4].

    Gonorrhea: Refer to physician if signs/symptoms. Possible oral lesions. No treatment modifications [4].

    Herpes: If patient has oral herpes ("cold sores"), delay treatment until the lesion is scabbed over or completely healed to minimize recurrences and spread of the infection. This is an occupational hazard to the dental team and to other patients. Use standard precautions, avoid manipulation of tissue infected with herpes simplex virus, and minimize use of aerosolizing agents (e.g. handpieces, ultrasonic scaler). May prescribe antivirals, topical anesthetics, and analgesics [54, 55]. Wear eye protection and gloves to avoid transmission to fingers and eyes. Localized genital infections pose no risk. Consult physician for systemic antivirals for prophylaxis a few days prior if recurrence is usual after dental treatment (trauma) [4]. Tell patient to avoid intimate contact/sharing saliva until cold sore is healed completely to prevent spread, although infection can spread even if no cold sores.

Human papillomavirus (HPV): Wear gloves to prevent transmission to fingers. Oral warts are infectious, so refer for biopsy [4]. Tell the patient to avoid intimate contact (i.e. sharing saliva) until the lesion is removed and biopsied to prevent spread. Assume any wart with finger-like projections in the mouth is contagious.

Syphilis: Oral lesions, blood and saliva are all contagious. Consult a physician if receiving treatment. Refer to physician if signs/symptoms [4].

Shingles: If oral ulcerations of shingles/herpes zoster are present, treat palliatively and possibly with antivirals [18]. Use standard precautions and avoid contact with fluid from blisters on patient's skin (causes transmission of varicella zoster virus) [56].

Sickle cell anemia: See *Anemia*.

Sinus trouble: Could be a source of nonodontogenic pain, or tooth could cause sinus infection. See Chapter 10.

Sleep apnea/obstructive sleep apnea: Caution with sedatives and opioids due to respiratory depression. Consult physician/pharmacist. Oral appliances (mandibular advancement devices and tongue-retaining devices) are an alternative to positive airway pressure (e.g. CPAP) [4]. Consult with patient's physician prior to treating with oral appliances because this requires a medical diagnosis.

Sleep disorder: Ranges from mild intermittent snoring to severe obstructive sleep apnea [4]. See *Snore* and *Sleep apnea*.

Snore: A symptom of sleep apnea. Ask the patient if they are experiencing excessive daytime sleepiness and/or breathing cessation during sleep; if so, refer to a physician. The patient may have undiagnosed sleep apnea (see *Sleep apnea*). Oral appliance can be used [4].

Splenectomy: Consult physician to determine the platelet function and recommend antibiotic premed due to possible decreased WBC.

Strep throat: If symptomatic, including fever or tonsillar exudate or malaise, refer to physician. Similar precautions as for flu [23] (see *Flu*).

Stroke/cerebrovascular accident (CVA): First six months after CVA, only undertake emergency treatment (including patients who have had transient ischemic attack [TIA] or reversible ischemic neurologic deficit [RIND]). Limit dosage of anesthetic with epinephrine to two cartridges. Short appointments, reduce stress, and consider nitrous. Be prepared to recognize and manage signs/symptoms of another stroke [4]. Determine the date of the stroke (document) and whether taking blood thinner.

Substance use disorder: See *Controlled substances*.

Syncope/fainting spells: Goal is to prevent syncope during the dental appointment. Determine severity (past trips to ER?), frequency, how it is managed, triggers (to avoid), and cause. If cause related to anxiety, see *Anxiety*. If severe/unstable, consult physician and postpone nonurgent dental treatment. Be prepared to manage syncope.

Systemic lupus erythematosus: See *Arthritis*.

T

Thrombocytopenia: Low platelets. See section Lab Values.

Thyroid problems: Evaluate the thyroid on all patients during the extraoral examination (see Chapter 2). Obtain a medical consult if poorly controlled, undiagnosed, or uncertain [4].

Hypothyroidism: Avoid narcotics and sedatives if poorly controlled, and reduce the dose if mild. Treat dental infections aggressively. Dental surgery or dental infection may precipitate a myxedema coma, so be prepared (major concern if poorly controlled and elderly). If a myxedema coma occurs, call EMS, check vitals, may need BLS (see Appendix B), inject 100–300 mg hydrocortisone, cover patient to conserve heat, and transport to ER [4].

Hyperthyroidism: If poorly controlled, avoid epinephrine in local anesthetics. Radioactive iodine is used to treat hyperthyroid conditions and thyroid cancer associated with salivary gland swelling, pain, loss of taste, sialadenitis, xerostomia, and dental caries. There is no risk of osteoradionecrosis of the jaw with radioactive iodine. Dental surgery or dental infection may precipitate a thyrotoxic crisis (major concern if poorly controlled). If thyrotoxic crisis occurs, call EMS, apply ice pack, inject 100–300 mg hydrocortisone, and transport to ER. **Graves' disease** is one of the main causes of hyperthyroidism.

Tobacco (cigarettes/cigars/hookah/chewing/bidis): Assess the quantity, duration, and the patient's level of interest in quitting. Warn patient that smoking is a risk factor for periodontal disease (tooth loss). When smoking <10 cigarettes/day, periodontal disease progresses at a moderate rate. When smoking >10 cigarettes/day, periodontal disease progresses at a rapid rate [56]. Warn the patient of an increased risk of oral cancer, delayed healing, and dry sockets. If suspicious oral lesions, refer for biopsy due to higher risk for oral and pharyngeal cancer [4] (see Chapter 2). Provide resources for quitting (e.g. 1800-QUIT-NOW or www.smokefree.gov) and refer to a physician. Document the discussion and recommendations. If chewing tobacco, establish same protocol and ask the patient the location of tobacco placement to assess soft tissue.

Transient ischemic attack: See *Stroke*.

Transplant [4] (Table 1.9).

Table 1.9 Transplants and dental treatment modifications.

Before organ/ bone marrow transplant	Consult with patient's physician. Determine the degree of organ dysfunction, need for antibiotic premedication, need for bleeding precautions, need to modify drug selection/ dosage (list anesthetics, analgesics, antibiotics, sedatives which may be prescribed), ability of patient to tolerate proposed dental treatment, and any need for supplemental corticosteroids. If surgery is planned, provide CBC with differential and PT and aPTT, and INR if on anticoagulant. Initiate an aggressive oral hygiene program to avoid complications of immunosuppression, oral diseases, infections, adverse reactions to stress, bleeding and healing complications post transplant. For patients with good dental status, emphasize aggressive oral hygiene program and warn of complications if dental disease develops. For patients with poor dental status, consider full mouth extractions and dentures. For patients with borderline dental status, evaluate dentition/periodontal status and whether patient is motivated to change diet/hygiene as risk of progression will complicate treatment post transplant. Goal is optimal oral health before surgery
After organ/ bone marrow transplant	First six months: only emergency treatment, as noninvasive as possible, with consultation with physician
After six months: obtain a medical consultation for any dental treatment. Determine stability of the transplant, need for antibiotic premedication, need for bleeding precautions, need to modify drug selection/dosage (list anesthetics, analgesics, antibiotics, sedatives which may be prescribed), ability of the patient to tolerate proposed dental treatment, and any need for supplemental corticosteroids. If surgery planned, provide a CBC with differential and PT and aPTT, INR if on anticoagulant
Chronic rejection period	Emergency dental treatment only with a medical consult obtaining same information as for After organ/bone marrow transplant

Tuberculosis (TB): Always use standard precautions.

Active infection: If aged six years or older patient must be treated in a hospital setting. If under six years old, can treat in dental office after medical consult.

History of TB: Obtain history of treatment, periodic chest radiographs, exams to rule out reactivation. If a questionable history, refer to physician and postpone treatment.

Signs/symptoms of active infection: Refer to physician and postpone treatment [4]. For healthcare providers, CDC recommends TB test upon hire and annual TB testing is not recommended unless there is a known exposure or ongoing transmission. If exposure by patient, get tested [57]. For TB, measles, and chickenpox, patients should be treated in hospital in a negative air pressure room and dentist wears an N95 mask.

U

Ulcerative colitis: See *Gastrointestinal disease.*

Ulcers (stomach/peptic ulcers): Use caution with ibuprofen (use lowest dosage for shortest period of time but consider alternatives). If also taking aspirin, there is a substantially increased risk of gastrointestinal complication (e.g. ulcers) [40].

V

Vision impaired: May need additional personalized oral hygiene instructions/assistance (see Chapter 5). Determine level of assistance patient requires. Use the patient's other senses, such as a warm handshake, to make patient feel comfortable. Face the patient, use descriptive language to explain upcoming steps (e.g. rinsing with water), and provide written instructions in large print (16 point or larger) [30].

Vitals: To establish a baseline and as a screening tool for abnormalities [4] (Table 1.10).

Table 1.10 Vitals summary.

Vital sign	Normal	Abnormal range	Additional info
Blood pressure	<120/80 mmHg [58]	<100/60 mmHg: hypotension [4]	Take BP at every dental appointment
		>140/90 mmHg: hypertension	Hypotension: place supine, administer oxygen, manage as syncope; if deterioration, call EMS [59]
			Hypertension: see *Hypertension*
Pulse rate [34]	60–90 beats/minute (bpm)	<60 or >110 bpm warrants a medical consult	If <60 bpm, the patient may become unconscious
			>110 bpm in nonanxious patient, seek medical consult
			Ask how the patient is feeling. Dizzy? Anxious? Just ran a long distance to get to appointment?
			Avoid epinephrine

Table 1.10 (Continued)

Vital sign	Normal	Abnormal range	Additional info
Respiratory rate [4]	12–16 breaths/minute	Any variation should be evaluated. Expect higher range in children [6]	By observation, normal for resting adult High may be fever, anxiety (see *Anxiety*) Labored/irregular may be cardiopulmonary Low may be due to opioids [6] Refer to a physician
Temperature [34]	96.8–99.4°F (36–37.4°C)	≥100.4°F (38°C) is a fever [60]	Fever is indication for antibiotics (if oral infection) Drink enough water [61]
Height and weight	Refer to body mass index (BMI) (not in book)	Refer to BMI (not in book)	Have scales for pediatric patients to calculate anesthetic/medication dosages (see Chapter 16) See *Severe or rapid weight loss* Inquire if recent changes. Rapid weight gain could be a sign of heart failure, edema, hypothyroidism, diabetes, or neoplasm
Blood oxygen level [62]	90–100%	<90%	Patient would require supplemental oxygen

Sources: Based on Little et al. [4], Malamed [6], Misch [34], and Centers for Disease Control and Prevention [60].

Von Willebrand disease: Similar precautions as hemophilia (see *Hemophilia*).

W

Wheelchair: Some dentists may feel comfortable assisting with transporting a patient (e.g. into the dental chair) while others do not for fear of liability if any falls or injuries occur and prefer to have the patient's caregiver involved with transporting the patient.

Medications

- Important to understand the dental implications of *every* medication your patient is taking (see Figure 1.4 and Table 1.11).
- Medications influence treatment modifications, can have oral manifestations, and may interact with a medication you prescribe.
- Recommend having a drug information book in the office, such as *Drug Information Handbook for Dentistry*.

SAFETY OF OUTPATIENT DENTAL TREATMENT FOR PATIENTS RECEIVING COUMARIN ANTICOAGULANT THERAPY.*

DENTAL TREATMENT[48]	SUBOPTIMAL INR RANGE[†]		NORMAL TARGET INR RANGE			OUT OF RANGE
				Mechanical Heart Valves		
	< 1.5	1.5 to < 2.0	2.0 to < 2.5	2.5 to 3.0	> 3.0 to 3.5	> 3.5
Examination, radiographs, study models						
Simple restorative dentistry, supragingival prophylaxis						
Complex restorative dentistry, scaling and root planing, endodontics					Probably safe (IR)[‡]	
Simple extraction, curettage, gingivoplasty				Local measures[§]	Local measures[§]	
Multiple extractions, removal of single bony impaction			Local measures[§]	Local measures[§]	Local measures[§]	
Gingivectomy, apicoectomy, minor periodontal flap surgery, placement of single implant	Probably safe (IR+)[**]	Probably safe (IR)[‡]	Probably safe (IR)[‡]			
Full-mouth/full-arch extractions	Probably safe (IR)[‡]	Local measures[§]				
Extensive flap surgery, extraction of multiple bony impactions, multiple implant placement	Probably safe (IR)[‡]	IR[‡]				
Open-fracture reduction, orthognathic surgey	Not advised[††]	Not advised[††]	Not advised[††]	Not advised[††]	Not advised[††]	Not advised[††]

* Green indicates that it is safe to proceed in a routine manner (local factors such as periodontitis/gingival inflammation can increase the severity of bleeding; the clinician should consider all factors when making a risk assessment). Yellow, use caution, but in many instances the procedure can be safely performed with judicious use of local measures. Red, procedure not advised at current INR level; refer to physician for adjustment.

† INR: international normalized ratio.

‡ IR: insufficient research to draw a conclusion.

§ Increased need for use of local measures such as sutures, oxidized cellulose, microfibrillar collagen hemostat, topical thrombin and tranexamic acid.

** IR+: insufficient research, but similar to other procedures for which research data are available.

†† Should not be performed in a dental office on a patient receiving anticoagulant therapy; this is a hospital procedure.

Figure 1.4   Dental treatment and INR ranges.

Table 1.11 Medications and precautions.

Medication (proprietary name)	Precautions
Warfarin (Coumadin, Jantoven)	• See Figure 1.4 • Obtain the INR within 24 hours for procedures involving bleeding • Avoid NSAIDs as these increase bleeding risk [40] • Patients that require INR: try combining appointments, such as SRP, complete half mouth per visit. And request a "standing order for [specific amount] INRs in the next 6 months" so the patient can go to laboratory and have the INR test within 24 hours
Heparin	• Risk of bleeding, obtain medical consult [40]
Antiplatelet or anticoagulants, such as apixaban (Eliquis), clopidogrel (Plavix), dabigatran (Pradaxa), rivaroxaban (Xarelto), cilostazol (Pletal)	• Patient should never discontinue without consulting physician. Serious risks with stopping. No lab tests available to determine risk. Consult physician prior to dental surgery [40] • Consider local measures for hemostasis
Aspirin 81 mg	• Can prolong bleeding. However, at this dose safe for extractions. 7–10 days for normal platelet function [40] • If taking higher dosage (e.g. 325 mg) expect more prolonged bleeding
Oral or IV bisphosphonates Antiresorptive medications Antiangiogenic medications	• Risk of MRONJ is higher with IV bisphosphonates (1–10%) vs. oral bisphosphonates (0.001–0.01%) • Consult physician [19] • Antiresorptive medications include Fosamax, Actonel, Atelvia, Boniva, Reclast, Prolia, Aredia, Zometa, Xgeva (see *Cancer*)
Denosumab (Prolia, Xgeva)	• Injectable medication with risk of MRONJ • Refer to OMFS for any invasive treatment (extractions) (see *Cancer*)
Antipsychotics	• May cause low WBC and thrombocytopenia [4] • Limit epinephrine to two cartridges
Lithium	• Avoid NSAIDs due to lithium toxicity, instead use acetaminophen (with or without opioids) [40]
Birth control pills	• Risk of dry socket and less effective when taking antibiotics (see *Birth control pills*)
Herbal/natural medications/vitamins/dietary supplements	• Can interfere with clotting.
Fish oil	• No scientific evidence to warrant discontinuance. Anticipate slower clotting time [40]
Long-term corticosteroids	• Consult with physician regarding need for supplemental steroids (i.e. the appropriate drug, dosage, and duration) if dental pain, infection, dental surgery, and/or postoperative pain
Nonselective beta-blockers Monoamine oxidase inhibitors Tricyclic antidepressants	• Vasoconstrictors (epinephrine in local anesthetic) are contraindicated [6]. If epinephrine is not needed for treatment, it is safest to avoid • Need to weigh the risks and benefits of using epinephrine. Always be sure to use proper technique (e.g. aspirate)
Digoxin	• Avoid vasoconstrictors, as may induce arrhythmia [4] • If epinephrine is not needed for treatment, it is safest to avoid. Need to weigh the risks and benefits of using epinephrine. Always be sure to use proper technique (e.g. aspirate)

MRONJ, medication-related osteonecrosis of the jaw; OMFS, oral and maxillofacial surgeon; SRP, scaling and root planing.

Sources: Based on Little et al. [4], American Dental Association [19], and Wynn et al. [40].

Table 1.12 Lab test information.

Lab test	Information
CBC with diff (WBC, absolute neutrophils, platelets)	CBC with differential. Screens for leukopenia, neutropenia, and thrombocytopenia. Obtain platelet count within one month if previously low. See *HIV*
HIV-1 RNA	See *HIV*
Absolute CD+	See *HIV*
Fasting blood glucose	See *Diabetes*
A1c	See *Diabetes*
AST	Aspartate aminotransferase
ALT	Alanine aminotransferase. If AST and ALT are available, gives a good picture of liver health
PT	Prothrombin time. Screen for bleeding disorder. Must be able to treat the area locally with various hemostatics
aPTT	Activated partial thromboplastin time. Screen for bleeding disorder
PTT	Partial thromboplastin time. Screen for bleeding disorder
TT	Thrombin time. Screen for bleeding disorder
Bleeding time	Screen for bleeding disorder. Rarely done. Difficult test and hard to standardize
INR	International normalized ratio. Obtain within 24 hours. See Figure 1.4

Lab Values

Miscellaneous Terms

- **CBC with diff**: Completed blood count with differential will include WBC, absolute neutrophils, and platelets. "CBC without diff" will not include absolute neutrophils.
  - **WBC**: Low count indicates immunocompromise, while high count indicates fighting infection.
  - **Leukopenia**: Low WBC, risk of infection.
- **Neutropenia**: Low neutrophils, risk of infection.
- **Thrombocytopenia**: Low platelet count, risk of uncontrolled bleeding.
- **Reference range**: the upper and lower limits of normal for each lab test result. These numbers can vary at different laboratories (Table 1.12).

ASA Physical Status Classification System

The American Society of Anesthesiologists (ASA) Physical Status Classification System is one method of categorizing patients into different risk levels (Figure 1.5).

ASA PS Classification	Definition	Adult Examples, Including, but not Limited to:	Pediatric Examples, Including but not Limited to:	Obstetric Examples, Including but not Limited to:
ASA I	A normal healthy patient	Healthy, non-smoking, no or minimal alcohol use	Healthy (no acute or chronic disease), normal BMI percentile for age	
ASA II	A patient with mild systemic disease	Mild diseases only without substantive functional limitations. Current smoker, social alcohol drinker, pregnancy, obesity (30<BMI<40), well-controlled DM/HTN, mild lung disease	Asymptomatic congenital cardiac disease, well controlled dysrhythmias, asthma without exacerbation, well controlled epilepsy, non-insulin dependent diabetes mellitus, abnormal BMI percentile for age, mild/moderate OSA, oncologic state in remission, autism with mild limitations	Normal pregnancy*, well controlled gestational HTN, controlled preeclampsia without severe features, diet-controlled gestational DM.
ASA III	A patient with severe systemic disease	Substantive functional limitations; One or more moderate to severe diseases. Poorly controlled DM or HTN, COPD, morbid obesity (BMI ≥40), active hepatitis, alcohol dependence or abuse, implanted pacemaker, moderate reduction of ejection fraction, ESRD undergoing regularly scheduled dialysis, history (>3 months) of MI, CVA, TIA, or CAD/stents.	Uncorrected stable congenital cardiac abnormality, asthma with exacerbation, poorly controlled epilepsy, insulin dependent diabetes mellitus, morbid obesity, malnutrition, severe OSA, oncologic state, renal failure, muscular dystrophy, cystic fibrosis, history of organ transplantation, brain/spinal cord malformation, symptomatic hydrocephalus, premature infant PCA <60 weeks, autism with severe limitations, metabolic disease, difficult airway, long term parenteral nutrition. Full term infants <6 weeks of age.	Preeclampsia with severe features, gestational DM with complications or high insulin requirements, a thrombophilic disease requiring anticoagulation.
ASA IV	A patient with severe systemic disease that is a constant threat to life	Recent (<3 months) MI, CVA, TIA or CAD/stents, ongoing cardiac ischemia or severe valve dysfunction, severe reduction of ejection fraction, shock, sepsis, DIC, ARD or ESRD not undergoing regularly scheduled dialysis	Symptomatic congenital cardiac abnormality, congestive heart failure, active sequelae of prematurity, acute hypoxic-ischemic encephalopathy, shock, sepsis, disseminated intravascular coagulation, automatic implantable cardioverter-defibrillator, ventilator dependence, endocrinopathy, severe trauma, severe respiratory distress, advanced oncologic state.	Preeclampsia with severe features complicated by HELLP or other adverse event, peripartum cardiomyopathy with EF <40, uncorrected/decompensated heart disease, acquired or congenital.
ASA V	A moribund patient who is not expected to survive without the operation	Ruptured abdominal/thoracic aneurysm, massive trauma, intracranial bleed with mass effect, ischemic bowel in the face of significant cardiac pathology or multiple organ/system dysfunction	Massive trauma, intracranial hemorrhage with mass effect, patient requiring ECMO, respiratory failure or arrest, malignant hypertension, decompensated congestive heart failure, hepatic encephalopathy, ischemic bowel or multiple organ/system dysfunction.	Uterine rupture.
ASA VI	A declared brain-dead patient whose organs are being removed for donor purposes			

Figure 1.5   ASA Physical Status Classification System. *Source:* Courtesy of the American Society of Anesthesiologists [63].

Medical Consultations

- Do not ask for a "medical clearance" from a medical provider but request a "medical consultation" instead.
- The dentist providing the dental treatment is liable for all treatment complications, even with a "medical clearance."
- Always make a copy of the medical consultation for your records as the patient may lose the form and you may have forgotten all the questions you listed on the form.

Sample Form

Medical Consultation for Dental Treatment

To: [physician name]   Fax: [physician's fax]

From: [dentist name]   Phone: [dentist's office number]

Regarding: [patient name]   Patient's date of birth: _____

Patient's signature authorizing exchange of information between the dentist and physician

_____

Date_____

Our mutual patient, _____, reports the following medical history:

Medical conditions:

_____

Medications:

_____

Allergies:

_____

Surgeries:

_____

Hospitalizations:

_____

Planned dental treatment and medications includes:

Local anesthetics:
- 20% Topical benzocaine
- 2% Lidocaine with epinephrine 1:100 000
- 4% Articaine with epinephrine 1:200 000
- 3% Mepivacaine (plain)
- 0.5% Bupivacaine with epinephrine 1:200 000

- Radiographs and exam
- Nitrous oxide and oxygen sedation
- Prophy (cleaning)
- Scaling and root planing (deep cleaning) fillings, crowns, bridges
- Extraction of _____ teeth
- Root canal treatment
- Implant placement
- Partials/dentures

- Antibiotics: penicillin, amoxicillin, amoxicillin/clavulanate, azithromycin, clindamycin, metronidazole, cephalexin
- Ibuprofen
- Acetaminophen
- Dietary fluoride supplements
- Other:

Dentist's Signature_____ Date_____

For the physician to complete:

1. Please confirm the medical history as stated above, and add any missing medical conditions, medications, allergies, surgeries, hospitalizations: (Please initial)
2. I have medical concerns about this patient's fitness for the planned dental treatment and request a consultation prior to treatment: (Please initial) YES_____ NO_____
3. Additional questions from the dentist:

_____
_____
_____
_____

_____   _____
Physician's Signature   Date

Return completed form to: [dentist's fax number]

Charting Template

- CC:
- Accompanied by [name and relationship]:
- Vitals:
- Patient denies: diabetes, CVA, MI, previous endocarditis, congenital heart disease, blood thinners, pacemaker, HIV, chemotherapy, IV bisphosphonates, radiation to head and neck, artificial joints, tobacco. *Women*: contraceptives, pregnant, nursing
- Reviewed medical history:
  - Medical conditions:
  - Medications:
  - Allergies: [may be no known drug allergies or NKDA]
  - Surgeries:
  - Hospitalizations:
  - Denies medical conditions, medications, allergies, surgeries, hospitalizations
- ASA level:
- No change in medical history since last visit:
- Health History form filled out on: [helps keep track as it should be filled out every two years]

Clinical Pearls

Troubleshooting

- Sometimes patients cannot recall all of their medical conditions. By asking the patient the reason for taking each individual medication, it can provide you with more information regarding their medical conditions.
- To find out about other medical conditions the patient may have, ask the patient "Are there any medications you are supposed to be taking but are not?"
- If you are concerned about the patient's ability to legally consent to treatment, you can:
  - Contact the patient's physician and ask if the patient has had a diagnosis of dementia, Alzheimer's, etc.
  - Find out if the patient has a court-appointed conservator or legal guardian.
  - Contact your lawyer or dental malpractice carrier for more guidance.

Tips

- Train your dental assistant to make sure *every* box is checked in the health history form before handing it to you.

- Follow your gut instinct if unsure about the patient's ability to report a thorough health history and consult with the patient's physician.
- Chart the year next to any surgeries, hospitalizations, or other significant events (e.g. heart attack in 2019, joint replacement 2012 and 2013). If you write "2 months ago" or "3.5 years ago" and then you treat the patient again, you will have to spend time going through your charts to determine when the actual incident occurred.
- Including medical alerts in the chart can be great reminders (e.g. antibiotic premed needed, limit epinephrine, breastfeeding). Be sure you don't write anything in the chart you wouldn't want your patient to read.
- When reviewing the health history with the patient, sit at eye level with them. Scan their hands and arms for bruises. This may indicate a possible blood disorder or blood thinners.
- If the paramedics are called for a patient, be prepared with the following information: patient name, date of birth, age, medical conditions, medications, allergies, surgeries, hospitalizations, vitals (with the time taken), time of incident, description, and any intervention you have provided.

Real-Life Clinical Questions Answered

Dental Student's Comment

- "My patient has asthma and is here for a filling."
  - I like to know how well controlled it is and if there is any chance the patient will have an asthma attack in the chair. See *Asthma*.

Dental Assistants' Questions

- "Doc, how often do we have the patient fill out the health history form?"
  - A new health history form must be filled out every two years [1].
  - And at every visit we need to ask the patient if there have been any changes to their health history, such as new medical conditions, new medications, recent hospitalizations or surgeries.
- "Doctor, the pulse is really high, is that OK?"
  - >110 beats/minute? Considered serious. See *Vitals*.
- "If I take his temperature, what temperature is considered a fever?"
  - ≥100.4°F (38°C). See *Vitals*.

Patient's Daughter's Comment

- "She [the patient] is my mother and I will translate for her."
  - Obtaining an accurate health history is critical for reducing complications.
  - Use a trained professional medical interpreter to ensure the patient understands the medical/dental terminology for accuracy [1]. In addition, having a relative or friend translate can breach medical confidentiality and add bias to the health history gathering.

Patients' Comments

- "Yeah I take medications but you don't need to know which ones I'm taking, you're just working on my teeth."

   – I understand how the two may not seem related, your medications and the dental treatment, but I need a full medical history including all the medications you are taking in order to provide you with the safest treatment possible. Some medications can affect your oral health and the treatment we provide. Without a full health history we are working in the dark.
- "I stopped my blood thinner medication a few days before this appointment."
   – Which medication? Was this recommended by the patient's physician?
      ○ The risks of stopping these medications can be very dangerous as there is a reason you were prescribed the medication [31]. I will have to consult with your physician before we proceed.
- "I took about 10 aspirin the last two days before today's extraction appointment."
   – An 81 mg daily dose is safe for extractions; however, if the patient took this many at once they will have prolonged bleeding.
   – Determine the urgency of the extraction. Can it be postponed one week?
   – If urgent, will need to use local measures (i.e. hemostatic agents).
   – With aspirin it takes 7–10 days for normal platelet function to return [40]. See section Medications.
- "My INR is always 2 so I'll be fine"
   – For invasive treatment we need your INR within 24 hours for accuracy as this number can fluctuate. This is in your best interest.
- "I have a newborn!"
   – Congratulations. Are you nursing now? See *Nursing*. Add a medical alert to the chart.
- "I have HIV but I'm undetectable."
   – No treatment modifications necessary, but for invasive treatment (SRP/oral surgery) it's a good idea to obtain recent lab results (i.e. WBC, neutrophils, platelets). See *HIV*.
- "I had radiation to my head"
   – Add medical alert to the chart. See *Cancer*.
- "I had a heart attack last week but don't worry about it, I'm fine just pull the tooth."
   – Determine the urgency of the extraction.
   – Are you taking any new medications? (May be on blood thinners.)
   – See *Heart conditions: Heart attack*.
- "I feel fine so I'm not going to the emergency room because of my blood pressure."
   – Determine if symptomatic.
   – See *Hypertension*.
   – Have a protocol in place for patient to sign an AMA form if patient declines to go to the ER. Contact lawyer/malpractice carrier for guidance and form.

Patients' Questions

- "I'm pregnant. Is it safe to get dental treatment?"
   – Add medical alert to the chart. See *Pregnancy*.
- "I'm just here for my denture, so why do you need to take my blood pressure?"
   – We screen all our patients at every visit. I've had patients with undiagnosed high blood pressure, patients whose blood pressure was poorly controlled, and blood pressures so high that the patient was referred to the ER. High blood pressure is considered a silent killer as you can be asymptomatic and putting you at high risk for heart attack, stroke, and other conditions.
- "I was diagnosed with cancer and I need a dental clearance signed."
   – The patient is asking you to sign a "dental clearance" to begin treatment which may include chemotherapy, radiation, IV bisphosphonates, etc.

- Consulting with the oncologist is beneficial.
- See *Cancer*.
- Once all the dental treatment is completed, recommend stating on the dental clearance form that "the patient is low risk," as there is no guarantee of zero risk.

References

1 ADA ebook (2019). *Guidelines for Practice Success: Managing Professional Risks.* American Dental Association.

2 USPS.COM (2019). What is general delivery? https://faq.usps.com/s/article/What-is-General-Delivery (accessed 28 April 2020).

3 Weber, M.L. Deaf patients in the dental office: how you can help. http://www.dmdtoday.com/news/deaf-patients-in-the-dental-office-how-you-can-help (accessed 8 April 2020).

4 Little, J.W., Falace, D.A., Miller, C.S., and Rhodus, N.L. (ed.) (2013). *Little and Falace's Dental Management of the Medically Compromised Patient*, 8e. St. Louis, MO: Elsevier Mosby.

5 Khalaf, M.W., Khader, R., Cobetto, G. et al. (2013). Risk of adrenal crisis in dental patients: results of a systematic search of the literature. *J. Am. Dent. Assoc.* 144 (2): 152–160.

6 Malamed, S.F. (2013). *Handbook of Local Anesthesia*, 6e. St. Louis, MO: Elsevier Mosby.

7 Shillingburg, H.T. Jr., Sather, D.A., Wilson, E.L. Jr. et al. (2012). *Fundamentals of Fixed Prosthodontics*, 4e. Chicago: Quintessence Books.

8 Horst, J.A., Ellenikiotis, H., UCSF Silver Caries Arrest Committee, and Milgrom, P.M. (2016). UCSF protocol for caries arrest using silver diamine fluoride: rationale, indications, and consent. *J. Calif. Dent. Assoc.* 44 (1): 16–28.

9 Rose, L.F. and Mealy, B.L. (2004). *Periodontics: Medicine, Surgery, and Implants*. St. Louis, MO: Elsevier Mosby.

10 American Dental Association (2020). Xerostomia. http://www.ada.org/en/member-center/oral-health-topics/xerostomia (accessed 8 April 2020).

11 University of Washington School of Dentistry (2012). Children with autism spectrum disorder. Oral Health Fact Sheet for Dental Professionals. https://dental.washington.edu/wp-content/media/sp_need_pdfs/Autism-Dental.pdf (accessed 9 April 2020).

12 University of California San Francisco (UCSF) (2020). Life after bariatric surgery. UCSF Patient Education. https://www.ucsfhealth.org/education/life-after-bariatric-surgery (accessed 8 April 2020).

13 Cummings, S. and Pratty, J. ((2015). Metabolic and bariatric surgery: nutrition and dental considerations. *J. Am. Dent. Assoc.* 146 (10): 767–772.

14 Kandray, D.P. (2014). Treating patients with Bell's palsy. Journal of Professional Excellence. Dimensions of Dental Hygiene. https://dimensionsofdentalhygiene.com/article/treating-patients-with-bells-palsy (accessed 10 April 2020).

15 American Dental Association. Mouth Healthy. Hormones and dental health: what every woman needs to know. https://www.mouthhealthy.org/en/az-topics/h/hormones (accessed 19 April 2020).

16 Crest Oral-B at dentalcare.com Continuing Education Course (2011), Revised 8 September 2011.

17 American Dental Association (ADA) (2020). Antibiotic prophylaxis prior to dental procedures. http://www.ada.org/en/member-center/oral-health-topics/antibiotic-prophylaxis (accessed 10 April 2020).

18 Newland, R.J., Meiller, T.F., Wynn, R.L. et al. (2013). *Oral Soft Tissue Diseases: A Reference Manual for Diagnosis and Management*, 6e. Hudson, OH: Lexicomp.

19 American Dental Association (ADA) (2019). Osteoporosis medications and medication-related osteonecrosis of the jaw. http://www.ada.org/en/member-center/oral-health-topics/osteoporosis-medications (accessed 25 April 2020).

20 American Dental Association (2020). Celiac disease. http://www.ada.org/en/member-center/oral-health-topics/celiac-disease (accessed 8 April 2020).

21 Jacobsen, P.L. (2013). *The Little Dental Drug Booklet: Handbook of Commonly Used Dental Medications*, 2e. Hudson, OH: Lexicomp.

22 University of Washington School of Dentistry Children with cerebral palsy (2012). Oral Health Fact Sheet for Dental Professionals. http://dental.washington.edu/wp-content/media/sp_need_pdfs/CP-Dental.pdf (accessed 8 April 2020).

23 Centers for Disease Control and Prevention (CDC) (2020). Influenza (flu). Cold versus flu. https://www.cdc.gov/flu/symptoms/coldflu.htm (accessed 9 April 2020).

24 O'Neil, M. (ed.) (2015). *The ADA Practical Guide to Substance Use Disorders and Safe Prescribing*. Hoboken, NJ: Wiley Blackwell.

25 American Academy of Periodontology (2016). Marijuana use linked to increased gum disease risk. http://www.perio.org/consumer/marijuana-use (accessed 10 April 2020).

26 Centers for Disease Control and Prevention (2020). About electronic cigarettes (E-cigarettes). http://www.cdc.gov/tobacco/basic_information/e-cigarettes/about-e-cigarettes.html (Accessed 4/10/2020).

27 U.S. Food and Drug Administration (2016). The facts on the FDA's new tobacco rule. http://www.fda.gov/consumers/consumer-updates/facts-fdas-new-tobacco-rule (Accessed 10 April 2020).

28 Centers for Disease Control and Prevention (2020). Electronic cigarettes: what's the

bottom line? https://www.cdc.gov/tobacco/basic_information/e-cigarettes/pdfs/Electronic-Cigarettes-Infographic-p.pdf (accessed 20 April 2020).

29 Waldron, R. (2018). Tips for communicating with deaf patients. http://www.colgateprofessional.com/education/professional-education/topics/patient-care/tips-for-communicating-with-deaf-patients (accessed 8 April 2020).

30 U.S. Department of Health and Human Services (2009). National Institutes of Health. National Institute of Dental and Craniofacial Research. Practical oral care for people with Down syndrome. https://www.nidcr.nih.gov/sites/default/files/2017-09/practical-oral-care-down-syndrome.pdf (accessed 27 April 2020).

31 American Academy of Oral Medicine (AAOM) (2007). Blood thinners and dental care. http://www.aaom.com/index.php?option=com_content&view=article&id=126:blood-thinners-and-dental-care&catid=22:patient-condition-information&Itemid=120 (accessed 10 April 2020).

32 American Academy of Periodontology (2018). Staging and grading periodontitis. http://www.perio.org/sites/default/files/files/Staging%20and%20Grading%20Periodontitis.pdf (accessed 21 April 2020).

33 University of Washington School of Dentistry (2012). Children with Down syndrome (trisomy 21). Oral Health Fact Sheet for Dental Professionals. http://dental.washington.edu/wp-content/media/sp_need_pdfs/Down-Dental.pdf (accessed 27 April 2020).

34 Misch, C.E. (2008). *Contemporary Implant Dentistry*, 3e. St. Louis, MO: Mosby.

35 Centers for Disease Control and Prevention (CDC) (2019). Influenza (flu). Preventive steps (updated 9 October 2019). http://www.cdc.gov/flu/prevent/prevention.htm (accessed 9 April 2020).

36 Centers for Disease Control and Prevention (CDC) (2018). Flu: what do do if you get sick (last updated 8 October 2018). https://www.cdc.gov/flu/treatment/takingcare.htm (accessed 9 April 2020).

37 MouthHealthy. Cold and flu season: 5 ways to care for your mouth when you're sick. http://www.mouthhealthy.org/en/az-topics/c/cold-and-flu-season (accessed 9 April 2020).

38 American Cancer Society. Esophageal cancer risk factors. http://www.cancer.org/cancer/esophagus-cancer/causes-risks-prevention/risk-factors.html (accessed 14 April 2020).

39 Bhattacharyya, I., Chehal, H., Gremillion, H., and Nair, M. (2010). Gout of the temporomandibular joint: a review of the literature. *J. Am. Dent. Assoc.* 141 (8): 979–985.

40 Wynn, R.L., Meiller, T.F., and Crossley, H.L. (2018). *Lexicomp*. In: *Drug Information Handbook for Dentistry*, 24e. Wolters Kluwer.

41 American Heart Association (2017). Managing high blood pressure medications. http://www.heart.org/en/health-topics/high-blood-pressure/changes-you-can-make-to-manage-high-blood-pressure/managing-high-blood-pressure-medications (accessed 19 April 2020).

42 American Dental Association (2015). Management of patients with prosthetic joints undergoing dental procedures. http://www.ada.org/~/media/EBD/Files/ADA_Chairside_Guide_Prosthetics.pdf?la=en (accessed 19 April 2020).

43 American Academy of Orthopedic Surgeons (AAOS) (2016). Appropriate use criteria. Management of patients with orthopedic implants undergoing dental procedures. https://aaos.webauthor.com/go/auc/terms.cfm?auc_id=224995&actionxm=Terms (accessed 9 April 2020).

44 Centers for Disease Control and Prevention (2019). Head lice. Prevention and control. http://www.cdc.gov/parasites/lice/head/prevent.html (accessed 8 April 2020).

45 Neville, B.W., Damm, D.D., Allen, C., and Chi, A. (2016). *Oral and Maxillofacial Pathology*, 4e. St. Louis, MO: Elsevier Saunders.

46 Zarb, G. and Bolender, C. (2004). *Prosthodontic Treatment for Edentulous Paienets: Complete Dentures and Implant-Supported Prostheses*, 12e. St. Louis, MO: Mosby.

47 Centers for Disease Control and Prevention (CDC) (2019). Methicillin-resistant *Staphylococcus aureus* (MRSA). General information (updated 26 June 2019). http://www.cdc.gov/mrsa/community/index.html#anchor_1548173148 (accessed 9 April 2020).

48 Skouteris, C.A. (ed.) (2018). *Dental Management of the Pregnant Patient*. Hoboken, NJ: Wiley Blackwell.

49 American Dental Association (2020). Cardiac implanted devices and electronic dental instruments. http://www.ada.org/en/member-center/oral-health-topics/cardiac-implanted-devices-and-electronic-dental-instruments (accessed 9 April 2020).

50 American College of Obstetricians and Gynecologists (ACOG) (2013). Oral health care during pregnancy and through the lifespan. http://www.acog.org/clinical/clinical-guidance/committee-opinion/articles/2013/08/oral-health-care-during-pregnancy-and-through-the-lifespan (accessed 19 April 2020).

51 Centers for Disease Control and Prevention (2020). Your risk of *C. diff*. https://www.cdc.gov/cdiff/risk.html (accessed 8 April 2020).

52 Centers for Disease Control and Prevention (2020). Prevent the spread of *C. diff*. https://www.cdc.gov/cdiff/prevent.html (accessed 8 April 2020).

53 Centers for Disease Control and Prevention (CDC) (2020). Scabies frequently asked questions (FAQs). http://www.cdc.gov/parasites/scabies/gen_info/faqs.html (accessed 10 April 2020).

54 American Academy of Oral Medicine (AAOM) (2016). Subject: Dental care for the patient with an oral herpetic lesion. https://www.aaom.com/index.php?option=com_content&view=article&id=161:clinical-practice-statement--dental-care-for-the-patient-with-an-oral-herpetic-

lesion&catid=24:clinical-practice-statement (accessed 18 April 2020).

55 Centers for Disease Control and Prevention (CDC) (2019). Shingles (herpes zoster). Transmission. http://www.cdc.gov/shingles/about/transmission.html (accessed 10 April 2020).

56 American Academy of Periodontology (2020). Classification of periodontal and peri-implant diseases and conditions. http://www.perio.org/sites/default/files/files/Classification%20at%20a%20glance.pdf (accessed 28 March 2020).

57 Centers for Disease Control and Prevention (CDC) (2019). Tuberculosis (TB) screening, testing, and treatment of U.S. health care personnel frequently asked questions (FAQs). http://www.cdc.gov/tb/topic/infectioncontrol/healthcarepersonnel-faq.htm (accessed 9 April 2020).

58 American Heart Association (2020). Understanding blood pressure readings. http://www.heart.org/en/health-topics/high-blood-pressure/understanding-blood-pressure-readings (accessed 19 April 2020).

59 Meiller, T.F., Wynn, R.L., McMullin, A.M. et al. (2012). *Dental Office Medical Emergencies*, 5e. Hudson, OH: Lexicomp.

60 Centers for Disease Control and Prevention (2017). Quarantine and isolation. http://www.cdc.gov/quarantine/maritime/definitions-signs-symptoms-conditions-ill-travelers.html (accessed 9 April 2020).

61 Centers for Disease Control and Prevention (2020). Water and nutrition. http://www.cdc.gov/healthywater/drinking/nutrition/index.html (accessed 9 April 2020).

62 American Lung Association (2020). Pulse oximetry. http://www.lung.org/lung-health-diseases/lung-procedures-and-tests/pulse-oximetry (accessed 9 April 2020).

63 American Society of Anesthesiologists (2021). ASA Physical Status Classification System. https://www.asahq.org/standards-and-guidelines/asa-physical-status-classification-system (accessed 8 May 2021).

64. Samhsa's national helpline: 1-800-662-HELP (4357). The substance use and mental health leadership counsil of RI. (2021). https://www.sumhlc.org/resources/samhsas-national-helpline-1800662-help/ (Accessed 19 December 2021).

2

Extraoral Exam, Intraoral Exam, and Oral Cancer Screening

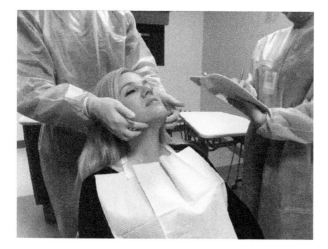

Figure 2.1 Palpation of the submandibular lymph nodes during an extraoral exam.

Chapter Outline

- Real-Life Questions and Comments
- Relevance
- Purpose of the EOE, IOE, and OCS
- Oral Cancer
  - Risk Factors
  - Signs and Symptoms
  - Prognosis
  - Treatment
  - Risk Reduction
- Screening Frequency
- Armamentarium
- Procedural Steps
- Detecting Oral Cancer Guide from the National Institute for Dental and Craniofacial Research (NIDCR)

Clinical Dentistry Daily Reference Guide, First Edition. William A. Jacobson.
© 2022 John Wiley & Sons, Inc. Published 2022 by John Wiley & Sons, Inc.

- Adjunctive Technologies
- The American Dental Association Evidence-Based Clinical Practice Guideline for the Evaluation of Potentially Malignant Disorders in the Oral Cavity
- Referral
- Informed Refusal
- Clinical Pearls: Tips
- Real-Life Questions and Comments Answered
- References

Real-Life Questions and Comments

Dental Student's Question

- "What is your sequence for conducting an oral cancer screening?"

Dental Assistant's Comment

- "Hey doc while you get started I'm going to get something from sterilization."

Patients' Questions

- "How can I lower my risk of oral cancer?"
- "I don't have oral cancer, right?"
- "I've heard some offices use a blue light to check for oral cancer."
- "Is this contagious?"
- "What causes that sound in my TMJ?"

Patients' Comments

- "I just got punched."
- "I know I'm healthy, I don't need a biopsy."

Relevance

You must conduct a thorough extraoral exam (EOE), intraoral exam (IOE), and oral cancer screening (OCS) on every patient at the initial and recall visits. You may only have the opportunity to meet the patient once. To avoid any oversights, it's important that you follow a systematic approach. You must also know what to do when an abnormality is detected.

Purpose of the EOE, IOE, and OCS

Some reasons include the following.

- Early detection of oral cancer. OCS is effective in reducing the mortality rate of oral cancer in high-risk individuals who use tobacco and/or alcohol [1].
- Identification of oral manifestations of systemic diseases and medications.

- Identification of treatment modifications, e.g. identifying a palatal tori, which may require surgical removal prior to fabricating a denture.
- Evaluation and documentation of trauma, e.g. patient was attacked at a bus stop and your records will be obtained later as part of a police report.
- Documentation of existing conditions, e.g. documenting temporomandibular joint (TMJ)-related conditions at the initial exam to prevent accusations in the future such as "After seeing you for a filling my TMJ started making noises."

Oral Cancer

Risk Factors

- Tobacco use
  - All tobacco products [2].
  - Cigarette smoking is the single largest risk factor for cancer including the head and neck [3].
  - Smoking risk is dose dependent.
  - Secondhand smoke may increase the risk of these cancers, but this has not yet been proved [3].
- Alcohol consumption: any type.
- Tobacco and alcohol consumption is synergistic.
- Human papillomavirus (HPV)
  - Most common sexually transmitted disease in the United States.
  - Causes cervical cancer in women, and vulvar, vaginal, penile, anal, and oropharyngeal cancers.
  - 70% of oropharynx cancers linked to HPV [2].
- Ultraviolet (UV) light is a major cause of cancer on lips.
- Men have twice the risk of women [2].
- Age: over 50 years [2].
- Occupational exposure: cancers of the nasopharynx if working in the construction, textile, ceramic, logging, and food processing industries, or if exposed to wood dust, formaldehyde, asbestos, nickel, and other chemicals [2].
- Being partially edentulous or edentulous: due to association with heavy alcohol and tobacco consumption, less education, lower socioeconomic status, and poor dental health [4].
- Ill-fitting dental prosthesis wearers:
  - "Chronic irritation caused by an ill-fitting prosthesis may promote carcinogenesis, particularly if other carcinogenic contributors (alcohol, tobacco) are involved. Persons with more than 15 missing teeth may be at greater risk for developing oral cancer, and they frequently wear dentures. Further, there is a four times greater risk of developing head and neck cancer if the denture is ill fitting" [5].
- Other: chewing betel quid, certain rare heritable conditions.

Signs and Symptoms

- Ulceration in the mouth that does not heal (most common sign).
- Persistent leukoplakia or erythroplakia on gingiva, tongue, tonsil, or oral mucosa.
  - Majority of leukoplakia does not progress to cancer.
  - Erythroplakia and lesions with erythroplakic components have greater potential for becoming cancerous [6].

- Painless lesion (initially) [7].
- Lump or thickening in the cheek (be sure to palpate).
- Increasing trismus (be sure to measure the range of motions).
- Decreasing tongue mobility.
- Sensory changes of tongue or other oral structures.
- Swelling of the edentulous areas causing the denture to fit poorly or become uncomfortable.
- Increasing tooth mobility or pain associated with teeth or jaw.
- Difficult chewing with or without dysphagia.
- Sore throat or feeling something is caught in the throat.
- Voice changes.
- Lump or mass in the neck.
- Weight loss [8].

Prognosis

- Localized disease: 83% five-year survival rate.
- Metastasized cancer: 36% five-year survival rate [6].

Treatment

- May involve surgery, radiation therapy, chemotherapy, or a combination [8].

Risk Reduction

- Do not smoke or use tobacco products.
  - History of smoking? Oral and oropharynx cancer risk declines and may approach that of non-smokers after 10 or more years of quitting [6].
- Limit alcohol consumption.
  - History of alcohol consumption? Risk of head and neck cancer declines and may approach that of individuals who have never consumed alcohol after 20 or more years [6].
- Lower your risk of developing an HPV-associated cancer.
  - Use condoms and dental dams during oral sex to lower risk of giving or getting HPV.
  - Discuss HPV vaccine inoculation with your physician.
    - ○ The HPV vaccine is recommended by the CDC, American Cancer Society, American Association of Oral and Maxillofacial Surgeons, ADA, and American Academy of Pediatric Dentistry [6, 9].
    - ○ The HPV vaccine is safe, for both males and females, and prevents infections associated with HPV associated with oral and oropharyngeal cancers.
    - ○ The HPV vaccine is recommended as early as age nine [9].
- Use lip balm with sunscreen, wear hats, and avoid indoor tanning.
- Wear masks if working around occupational hazards.
- Visit the dentist regularly [2].

Screening Frequency

- Initial and recall visits for all patients [10].

Armamentarium

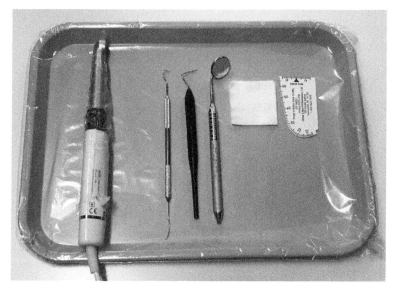

Figure 2.2 Armamentarium for the extraoral, intraoral, and oral cancer screening exams.

Armamentarium for conducting extraoral, intraoral, and oral cancer screening exams (See Figure 2.2):

- Intraoral camera for documentation of any abnormal findings.
- Exam kit including a mouth mirror, periodontal probe, and explorer.
- Gauze (2×2 inch) to retract the tongue, dry and wipe off any debris.
- Range of motion scale for baseline findings.

Procedural Steps

1) Review the health history:
   a) Consider any risk factors for oral cancer. Inform your patient of these risk factors and their association with oral cancer. See section Risk Factors.
2) Utilize your dental assistant as both a witness and to record the findings during the exam (See Figure 2.1).
3) Obtain verbal consent from the patient:
   a) "I will perform a thorough evaluation checking for any abnormalities and conducting an oral cancer screening. This involves touching your face and neck. May I have your permission to do so?"
4) Request the patient to remove any eyewear, scarf, lipstick, and removable oral appliances (Figure 2.3).
5) Conduct the EOE, IOE, and OCS, and end by checking occlusion.
   a) Use a systematic approach to avoid any oversights (underdiagnosing) (Figure 2.4).
6) Discuss the findings with the patient:
   a) If no abnormal findings, inform the patient "no abnormalities detected."
   b) If abnormal findings:

    i) Take intraoral photos as baseline findings for the patient's records.

    ii) If a white or red patch/lesion, schedule a two-week follow up for reevaluation [6].

    iii) If a lesion is suspected to be a potentially malignant disorder, "perform a biopsy of lesion or provide immediate referral to a specialist" [11] (see Figure 2.9).

7) Document findings in the patient record.

8) Additional site-specific considerations during EOE/IOE/OCS are listed in Table 2.1.

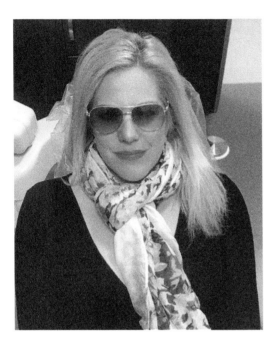

Figure 2.3 The patient's sunglasses, lipstick, and scarf will have to be removed prior to the EOE/IOE/OCS.

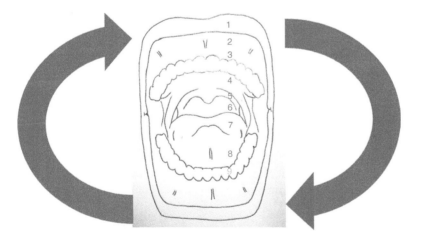

Figure 2.4 My systematic clockwise approach for examining (1) lips; (2) labial mucosa, vestibule, and buccal mucosa; (3) gingiva; (4) hard palate; (5) soft palate, uvula, palatoglossal arch, palatine tonsils, and palatopharyngeal arch; (6) posterior pharyngeal wall; (7) tongue: dorsal, lateral, tip, ventral; (8) floor of the mouth; (9) dentition (different color to emphasize teeth are examined last).

Table 2.1 Site-specific additional considerations during the EOE/IOE/OCS.

Site	Additional considerations
Face	• Look for symmetry and for facial swelling from an odontogenic infection • Refer to the ER for IV antibiotics if swelling causes difficult breathing/swallowing, cellulitis lower than inferior border of the mandible, involves the eye, or if anatomy is distorted (patient does not look human) • Document any trauma, scars, piercings • Look for yellowing of the skin or eyes (jaundice)
Sinuses	• Not all the sinuses can be palpated and no tenderness on palpation does not rule out sinus congestion. An increase in pain bending forward may predict sinus congestion. Can try a trial period of decongestants or referral to medical provider [12]
Skin	• Evaluate for changes in color, contour, and consistency • Evaluate moles on face • Look for the ABCDE of melanoma: A, asymmetry; B, border (irregular); C, color (uneven); D, diameter (>6 mm); E, evolving [13]
Salivary glands	• Evaluate the submental, submandibular, parotid, and minor salivary glands
Lymph nodes	• Evaluate the lymph nodes for size, consistency, and tenderness. The face and neck must be relaxed to prevent palpating the muscles. If the lymph nodes are palpable, they are considered enlarged • Evaluate the submental, submandibular, tonsillar, parotid, preauricular, posterior auricular, occipital, superficial cervical, deep cervical, posterior cervical, and supraclavicular lymph nodes (Figure 2.5) • Healthy: small, soft, free/mobile, cannot be visualized or palpated • Enlarged lymph nodes due to infection/inflammation: soft, movable, painful [7] • Enlarged lymph nodes due to primary or malignant neoplasm: firm, fixed, not painful [7]
Thyroid	• The thyroid rises when the patient swallows • Evaluate size and palpate for diffuse or nodular enlargements, firmness, or tenderness and refer to medical doctor if detected [14]
TMJ	• For more details see section Clinical and Radiographic Exam in Chapter 15
Range of motions	• For more details see section Clinical and Radiographic Exam in Chapter 15
Muscles	• For more details see section Clinical and Radiographic Exam in Chapter 15
Oral region	• In children may note lip licker's dermatitis
Lip: vermilion border	• Common site of herpes simplex virus
Lip: commissures	• Look for angular cheilitis
Lips	• Fordyce granules
Labial mucosa	• Look for mucoceles and aphthous ulcers.
Buccal mucosa	• Palpate for any lumps or thickening. If leukoedema confirm with the stretch test • Site of Stenson's duct and Fordyce granules
Gingiva	• Note physiologic pigmentation, gingivitis, parulis, buccal exostosis, amalgam tattoo
Vestibule	• Check for epulis fissuratum in denture/partial wearers • If the patient chews tobacco, ask the location of tobacco placement and evaluate tissue
Hard palate	• Check for palatal tori. In smokers check for nicotine stomatitis
Soft palate	• Determine the Mallampati score (significance: as it increases, the patient is harder to intubate and increased risk of sleep apnea) (Figure 2.6)
Uvula	• May be missing due to surgical removal for obstructive sleep apnea

(*Continued*)

Table 2.1 (Continued)

Site	Additional considerations
Palatine tonsils	• Evaluate for the size of tonsils (if present), which can differ on the left and right • Grade: 0 (previous tonsillectomy), 1 (hidden in pillars), 2 (visible beyond pillars), 3 (extending 50–75% to midline), 4 (occupy >75% pharyngeal space, or "kissing") [15] • Tend to decrease in size after age nine and shrink rapidly during the teen years. If enlarged can obstruct the airway and cause sleep apnea and breathing difficulty [16] (Figure 2.7)
Floor of mouth	• Palpate to locate any mandibular tori
Tongue: dorsal	• Evaluate mobility/function. Common findings: scalloped tongue, fissured tongue, geographic tongue • Papillae present: vallate, fungiform papillae, filiform papillae
Tongue: lateral	• Site of foliate papillae • Don't forget to evaluate the tip of the tongue (often covered in gauze when retracting tongue)
Tongue: ventral	• Site of lingual varicosities
Occlusion	• Molar Class I (normal or malocclusion), II (malocclusion), III (malocclusion) • Canine Class I, II, III • Overbite (%) and overjet (mm) • Midline on/off • Edge-to-edge, anterior/posterior open bite (mm) • Crossbite (unilateral/bilateral) • Buccal crossbite/Brodie bite • Crowding, supraerupted, intruded

Sources: based on Wright [12], American Academy of Dermatology [13] and Little et al. [14].

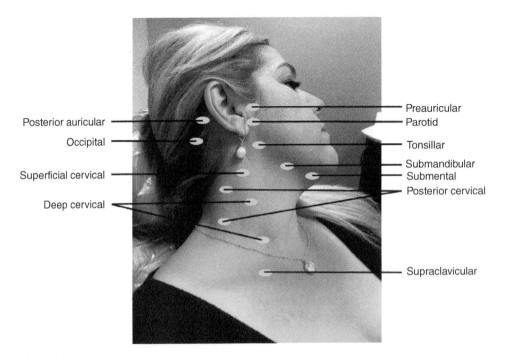

Figure 2.5 Lymph nodes.

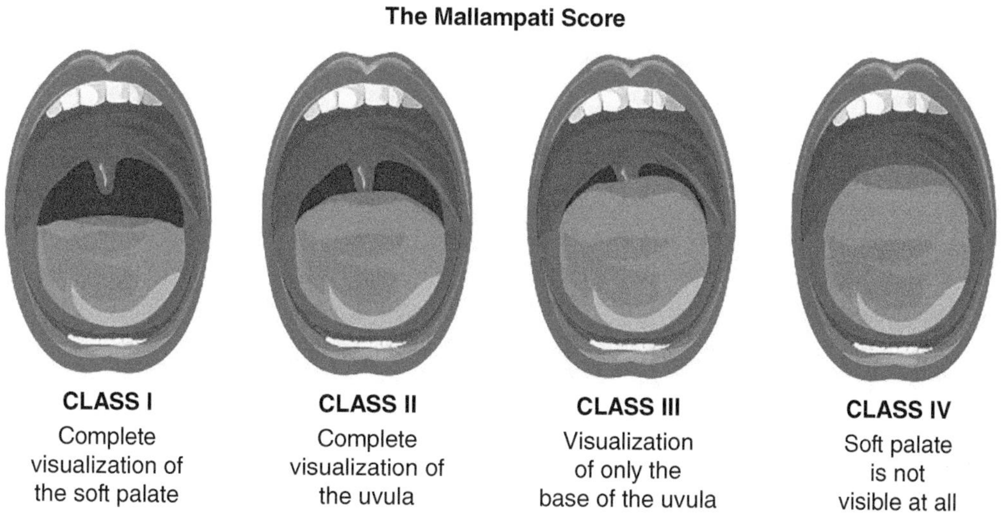

The Mallampati Score

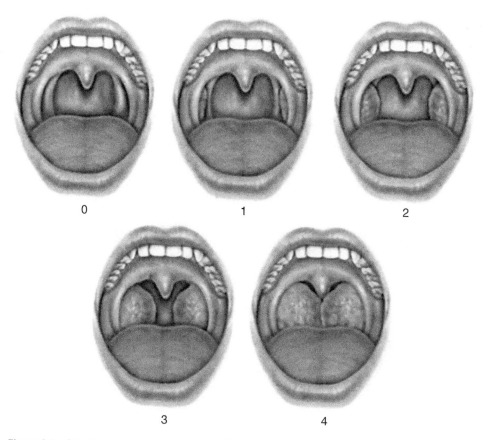

CLASS I	CLASS II	CLASS III	CLASS IV
Complete visualization of the soft palate	Complete visualization of the uvula	Visualization of only the base of the uvula	Soft palate is not visible at all

Figure 2.6 Mallampati score. Source: O'Brien, S.M. (2016). Understanding the Mallampati score. https://www.clinicaladvisor.com/home/the-waiting-room/understanding-the-mallampati-score/.

0   1   2

3   4

Figure 2.7 Brodsky grading scale for tonsils. *Source:* Lu et al. [15]. Licensed under CC BY 4.0.

Detecting Oral Cancer Guide from the National Institute for Dental and Craniofacial Research (NIDCR) [17]

An oral cancer screening guide for health care professionals developed by the National Institute for Dental and Craniofacial Research (NIDCR). See Figure 2.8.

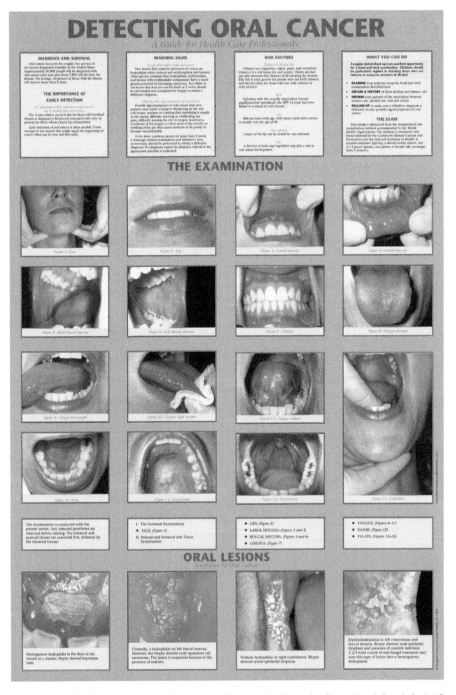

Figure 2.8 NIDCR oral cancer guide. *Source:* National Institute for Dental and Craniofacial Research [17].

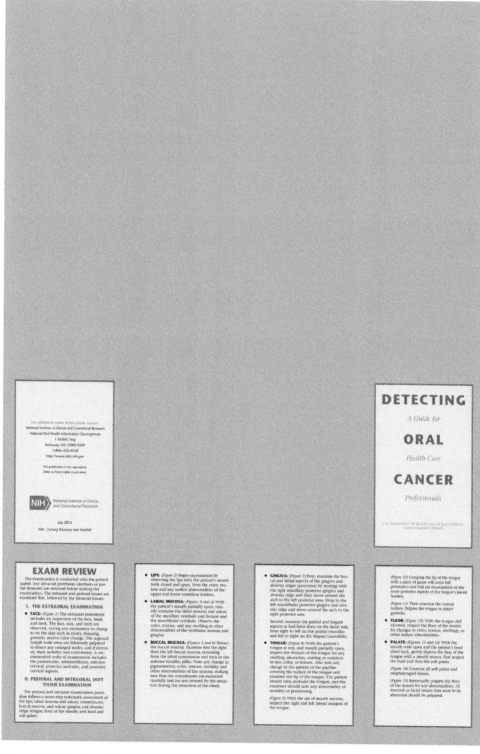

Figure 2.8 (Continued)

Adjunctive Technologies

"Adjunctive technologies – such as toluidine blue, cytologic testing, autofluorescence, tissue reflectance and salivary adjuncts have demonstrated limited diagnostic accuracy to routinely be used as a screening tool for head and neck cancer" according to the American Association of Oral and Maxillofacial Surgeons [1].

The American Dental Association Evidence-Based Clinical Practice Guideline for the Evaluation of Potentially Malignant Disorders in the Oral Cavity

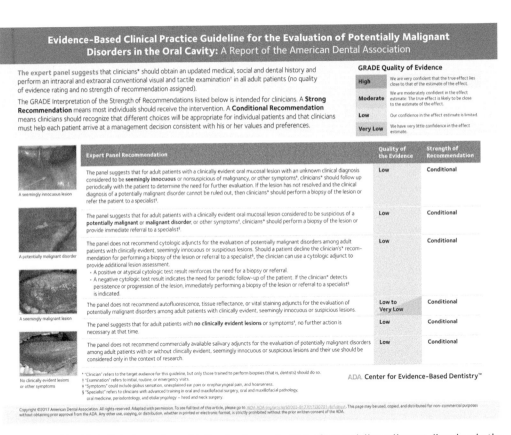

Figure 2.9 The ADA clinical practice guideline for the evaluation of potentially malignant disorders in the oral cavity.

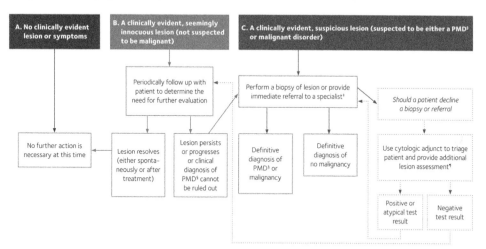

Evidence-Based Clinical Practice Guideline for the Evaluation of Potentially Malignant Disorders in the Oral Cavity: A Report of the American Dental Association

Clinical Pathway for the Evaluation of Potentially Malignant Disorders in the Oral Cavity
Clinicians* should obtain or update patient history† and perform an intraoral and extraoral conventional visual and tactile examination in all adult patients. If during initial, routine or emergency examinations, a patient has:

A. No clinically evident lesion or symptoms

B. A clinically evident, seemingly innocuous lesion (not suspected to be malignant)

C. A clinically evident, suspicious lesion (suspected to be either a PMD§ or malignant disorder)

Periodically follow up with patient to determine the need for further evaluation

Perform a biopsy of lesion or provide immediate referral to a specialist‡

Should a patient decline a biopsy or referral

No further action is necessary at this time

Lesion resolves (either spontaneously or after treatment)

Lesion persists or progresses or clinical diagnosis of PMD§ cannot be ruled out

Definitive diagnosis of PMD§ or malignancy

Definitive diagnosis of no malignancy

Use cytologic adjunct to triage patient and provide additional lesion assessment¶

Positive or atypical test result

Negative test result

* "Clinician" refers to general dentists, specialists, and hygienists.
† Along with evaluation of lesions, clinicians should take a comprehensive history that considers signs and symptoms of disease. Symptoms could include globus sensation, unexplained ear or oropharyngeal pain, and hoarseness.
‡ Specialists have advanced training in oral and maxillofacial surgery, oral and maxillofacial pathology, oral medicine, periodontology, and otolaryngology – head and neck surgery (ENT).
§ "PMD" refers to potentially malignant disorder.
¶ If cytologic adjunct is used, downstream consequences of true-positive, false-positive, true-negative, and false-negative test results should be considered. In particular, clinicians need to periodically monitor patients who test negative for the target condition via cytologic testing to minimize the downstream consequences of a potential false-negative result (that is, to avoid a delayed definitive diagnosis or treatment).

Figure 2.9 (Continued)

Referral

- Patient's chief complaint
- History of present illness: onset, changes in size, symptoms
- Symptoms of the lesion: Is the patient aware of the lesion?
- Prior treatment and response to treatment
- Familial history
- Is medical history contributory?
- Is dental history contributory?
- Oral habits
- Photos (and radiographs if applicable)
- Clinical diagnosis/impression: can include differential diagnosis (list of about four or five diseases in decreasing order of your likely diagnosis)
- Description of the abnormality
  - Size: length, width, and height (mm)
  - Appearance
  - Color
  - Configuration: flat or raised
  - Surface: smooth or rough
  - Mobility: fixed or movable
  - Attachment: broad or narrow stalk
  - Consistency: soft or firm

Oral Cancer Screening

- – Quantity: solitary or multiple
- – Symmetrical or asymmetrical [7]
- The referral may be sent to an:
  - – Oral medicine specialist
  - – Orofacial pain specialist
  - – Oral and maxillofacial surgeon
  - – Oral and maxillofacial pathologist
  - – Oral and maxillofacial radiologist
  - – Otolaryngologist/ear, nose, and throat (ENT) doctor
  - – Dermatologist (extraoral)
  - – PCP (who may refer to a specialist)

Informed Refusal

Contact your professional liability carrier and/or attorney for specific guidance and forms. Legally and ethically a patient cannot consent to substandard care and you can be accused of "supervised neglect."

Clinical Pearls: Tips

- EOE:
  - – EOE before IOE to avoid spreading saliva to the face.
  - – Learn the anatomic names of regions of face and lymph nodes for documentation and for referrals to specialists.
  - – Detecting facial swelling: Look at the patient face to face and also look from behind and above the patient's head (Figure 2.10).
  - – If the lips appear dry, apply lubricant prior to procedures to prevent cracking.

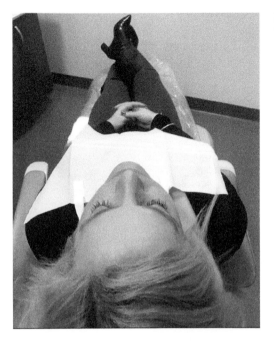

Figure 2.10 Vantage point to evaluate for any facial swelling.

- IOE:
  - Always verify the mouth mirror is securely tightened in the handle prior to placing in the patient's mouth.
  - Scan slowly; if you go too fast you can underdiagnose.
  - If oral soft tissue is supported by bone, palpate against the bone [7].
  - If oral soft tissue is not supported by bone, palpate between fingers [7].
  - Can apply pressure with the side of an explorer to extrude suppuration to confirm the presence of a fistula (Figures 2.11 and 2.12).

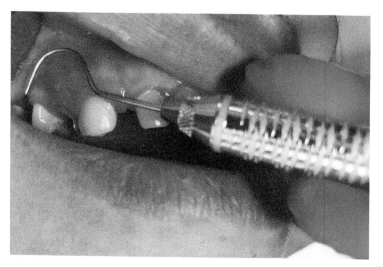

Figure 2.11 A small swelling noted on the gingiva adjacent to a severely decayed and fractured tooth #5.

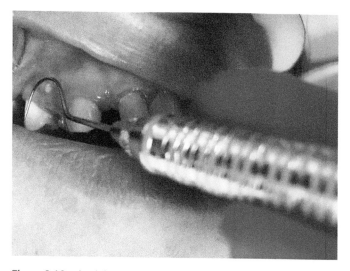

Figure 2.12 Applying pressure to the gingiva with the side of the explorer resulted in the extrusion of suppuration, confirming the presence of a fistula.

– The reason we tell the patient to "Say aah" for better visualization (Figures 2.13 and 2.14).

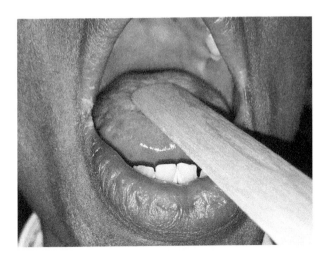

Figure 2.13 The patient was asked to open her mouth. The tongue is obstructing the view of the soft palate, uvula, palatine tonsils, palatoglossal arch, palatopharyngeal arch, and posterior pharyngeal wall.

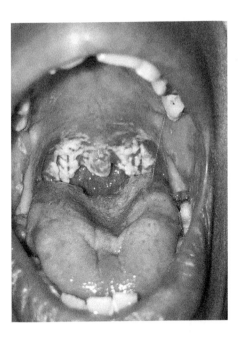

Figure 2.14 The same patient was told "Say aah" and to "yawn" for better visualization of her anatomy. White patches were noted on the soft palate, uvula, palatoglossal arch, and palatopharyngeal arch.

– If you see an ulceration in mouth, try to determine the etiology (e.g. sharp tooth adjacent to ulceration).
– Don't forget to evaluate the tip of the tongue for abnormalities. Oftentimes it is covered in gauze when you are holding it to evaluate the lateral borders.
– For any abnormalities, take an intraoral photo with a periodontal probe as a reference for size. Measure and document the length, width, and height (Figure 2.15).

Figure 2.15 A periodontal probe adjacent to a soft tissue lesion as a reference for size.

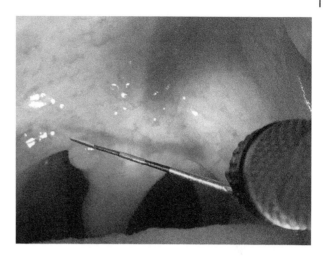

- – "If [you] see unilateral tonsil swelling in an adult, until proven otherwise it is cancer, inflammatory process usually bilateral" – this is a quote from a continuing education speaker.
- – Detecting dry mouth: if the buccal mucosa sticks to mirror the mucosa is very dry.
- Figure 2.16 is my collage of abnormal findings on EOE/IOE/OCS that emphasize the importance of examining *every square inch* in the mouth.

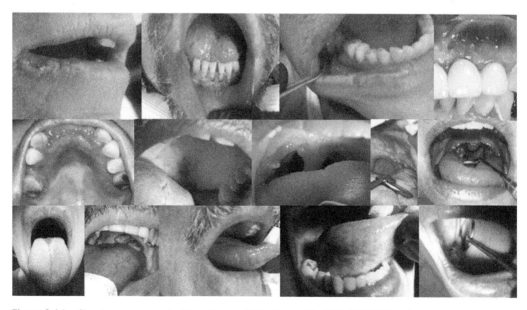

Figure 2.16 Check *every square inch* for abnormalities during the EOE/IOE/OCS as these can appear anywhere.

- Recommend keeping oral pathology books in your dental office to reference when evaluating pathology. Useful books include:
  - Newland, J.R., Meiller, T.F., Wynn, R.L. and Crossley, H.L. (2013). *Oral Soft Tissue Diseases: A Reference Manual for Diagnosis and Management*, 6th edn. Hudson, OH: Lexicomp.
  - Newland, J.R. (2012). *Oral Hard Tissue Diseases: A Reference Manual for Radiographic Diagnosis*, 3rd edn. Hudson, OH: Lexicomp.
  - Neville, B.W., Damm, D.D., Allen, C.M. and Chi, A.C. (2016). *Oral and Maxillofacial Pathology*, 4th edn. St. Louis, MO: Saunders Elsevier.
- Medicolegal considerations:
  - It can be easy to forget to follow up on a lesion. Do not allow a year to go by and then realize that you wrote on the patient's record "Follow up on tongue lesion." If it ended up being oral cancer, by the time you see the patient the cancer could have metastasized. Be sure to schedule a follow-up appointment.
  - Malpractice litigations have been due to failure to reexamine lesions and failure to biopsy.
- CDT billing codes: D0150 (Comprehensive Oral Evaluation), D0120 (Periodic Oral Evaluation), and D0180 (Comprehensive Periodontal Evaluation) all include "oral cancer evaluation" in the description [18].
- Documentation:
  - If there are no abnormal findings during the OCS, document "Oral cancer screening: no abnormalities detected."
  - Some people advise against writing "WNL" (i.e. within normal limits) and refer to it jokingly as "we never looked" as it is ambigous.

Real-Life Questions and Comments Answered

Dental Student's Question

- "What is your sequence for conducting an oral cancer screening?"
  - See section Procedural Steps.

Dental Assistant's Comment

- "Hey doc, while you get started I'm going to get something from sterilization."
  - Inform the assistant that you need him or her present as a witness during the oral cancer screening (to avoid being accused of any inappropriate behavior by the patient).

Patients' Questions

- "How can I lower my risk of oral cancer?"
  - See section Oral Cancer: Risk Reduction.
- "I don't have oral cancer, right?"
  - I have not detected any abnormalities today. I will check routinely, every year. However without a biopsy I cannot provide a definitive diagnosis.
- "I've heard some offices use a blue light to check for oral cancer."
  - See section Adjunctive Technologies.

- "Is this contagious?"
  - You should be familiar with common abnormalities in the mouth to answer questions like this. Also having an oral pathology book in the office as a reference is valuable. If uncertain, inform the patient that until we have a definitive diagnosis it is better to err on the side of caution. Tell the patient to avoid sharing saliva with people.
- "What causes that sound in my TMJ?"
  - See section Clinical and Radiographic Exam in Chapter 15.

Patients' Comments

- "I just got punched."
  - Ask the patient if they are in danger. If they are, provide resources (e.g. directing the patient to a social worker).
- Depending on the state you live in, you may be a mandated reporter whereby you are legally required to report child abuse (under age 18) and elderly abuse (65 and older).
- Take extraoral/intraoral photos for documentation.
- "I know I'm healthy, I don't need a biopsy."
  - See section Informed Refusal

References

1 American Association of Oral and Maxillofacial Surgeons (2020). Head and neck cancer screening and prevention. Position paper. https://www.aaoms.org/docs/govt_affairs/advocacy_white_papers/HeadNeckCancerScreening_PositionPaper.pdf (accessed 28 June 2020).

2 Centers for Disease Control and Prevention (CDC) (2018). Head and neck cancers. https://www.cdc.gov/cancer/headneck/index.htm (accessed 28 June 2020).

3 American Association of Oral and Maxillofacial Surgeons (2020). Tobacco and electronic cigarettes. Position paper. https://www.aaoms.org/docs/govt_affairs/advocacy_white_papers/TobaccoEcigarettes_PositionPaper.pdf (accessed 28 June 2020).

4 Zarb, G. and Bolender, C. (2004). *Prosthodontic Treatment for Edentulous Patients: Complete Dentures and Implant-Supported Prostheses*, 12e. St. Louis, MO: Mosby.

5 American College of Prosthodontists (2018). The frequency of denture replacement. https://www.prosthodontics.org/about-acp/position-statement-the-frequency-of-denture-replacement (accessed 1 December 2019).

6 American Dental Association (ADA) (2019). Cancer (head and neck). https://www.ada.org/en/member-center/oral-health-topics/cancer-head-and-neck (accessed 28 June 2020).

7 Newland, J.R., Meiller, T.F., Wynn, R.L., and Crossley, H.L. *Oral Soft Tissue Diseases: A Reference Manual for Diagnosis and Management*, 6e. Hudson, OH: Lexicomp.

8 American College of Prosthodontists (2015). Oral cancer screening. Position statement. https://www.prosthodontics.org/about-acp/position-statement-oral-cancer-screening (accessed 28 June 2020).

9 American Association of Oral and Maxillofacial Surgeons (2020). Human papillomavirus vaccination. Position paper. https://www.aaoms.org/docs/govt_affairs/advocacy_white_papers/HPV-vaccination_PositionPaper.pdf (accessed 28 June 2020).

10 American Academy of Oral Medicine (AAOM) (2016). Subject: oral cancer screening. https://www.aaom.com/clinical-practice-statement--oral-cancer-screening (accessed 28 June 2020).

Oral Cancer Screening

11 American Dental Association (2017). Evidence-based clinical practice guidelines for the evaluation of potentially malignant disorders in the oral cavity: a report of the American Dental Association. https://ebd.ada.org/~/media/EBD/Files/10870A_Chairside_Guide_OralCancer_FINAL.pdf?la=en (accessed 21 July 2020).

12 Wright, E.F. (2005). *Manual of Temporomandibular Disorders*. Ames, IA: Blackwell Munksgaard.

13 American Academy of Dermatology (2020). What to look for: ABCDEs of melanoma. https://www.aad.org/public/diseases/skin-cancer/find/at-risk/abcdes (accessed 28 June 2020).

14 Little, J.W., Falace, D.A., Miller, C.S., and Rhodus, N.L. (2013). *Little and Falace's Dental Management of the Medically Compromised Patient*, 8e. St. Louis, MO: Elsevier Mosby.

15 Lu, X., Zhang, J., and Xiao, S. (2018). Correlation between Brodsky tonsil scale and tonsil volume in adult patients. *BioMed Res. Int.* 6434872. https://doi.org/10.1155/2018/6434872 (accessed 28 June 2020).

16 Maddern, B.R. (2021). When a child's tonsils need to come out. Stanford Children's Health. https://www.stanfordchildrens.org/en/topic/default?id=when-a-childs-tonsils-need-to-come-out-1-1683 (accessed 21 May 2021).

17 National Institute for Dental and Craniofacial Research (2013). Detecting oral cancer: a guide for health care professionals. https://www.nidcr.nih.gov/sites/default/files/2017-09/detecting-oral-cancer-poster.pdf (accessed 28 June 2020).

18 American Dental Association (2016). CDT Code Check phone app.

3

Radiographs and Interpretation

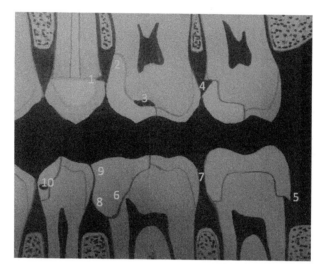

Figure 3.1 Evaluating restorations on a bitewings.

Chapter Outline

- Real-Life Clinical Questions
- Relevance
- Types of Radiographs
  – Bitewing
  – Periapical
  – Panoramic
  – Occlusal
  – Cone Beam Computed Tomography (CBCT)
- Treatment Planning
  – Recommendations for Prescribing Dental Radiographs
- Informed Consents
  – Informed Refusal
  – Verbal Consents

Clinical Dentistry Daily Reference Guide, First Edition. William A. Jacobson.
© 2022 John Wiley & Sons, Inc. Published 2022 by John Wiley & Sons, Inc.

Real-Life Clinical Questions

Dental Assistant's Question

- "Hey doc, what type of X-rays do you want me to take on this 5-year-old?"

Patients' Health Concerns

- "How much am I getting radiated?"
- "I'm pregnant and was told not to get X-rays."
- "I've had radiation treatment for cancer to my head. Is it bad to get more radiation?"
- "Where should I move the stroller to so that my baby is not radiated when you take my X-rays?"

Patients' Questions

- "I just want you to do an exam without taking X-rays."
- "I just had X-rays taken one month ago at another office. Can they send you those?"
- "What is a bitewing and a PA?"
- "What is a lead apron and thyroid collar?"
- "Why can't you check for cavities in the pano? Why do you have to take more X-rays?"
- "Does the X-ray show the tooth fracture?"
- "I have a cavity on the X-ray you want to watch? Why aren't you going to remove it?"
- "How long will it take for that cavity in the X-ray to get bigger? Can I wait until I'm back from out of town?"
- "Why can't you see which tooth is infected from the X-ray?"
- "I fell and chipped my tooth and cut my lip."

Relevance

It's important to know how often to prescribe radiographs, the type of radiographs indicated, and how to interpret these radiographs for a timely diagnosis. You should also understand the risks and benefits of taking radiographs to address patients' concerns about their amount of radiation exposure.

Types of Radiographs

A complete series of radiographic images/full-mouth radiographic series/full-mouth examination (FMX) typically consist of 18 images, including four bitewing (BW) and 14 periapical (PA) images.

Bitewing

- For posterior teeth, used to check alveolar crest height, calculus, interproximal decay, and integrity of restorations.
- Vertical BWs:
  - Same as a BW except oriented vertically in order to capture the crestal bone when there is bone loss for diagnosing.
  - Due to the narrower mesial–distal length when the sensor is oriented vertically, six BWs would be required instead of four BWs.

Periapical

- For anterior and posterior teeth, used to evaluate the roots, and the adjacent structures. including periodontal ligament (PDL), lamina dura (cortical bone), cancellous bone (spongy bone), any PA pathosis.
- Used to diagnose caries in anterior PAs, but not in posterior PAs due to distortion.

Panoramic

- A single image which includes both the maxillary and the mandibular dental arches and their supporting structures. Useful for detecting trauma, third molars, extensive dental and periodontal disease, large lesions, tooth development, retained teeth or root tips, TMJ, carotid artery calcifications, and developmental anomalies.
- The main disadvantage is that it lacks fine detail for detecting small carious lesions, changes in periodontium, and PA disease, and the anterior region has the most distortion and superimposition from the cervical vertebrae [1].

Occlusal

- May be used in children instead of PA due to the small size.
- Can be used to evaluate impacted, missing, or supernumerary teeth, or abnormally positioned teeth.

Cone Beam Computed Tomography (CBCT)

- Allows a three-dimensional view of the anatomy versus a two-dimensional view.
- Can view cross-sections of the anatomy (think of sliced bread).
- May be used in cases involving the evaluation of failing endodontic treatment, pathology, root resorption, trauma, distance to the inferior alveolar nerve or sinuses, implant treatment planning, etc.
- Regarding usage in endodontics, see Chapter 8.

Treatment Planning

Recommendations for Prescribing Dental Radiographs

"These recommendations are subject to clinical judgment and may not apply to every patient. They are to be used by dentists only after reviewing the patient's health history and completing a clinical examination. Even though radiation exposure from dental radiographs is low, once a decision to obtain radiographs is made it is the dentist's responsibility to follow the ALARA Principle (As Low as Reasonably Achievable) to minimize the patient's exposure" (American Dental Association and Food and Drug Administration [2]) (Table 3.1).

Table 3.1 Recommendations for prescribing dental radiographs.

	Patient age and dental developmental stage				
Type of encounter	Child with primary dentition (prior to eruption of first permanent tooth)	Child with transitional dentition (after eruption of first permanent tooth)	Adolescent with permanent dentition (prior to eruption of third molars)	Adult, dentate, or partially edentulous	Adult, edentulous
New patient[a] being evaluated for oral diseases	Individualized radiographic exam consisting of selected PA/occlusal views and/or posterior BWs if proximal surfaces cannot be visualized or probed. Patients without evidence of disease and with open proximal contacts may not require a radiographic exam at this time	Individualized radiographic exam consisting of posterior BWs with panoramic exam or posterior BWs and selected PA images‛	Individualized radiographic exam consisting of posterior BWs with panoramic exam or posterior BWs and selected PA images. An intraoral FMX is preferred when the patient has clinical evidence of generalized oral disease or a history of extensive dental treatment		Individualized radiographic exam based on clinical signs and symptoms
Recall patient[a] with clinical caries or at increased risk for caries[b]	Posterior BW exam at 6–12 month intervals if proximal surfaces cannot be examined visually or with a probe			Posterior BW exam at 6–18 month intervals	Not applicable
Recall patient[a] with no clinical caries and not at increased risk for caries[b]	Posterior BW exam at 12–24 month intervals if proximal surfaces cannot be examined visually or with a probe		Posterior BW exam at 18–36 month intervals	Posterior BW exam at 24–36 month intervals	Not applicable
Recall patient[a] with periodontal disease	Clinical judgment as to the need for and type of radiographic images for the evaluation of periodontal disease. Imaging may consist of, but is not limited to, selected BW and/or PA images of areas where periodontal disease (other than nonspecific gingivitis) can be demonstrated clinically				Not applicable
Patient (new and recall) for monitoring of dentofacial growth and development, and/or assessment of dental/skeletal relationships	Clinical judgment as to need for and type of radiographic images for evaluation and/or monitoring of dentofacial growth and development or assessment of dental and skeletal relationships		Clinical judgment as to need for and type of radiographic images for evaluation and/or monitoring of dentofacial growth and development, or assessment of dental and skeletal relationships. Panoramic or PA exam to assess developing third molars	Usually not indicated for monitoring of growth and development. Clinical judgment as to the need for and type of radiographic image for evaluation of dental and skeletal relationships	

(Continued)

Table 3.1 (Continued)

Type of encounter	Patient age and dental developmental stage				
	Child with primary dentition (prior to eruption of first permanent tooth)	Child with transitional dentition (after eruption of first permanent tooth)	Adolescent with permanent dentition (prior to eruption of third molars)	Adult, dentate, or partially edentulous	Adult, edentulous
Patient with other circumstances, including, but not limited to, proposed or existing implants, other dental and craniofacial pathoses, restorative or endodontic needs, treated periodontal disease and caries remineralization	Clinical judgment as to need for and type of radiographic images for evaluation and/or monitoring of these conditions				

^a Clinical situations for which radiographs may be indicated include, but are not limited to:

A) Positive Historical Findings
   1) Previous periodontal or endodontic treatment
   2) History of pain or trauma
   3) Familial history of dental anomalies
   4) Postoperative evaluation of healing
   5) Remineralization monitoring
   6) Presence of implants, previous implant-related pathosis or evaluation for implant placement
B) Positive Clinical Signs/Symptoms
   1) Clinical evidence of periodontal disease
   2) Large or deep restorations
   3) Deep carious lesions
   4) Malposed or clinically impacted teeth
   5) Swelling
   6) Evidence of dental/facial trauma
   7) Mobility of teeth
   8) Sinus tract ("fistula")
   9) Clinically suspected sinus pathosis

10) Growth abnormalities
11) Oral involvement in known or suspected systemic disease
12) Positive neurologic findings in the head and neck
13) Evidence of foreign objects
14) Pain and/or dysfunction of the temporomandibular joint
15) Facial asymmetry
16) Abutment teeth for fixed or removable partial prosthesis
17) Unexplained bleeding
18) Unexplained sensitivity of teeth
19) Unusual eruption, spacing, or migration of teeth
20) Unusual tooth morphology, calcification, or color
21) Unexplained absence of teeth
22) Clinical tooth erosion
23) Peri-implantitis.

[b] Factors increasing risk for caries may be assessed using the ADA Caries Risk Assessment Forms (0–6 years of age and over 6 years of age) [2] (see Chapter 5).

Source: Copyright © 2012 American Dental Association. All rights reserved. Reprinted with permission.

Informed Consents

Informed Refusal

If a patient is refusing radiographs when the dentist determines radiographs are necessary, the dentist should:

- Seek to understand why the patient is refusing radiographs (e.g. financial, concerns about radiation exposure).
- Explain why the radiographs are necessary (e.g. "It is like doing an exam in the dark").
- Do not allow the patient to sign an informed refusal consent form as he or she would be consenting to substandard treatment (i.e. below the standard of care, considered negligence) and dentists must practice within the standards of care. It is in the dentist's best interest to terminate the dentist–patient relationship and follow protocols recommended by the dentist's dental liability insurance company and/or consult with an attorney [3].

Verbal Consents

Be sure to discuss (and document) the radiographic findings with your patient.
Two common scenarios include:

- Deep decay planned for a filling: inform the patient that the goal is to save the teeth. However, the decay appears deep and the tooth may require more treatment or not be savable. The tooth may require root canal treatment, crown lengthening, post and core, core buildup, and a crown, or extraction and tooth replacement.
- A defective crown planned for replacement: inform the patient the crown is defective and the reason (e.g. open margin, recurrent decay, fracture, open proximal contact, shade). The goal is to replace the crown. The condition of the tooth beneath the crown cannot be determined radiographically and can only be discovered once the crown is removed. Since we do not know the condition of the tooth at this point, there is a possibility the tooth may require more treatment or not be savable. The tooth may require root canal treatment, crown lengthening, post and core, core buildup, and a crown, or extraction and tooth replacement. If there is an existing post, then assume the tooth is even more compromised (less chance of being restorable).

Procedural Steps

1) Review the health history.
2) Examine the mouth to determine the radiographs needed (see section Recommendations for Prescribing Dental Radiographs).
3) Dental assistant takes radiographs: review X-rays for any retakes necessary *prior* to the assistant saving X-rays and putting the equipment away.
4) Interpret and document the radiographic findings in the odontogram.
5) Clinical examination:
    a) Perform the EOE, IOE, and OCS (see Chapter 2).
    b) Check *every* surface of *every* tooth for additional findings, and to confirm radiographic findings. Add findings to the odontogram.

6) Take intraoral photos: if findings do not appear radiographically (e.g. caries, open margins, defective restorations), it is a good idea to take intraoral photos for documentation. The dental insurance company could do an audit and accuse you of "overtreatment" if the radiographs do not show the findings which appear only clinically. Also useful for patient education and as your documentation in any future malpractice claims.
7) Show the patient the radiographs and intraoral photos and communicate the findings.
8) Discuss the proposed treatment plan and answer any questions.
9) Document.

Radiographic Interpretation

Diagnostic Image Criteria

- Good image quality?
- BW radiographs: find out if the following are present:
  - Posterior contacts open (if overlapping, retake unless open contacts on another BW).
  - Distal of canine visible (to diagnose distal caries on the canine and mesial caries on the first premolar).
  - Distal of last molar (to diagnose distal caries).
  - Visible crestal bone on maxillary and mandibular arches (to diagnose bone loss).
- PA radiographs: find out if the following are present:
  - 2 mm beyond the apex (to check for periapical radiolucency [PARL]).
    - On an anterior PA, the entire incisal edge captured (important to capture as the patient can blame you for chipping the edge during treatment when it was already present).
    - If present, the entire PA pathosis captured in image (if large, consider panoramic radiograph).

Diagnosis

- Do not simply look at the radiographs. You must interpret the image.
- When viewing bitewings (BWs) outline the crestal bone and the teeth. See Figure 3.2
- Be on the lookout for potential findings. See Figure 3.3
- When viewing periapicals (PAs) outline the entire roots. See Figure 3.4
- Be on the lookout for potential findings. See Figure 3.5

Figure 3.2 With your eyes, outline the clinical crown from the crestal bone on one side of the tooth to the crestal bone on the other side of the tooth (numbers correspond to the sequence of examination).

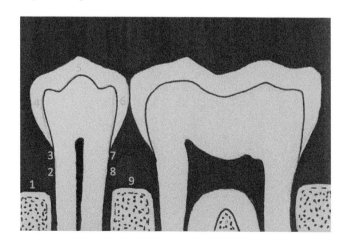

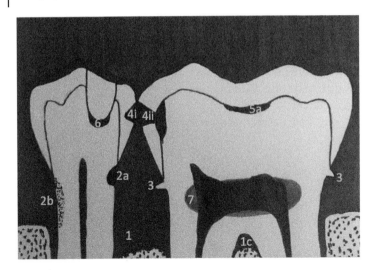

Figure 3.3 Potential findings on the BW radiograph (numbers refer to the list in section Bitewing Radiographs).

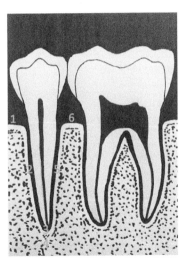

Figure 3.4 With your eyes, outline the root(s) of the tooth (numbers correspond to the sequence of examination).

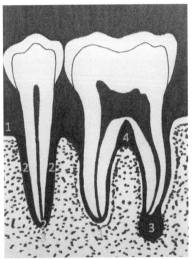

Figure 3.5 Potential findings on the PA radiograph (numbers refer to the list in section Periapical Radiographs).

Bitewing Radiographs

1) Crestal bone
   a) Measure the distance from the cementoenamel junction (CEJ) to crestal bone (in health ≤1.5 mm [1]; range 0.5–2 mm).
   b) Horizontal or vertical bone loss?
   c) Furcation involvement?
2) Cementum
   a) Root caries present?
   b) Cervical burnout present (apical to CEJ)?
3) CEJ: calculus?
4) Enamel
   a) Any breaks in enamel?
      i) Decay to enamel?
      ii) Decay to dentin?
      iii) Decay to pulp?
5) Dentin: decay?
6) Restorations: recurrent decay?
7) Cervical decay?

Periapical Radiographs

1) Determine the crown/root ratio.
2) Follow the PDL around the entire root(s):
   a) Check for presence of lamina dura.
   b) Check for presence of PDL:
      i) Widened PDL (occlusal trauma, PA pathosis)
      ii) Missing PDL (ankylosed)
3) Check for any PA pathosis (radiolucency, radiopacities, or combination).
4) Check for furcation involvement (hard to detect at initial stages).

Additional Considerations

- When evaluating for vertical bone loss, create an imaginary line connecting the CEJs. This line should be parallel to the crestal bone [1] (Figure 3.6).

Figure 3.6 This image may appear as vertical bone loss initially, but the CEJs are parallel to the crestal bone.

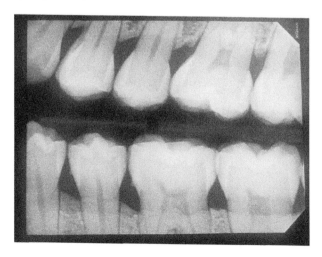

- Radiographic calculus: absence radiographically does not mean absence clinically (Figure 3.7).
- Root caries (Figure 3.7).
- Evaluating unsatisfactory restorations (Figure 3.8, same as Figure 3.1):
  1) Open margins
  2) Subgingival restoration (not unsatisfactory unless it violates the biologic width causing bone loss; may be impossible to replace if recurrent decay without crown lengthening)
  3) Recurrent decay
  4) Under-contoured
  5) Overhang
  6) Deep restoration (not unsatisfactory, may have pulpal exposure if replaced)
  7) Open contact
  8) Over-contoured
  9) Poorly contoured
  10) Voids.

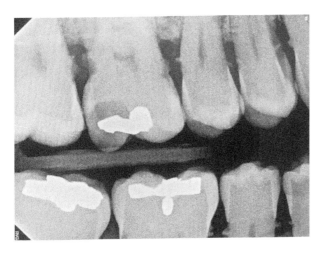

Figure 3.7   Subgingival calculus on every tooth and root caries on the distal of #3.

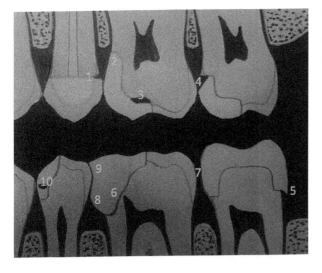

Figure 3.8   Rendition of unsatisfactory restorations (numbers refer to the list under Evaluating unsatisfactory restorations in section Additional Considerations).

- Actual unsatisfactory restorations:
  - BW radiograph reveals deep subgingival decay on lingual of #14. Note that you cannot determine if the decay is buccal or lingual from a single BW (Figure 3.9).
  - BW radiograph of #12 DO composite with recurrent decay (Figure 3.10).
  - PA radiograph of #30 and #31 zirconia crowns with deep subgingival recurrent decay on the buccal. Keep in mind that PA radiograph can distort the image; however, this image has excellent paralleling technique (Figure 3.11).
  - BW radiograph of #30 and #31 PFM crowns with deep recurrent decay (Figure 3.12).
  - PA radiograph in which #30 appears to have a deep cavity to the pulp. Clinically the mesiolingual cusp is fractured and not close to pulp. Note how the PA image creates distortion (Figure 3.13).

Figure 3.9 Subgingival decay on lingual of #14.

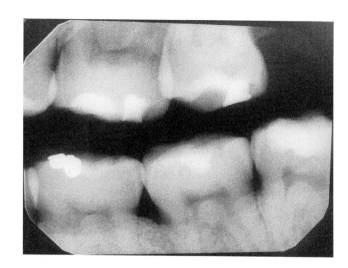

Figure 3.10 Recurrent decay on #12.

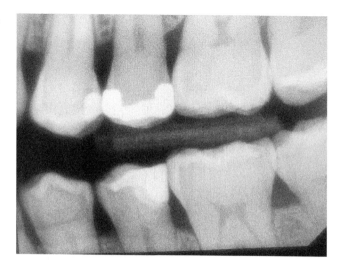

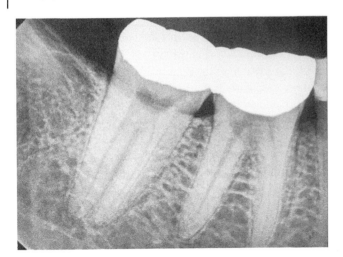

Figure 3.11 Crowns with recurrent decay.

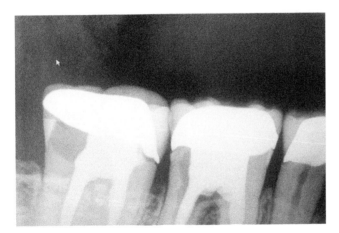

Figure 3.12 Crowns with recurrent decay.

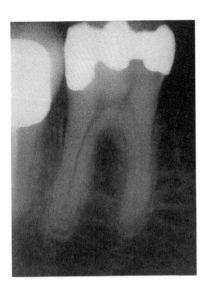

Figure 3.13 Example of distortion with PAs.

- Evaluation of the roots: look for evidence of the following.
  - Crown/root ratios (Figure 3.14)
    - <1 : 1 (favorable; 2 : 3 ratio is optimal) (Figure 3.14, tooth #23)
    - 1 : 1 (minimum) (Figure 3.14, tooth # 25) [4]
    - >1 : 1 (unfavorable) (Figure 3.14, tooth #24)
  - Visible PDL
  - Widened PDL (suggests tooth mobility from occlusal trauma or bone loss)
  - Ankylosed (no visible PDL)
  - PARL (Figure 3.15)
  - PA radiopacity
  - Internal root resorption (Figure 3.16)
  - External root resorption (Figure 3.17)
  - Hypercementosis
  - Curved

- Evaluation of the pulp chamber
  - Large (typically in children)
  - Receded (typically in older adults)
  - Pulp stones
  - Calcified canals

- Previously root canal treated teeth
  - Overfilled
  - Underfilled
  - PARL
  - Post
- Dental implants: See Chapter 14

Figure 3.14 Evaluating crown/root ratios.

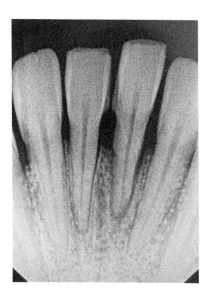

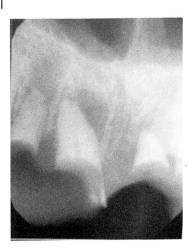

Figure 3.15   Periapical radiolucencies.

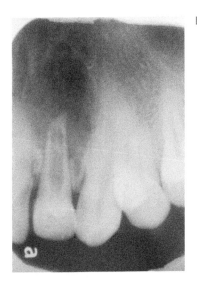

Figure 3.16   Internal root resorption of #10.

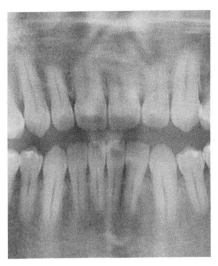

Figure 3.17   External root resorption of upper and lower incisors due to orthodontic treatment. Emphasize oral hygiene to this patient to prevent periodontal disease as any bone loss could be catastrophic.

Panoramic Anatomy

(a)

(b)

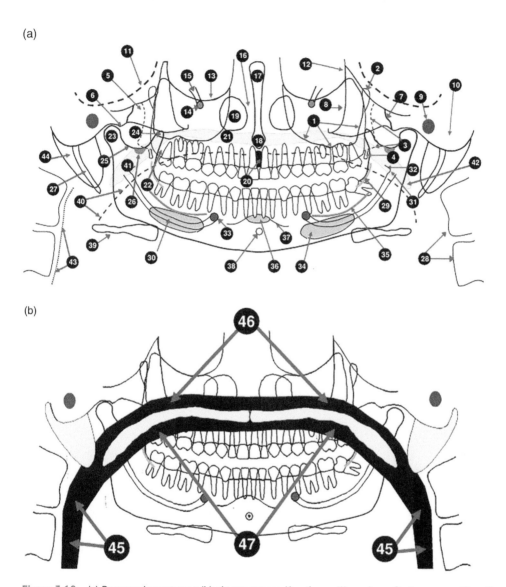

Figure 3.18   (a) Panoramic anatomy; (b) airway spaces. Key: 1, maxillary sinus; 2, pterygomaxillary fissure; 3, pterygoid plates; 4, hamulus; 5, zygomatic arch; 6, articular eminence; 7, zygomaticotemporal suture; 8, zygomatic process; 9, external auditory meatus; 10, mastoid process; 11, middle cranial fossa; 12, lateral border of the orbit; 13, infraorbital ridge; 14, infraorbital foramen; 15, infraorbital canal; 16, nasal fossa; 17, nasal septum; 18, anterior nasal spine; 19, inferior concha; 20, incisive foramen; 21, hard palate; 22, maxillary tuberosity; 23, condyle; 24, coronoid process; 25, sigmoid notch; 26, medial sigmoid depression; 27, styloid process; 28, cervical vertebrae; 29, external oblique ridge; 30, mandibular canal; 31, mandibular foramen; 32, lingula; 33, mental foramen; 34, submandibular gland fossa; 35, internal oblique ridge; 36, mental fossa; 37, mental ridges; 38, genial tubercles; 39, hyoid bone; 40, tongue; 41, soft palate; 42, uvula; 43, posterior pharyngeal wall; 44, ear lobe; 45, glossopharyngeal air space; 46, nasopharyngeal air space; 47, palatoglossal air space. *Source:* Courtesy of Robert Jaynes, DDS, MS.

Use a systematic approach to avoid oversights when interpreting panoramic radiographs. If unsure of the anatomy, see Figure 3.18 for guidance.

- Compare the left and ride side for symmetry.
- Evaluate the periphery and corners of the film (often overlooked): orbits, skull base, articular process of the temporal bone, cervical spine, styloid process, pharynx, submandibular gland (check for calcifications), and hyoid [5]. Check for any radiopacity at a 45° angle from the angle of the mandible adjacent to cervical vertebrae 3 and 4. This could indicate a carotid atheroma, with an increased risk for stroke, and warrants a referral to the patient's PCP [5]. Consider differential diagnosis such as triticeal cartilage or tonsilolith [3]. Tonsiloliths are usually located mid-ramus.
- Outline the mandible: check for fractures, asymmetries.
- Outline the maxilla:
  - Outline the sinuses and compare sinus densities.
  - Zygomatic process to the temporal bone.
  - Nasal cavity, nasal spine, nasal septum, and nasal floor.
  - Hard palate to the soft palate.
- Evaluate the bone pattern of the maxilla and mandible:
  - Compare the left and right: submandibular and sublingual gland depressions appear more radiolucent on the panoramic [1].
  - Locate the inferior alveolar nerve canal and mental foramina.
  - PA radiopacities and radiolucencies.
- Evaluate the alveolar process: bone height, PDL, lamina dura, horizontal/vertical defects, furcation.
- Evaluate the dentition: existing, missing, unerupted, impacted, decayed, restorations, etc.

Periapical Anatomy

It is important to keep in mind anatomic findings to differentiate anatomy from pathology when interpreting PAs (Table 3.2).

Table 3.2 Periapical anatomy.

Periapical location	Anatomy	Description
Posterior maxilla	Coronoid process	Radiopaque triangular shape around maxillary third or second molar in a PA when the mouth is open wide. Can interfere with diagnosis. Have the patient open minimally. Can be confused for a root tip
	Maxillary sinus	Thin radiopaque line usually from the distal of the canine to the posterior wall of maxilla above the tuberosity. On canine PAs, the floors of the sinus and nasal cavity may be superimposed forming an inverted Y. Typically, with loss of molars the floor of the sinus will appear very close to the alveolar ridge (i.e. a pneumatized sinus)
		Septa: the radiopaque lines in maxillary sinus, which are folds of cortical bone that may project a few millimeters or cross the sinus. Rarely do they separate the sinus into different compartments
	Zygomatic process	U-shaped radiopacity around apices of first and second molar
Anterior maxilla	Nasal fossa	A radiolucent oblong shape superior to maxillary anteriors and the floor of the nasal fossa extends to posterior maxilla PAs
	Intermaxillary suture/median suture	A thin radiolucent line between maxillary central incisors from the crestal bone to the posterior hard palate. May be confused for a fracture
	Lateral fossa	A diffuse radiolucency around the apex of the maxillary lateral incisor apex due to a depression on the maxilla. Can be confused for pathology, so look for intact lamina dura around the root
Posterior mandible	Mandibular canal	Radiolucent with thin radiopaque superior/inferior borders typically in contact with apex of lower third molar and further from the apex going anteriorly seen in mandibular PAs. When overlap exists between apices and mandibular canal radiographically, the PDL appears thickened and the lamina dura appears missing. Can be confused for a PARL
	Submandibular gland fossa	Poorly defined radiolucency and minimal trabecular bone located inferior to mandibular molars. Due to a depression on the lingual surface of the mandible accommodating the submandibular salivary gland [1]. May be confused for pathology
	Mental foramen	Radiolucency typically around the apex of mandibular second premolar, visible radiographically half the time. In one study "average foramen of white people was below or in front of the second premolar (89.3%) and the average foramen in blacks was below or distal to the second premolar (85.9%)" [6]. To rule out pathosis take angled PAs. See section Clinical Pearls: Troubleshooting for the SLOB rule
Anterior mandible	Genial tubercles	Radiopaque mass inferior to mandibular central incisor, serves as a muscle attachment
	Lingual foramen	A single round radiolucency in the center of the genial tubercles
	Nutrient canals	Radiolucent lines running parallel from incisive nerve to teeth apices or spaces between teeth
	Mental fossa	Diffuse radiolucency around the mandibular centrals/laterals due to a depression on the labial surface of the mandible [1]

Radiographs and Interpretation

Referrals

- Abnormal findings may be identified on radiographs, including:
  - Radiolucent lesions from diseases that destroy bone.
  - Radiopaque lesions from diseases which produce calcified material.
  - Mixed radiolucent/radiopaque lesions

- *Standard of care*: if it looks abnormal, inform the patient, write a referral to a specialist (e.g. oral and maxillofacial surgeon, oral medicine specialist, oral and maxillofacial pathologist, or oral and maxillofacial radiologist), and document the findings, discussion, and referral.
- A detailed evaluation and referral would include:
  - Investigate:
    - Patient's chief complaint.
    - History of present illness: onset, changes in size, symptoms.
    - Is medical history contributory?
    - Is dental history contributory?
  - Determine:
    - Lesion:
      - Radiolucent: unilocular, multilocular, honeycomb, or soap bubble.
      - Radiopaque: cotton wool, ground glass, or orange peel.
      - Mixed in appearance.
    - Margins:
      - Circumscribed (defined) or poorly circumscribed (poorly defined).
      - Corticated (thin radiopacity), sclerotic (thick radiopacity), or punched out (no margin).
      - Regular, irregular, or scalloped.
    - Location: maxilla, mandible, anterior, posterior, unilateral, bilateral, focal, diffuse, adjacent structures.
    - Associated with tooth root, tooth apex, or crown.
    - Adjacent structures displaced, eroded/destroyed [7].
  - Example of a referral to an oral maxillofacial surgeon:
    [Patient's name] presented for a new patient exam on December 2, 2019. A panoramic and FMX were taken. On the panoramic noted a circumscribed unilocular radiolucent lesion with corticated margins in the left posterior mandibular body distal to roots of tooth #18. Patient was unaware of this lesion and is asymptomatic at this time. Please evaluate and treat as deemed necessary and send report. Thank you.

Charting Template

Figure 3.19   At minimum, you must document all three parts of the tooth: the clinical crown (decay?), the bone level (bone loss?), and PA findings (PA pathosis?).

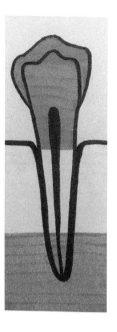

- Radiographs taken:
  - Panoramic
  - FMX
  - __ BWs
  - __ PAs

- Radiographic findings (See Figure 3.19):
  - Tooth decay (none, caries to enamel/dentin/pulp, root caries, recurrent decay)
  - Bone loss (none, generalized, localized, vertical, horizontal)
  - PA pathosis (none, PARL, PA radiopacity)
  - Teeth (missing, unerupted, impacted, supernumerary)
  - Crown/root ratio
  - Radiographic calculus
  - RCT
  - Other findings (e.g. resorption, plate, and screws)
- Discussed the radiographic findings with the patient

Billing Clarifications

- Bill the radiograph codes when used for diagnosing.
- When taking only a BW and a PA:
  - D0270: BW – single radiographic image.
  - D0220: Intraoral – PA *first* radiographic image.
  - Any more PAs would be considered *additional* PAs (D0230).

- When taking only PAs:
  - D0220: Intraoral – PA *first* radiographic image.
  - D0230: Intraoral – PA each *additional* radiographic image.
- When taking PAs during the RCT:
  - Do not bill the PA codes.
  - "Working and post-treatment" images associated with endodontic treatment are part of the global endodontic fee. Post-treatment within 30 days [8].
- When taking a crown pre-cementation BW or PA:
  - Do not bill the BW as it is part of the global crown fee.

Clinical Pearls

Troubleshooting

- Determining how many retakes: complete the series (e.g. FMX or four BWs) prior to determining which retakes are necessary as the anatomy required may be captured in a different radiograph. At Case Western Reserve University School of Dental Medicine, dental students were only allowed five retakes for an FMX and two retakes for four BWs.
- Determining why you're getting blurry radiographs: if the patient moves or the X-ray tube is moving, it will result in a blurry image.
- Determining which settings to change.
  - May need to change the settings which affect the contrast and density (Figure 3.20).
    - Density: degree of blackening.

Figure 3.20   Radiograph settings.

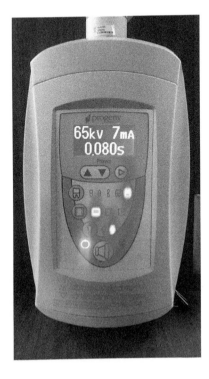

- Milliampere (mA): determines the amount of heat applied to the filament and the quantity of electrons released. The higher the mA, the darker the image.
  - Distance affects density [9].
  - ○ Contrast: the differences between the densities in the film.
    - Kilovolt peak (kVp): affects the acceleration of the electrons. The higher the kVp, the lower the contrast.
    - Seconds (s): the longer the exposure time, the darker the image.
  - – Consider contacting the X-ray equipment manufacturer.
- Diagnostic challenges
  - – Diagnosing caries.
    - ○ Always diagnose caries from a BW for posteriors and a PA for anteriors.
    - ○ Zoom out (making the image smaller) and darken to find decay (Figures 3.21 and 3.22).
    - ○ Note in the smaller darker image that teeth #2 and #31 have O decay.
    - ○ Look carefully at proximal surfaces adjacent to crowns. These are often nicked and become plaque traps that develop caries.
  - – Things that appear similar to cavities
    - ○ Tooth wear, abfraction, pits and fissures, cervical burnout, existing radiolucent dental materials, root resorption, anatomical concavity, and Mach band effect (an optical illusion that occurs when there is a sharply defined density difference, so that the more radiolucent region may appear immediately adjacent to the more radiopaque region [1]).

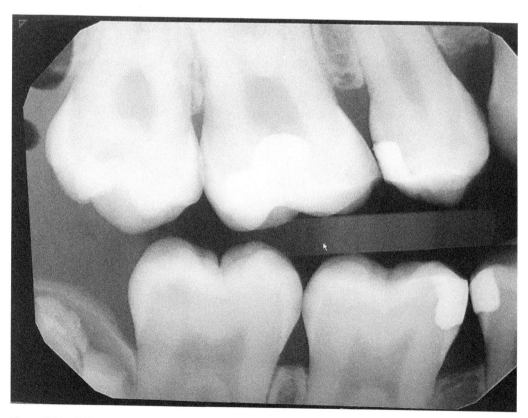

Figure 3.21   Difficult to see any radiographic caries.

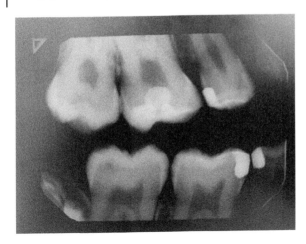

Figure 3.22   Zoomed out and darkened, teeth #2 and #31 appear have O decay..

- ○ When unsure, check clinically to confirm the diagnosis.
- ○ Older composites and dental materials may be radiolucent but are usually geometric in shape.
- – Differentiating cervical burnout versus root caries
  - ○ Cervical burnout: radiolucent band around necks of teeth should be anticipated, due to decreased X-ray absorption/overexposure.
  - ○ Root caries: only present if bone loss. Confirm clinically with an explorer and visually.
  - ○ Typically, interproximal decay occurs at the contact points, not the root surface, but if root caries will require more tooth removal to access.
- – Differentiating anatomic variation versus pathology: check for symmetry on the contralateral side radiograph.
- – Determining restorability (Figures 3.23 and 3.24): to determine the amount of tooth structure remaining after removing decay, try covering the decay on the X-ray with your hand (in Figure 3.24 it is blacked out). Does it appear that there is adequate tooth structure left to save the tooth?

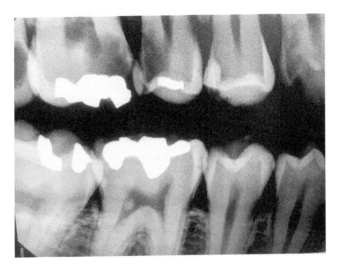

Figure 3.23   Teeth #3 and #4 have deep cavities.

Figure 3.24 By blocking out the decayed portion with your hand (or in this case by black marker) you can visualize how much tooth structure would remain after excavating the decay. This clinical pearl can help you quickly determine if the tooth is restorable.

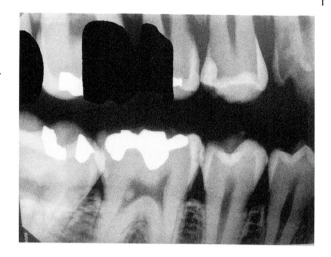

- Differentiating sealants versus composites: sealants may not be visible radiographically and are superimposed with the enamel. Composites (unless limited to enamel) are deeper and involve dentin and do not follow the external anatomy of the enamel.
- Determining the location of a radiolucency or radiopacity.
  - o Use the SLOB (same lingual opposite buccal) rule to determine the buccal or lingual position of an object.
  - o If the image moves in the same direction as the X-ray tube (e.g. mesial), then the object is located lingually. If the object moves in the opposite direction to the tube head (e.g. distal), then the object is located buccally [10].
  - o This rule can be used if unsure if a PARL is associated with a tooth (e.g. mental foramen) or to determine the location of external root resorption.
- Differentiating recurrent decay beneath a composite from bonding agent or a void (Figure 3.25).

Figure 3.25 Voids in composite #2 MO and #3 MOD.

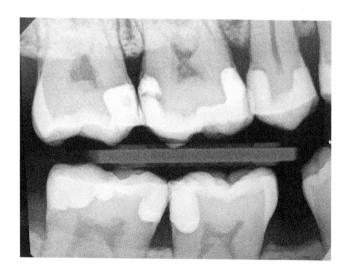

- ○ A radiolucency beneath a composite could be recurrent decay, excess bonding agent, radiolucent dental material, or a void (air bubble).
  - ○ If you completed the restoration recently and you know you did not leave any decay, you can monitor the tooth. If the restoration is from another provider, better to redo as there could be recurrent decay.
- – Differentiating a post from a cast post and core.
  - ○ It can be a challenge to predict if beneath the crown there is a cast post and core or a post with separate buildup.
  - ○ If planning on replacing the defective crown, you can assume the tooth is already compromised as a post was previously necessary. Warn the patient that the tooth may not be restorable.

Tips

- Advice for your dental assistant.
  - – Ergonomics: position the patient upright in the chair with their back and head well supported. Position chair low for maxillary X-rays and elevated for mandibular X-rays [1].
  - – Taking radiographs on a patient with a strong tongue: ask the patient to swallow deeply before opening, which will relax tongue and position it on the floor. Avoid mentioning tongue position as the patient will become more conscious and more tongue movements will occur [1].
  - – Patient unable to bite down for a BW due to missing teeth: place cotton rolls.
  - – Taking radiographs on a patient with a strong gag reflex:
    - ○ It is worse when the patient is tired.
    - ○ Limit the time the patient has the sensor in their mouth by first positioning the X-ray tube and then inserting the sensor.
    - ○ Avoiding contacting the posterior tongue or soft palate.
    - ○ Use distraction techniques: have the patient lift their feet, curl their toes, breathe through their nose, make a fist, etc. [1].
    - ○ Consider topical anesthetic spray (e.g. Cetacaine).
  - – Overlapping teeth on BWs: one trick to prevent overlapping is to have the patient bite on the cotton end of a cotton tip applicator placed between the teeth where you want open proximal contacts. Carefully position the X-ray tube with the stick in the center (imagine the stick being the central X-ray beam). Without the patient moving their head, remove the cotton tip applicator and insert the X-ray sensor and move the X-ray tube closer to the teeth [9] (Figure 3.26).

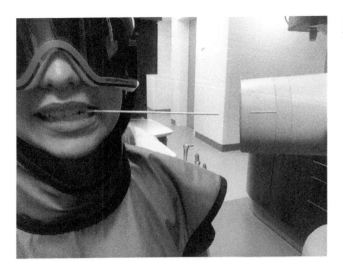

Figure 3.26 Cotton tip applicator technique for preventing overlapping contacts on BWs.

- During RCT on molars, to separate the canals for visibility and less overlap.
  - For maxillary molars, separate the MB1 and MB2 canals by a mesial cone angle.
  - For mandibular molars, separate the MB and ML canals by a distal cone angle [11].
- Count the teeth to verify all the teeth planned for radiography were captured.
- Do not save the radiographs and put all the equipment away until the dentist checks the radiographs for any necessary retakes or additional radiographs.
- Foreshortening and elongation results in radiographs that are not diagnostic.
  - Foreshortening is caused by the vertical angulation of the X-ray cone being positioned too steep. Foreshortening creates distortion of root shape/length and therefore cannot properly diagnose crown/root ratio, pulpal morphology for evaluating endodontic difficulty, can overlap PARL (underdiagnose), and distort distance of the crown margin to bone (insurance may reject crown if too close to bone).
  - Elongation is caused by the vertical angulation of X-ray cone being positioned too shallow.
- Treatment planning for occlusal fillings: keep in mind that an occlusal cavity can extend to the proximal contact even though the classic-looking break in enamel or triangle is not seen radiographically.
- Determining depth of decay to the pulp: can be visualized from the mesial, distal, occlusal, and incisal but cannot be determined if facial/buccal or lingual, which requires clinical evaluation.
- Counting teeth: always count teeth (Figure 3.27) as the patient could be missing teeth, have supernumerary teeth, or have malpositioned teeth with overlap, fusion, gemination (Figure 3.28), or concrescence.

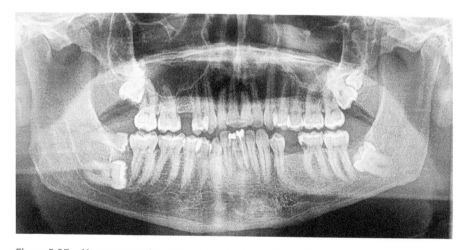

Figure 3.27 Always count the teeth when viewing radiographs: supernumerary and missing teeth.

Radiographs and Interpretation

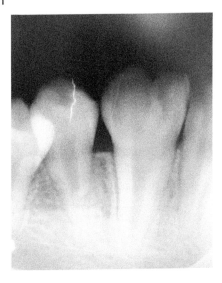

Figure 3.28 Count the teeth: gemination.

- Numbering supernumerary teeth.
  - Permanent dentition: instead of teeth 1–32, the numbers are 51–82.
  - Primary dentition: add letter "S" after tooth letter A–T [12].

- Before *any* dental treatment (e.g. fillings, crowns), carefully examine both the BW and PA.
  - Check for any PA pathology, as RCT may be necessary.
  - Check distance of the planned restorative margin to the crestal bone, as crown lengthening may be necessary. Of note, the radiograph will only give you an idea if the biologic width would be invaded interproximally, not buccolingually.

- Evaluate every radiograph carefully without bias and do not rush. Even a patient with excellent oral hygiene (who you assume will be caries free) may have pathosis.
- In primary molars look for radiolucencies in the furcation (unlike permanent molars at the apices).
- Do not take BWs or PAs on a patient wearing orthodontic wires as the wire is superimposed on the image preventing diagnosis of interproximal caries. Request in writing (and document) for the patient's orthodontist to remove the orthodontic wires for the radiographic exam and cleaning (Figure 3.29).

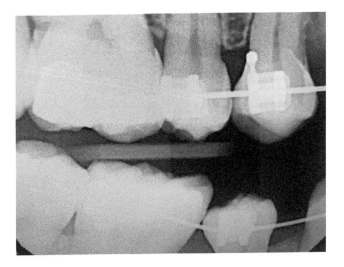

Figure 3.29 With braces you cannot determine if there is interproximal decay.

- Sometimes a suspected amalgam tattoo seen clinically on the gingiva appears radiographically, confirming the diagnosis (Figures 3.30 and 3.31).

Figure 3.30 Discoloration noted on the gingiva during oral cancer screening.

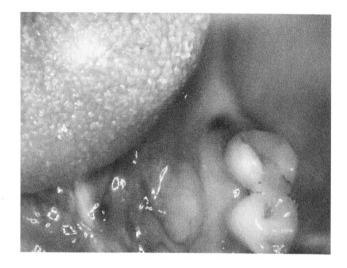

Figure 3.31 The BW confirms the cause of the discoloration, an amalgam tattoo.

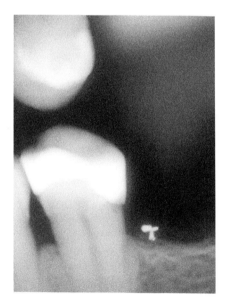

- A useful term is "radiographic artifact." This means "any distortion or error in the image that is unrelated to the subject being studied" [1].
- If you place a deep restoration with an indirect or direct pulp cap, recommend taking a PA at the recall visit to monitor for development of a PARL.

Real-Life Clinical Questions Answered

Dental Assistant's Question

- "Hey doc, what type of X-rays do you want me to take on this 5-year-old?"
  - Consider the following.
    - Is this a new patient?
    - Any chief complaint?
    - Does the patient only have primary teeth?
    - Are the contacts between teeth closed?
    - Is the patient high or low caries risk? If the patient is low risk and there are no clinical signs/symptoms and the interproximals are all accessible with an explorer, the patient may not require X-rays at this time.

Patients' Health Concerns

- "How much am I getting radiated?"
  - The relatively small exposure to radiation "poses a far smaller risk to your health than an undetected and untreated dental problem. An X-ray is essential to the diagnosis of not just cavities but other serious health conditions, such as bone infections and tumors" [13].
  - I can assure you that dental radiographs are very safe. We use digital radiographs and a lead apron/thyroid collar to reduce your exposure. A digital full mouth series (18 images) is about the same amount of radiation you're exposed to if you fly roundtrip from California to New York.
  - Let me share with you a radiation dosage chart (Figure 3.32).
  - Units are in microsieverts. A sievert is the "SI unit of dose equivalent equal to the product of a dose of one Gray, the quality factor, and any other applicable modifying factors (1Sv = 100 rem)" [10].
- "I'm pregnant and was told not to get X-rays."
  - According to the American Dental Association and American College of Obstetricians and Gynecologists Committee on Health Care for Underserved Women "Patients often need reassurance that prevention, diagnosis, and treatment of oral conditions, including dental X-rays (with shielding of the abdomen and thyroid). . .[is] safe during pregnancy" [14].
    - Without an X-ray I cannot properly diagnose and treat you.
    - Consider obtaining a medical consultation from their obstetrician/gynecologist if a high-risk pregnancy.
- "I've had radiation treatment for cancer to my head. Is it bad to get more radiation?"
  - I understand your concern about having further radiation. However, the dental radiographs we take are an insignificant amount compared to the radiation treatment which you have had. Due to your previous radiation treatment you are at high risk for developing radiation caries which can have serious consequences if not diagnosed and treated promptly. The X-rays will allow us to diagnose and treat you [1].
- "Where should I move the stroller to so that my baby is not radiated when you take my X-rays?"
  - Your baby will not be exposed to radiation as long as the child is not in the path of the X-ray beam (between 90 and 135°) and at least 6 feet (~2 m) away [10].

Radiation Dosage Chart
Micro-Sieverts (µSv) effective dose

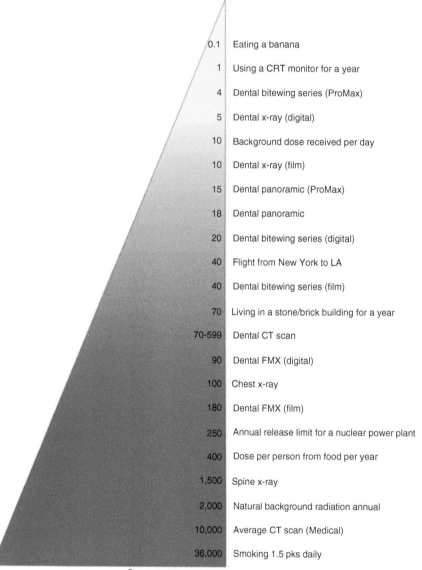

0.1	Eating a banana
1	Using a CRT monitor for a year
4	Dental bitewing series (ProMax)
5	Dental x-ray (digital)
10	Background dose received per day
10	Dental x-ray (film)
15	Dental panoramic (ProMax)
18	Dental panoramic
20	Dental bitewing series (digital)
40	Flight from New York to LA
40	Dental bitewing series (film)
70	Living in a stone/brick building for a year
70-599	Dental CT scan
90	Dental FMX (digital)
100	Chest x-ray
180	Dental FMX (film)
250	Annual release limit for a nuclear power plant
400	Dose per person from food per year
1,500	Spine x-ray
2,000	Natural background radiation annual
10,000	Average CT scan (Medical)
36,000	Smoking 1.5 pks daily

Source: BBC, Guardian Datablog, Mayo Clinic, XKCD
UNC Chapel Hill...Ludlow John, B Technical Paper June 2C08
Dr. Juha Koivisto, Physicist, Univ of Helsinki, Finland

Figure 3.32   Radiation dosage chart. Source: Courtesy of Dr. Juha Koivisto with Planmeca Oy.

- The baby and "dental personnel who perform dental radiography should stand behind a protective barrier. In situations where dental personnel cannot stand behind a protective barrier, they must stand at least 6 ft [2 m] away from the patient and the X-ray tube, not in the path of the primary beam but preferably behind a fixe or mobile barrier such as a lead-shielded wall or movable leaded Plexiglass shield" [15].

Patients' Questions

- "I just want you to do an exam without taking X-rays."
  - May I ask why you do not want any X-rays taken?
    - ○ Seek to understand and ask open-ended questions. Patient's concerns could be financial, time constraints, fear of radiation.
    - ○ If patient refuses, state "While I would like to help, I cannot do my job properly if I am unable to diagnose and see the entire picture, so I may not be the right provider for you."
    - ○ Follow your gut. Don't get pressured into rendering any treatment you are not comfortable with. A patient cannot consent to treatment below the standards of care. When in doubt, refer out!
    - ○ Alternative response: "Trying to diagnose without X-rays is like trying to do an exam with the lights off. I can't see everything necessary to get a complete picture of your dental health" [13].
    - ○ See section Informed Consents.
- "I just had X-rays taken one month ago at another office. Can they send you those?"
  - May I ask why you changed dental offices? (The reason can provide insight.)
  - With your permission (may require a signature or a patient contacting the previous dental office) we can try to obtain a copy of your radiographs from the previous office. However, if the radiographs are not of diagnostic quality we will have to take our own set of radiographs.
- "What is a bitewing and a PA?"
  - A BW refers to the radiograph we take of your back teeth. This allows us to diagnose cavities between the teeth, check for bone loss, and check the condition of any restorations you may have. A PA allows us to see below the gumline to diagnose the roots of your teeth and the adjacent structures.
- "What is a lead apron and thyroid collar?"
  - "The function of leaded aprons and thyroid collars is to reduce radiation exposure to the gonads and thyroid gland" [1].
- "Why can't you check for cavities in the pano? Why do you have to take more X-rays?"
  - Different radiographs serve different purposes. With the panoramic we see the big picture, like a forest, and with the BWs and PAs we see the individual trees. The panoramic image is not detailed enough to diagnose smaller cavities but allows us to see parts of the mouth we cannot reach with the intraoral sensors.
- "Does the X-ray show the tooth fracture?"
  - Fractures can be a challenge to diagnose and oftentimes are not visible on dental X-rays. Sometimes diagnosing fractures requires other forms of radiographs, exploratory periodontal surgery, or accessing the tooth for RCT to determine if there is a fracture once inside the tooth.
  - "Signs and symptoms often are not present early but manifest months, years, or decades after fracture initiation" [11].
- "I have a cavity on the X-ray you want to watch? Why aren't you going to remove it?"
  - Let me show you the radiograph. Some cavities are very small and limited to enamel which is the outer layer of the tooth. When I see this I prefer to monitor the tooth and not remove the decay in order to preserve tooth structure. There are three potential outcomes with these small cavities:
    - ○ The cavity could remineralize and reverse (best outcome).
    - ○ The cavity could stay this size for years, and we continue to monitor it.
    - ○ The cavity could progress. If this occurs we will remove the decay and place a restoration.

- In order to determine if the lesion is active and will progress, we will take follow-up radiographs in one year and compare the radiographs [1].
- "How long will it take for that cavity in the X-ray to get bigger? Can I wait until I'm back from out of town?"
  - When will you be back in town?
  - Progression of a cavity can vary depending on many factors, such as diet, medications, hygiene, oral habits, and recreational drug use, and these are all related to your caries risk. It is also impossible to predict when an asymptomatic tooth with a deep cavity may become symptomatic.
  - The radiographs in Figures 3.33 and 3.34 were taken 12 months apart on a patient with a extreme caries risk. Note the extent of destruction in one year. The patient had dry mouth and used recreational drugs.

Figure 3.33   Note the decay on teeth #2, #3, and #31.

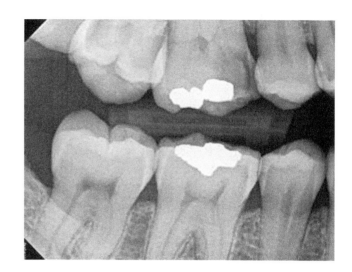

Figure 3.34   Note the decay on teeth #2, #3, and #31 one year later.

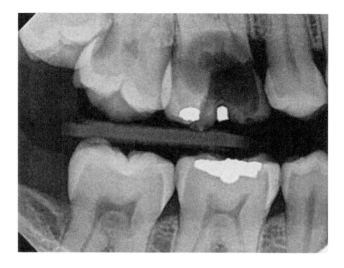

- "Why can't you see which tooth is infected from the X-ray?"
  - Signs of an infected tooth do not always appear radiographically.
  - "In addition, 30–60% of mineralization must be lost before the bone destruction (or cavity) shows radiographically, so the radiographic image can lag behind the clinical picture" [15].
- "I fell and chipped my tooth and cut my lip."
  - To verify that there are no tooth fragments embedded in your lip we will take a radiograph of your lip, in addition to a radiograph of the tooth (Figure 3.35).
  - I also recommend vitamin E oil. If the lip laceration is deep, refer to an OMFS or plastic surgeon.

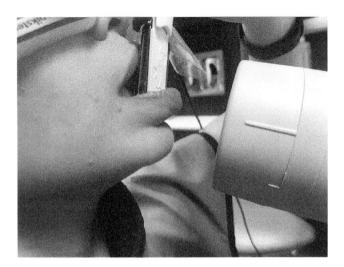

Figure 3.35 Checking for tooth fragments embedded in the lip.

References

1 White, S.C. and Pharoah, M.J. (2009). *Oral Radiology Principles and Interpretation*. St. Louis, MO: Mosby Elsevier.

2 American Dental Association and Food and Drug Administration (2012). Recommendations for prescribing dental radiographs. Revised 2012. http://www.ada.org/~/media/ADA/ Publications/ADA%20News/Files/Dental_ Radiographic_Examinations_2012.pdf?la=en (accessed 3 January 2020).

3 Henriques, J.C.G., Kreich, E.M., Baldani, M.H. et al. (2011). Panoramic radiography in the diagnosis of carotid artery atheromas and the associated risk factors. *Open Dent. J.* 5: 79–83.

4 Shillingburg, H.T., Sather, D.A., Wilson, E.L. Jr. et al. (2012). *Fundamentals of Fixed Prosthodontics*, 4e. Chicago: Quintessence Publishing Co.

5 Little, J.W., Falace, D.A., Miller, C.S., and Rhodus, N.L. (2013). *Little and Falace's Dental Management of the Medically Compromised Patient*, 8e. St. Louis, MO: Mosby Elsevier.

6 Cutright, B., Quillopa, N., and Schubert, W. (2003). An anthropometric analysis of the key foramina for maxillofacial surgery. *J. Oral Maxillofac. Surg.* 61 (3): 354–357.

7 Newland, J.R. (2012). *Oral Hard Tissue Diseases: A Reference Manual for Radiographic Diagnosis*, 3e. Lexicomp: Hudson, OH.

8 Blair, C. (2020). *Coding with Confidence: The "Go to" Dental Coding Guide*. CDT 2020. Belmont, NC: Dr. Charles Blair & Associates, Inc.

9 Carson, J. (2013). Improve your bitewings with a cotton tip applicator. http://www. speareducation.com/spear-review/2013/06/ improve-your-bitewings-with-a-cotton-tip-applicator (accessed 20 January 2020).

10 California Dental Association. (2014). Radiation safety in dental practice. http:// www.cda.org/Portals/0/pdfs/practice_support/ radiation_safety_in_dental_practice.pdf (accessed 2 February 2020).

11 Torabinejad, M. and Walton, R.E. (2009). *Endodontics Principles and Practice*, 4e. St. Louis, MO: Elsevier Saunders.

12 American Dental Association (2012). ADA dental claim form. Completion instructions. http://www.ada.org/~/media/ADA/ Member%20Center/FIles/ada_dental_claim_ form_completion_instructions_2012.ashx (accessed 21 January 2020).

13 Wright, R. *Tough Questions, Great Answers. Responding to Patient Concerns about Today's Dentistry*. Chicago: Quintessence Books.

14 American Dental Association. Oral health topics. X-rays/radiographs. http://www.ada. org/en/member-center/oral-health-topics/x--rays (accessed 2 February 2020).

15 Soxman, J.A. (ed.) (2015). *Handbook of Clinical Techniques in Pediatric Dentistry*. Ames, IA: Wiley Blackwell.

Radiographs and Interpretation

4

Treatment Planning

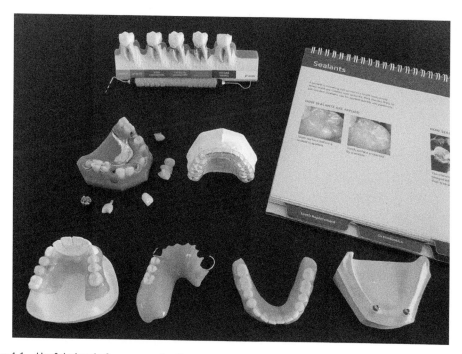

Figure 4.1 Useful visuals for communicating treatment plans with patients.

Chapter Outline

- Real-Life Clinical Questions
- Relevance
- Treatment Planning Phases
- Special Sequencing Considerations
- Tooth Replacement Options
- Pediatric Treatment Planning

Clinical Dentistry Daily Reference Guide, First Edition. William A. Jacobson.
© 2022 John Wiley & Sons, Inc. Published 2022 by John Wiley & Sons, Inc.

- Referrals
- Treatment Plan, Refusal, and Informed Consent Forms
- Charting Template
- Clinical Pearls
  - Troubleshooting
  - Tips
  - Miscellaneous

- Real-Life Clinical Questions Answered
- References

Real-Life Clinical Questions

Patients' Comments

- "I want you to replace my missing teeth and then you can work on my fillings."
- "You should have prioritized this tooth instead of working on those small cavities because now I have to get this tooth pulled."

Patients' Questions

- "Which type of crown will last the longest?"
- "Did my dentist do a bad job on the work in my mouth?"

Relevance

As a dentist you create treatment plans for every patient. Treatment planning is the process of "formulating a rational sequence of treatment steps designed to eliminate disease and restore efficient, comfortable, esthetic masticatory function to a patient" [1]. The treatment plan takes into consideration many variables, including the patient's chief complaints, expectations, health history treatment modifications, psychological and/or behavioral status, radiographic and clinical findings, caries and periodontal status and risk level, plaque control and motivation for improving, occlusion, oral habits, esthetics, and functionality.

First present your patient with the radiographic and clinical findings. For clinical findings, it is useful to show the patient their introaral photographs.

Presenting the treatment plan to your patient involves a discussion of the risks, benefits and alternatives (including the risks of no treatment). Audiovisuals such as brochures, flip charts, videos, and dental models are helpful (see Figure 4.1). The discussion and the treatment plan must be documented in the patient's chart.

Time frame, including number of visits to complete the treatment, and costs should be addressed. Dentists are responsible for ensuring the patient completes the treatment plan once it has been initiated. Therefore, it's important to have a system in place for following up with patients and to document all follow-up communications.

Treatment Planning Phases

Table 4.1 provides an overview of the dental treatment planning phases.

Table 4.1   Treatment planning phases.

Treatment phase	Description (may or may not apply)
Emergency phase	• Urgent treatment of pain, infection, trauma, and/or esthetic emergency
Data gathering phase	• Comprehensive oral evaluation • Medical history: medical consultation • EOE, IOE, and OCS • Full mouth debridement (if necessary for diagnosing) • Radiographs and interpretation • Clinical findings • Periodontal evaluation • Intraoral photographs • Endodontic diagnostic testing • Caries and periodontal risk assessment • Parafunction and/or habits • Patient expectations • Referrals to specialists • Treatment plan discussion

Stabilization phase (to control disease)	• Extraction of hopeless teeth
	• Hygiene
	  - Prophyylaxis
	  - SRP: one-month reevaluation
	  - Oral hygiene instructions, nutritional counseling, motivational interviewing, tobacco counseling
	• Caries control (bleaching if desired prior)
	  - Silver diamine fluoride
	  - Symptomatic teeth > larger cavities > smaller cavities
	• Replacement of defective restorations

Definitive phase	• Orthodontics
	• Crowns (if a survey crown, design the RPD prior)
	• Tooth replacement
	  - Fixed partial denture (bridge)
	  - Implant
	  - RPD
	  - Complete denture
	• Veneers
	• Occlusal guard

Maintenance phase	• Prophylaxis or periodontal maintenance, oral hygiene instructions, fluoride varnish • Recall exam/periodic oral evaluation including OCS, caries risk assessments, radiographs, reevaluation of "monitors" (e.g. incipient caries), clinical findings, periodontal evaluation • Evaluation of removable appliances (possible adjustments, repairs, relines, and replacements)

Special Sequencing Considerations

Table 4.2 addresses special sequencing considerations.

Table 4.2 Special sequencing considerations.

Abnormal intraoral findings	See section Evidence-Based Clinical Practice Guidelines for the Evaluation of Potentially Malignant Disorders in the Oral Cavity in Chapter 2
Bleaching before treatment	After completing the bleaching treatment, wait two weeks before definitive treatment (composites, crowns, veneers) or removable treatment (RPD) for the optimal shade match and composite bond strength [2]. Color often comes back halfway (regresses)
RCT follow-up visits	At six months and additional follow-ups as necessary until healing is complete. This involves clinical and radiographic examinations and diagnostic tests
Restoration after RCT	• If the RCT was completed by the endodontist, obtain the endodontic report prior to restoring the tooth and take an updated radiograph • Any delay in restoration can result in the tooth fracturing and becoming nonrestorable and/or contamination of the gutta percha requiring retreatment
Crown lengthening	• (i) Determine restorability, (ii) RCT (if indicated), (iii) core buildup (if RCT), (iv) fabricate a temporary crown, (v) crown lengthening, (vi) healing time, and (vii) definitive crown • Rationale for RCT (if indicated) prior to crown lengthening: the RCT could deem the tooth nonrestorable (e.g. root fracture, endodontic complication or procedural accident) and then crown lengthening would not be necessary • Rationale for placing a temporary crown prior to crown lengthening is to help the periodontist by improving access/visibility and to determine where to position the bone level
Periodic oral evaluation	Whether the recall exams are annually or every six months, when scheduling add the number of months and add one day for billing purposes. Exam frequency varies based on caries risk, periodontitis risk, with children, and varies with insurance
Annual radiographs	See section Recommendations for Prescribing Dental Radiographs in Chapter 3
Health history form	Every two years [3]
Six-month prophys	For billing purposes to the dental insurance, schedule six months and one day from the previous prophy

Healing times	• Crown lengthening: 8–12 weeks (restorative), 4–6 months (esthetic)
	  – Contact the surgeon
	  – May choose to wait two months, temporarily cement the permanent crown for one month to make sure it is stable and then permanently cement crown. "Stable" means tissue level has not changed, papillae ideal, no black triangles (or space below pontics), patient happy with esthetics and occlusion and comfortable (asymptomatic, no need for RCT). Sand blast temporary cement and use Ivoclean for ceramic crowns
	• Extraction with or without socket preservation before a bridge: four to six months
	  – Debatable, some say two months, preferably three
	  – May choose to wait three months, temporarily cement bridge for one month to make sure stable (no RCT needed), and then permanently cement bridge
	• Extractions and alveoplasty before a cast metal RPD or a complete denture: three months. Soonest time for a hard reline at six months. For more information, see Chapter 12, Table 12.1
	• Implant: three to six months, possible immediate loading, contact the surgeon
	• Socket preservation and implant: six to nine months, contact the surgeon
	• Extraction and socket preservation (by general dentist) before implant placement (by specialist): ideally provide the surgeon with the option of performing the extraction with the immediate placement of an implant

Tooth Replacement Options

Table 4.3 provides a summary of the advantages, disadvantages, risks, and costs for various tooth replacement options.

Table 4.3   Tooth replacement options.

Treatment option	Advantages	Disadvantages	Risks	Costs
Bridge (fixed partial denture)	• Fixed option • Prevents tooth migration • Esthetic (highly dependent on the pontic-to-ridge relationship and visibility) • Provides function • An option when an implant is not indicated, such as inadequate bone height and/or width, inadequate space between adjacent roots, lack of interocclusal space	• Typically requires a distal and mesial abutment • Challenging to maintain proper oral hygiene (requires motivation and manual dexterity) • Multiple visits • Typically, cannot repair and may require replacement • Removal of healthy tooth structure on virgin teeth	• Need for RCT, crown lengthening, post and core, and/ or core buildup • Abutment teeth can fracture and/or become decayed • If not well maintained can lead to loss of abutment teeth • May increase periodontitis and caries risk	• Could be similar to implants
Implant	• Fixed option • Conserves tooth structure (vs. a bridge)	• May require a sinus lift and/or a bone graft • Multiple healing times may be required • Multiple visits over a much longer time frame • May require replacement	• Implant failure (no guarantee as with all dentistry) • Risks related to surgery	• Could be similar to bridges
Removable partial denture	• Option for patients who do not want surgery (implants) or surgery is contraindicated • Conserves tooth structure (vs. a bridge) • Prevents tooth migration • Esthetics • Function • Can add teeth to appliance if more teeth are lost • For removable appliance types, See Table 13.1	• Removable • Patient's adaptability plays a major role • May require preparation of teeth, surgery, and crowns • Multiple visits • Will require replacement, relines, repairs • Need for maintaining oral hygiene and partial denture hygiene • Discomfort beneath partial • Sore spots, gagging, decreased chewing efficiency, food beneath the prosthesis, looseness, functional problems, need for denture adhesives	• Increased caries risk • Lack of adaptability to the appliance	• Significantly lower cost than implants or bridges

Treatment Planning

(Continued)

Table 4.3 (Continued)

Treatment option	Advantages	Disadvantages	Risks	Costs
Orthodontics (to close the space)	• Conserves tooth structure (vs. a bridge) • No removable appliance • Proprioception maintained	• May not be an esthetic or functional option • Time commitment • Lifelong commitment of wearing a retainer • If a fixed retainer, requires manual dexterity for hygiene	• Root resorption • Increased caries (plaque traps) and periodontitis risk during treatment • Pulpal reactions	• Cost will vary
Complete denture	• Option for edentulous patients • Esthetics • Function (if the patient can adapt) • Can add teeth, adjust, repair, reline, replace	• Removable • Patient's adaptability plays a major role • May require surgeries • Multiple visits • May require adjustments, repairs, relines, and replacements • Sore spots, gagging, decreased chewing efficiency, food beneath the prosthesis, looseness, functional problems, need for denture adhesives, lack of proprioception	• Fungal infections • Lack of adaptability to the dentures	• Lower cost than implants
No treatment	• Short term: no cost and no multiple visits	• Compromised esthetics • Compromised function • Tooth migration	• Overloading of other teeth (occlusal trauma) • Long term: more treatment necessary including surgery	• Short term: no cost • Long term: more cost

Pediatric Treatment Planning

See Chapter 17.

Referrals

Work with specialists if the treatment is beyond your scope. For complex restorative treatment consider referring to a prosthodontist (collapsed vertical dimension of occlusion [VDO], full-mouth rehabilitation, high esthetic demands, complex implant-supported restorations, severely resorbed ridges, TMJ problems, and/or congenital abnormalities).

Treatment Plan, Refusal, and Informed Consent Forms

Contact your professional liability carrier and/or attorney for specific guidance and forms.

Treatment Plan Form

- Have the patient sign the treatment plan to acknowledge:
  - He or she has reviewed and accepts it, *or*
  - He or she has reviewed and rejects it.
- If changes to the original treatment plan are made, have the patient sign the updated treatment plan.

Treatment Plan Refusal Form

- The form should follow the layout below:
  - Patient advised to:
  - Reason for refusal:
  - Risks, benefits, and alternatives reviewed including: (worst-case scenario)
    - Examples of worst-case scenarios include: "serious health issues or possibly death" if refusing biopsy, or "loss of teeth" if refusing periodontal treatment.
  - Date:
  - Patient signature:
  - Witness:

- If the patient does not agree with your recommended treatment plan, he or she is entitled to a second opinion (or more) with another provider.
- If the treatment plan refusal will impact your ability to provide treatment which meets the standard of care, consider discontinuing the doctor–patient relationship. A patient cannot consent to substandard care and you can be accused of "supervised neglect." Contact your malpractice carrier/lawyer for assistance so it is not considered patient abandonment.
- Patient refuses radiographs (see Chapter 3).

Informed Consent Forms

Informed consent is governed by state law.

Charting Template

1) Document the procedure.
2) Include the following: "The treatment plan was discussed and reviewed with the patient. All questions were answered and the patient verbalized an understanding of the nature of the treatment/procedures including the risks and benefits."
3) Copy/paste the treatment plan from the previous note and update it by inserting "Completed" next to each treatment. See Figure 4.2 as an example.

Treatment Planning

TREATMENT PLAN

Emergency visit: #19 referred to endodontist for RCT (necrotic, acute apical abscess) [sent]

Review of endodontic report [reviewed]
#19 O core buildup [completed]

New patient exam [Date completed]

Full mouth series [Date completed]

Two-week follow-up of intraoral lesion [completed]

Prophy/OHI/F varnish [Date completed]

#18 MO/direct pulp cap (deep decay) [completed]

Possible: RCT, crown lengthening, post and core, buildup, crown or extraction

#2 MO composite (decay to dentin) [completed]

#3 DO composite (recurrent decay) [completed]

#19 PFM crown (previous RCT and core buildup, prevention of tooth fx)
[in progress]

Occlusal guard (nighttime bruxism)

Prophy/OHI/F varnish
[Date due]

Periodic oral evaluation (monitor #8 M incipient caries, #30 M incipient caries)
[Date due]

Figure 4.2 An example of a treatment plan within the patient's chart note. At each subsequent visit this treatment plan is copy and pasted and updated in future chart notes.

Clinical Pearls

Troubleshooting

- Are many extractions required? Inform the patient "It is in your best interest to see an oral surgeon to have all the extractions completed in one appointment. This way you have one recovery and less chances of postoperative complications."
- *Potential dilemmas with restorability (and sequencing) you may face*: a patient shows up with a severe toothache on a tooth with an existing crown and you want to refer the patient to the endodontist immediately for RCT. How do you know if the tooth is restorable?
  - Did you place the crown recently and you know there was an adequate amount of tooth structure beneath the crown? If so, the tooth is likely restorable and can be referred to the endodontist.
  - Are there clinical/radiographic signs of caries or of an open margin?
    - In this case, it is best to remove the crown and determine the restorability prior to referring to the endodontist as the tooth may require extraction instead of RCT.
    - If the patient is referred to the endodontist for RCT and it is completed on a nonrestorable tooth, the patient may blame the endodontist and demand a refund for the RCT, putting the endodontist in a difficult position.
  - If you did not place the crown and there are no clinical/radiographic signs of caries or an open margin, then restorability is questionable.

○ The tooth may only require a permanent seal after the RCT is completed.
○ Warn the patient of potential risks including:
  ■ A new crown may be necessary.
  ■ The tooth may not be restorable and require extraction once the RCT is attempted or when the crown is sectioned for removal and replacement.
  ■ The tooth may require crown lengthening, post and core, and crown or extraction.

Tips

- At the new patient exam, "explain what you are looking for as you proceed through the examination and provide the patient with a summary of your findings when you are finished. Encourage patients to ask questions so they feel they are an active member of the oral health team" [4].
- If the diagnosis is not visible radiographically, take intraoral photos and save these in the chart. Sometimes decay, unsatisfactory restorations (e.g. open margins), and tori are not visible radiographically. These photos are useful for:
  – Your defense if audited by a dental insurance company to avoid being accused of overtreating.
  – Your defense in a legal dispute.
  – Patient education.
- Do not let the dental insurance dictate the treatment plan. Provide the ideal treatment plan and alternatives.
- Inform the patient that sometimes more treatment is recommended mid-treatment. For example, after a deep cleaning a cavity may be discovered which was hidden beneath calculus, or after removal of an unsatisfactory crown a cavity may be discovered on the adjacent tooth.
- At the recall exam, don't forget to reevaluate anything on which you placed a "monitor" or "watch" for progression and document the new status. The new status may remain unchanged and you may continue to monitor it.
- Referring patients to specialists: whenever you refer a patient to a specialist for treatment, emphasize that "If you have *any* complications or pain afterwards be sure to follow up with the specialist." If this is not communicated, the patient will show up in your chair for treatment and will have to be informed to return to the specialist. This will delay follow-up with the specialist and frustrate the patient.
- Referring patients to endodontists:
  – Inform the patient you cannot replace the temporary filling with a permanent filling until you receive the report from the endodontist. The report will provide you with:
    ○ The prognosis.
    ○ Recommendations (such as RCT not indicated at this time, instead make a temporary crown and if symptoms subside fabricate a permanent crown, or if symptoms don't subside refer back for RCT).
    ○ If decay was found inside a crown.
    ○ What materials were used to seal the access (permanent orifice barrier, temporary filling, foam, cotton, core buildup, etc.). Many materials are used and you may not recognize those used.
- Useful one-liners and analogies:
  – Our goal is prevention and treatment when necessary. It is easier to prevent disease than to treat later on.

Treatment Planning

- An analogy that helps patients understand a questionable restorability prior to treating is telling them there is a "50/50 chance" that we can save the tooth.
- Sequencing analogy: "Let's say you want the front door of your house repainted white and your backyard is on fire. We first need to put out the fire to prevent it from destroying your backyard, your house and your entire neighborhood. Once we put out the fire, then we can repaint your front door. We would not prioritize repainting the front door while allowing the fire to grow."
- We need to address the periodontal disease so that we have a solid foundation to work on.
- Short cuts can end up causing more delays.
- With heroic dentistry, inform the patient this is a last ditch effort or last hurrah.
- The goal is to add mileage to the teeth.

Miscellaneous

ICD-10-CM versus CDT:
- ICD refers to "International Classification of Diseases," CM refers to "Clinical Modifications," and 10 refers to the "10th revision" [5]. These codes refer to the diagnosis related to the treatment.
- CDT, or "Current Dental Terminology," refers to the procedure codes used to inform the dental payer which procedure was performed [6].

Real-Life Clinical Questions Answered

Patients' Comments

- "I want you to replace my missing teeth and then you can work on my fillings."
  - I understand you are eager to have the partial made. We want to make sure the foundation is strong before we replace any teeth so I always recommend we take care of active disease first. If we make your partial first and then clean out the cavities, we may find that one or more of the anchor teeth for the partial has to be extracted. Once it is extracted the partial will no longer fit and you will have to pay for a new partial (or the insurance will not cover a new partial for another five years). I've been burned by taking shortcuts before so this is what I recommend.
  - If an esthetic emergency, consider fabricating an Essex appliance or stayplate prior to caries control (see Chapter 13).
- "You should have prioritized this tooth instead of working on those small cavities because now I have to get this tooth pulled."
  - This is a tough lesson to learn about the importance of properly sequenced treatment plans. Prioritize the teeth in order of urgency (symptomatic teeth > teeth that may soon become symptomatic, i.e. the largest cavities > smallest cavities) to prevent being in this situation (see section Treatment Planning Phases).

Patients' Questions

- "Which type of crown will last the longest?"
  - See section Real-Life Clinical Questions Answered in Chapter 11.
- "Did my dentist do a bad job on the work in my mouth?"
  - "I can only report to you what I see today, based on your radiographic and clinical findings. Also, since I was not there at the time of the procedure, and time has lapsed since, it is hard to make that determination."
  - Do not speak poorly of other dentists and their work to patients. What you say could be used in court against another dentist and create distrust among other problems. Be objective and only report on what you see on that day. You do not know the circumstances under which the dentist was working (e.g. moving patient, limited mouth opening, bleeding, a hot tooth, uncooperative patient). Instead focus on correcting the problem.

References

1 Hook, C.R., Comer, R.W., Trombly, R.M. et al. (2002). Treatment planning processes in dental schools. *J. Dent. Educ.* 66 (1): 68–74.

2 Topcu, F.T., Erdemir, U., Ozel, E. et al. (2017). Influence of bleaching regimen and time elapsed on microtensile bond strength of resin composite to enamel. *Contemp. Clin. Dent.* 8 (3): 451–458.

3 ADA ebook (2019). *Guidelines for Practice Success: Managing Professional Risks.* American Dental Association.

4 Alberta Dental Association and College (2021). Patient communication guide. https://www.dentalhealthalberta.ca/wp-content/uploads/2021/01/ADAC-Patient-Communication-Guide.pdf (accessed 31 March 2021).

5 American Dental Association (2020). Answers to frequently asked questions about ICD-10-CM. http://www.ada.org/en/member-center/member-benefits/practice-resources/dental-informatics/standard-terminologies-and-codes/faq-icd-10-cm (accessed 12 May 2020).

6 Silverman, W.S. and Bone, J.J. (2016). What to know about the CDT code. http://www.agd.org/docs/default-source/policies-and-white-papers/impact-and-gd-articles/what-to-know-about-hte-cdt-code.pdf?sfvrsn=2 (accessed 12 May 2020).

Treatment Planning

5

Preventive Dentistry

An ounce of prevention is worth a pound of cure

Benjamin Franklin [1]

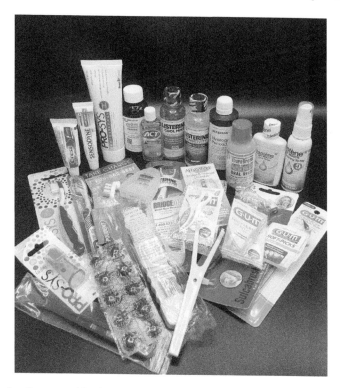

Figure 5.1   Example of some oral hygiene products.

Chapter Outline

- Real-Life Clinical Questions
- Relevance
- Treatment Planning
- Armamentarium
- Clinical/Radiographic Exam

Clinical Dentistry Daily Reference Guide, First Edition. William A. Jacobson.
© 2022 John Wiley & Sons, Inc. Published 2022 by John Wiley & Sons, Inc.

- Caries Management by Risk Assessment (CAMBRA)
  - Background
- Oral Hygiene Instructions
  - Motivational Interviewing
  - Basics
  - Specific Populations
- Nutritional Counseling
  - Background
  - Nutritional Counseling for Oral Health
  - Additional Nutritional Counseling for Specific Populations
- Tobacco Cessation
- Procedural Steps
  - Infant Prophylaxis
  - Child Prophylaxis
  - Adult Prophylaxis
  - Sealants
  - Preventive Resin Restoration
  - Fluoride Varnish
  - Silver Diamine Fluoride (SDF)
  - Postoperative Instructions
- Erosion, Abrasion, and Attrition Prevention
- Xerostomia
- Thumb-sucking and Pacifiers
- Sports Injuries
- Clinical Pearls
  - Tips
- Real-Life Clinical Questions Answered
- References

Real-Life Clinical Questions

Dental Hygienist's Question

- "When do we bill a child prophy versus an adult prophy?"

Patients' Demands

- "I want a deep cleaning not a regular one."
- "I don't want my daughter to have any fluoride."

Patients' Comments

- "I brush every morning before breakfast."
- "I have arthritis so it is difficult for me to brush my teeth."
- "I don't floss because it makes my gums bleed."
- "I only floss if there is a piece of meat stuck between my teeth."
- "I use hard bristles because the soft doesn't clean my teeth as well."
- "I use an all-natural toothpaste so it's fluoride free."
- "I always rinse with hydrogen peroxide."

Patients' Questions

- "Is fluoride safe for my baby?"
- "I don't know how to brush my child's teeth because she's three years old, she is my first kid and when I try she runs out of the room with the toothbrush."
- "Why do I have so many cavities? I don't eat sweets and I drink diet soda."
- "I'll do whatever you say doctor. How can I lower my risk of getting cavities?"
- "What can I do to get rid of bad breath?"
- "What mouthwash do you recommend?"
- "Should I buy a Waterpik?"
- "I read that oil pulling is really healthy for your teeth and that charcoal toothpaste will whiten your teeth."
- "I read that there is no benefit to flossing."
- "Do I really have to brush for two minutes?"
- "I want a refill of that mouthwash in the brown bottle."
- "I need a mouthguard for football, what do you recommend?"

Relevance

As a dentist, providing preventive dentistry encompasses both treatment and patient education. It is your responsibility to educate and empower the patients to prevent the development or progression of oral health problems such as caries, gingivitis, periodontal disease, erosion, abrasion, occlusal wear, trauma, and oral cancer. Oral health is crucial as it affects one's ability to eat, speak, and smile, and affects one's self-esteem, school performance, and work or school attendance [2]. In addition, studies have linked poor oral health with cardiovascular diseases, poor glycemic control in diabetics, preterm births, low birthweight, and a variety of other conditions [3].

Treatment Planning

For treatment planning related to preventive dentistry, see Table 5.1

Table 5.1 Treatment planning phases.

Treatment phase	Description (may or may not apply)
Emergency phase	Not applicable
Data gathering phase	• Medical history • Caries and periodontal risk assessment • Parafunction and/or habits

Stabilization phase (to control disease)	• Hygiene
	  – Prophylaxis
	  – SRP: one-month reevaluation
	  – Oral hygiene instructions, nutritional counseling, motivational interviewing, tobacco counseling
	• Caries control (bleaching if desired prior)
	  – Silver diamine fluoride
	  – Symptomatic teeth > larger cavities > smaller cavities
	• Replacement of defective restorations
	• Sealants
	• Preventive resin restorations

Definitive phase	• Occlusal guard (athletic mouthguards)
Maintenance phase	• Prophylaxis or periodontal maintenance, oral hygiene instructions, fluoride varnish • Caries risk assessments • Evaluation of removable appliances (possible adjustments, repairs, relines, and replacements)

Armamentarium

See Chapter 6 for hand instruments, instrument advice, rubber cup/polishing paste, and ultrasonic scaler (USS).

Clinical/Radiographic Exam

The clinical and radiographic exam is completed as part of the comprehensive oral evaluation (COE/new patient exam) and at the periodic oral evaluation (POE). This involves:

• Addressing the chief complaint.
• Reviewing the medical history (see Chapter 1).
• Performing the EOE, IOE, OCS, and occlusion (see Chapter 2).
• Determining if radiographs are indicated and the type (see Chapter 3).
• Interpreting the radiographic findings (see Chapter 3).
• Assessing and documenting the tooth findings on the odontogram.

- Completing a comprehensive periodontal evaluation (see Chapter 6): full-mouth debridement if necessary, for accurate diagnosing.
- Completing a caries risk assessment (see section Caries Management by Risk Assessment).
- Combining all the findings to formulate a diagnosis, prognosis, and treatment plan (see Chapter 4).
- Discussing with the patient the findings, diagnosis, prognosis, and recommendations,
- And lastly, documenting.

Caries Management by Risk Assessment (CAMBRA)

Background

- Risk assessments are used to estimate the likelihood that an event will occur in the future.
- CAMBRA is an evidence-based approach to preventing, reversing, and treating dental caries.
- One major takeaway from the CAMBRA studies is that simply placing restorations (aka "drilling and filling") did not lower the caries risk level of an individual.
- In order to reduce the caries risk level, it requires minimally invasive restorative work, chemical therapy (see Chapter 16), and behavioral change.
- CAMBRA intervention studies showed a significant reduction in the caries risk level and caries disease indicators (i.e. new caries lesions) in thousands of patients.
- A caries risk assessment should be performed on all patients in order to provide individualized recommendations.
  - For age 0–5 years (Figure 5.2).
  - For age 6 through adult (Figure 5.3).
  - Have the patient (or parent/guardian) select two caries self-management options (Figure 5.4).
- My recommendation is to create a personalized goody bag for your patients containing:
  - Prescription-strength fluoride toothpaste (first toothpaste as a sample and then by prescription only) (see Chapter 16).
  - Chlorhexidine (alcohol free) (first as a sample and then by prescription only) (see Chapter 16).
  - Soft bristled toothbrush, toothpaste, floss.
  - Written recommendations based on the patient's risk level.
  - Miscellaneous adjunctive recommendations (e.g. tongue scraper, Superfloss, saliva substitute) (Figure 5.1).

Updated CAMBRA*** Caries Risk Assessment Form for Patients Aged 0 to 5 (January 2019)
(Refer to the second page of this form for instructions for use.)

Patient name: Reference number:

Provider name: Date:

Caries risk component	Column 1	Column 2	Column 3
Biological or environmental risk factors*		Check if Yes**	
1. Frequent snacking (more than three times daily)			
2. Uses bottle/nonspill cup containing liquids other than water or milk			
3. Mother/primary caregiver or sibling has current decay or a recent history of decay (see high-risk description on next page)			
4. Family has low socioeconomic/health literacy status			
5. Medications that induce hyposalivation			
Protective factors**			Cheek if Yes**
1. Lives in a fluoridated drinking water area			
2. Drinks fluoridated water			
3. Uses fluoride-containing tooth paste at least two times daily — a smear for ages 0–2 years and pea sized for ages 3–6 years			
4. Has had fluoride varnish applied in the last six months			
Biological risk factors — clinical exam*		Check if Yes**	
1. Cariogenic bacteria quantity — Not currently available			
2. Heavy plaque on the teeth			
Disease indicators — clinical exam	Check if Yes**		
1. Evident tooth decay or white spots			
2. Recent restorations in last two years (new patient) or the last year (patient of record)			
	Column I total	Column 2 total	Column 3 total
Yes in Column 1 indicates high risk **Yes In columns 2 and 3: Consider the caries balance as illustrated on next page**			

Final overall caries risk assessment category (check) determined as per guidelines on next page

HIGH ☐   MODERATE ☐   LOW ☐

*Biological and environmental risk factors are split into (a) question items, (b) clinical exam.
**Check the "yes" answers in the appropriate column. Shading indicates which column to place the appropriate "yes."

Figure 5.2 Caries risk assessment form for patients aged 0–5 [4]. *Source:* CDA CAMBRA Guide 2019.

Caries Risk Assessment Form for Patients Aged 0 to 5 (continued)

<u>Determining the caries risk as high, moderate or low</u>

1. *High risk.* If there is a "yes" in Column 1 (one or both disease indicators), the patient is at high risk. Even if there are no "yes" disease indicators the patient can still be at high risk if the risk factors definitively outweigh the protective factors. Mother or caregiver with current or recent dental decay most likely indicates high caries risk for the child. Use the "yes" checks for each of the risk factor and protective factor columns to visualize the caries balance as illustrated below. The balance clearly to the left indicates high caries risk, whereas clearly to the right the risk level is low.

2. *Moderate risk.* If there are no disease indicators and the risk factors and protective factors appear to he balanced, then a moderate caries risk determination is appropriate. If in doubt, move the moderate to a high classification.

3. *Low risk.* If there are no disease indicators, very few or no risk factors and the protective factors prevail, the patient is at low risk.

Any items checked "yes" may also be used as topics to modify behavior or determine additional therapy. Use the following modified caries balance to visualize the overall result and determine the risk level:

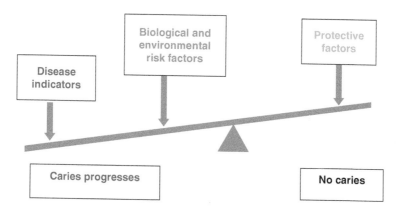

Additional caries-related components for caregiver/patient counseling
Frequency of use of fluoride toothpaste and amount
Use of silver diamine fluoride in appropriate cases
Dietary counseling to reduce frequency and amount of fermentable carbohydnues, especially sucrose, fructose (high-fructose corn syrup) and continual fruit juice (e.g., apple juice)
Bottle used continually, bottle used in bed or nursing on demand
Child has developmental problems/child has special care needs (CHSCN)
Inadequate saliva flow and related medications, medical conditions or illnesses

Self-management goals (discussed and agreed with parent/caregiver)

1. _____
2. _____

***CAMBRA is a registered trademark of the University of California

Figure 5.2   (Continued)

Updated CAMBRA* Caries Risk Assessment Form for Patients Aged 6 Through Adult (January 2019) (Refer to the second page of this form for details and instructions for use.)

Patient name: Reference number:

Provider name: Date:

Caries risk component			
Disease indicators	Check if Yes		
1. New cavities or lension (s) into dentin (radiographically)			
2. New white spot lesions on smooth surfaces			
3. New noncavitated lesion(s) in enamel (radiographically)			
4. Existing restorations in last three years (new patient) or the last year (patient of record)			
Biological or environmental risk factors		Check if Yes	
1. Cariogenic bacteria quantity — **not currently available**			
2. Heavy plaque on the teeth			
3. Frequent snacking (> 3 times daily)			
4. Hyposalivatory medications			
5. **Reduced salivary function (measured low flow rate)****			
6. Deep pits and fissures			
7. Recreational drug use			
8. Exposed tooth roots			
9. Orthodontic appliances			
Protective factors			Check if Yes
1. Fluoridated water			
2. F toothpaste once a day			
3. F toothpaste 2X daily or more			
4. 5000 ppm F toothpaste			
5. F varnish last six months			
6. 0.05% sodium fluoride mouthrinse daily			
7. 0.12% chlorhcxidine gluconate mouthrinse daily seven days monthly			
8. Normal salivary function			
	Column 1	Column 2	Column 3
Final Score: **Yes in Column 1: Indicates high or extreme risk** **Yes in columns 2 and 3: Consider the caries balance** **** Hyposalivation plus high risk factors = extreme risk**			

Final overall caries risk assessment category (check) determined as per guidelines on next page

EXTREME ☐   HIGH ☐   MODERATE ☐   LOW ☐

***CAMBRA is a registered trademark of the University of California

Figure 5.3   Caries risk assessment form for patients aged 6 through adult [5]. *Source:* CDA CAMBRA Guide 2019.

Caries Risk Assessment Form for Patients Aged 6 Through Adult (continued)

Determining the caries risk as low, moderate, high or extreme

Add up the number of "yes" checks for each of the disease indicators (Column 1) and risk factors (Column 2). Offset this total by the total number of "yes" checks for protective factors (Column 3). Use these numbers to determine whether the patient has a higher risk factor score than a protective factor score or vice versa. Use the caries balance to visualize the overall result and determine the risk level:

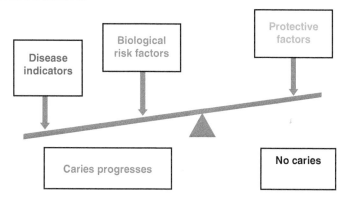

This enables a determination of low, moderate or high risk determined by the balance between disease indicators/risk factors and protective factors. The "yes" indications are also used to modify behavior or determine additional therapy.

In addition to counting the "yes" checks as described above, the following three modifiers apply:

1. *High and extreme risk*. One or more disease indicators signals at least high risk. If there is also hyposalivation, the patient is at extreme risk. Even if there are no positive disease indicators the patient can still be at high risk if the risk factors definitively outweigh the protective factors. Think of the caries balance: Visualize the balance diagram as illustrated above.
2. *Low risk*. If there are no disease indicators, very few or no risk factors and the protective factors prevail, the patient is at low risk. Usually this is obvious.
3. *Moderate risk*. If the patient is not obviously at high or extreme risk and them is doubt about low risk, then the patient should be allocated to moderate risk and followed carefully, with additional chemical therapy added. An example would be a patient who had a root canal as a result of caries four years ago and has no new clinical caries lesions, but has exposed tooth roots and only uses a fluoride toothpaste once a day.

***CAMBRA is a registered trademark of the University of California

Figure 5.3 (Continued)

Caries Self-Management Menu of Options

Protective factors

- Use an antibacterial mouthrinse/fluoride mouthwash
- Drink fluoridated tap water or fluoridated bottled water
- 2 tsp. baking soda in 8 oz. water for buffering
- Brush at least 2x daily with a fluoridated toothpaste

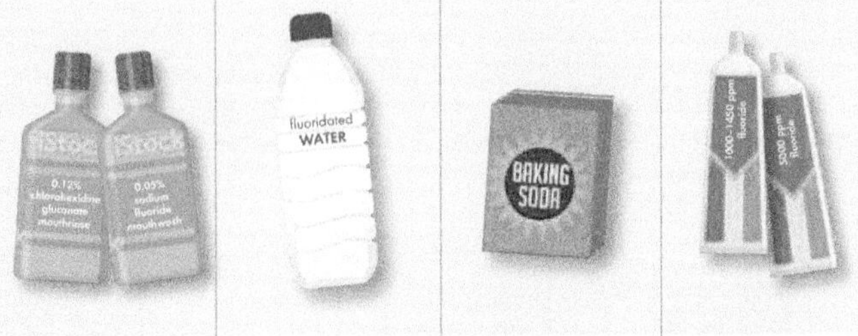

Fermentable carbohydrate changes

- Reduce frequency of processed starchy snacks
- Substitute xylitol-based products for fermentable carbohydrates
- Limit snacking on fermentable carbohydrates to 2x or less outside of meal time
- Reduce frequency of sugary snacks

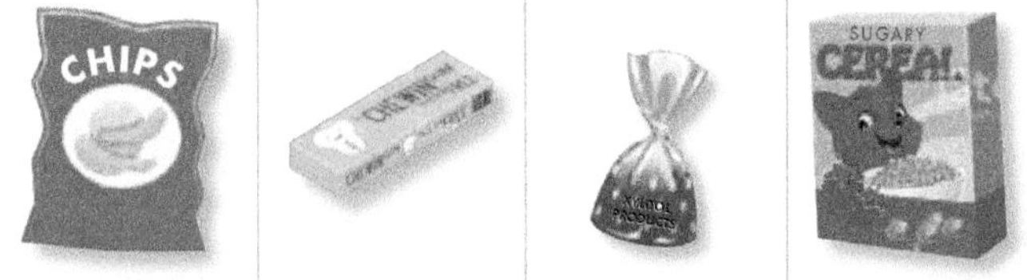

Sugar control options

- Drink water or milk instead of sugar-sweetened beverages; limit to meal time if at all
- Do not add sugar to beverages
- Dilute juice with water; exercise portion control; limit to meal time if at all
- Read nutrition labels for sugar content

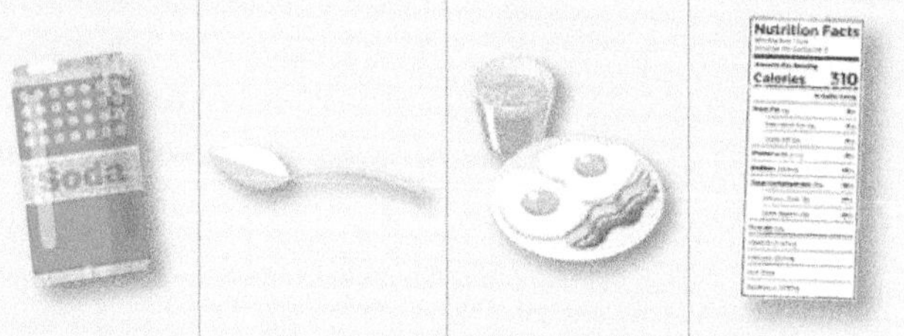

Oral health lifestyle reinforcements

- Daily plaque removal
- Choose healthful snacks
- Keep all oral health appointments
- Track goal progress

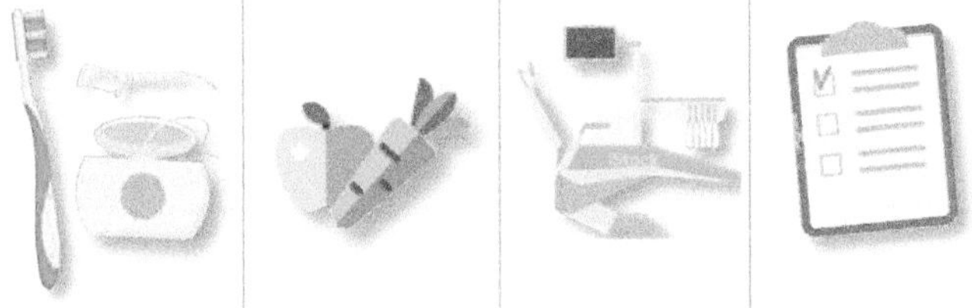

Self-management goals

Select two goals, such as buffering or limiting sugary drinks, and number each goal.

- Goal 1: How important it is _____ (1–10)   How likely to accomplish it _____ (1–10)
- Goal 2: How important it is _____ (1–10)   How likely to accomplish it _____ (1–10)

Figure 5.4   Caries self-management menu of options [5]. *Source:* CDA CAMBRA Guide 2019.

Oral Hygiene Instructions

Motivational Interviewing

- Motivational interviewing provides strategies to move patients from inaction to action [6].
- I like to find out what would motivate patients to improve their oral hygiene, such as:
    - Improved overall health (both oral and systemic)
    - Prevention of cavities
    - Prevention of gum disease or the progression of bone loss
    - Maintaining a nice smile
    - Maintenance of costly dental work
    - Fresh breath
    - Whiter teeth
    - Pleasing the dental professionals
    - Avoiding the dentist and dental procedures
    - Save time by only seeing the dentist for checkups and cleanings
    - Avoiding toothaches
    - Avoiding costly dental procedures
- Have the patient (or parent/guardian) select two caries self-management options (see Figure 5.4).

Basics

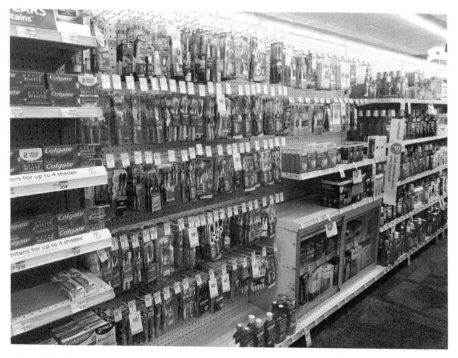

Figure 5.5 It can be overwhelming figuring out which oral hygiene products to purchase at the drug store if you do not know how to narrow down your search.

When deciding which oral hygiene products to purchase (See Figure 5.5), I recommend to choose those with the ADA stamp of approval, which have scientific evidence demonstrating both safety and efficac [7, 8].

Toothbrushes

- Hard, medium, or soft bristles: use soft bristles to minimize gingival abrasion.
- Replacement frequency: replace every three to four months or more if bristles are frayed.
- Electric versus manual: either is acceptable. Those with dexterity problems may find a powered toothbrush easier to use.
- Storage: rinse after brushing and store upright and allow to air dry [9]
- Sanitizing: soak in 3% hydrogen peroxide or Listerine for seven minutes to reduce bacterial load, as brushes can harbor bacteria (including fecal coliforms released into the air from toilet flushing) [10].

Toothpastes

- Types
  - Fluoridated versus nonfluoridated: choose fluoridated.
  - Whitening: choose products with the ADA stamp of approval.
  - Baking soda: not currently approved by the ADA. However, most baking soda toothpastes have low abrasivity, have whitening properties, reduce gingivitis, neutralize plaque acids, and most contain fluoride [11].
  - Charcoal: no evidence this is safe or effective. In addition, if too abrasive the teeth can appear more yellow (by exposing dentin) [12].
  - Desensitizing: usually requires several applications before sensitivity is reduced. Choose products with the ADA stamp of approval [13]. Can take up to two weeks to work.
  - Prescription-strength fluoride toothpaste (see Chapter 16).
- Amount of toothpaste:
  - First tooth eruption to age 3: apply only a smear of toothpaste, the size of a grain of rice.
  - Age 3–6: pea-sized amount [7].
  - Age 6+: can use a pea-sized amount. Using too much toothpaste can falsely convince a person their teeth are cleaner. Some suggest brushing teeth without toothpaste initially, and then brushing with toothpaste for maximum benefit [14].

Brushing

- When?
  - Brush *after* breakfast.
  - Brush before bed (after flossing).
- Duration:
  - Two minutes to achieve clinically significant plaque removal [9].
  - If 20 teeth, roughly six seconds per tooth.
  - If 28 teeth, roughly four seconds per tooth.
- Technique: brush all surfaces, aiming at the gumline (45°) to remove plaque above and below the gumline. Short back and forth strokes (tooth-wide strokes). Up-and-down strokes vertically for anterior linguals [9].
- Rinse with water after? Rinsing after brushing should be kept to a minimum or eliminated altogether [15].

Floss

Floss (and other interdental cleaners) reduce the likelihood of gum disease and tooth decay as toothbrush bristles cannot clean efficiently between tight spaces [16].

- Type: floss or tape, waxed or unwaxed, demonstrate equal effectiveness in cleaning proximal surfaces [17].
- Flossing: use 18 inches (46 cm) of floss and wind most around the middle or index finger. This way the floss is long enough to permit clean portions of floss to be used as you slide the dirty/used portions. Guide floss between teeth in rubbing motion. Don't snap the floss between the teeth as this causes pain/trauma. Curve the floss into a C-shape against one tooth, gently slide beneath the gumline (floss should disappear), and repeat against neighboring tooth with up-and-down motions [18] (Figure 5.6).
- Floss before or after brushing: floss to loosen bacteria and debris between teeth before brushing [19].
- Reuse of floss:
  - Discard after flossing the mouth.
  - Do not reuse the floss strand more than once [16].

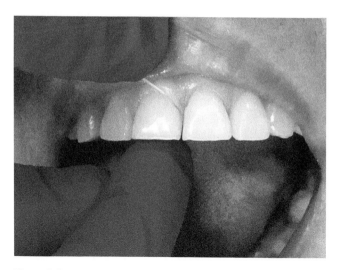

Figure 5.6 Demonstrate how to properly floss while the patient holds the mirror and watches. Show the patient how the floss should hug the tooth and disappear beneath the gumline, going up and down to remove the plaque and then repeating on the adjacent tooth.

Mouthrinses

- Various types for various indications.
- Indications include:
  - High caries risk (fluoride or chlorhexidine): fluoride mouthrinses should not be used in those aged under 6 years or until they can spit.
  - Plaque and gingivitis control.
  - Halitosis.
  - Dry mouth symptoms.
  - Gingivitis and caries (e.g. Listerine Total Care Zero Alcohol).
- Alcohol-free mouthrinse: for those with religious contraindications, xerostomia, or in alcohol recovery.

Specific Populations

Infant and Toddler
- Before teeth erupt: clean infant's mouth with a wet washcloth or cotton finger cloths to introduce oral cleansing at a young age.
- Once the first tooth erupts:
  - Use a soft toothbrush with fluoridated toothpaste.
  - Use only a grain-of-rice amount of toothpaste [7].
- Flossing is not necessary until interdental contacts have been established.
- Don't share toothbrush or utensils, or lick the pacifier [20] as this transfers cavity-causing bacteria (also avoid kissing on the mouth).
- For advice on brushing, see section Real-Life Clinical Questions Answered.

Age Three to Six Years
- Use only a pea-sized amount of toothpaste [7].
- Once spaces have closed, dental floss is indicated: children this age don't have the fine motor skills to floss, so caregiver can use floss holders.
- A power toothbrush can be more fun for a child than a manual toothbrush.
- Brushing is especially important at night, with reduction in saliva production and increase in acid production.
- Gums may be sore from "loosening" of teeth, so gently wipe with brush [20].

Age 6–12 Years
- At this age children are still developing fine motor skills, so those closer to 12 years old may be able to floss.
- At school, swish vigorously with water after lunch if unable to brush.
- Weekly use of disclosing tablet or solution with parent's supervision to improve flossing/brushing.
- Gums may be sore from "loosening" of teeth, so gently wipe with brush.
- Child's social activities may involve sleeping outside of the home (e.g. sleepovers) so be sure to pack oral hygiene products in overnight bag [20].
- Supervise children's toothbrushing up to around age 8.

Adolescent
- Nagging adolescents about oral hygiene can have a negative response.
- Fine motor skills should be well developed for brushing/flossing.
- After meals swish vigorously with water.
- If orthodontic appliances, additional time is needed.
- Consider plaque control agents if there are orthodontic appliances and gingivitis is present.
- Discuss complications of oral piercings if the patient is contemplating their use, or if oral piercings are present. Consider shorter recalls if present.
- Emphasis on oral hygiene education versus an authoritarian approach may be better accepted. Appeal to the adolescent's focus on appearance, hygiene, and ability to be autonomous.
- May require smoking cessation at this age [20].

Pregnant Patients
- More prone to periodontal disease and caries. Poor oral health can lead to poor outcomes for the mother and baby.
- Oral hygiene is very important as the gums will overreact to plaque due to hormonal changes.

- Increased caries risk due to behavior changes, such as eating habits. Cariogenic bacteria can be passed to a baby from saliva [21].
- Women with periodontal disease may be at risk of adverse pregnancy outcomes, e.g. preterm birth or low birthweight baby. These two outcomes are associated with other health problems for the baby [22].
- If vomiting, avoid brushing immediately after, instead swish with baking soda (two teaspoons of baking soda in one cup of water) to neutralize the acid.
- See Chapter 1.

Breastfeeding Patients

- Stay hydrated to prevent xerostomia, which increases risk of gum disease and cavities.
- Clean baby's gums with wet gauze or washcloth daily. Once the first tooth erupts, brush twice a day with grain-sized amount of fluoridated toothpaste.
- Don't neglect your own oral hygiene while taking care of a baby [23].

Other Special Cases

- Patients with a history of bariatric surgery: see Chapter 1.
- Patients with bulimia: see Chapter 1.
- Patients with special needs
  - Includes those with glaucoma, impaired vision, schizophrenia, autism, Down syndrome, cerebral palsy, arthritis, dementia, Alzheimer's (see Chapter 1).
  - Variety of products to help:
    - Electric toothbrush may be indicated.
    - Flossaid.
    - Open Wide mouth props.
    - DenTrust: a three-sided toothbrush.
    - Surround toothbrush: another three-sided toothbrush.
    - Collis Curve toothbrush: has curved bristles.
  - Techniques for brushing someone else's teeth:
    - Hand-over-hand technique.
    - If difficulty expectorating, a bulb syringe can be used.
    - If the patient is in bed:
      - Sit patient up, place towel over chest, and provide a glass of water and a bowl to spit.
      - If risk of aspiration with water, swab mouth with wet gauze or cloth [24].
- Patients with braces, bridges, implants, isolated deep pocket, or permanent retainers:
  - Floss threaders.
  - Superfloss (similar to shoelaces because the end is stiff to thread beneath the bridge or metal wire).
  - Oral irrigation systems (e.g. Waterpik) as an adjunctive aid.
- Patients with dental implants: to reduce the risk of periodontal disease it is necessary to brush (electric or manual) and floss, and to use end-tufted brushes, interdental brushes, toothpicks, and oral irrigators (on the lowest setting and aimed interproximally to avoid pressure on the tissue cuff can alter tissue and induce bacteremia). Chlorhexidine can be rinsed or applied to area with swab/brush [25].
- Patients with tongue debris: recommend a tongue scraper.
- Patients with sensitive teeth: ADA-approved desensitizing toothpastes. Some may take up to 2 weeks to work. Avoid abrasive whitening toothpastes.

Preventive Dentistry

- Patients with partials and dentures: see Chapters 12 and 13.
- Patients with crowns or hard-to-reach cervical areas (furcations, lower lingual cervical areas): gum stimulator.
- Patients with black triangles/larger spaces between teeth:
  - Interdental brushes.
  - Use a double length of floss and fold it in half.
- Patients not brushing adequately: have the patient floss and brush and then rinse their mouth with water, and then chew a plaque disclosing tablet (e.g. GUM Red-Cote) for 30 seconds without swallowing. This will turn plaque red, showing areas missed with flossing and brushing. Then floss and brush until the teeth are no longer red [26]. The plaque disclosing tablets can be used to "train" patients on how to properly floss and brush.

Nutritional Counseling

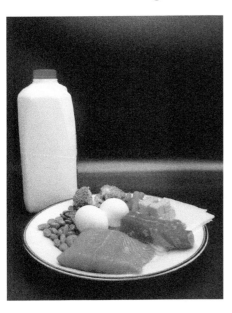

Figure 5.7 Nonacidogenic or low-acidogenic (cariostatic) foods.

Dietary counseling is a component of CAMBRA.

Background

The Stephan Curve and Critical pH

- After consuming fermentable carbohydrates, the pH in the mouth decreases within 5–10 minutes. This is followed by a gradual increase which may take 30–60 minutes or longer to return to the pH of dental plaque under resting conditions. The critical pH of enamel is the highest pH at which there is demineralization, i.e. 5.5 [27, 28]. In people with low salivary concentrations of calcium and phosphate the critical pH may be 6.5 [29]. The critical pH of dentin is 6.6 and of cementum 6.0–6.7.
- Wait 60 minutes before brushing teeth after eating, especially following acidic food or an acidic drink [30].

Nutritional Counseling for Oral Health

- Meals and snacks
  - Eat nonacidogenic or low-acidogenic foods (Figure 5.7):
    - Raw vegetables
    - Meat, fish, poultry (e.g. eggs)
    - Beans, peas, nuts, natural peanut butter
    - Milk and cheeses
    - Nonsugar sweetener stevia [31].
  - Choose healthy snacks: a diet with fruits and vegetables is associated with a lower risk of head and neck cancers [32].
  - Limit carbohydrates:
    - Reduce the frequency and amount of fermentable carbohydrates, especially sucrose, fructose, and continual fruit juice.
    - Reduce the frequency of processed starchy snacks (e.g. chips).
    - Limit snacking on fermentable carbohydrates to two or less occasions outside mealtimes [4, 5].
    - Avoid sucking on sugary hard candies or mints [33].
    - Avoid dried fruits, which are sticky, acidic and sweet [34].
- Drinks
  - Overconsumption of unhealthy beverages coupled with the underconsumption of healthy beverages during early childhood can lead to diabetes, obesity, and dental caries [35].
  - Drink water or milk instead of sugary beverages.
    - Limit bottled water consumption: the majority do not contain optimal levels of fluoride [36] and some have no fluoride [35]. Many popular bottled water brands are acidic [37].
    - Check if your (tap) water filter has the ADA Seal of Acceptance. Some filters remove fluoride [36], but note that the Britta Faucet filter removes only a trace amount of fluoride over the life of the filter [38].
  - Avoid soda, sports drinks, and energy drinks: if you indulge, use a straw and do not swish or hold it in your mouth longer than you need to [34].
  - Limit alcohol: heavy alcohol consumption is associated with an increased risk of developing oral cancer [39].
  - After the acidic meal or beverage: buffer the acids by rinsing your mouth with water or milk, or snack on cheese as dairy will neutralize the acid [34].
- Calcium intake
  - Important for the bones supporting teeth and for teeth themselves, in addition to phosphorus and vitamin D.
  - Age 1–3: intake of 700 mg calcium daily.
  - Age 4–8: intake of 1000 mg calcium daily.
  - Adults: intake 1000 mg daily [39].
- Children and vitamins
  - Many OTC medications have high sugar content.
  - The American Academy of Pediatrics (AAP) recommends that the optimal way to obtain the adequate amount of vitamins is to consume a healthy and well-balanced diet [40].

Preventive Dentistry

Additional Nutritional Counseling for Specific Populations

- Infants
  - The American Academy of Pediatric Dentistry (AAPD) recommends "breast-feeding of infants prior to 12 months to ensure the best possible health and developmental and psycho-social outcomes for infants" [40].
  - The AAPD recommends weaning off bottle feeding by 12–14 months to reduce risk of early childhood caries [41].
  - Avoid continual bottle use, or bottle in bed with anything other than water, or nursing on demand.
  - Don't dip the pacifier in sugar or honey, or place it in your mouth prior to inserting in the infant's mouth.
  - Don't share utensils [20] as this transfers cavity-causing bacteria to the infant.
  - Encourage drinking from a cup by age one year versus frequent prolonged use of sippy cups [42].

- Children and beverages
  - The Committee on Nutrition of the AAP stated that 100% juice and juice drinks have no essential role in a healthy diet for children and contribute to excessive calorie intake and risk of dental caries in children [40].
  - Age 0–6 months:
    ○ No supplemental drinking water is necessary [35].
    ○ Do not put children to bed with a bottle containing anything but water [35].
  - Age 0–1: 100% fruit juice is not recommended [35].
  - Age 0–5:
    ○ Should not consume sugar-sweetened beverages, including soft drinks/soda, fruit drinks, fruit-flavored drinks, sports drinks, energy drinks, sweetened waters, and sweetened coffee and tea beverages [35].
    ○ Wean child from a bottle by age one year [35].
    ○ Encourage to consume plain drinking water (i.e. unflavored, unsweetened, uncarbonated, fluoridated drinking water) particularly for beverages consumed outside of meals and snacks [35].
  - Age 1–5: while fruit juice is not recommended, whole fruit is preferred. No more than 4 ounces (113 g or ½ cup) per day of 100% juice [35].

- Adults with dry mouth
  - Alcohol, caffeine, acidic foods, dry foods, and salty foods contribute to dry mouth [39, 43].
  - Xylitol is no longer recommended in CAMBRA as a protective factor due to limited evidence [4, 5].

- Denture wearers
  - Typically, intake of hard foods (e.g. raw vegetables, nuts, meats) is reduced while soft foods (bread, pastries, canned fruits) is increased. The change may affect nutritional status if foods are not nutrient dense. Often soft foods are lower in nutrient density and fiber. Nutritional goals include a variety of foods, protein, dairy, fruits, vegetables, grains, and cereals, while limiting salt, fat, and sugar [43].
  - Recommend the patient meets with a registered dietitian or a family primary care provider.
  - To eat nuts, try soaking overnight in a cup of water (e.g. almonds).
- Additional resources: www.choosemyplate.gov is a nutrition education tool from the US Department of Agriculture [44].

Tobacco Cessation

The oral health risks of tobacco include oral and pharyngeal cancers (see Chapter 2), increased prevalence and severity of periodontal disease, poorer prognosis of periodontal treatment, increase risk of dental implant failure [45], delayed wound healing, and staining of teeth.

Dentists are in a unique position to help with tobacco cessation as they can identify the oral consequences of tobacco usage and intervene.

The "5 A's" model for treating tobacco use and dependence comprises the following.

- *Ask* about tobacco use (type, amount, frequency, duration): find out if patient is a current or former smoker, or has never smoked. For former smoker, provide relapse prevention.
- *Advise* to quit.
- *Assess* willingness to quit.
- *Assist*: offer medication and provide or refer for counseling.
  - Provide materials such as 1800-QUIT-NOW, a US Quitline database operated by the National Cancer Institute with trained counselors who will direct patients to the state's Quitline. No cost to US residents in each state, District of Columbia, Guam, and Puerto Rico. The Quitline offers free counseling and referral to other cessation resources, and may offer free or discounted cessation medications [46].
  - Provide other local/state resources.
  - Inform the patient that the combination of counseling and medication is more effective than either treatment modality alone.
- *Arrange* a follow-up [47].

It is recommended that patients quit all forms of smoking, including tobacco, marijuana, and vaping (see *Tobacco*, *Marijuana*, and *Vaping* in Chapter 1). Chewing tobacco is associated with root caries (high sugar level), gingival recession, oral cancer risk, and enamel wear [48].

Procedural Steps

Infant Prophylaxis

- Explain to the parent/guardian the plan:
  - A knee-to-knee exam (Figure 5.8).
  - A toothbrush cleaning.
  - Application of fluoride varnish.

- Warn the parent/guardian that children at this age typically cry and that the procedure is fast, does not hurt the child, and that crying is fine as the dentist will be able to see all the teeth.
- Assume the knee-to-knee position.
- Provide a toothbrush prophylaxis (demonstrating proper oral hygiene instructions) and apply fluoride varnish.
- Complete the caries risk assessment (for ages 0–5) and determine the risk level.
- Provide oral hygiene instructions and nutritional counseling.
- Help the parent/guardian set one to two goals for home care [49].

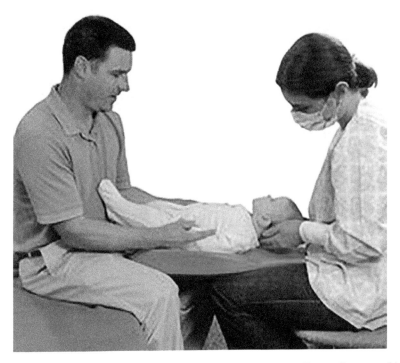

Figure 5.8   A knee-to-knee examination using a lap support. *Source:* Courtesy of http://Specializedcare.com

Child Prophylaxis

1) USS (if indicated). Caution: don't contact any white spots/incipient lesions or it will create a cavitation (see Chapter 6).
2) Hand instruments, if indicated (see Chapter 6).
3) Oral hygiene instructions/nutritional counseling.
4) Polish (see Chapter 6).
5) Floss.
6) Fluoride varnish.

Adult Prophylaxis

Typically, if the pocket depths are less than 5 mm, then a prophylaxis is indicated. If 5 mm or greater, SRP is indicated (see Chapter 6).

1) USS. Caution: don't contact any white spots/incipient lesions or it will create a cavitation (see Chapter 6).
2) Hand instruments (see Chapter 6).
3) Oral hygiene instructions/nutritional counseling/tobacco counseling.
4) Polish (see Chapter 6).
5) Floss.
6) Rinse with a mouthrinse (to remove the taste of blood).
7) Fluoride varnish.

Sealants

Background

- Some teeth have pits and fissures that are so deep that the toothbrush bristles cannot reach and clean these surfaces. These surfaces can trap food and promote the presence of bacterial biofilm, increasing the risk of caries. Sealants form a physical barrier that prevents and arrests caries (noncavitated carious lesions) of primary and permanent molars in children and adolescents.
- Sealants on permanent molars reduce the risk of cavities by 80% [50].
- Permanent molars are highly porous at the time of eruption and susceptible to caries [51].
- Prognosis: 5–10% fail annually. Reasons include poor isolation during placement, poor oral hygiene, bruxism, hard candy, or high caries risk [51].

Indications

- Sound teeth and incipient caries: if you are unsure whether the tooth in question has an occlusal stain or incipient caries on the occlusal surface, place the sealant. The AAPD and ADA "concluded that sealants could minimize the progression of non-cavitated occlusal carious lesions (also referred to as initial lesions) that receive a sealant" [52].
- Primary teeth and permanent teeth: "Sealants are effective in preventing and arresting pit-and-fissure occlusal carious lesions of primary and permanent molars in children and adolescents compared with the nonuse of sealants or use of fluoride varnishes. They also concluded that sealants could minimize the progression of non-cavitated occlusal carious lesions (also referred to as initial lesions) that receive a sealant" [52].
- Molars, premolars, any tooth at risk.
- Maxillary molar (occlusal and lingual grooves).
- Mandibular molar (occlusal and buccal grooves).
- Deep retentive pits and fissures which cause wedging/catch of explorer.
- No radiographic evidence of interproximal caries.
- When the gingival tissue is at or below the marginal ridge (no operculum).
- Cooperative patient and ability to isolate from salivary contamination [20].

Steps

- Clean the fissures with water and flour of pumice using a prophy angle tapered brush (plaque must be removed for bonding).
- Rinse well.
- Isolate the teeth (primary loss is due to moisture) [51].
- Dry.
- Etch (e.g. 35% phosphoric acid) for 15–20 seconds, rinse, and dry. The enamel should appear chalky/frosted; if not, etch for longer (unlike restorative dentistry in which dentin should not be desiccated) [20].
- Isolate the teeth: place dry angles and cotton rolls to isolate teeth and keep the suction near the tooth (saliva contamination lowers bond strength) [20].
- Place bonding agent: apply a thin layer and dry (do not light cure until the sealant is added) [51].
- Place the sealant material:
  - Use a composite-based sealant material for longevity, unless a partially erupted tooth (use resin-modified glass ionomer [RMGI]).
  - Apply to the pits and fissures.
  - Remove excess with cotton tip applicator.
  - Tease out any bubbles with the explorer.

Preventive Dentistry

- Light cure (with the light touching the cusp tips) [51].
- Check the sealant with explorer for retention, sealed margins, and voids: if deficient, material can be added at this time if sealant is undisturbed/isolated [20].
- Check occlusion: depending on the sealant material type, occlusion may require adjusting (some sealants are "self-adjusting" while some require the handpiece) [20].
- Floss to remove any excess bond or sealant material.
- Follow-up: evaluate the sealant at every recall for repair or replacement
  - If a portion is missing, remove the remaining portion with an explorer or follow procedural steps to add additional sealant [20].
  - Check for shadowing underneath (i.e. caries), open margins, loss of retention [51].

Preventive Resin Restoration

- Now known as conservative adhesive restoration (CAR).
- A conservative approach in which the preventive resin restoration (PRR)/CAR limits cavity preparation to the area of decay while sealing the pits and fissures.

Steps

- Decay to enamel:
  - Remove decay with the high-speed bur.
  - Place sealant material (following manufacturer's guidelines) into the cavity preparation and over susceptible pits and fissures [20].
  - Check occlusion and adjust as needed.
- Decay to dentin:
  - Remove decay with the high-speed and slow-speed bur.
  - Restore the cavity preparation with composite.
  - Place sealant material (following manufacturer's guidelines) over the susceptible pits and fissures [20].
  - Check occlusion and adjust as needed.

Fluoride Varnish

- Background
  - Fluoride ions are found naturally in all bodies of water, and as minerals in rocks, sand, and soil. Some bodies of water have excessive fluoride, such as deep well water.
  - Water fluoridation is the process of controlling the amount of fluoride in the water to an optimal beneficial level (0.7–1.2 ppm).
  - Water fluoridation reduces dental decay by 20–40%.
  - Fluoride-containing water is analogous to micronutrient-fortified foods such as orange juice (vitamin C and calcium), milk (vitamin D), and salt (iodine).

- – Fluorosis occurs when an excessive amount of fluoride is ingested during tooth development. Fluorosis does not pose a threat at age six years or older once the enamel has formed.
- – Fluoride varnish is safe and effective in preventing tooth decay in children and adults and can be applied after a toothbrushing or prophylaxis [20].
- Indications
  - – For those with moderate, high, or extreme caries risk.
  - – For those with low caries risk in the presence of tooth sensitivity or excessive root exposure [53].
- Frequency: at least every six months [15]. Max every 3 months.
- Steps
  - – Mix 2.26% fluoride varnish [54] to a homogeneous consistency.
  - – Dry the patient's teeth with gauze or air.
  - – Apply one thin layer of fluoride varnish to *all* the tooth surfaces [20].
    - ○ Avoid applying more than one coat on the same tooth as it will become thick and bumpy.
    - ○ Have the patient bite down, retract the cheek and lips and swipe across the teeth, then have the patient open to swipe the linguals.
  - – Provide a cup for the patient to expectorate if they would like. Do not use the saliva ejector as the fluoride varnish can harden and clog the lines.

Silver Diamine Fluoride (SDF)

- The FDA has approved SDF for reducing tooth sensitivity.
- SDF is used off-label for caries arrest and prevention.
- Components: 38% silver and 5–5.9% fluoride.
  - – Silver: antimicrobial action.
  - – Fluoride: promotes remineralization.
- Obtain verbal and written consent (Figure 5.9). Over time, SDF will permanently stain the decay black. Warn the patient that SDF can also "leach" onto other surfaces that are decalcified and stain those too [54].
- Steps (see Figure 5.10)
- Follow-up: check if the sites the SDF was applied to appear arrested (dark and hard).
- Frequency: once or twice annually until the tooth is restored or exfoliates, or indefinitely. Research is needed for results beyond two to three years [55]. Application three times per year showed highest arrest rates [55].
- Interproximal decay: interproximal application is a challenge as applying SDF to floss becomes contaminated with saliva and there is a risk of gingival bleeding contaminating the solution. For the solution to be effective it must contact tooth structure for an extended period [54].

UCSF DENTAL CENTER INFORMED CONTEST FOR SILVER DIAMINE FLUORIDE

Fads for consideration:

- Silver diamine fluoride (SDF) is an antibiotic liquid. We use SDF on cavities to help stop tooth decay. We also use it to treat tooth sensitivity. SDF application every 6-12 months is necessary.
- The procedure: 1) Dry the affected area, 2) Place a small amount of SDF on the affected area, 3) Allow SDF to dry for one minute, 4) Rinse.
- **Treatment with SDF does not eliminate the need for dental fillings or crowns to repair function or esthetics. Additional procedures will incur a separate fee.**
- I should not be treated with SDF if: 1) I am allergic to silver. 2. There are painful sores or raw areas on my gums (i.e., ulcerative gingivitis) or anywhere in my mouth (i.e., stomatitis).

Benefits of receiving SDF:

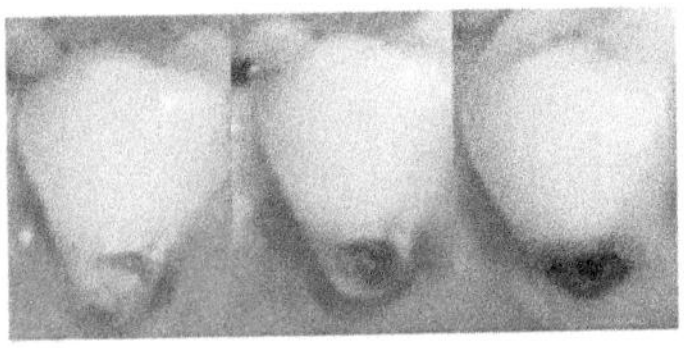

- SDF can help stop tooth decay.
- SDF can help relieve sensitivity.

Risks related to SDF include, but are not limited to:

- **The affected area will stain black permanently.** Healthy tooth structure will not stain. Stained tooth structure can be replaced with a filling or a crown.
- Tooth-colored fillings and crowns may discolor if SDF is applied to them. Color changes on the surface can normally be polished off. The edge between a tooth and filling may keep the color.
- If accidentally applied to the skin or gums, a brown or white stain may appear that causes no harm, cannot be washed off and will disappear in 1-3 weeks.
- You may notice a metallic taste. This will go away rapidly.
- If tooth decay is not arrested, the decay will progress. In that case the tooth will require further treatment, such as repeat SDF, a filling or crown, root canal treatment or extraction.
- These side effects may not include all of the possible situations reported by the manufacturer. If you notice other effects, please contact your dental provider.
- Every reasonable effort will be made to ensure the success of SDF treatment. There is a risk that the procedure will not stop the decay and no guarantee of success is granted or implied.

Alternatives to SDF, not limited to the following:

- No treatment, which may lead to continued deterioration of tooth structures and cosmetic appearance. Symptoms may increase in severity.
- Depending on the location and extent of the tooth decay, other treatment may include placement of fluoride varnish, a filling or crown, extraction or referral for advanced treatment modalities.

I CERTIFY THAT I HAVE READ AND FULLY UNDERSTAND THIS DOCUMENT, AND ALL MY QUESTIONS WERE ANSWERED:

_____ (signature of patient)   _____ (date)

_____ (signature of witness)   _____ (date)

Figure 5.9 UCSF dental center informed consent for silver diamine fluoride. *Source:* Horst et al. [55].

<u>Silver Diamine Fluoride (SDF)</u>
<u>UCSF Protocol for Arresting Dental Carious Lesions or Treating Tooth Sensitivity</u>

Material: Advantage Silver Arrest (38% SDF, purified water) from Elevate Oral Care.
Shelf life: 3 years unopened. Do not refrigerate. Avoid freezing or extreme heat.

Indications:
1. Extreme caries risk (Xerostomia or severe early Childhood Caries).
2. Treatment challenged by behavioral or medical management.
3. Patients with carious lesions that may not all be treated in one visit.
4. Difficult to treat dental carious lesions.
5. Patients without access to dental care.

Maximum dose: 25 μL (1 drop) / 10kg per treatment visit.
SDF Contraindication: Silver allergy.
SDF Relative Contraindications: Ulcerative gingivitis, Stomatitis.
SSKI Contraindications: Pregnancy, Breastfeeding.

Considerations:
- Decayed dentin will darken as the caries lesions arrest. Most will be dark brown or black
- SDF can stain the skin, which will clear in two to three weeks without treatment.
- SDF can permanently stain operatory surfaces and clothes.
- A control restoration (e.g., GI via ART or other material) may be considered after SDF treatment.
- Saturated solution of potassium iodide (SSKI, Lugol's Solution, various sources) can be used after SDF to decrease color changes.
- Re-application is usually recommended, biannually until the cavity is restored or arrested or the tooth exfoliates.

Procedure:
1. Plastic-lined cover for counter, plastic-lined bib for patient.
2. Standard personal protective equipment (PPE) for provider and patient.
3. One drop of SDF into the deep end of a plastic dappen dish
   (also obtain one drop of SSKI in a separate dappen dish if selected).
4. Remove bulk saliva with saliva ejector.
5. Isolate tongue and cheek from affected teeth with 2-inch by 2-inch gauze or cotton rolls.
6. If near the gingiva, consider applying petroleum jelly with a cotton applicator for safety.
7. Dry affected tooth surfaces with triple syringe or if not feasible dry with cotton.
8. Bend microsponge, immerse into SDF, remove excess on side of dappen dish.
9. Apply directly onto the affected tooth surface(s) with microsponge.
10. Allow SDF to absorb for up to one minute if reasonable, then remove excess with gauze or cotton roll.

    (If using SSKI, apply with a different microsponge. Repeat one to three times until no further white precipitates are observed. Wait five to 10 seconds between applications. Remove excess with cotton.)
11. Rinse with water.
12. Place gloves, cotton and microbrushes into plastic waste bags.

Figure 5.10   Silver diamine fluoride: UCSF protocol for arresting dental carious lesions or treating tooth sensitivity. *Source:* Horst et al. [55].

Postoperative Instructions

Prophylaxis

- For gums that are sensitive, rinse with warm saline (one teaspoon of salt in one cup of water) to reduce inflammation multiple times a day until the gums are no longer sore.
- If tooth sensitivity, use an OTC desensitizing toothpaste.

Sealants

- If a "self-adjusting" sealant material was used, the bite may feel high but it will return to normal.
- The sealant helps protect the pits and fissures of the teeth but it is still necessary to clean all the surfaces of all teeth by brushing twice a day and flossing daily.
- The status of the sealants should be monitored at future visits as they may require repair or replacement.

Fluoride Varnish

- The goal is to keep the fluoride varnish contacting the teeth for as long as possible.
  - No eating or drinking for 30 minutes.
  - Recommend a soft diet on day of treatment (avoid hot, hard, crunchy, sticky foods).
  - Resume toothbrushing and flossing the following day to increase varnish contact time with teeth [20].
- Recommend reapplication every six months, and every three months if high caries risk [20].

Erosion, Abrasion, and Attrition Prevention

Erosion Prevention

- Tooth erosion is the loss of tooth structure due to a nonbacterial chemical process that causes yellow tooth discoloration (i.e. dentin exposed), tooth transparency (thin enamel), enamel fractures (thin brittle enamel), tooth sensitivity (dentin exposed), and makes the tooth more susceptible to decay [56].
- Clinically erosion has a "melted candle" appearance and cupping on cusp tips.
- Identify the cause in order to reduce the culprit.
  - Xerostomia (a symptom with its own cause, less bicarbonate/buffering capability) increases susceptibility to acid erosion [56].
  - Acidic foods, drinks, and medications. Drinks include carbonated beverages (including sugar-free), sports drinks, energy drinks, alcohol (e.g. wine), coffee, and tea [56].
  - Regurgitation (e.g. pregnancy, alcoholism, bulimia, bariatric surgery, GERD).
  - Chlorinated swimming pools.
  - Industrial environmental exposure [57].
- Treatment/prevention
  - If drinking acidic drinks, use a straw and minimize contact time with teeth [56].
  - Treat xerostomia (see section Xerostomia).
  - Buffer acids after exposure. If the patient vomited, recommend immediately rinsing with a freshly made baking soda mouthrinse (two teaspoons of baking soda in 8 ounces [226 ml] of water) and avoid brushing teeth for 40 minutes (to prevent abrasion).
  - See section Nutritional Counseling.

Abrasion Prevention

- Loss of tooth structure from mechanical action of an external source.
- Avoid the cause, such as toothbrushing with heavy pressure and abrasive toothpaste [57].
- If the patient vomited, recommend immediately rinsing with a freshly made baking soda mouthrinse (two teaspoons of baking soda in 8 ounces [226 ml] of water) and avoid brushing teeth for 40 minutes (to prevent abrasion).

Attrition Prevention

See Chapter 15.

Xerostomia

- Dry mouth is a symptom of a medical disorder or a side effect of medications and medical treatment [58].
- Identify dry mouth based on patient's complaint and/or during the oral examination.
- Discuss with the patient the benefits of saliva:
  - Lubricates and protects mucosa from chemical, microbial and physical injury (e.g. denture sore spots).
  - Helps digest food (digestive enzymes).
  - Cleanses the oral cavity.
  - Neutralizes acid from bacteria in the mouth.
  - Defends the body (e.g. antimicrobial enzymes).
- Discuss with the patient the oral health complications of having dry mouth.
  - Dry mouth, in addition to a high-risk factor, places a patient at "extreme risk" for caries [4, 5]. Caries often found at the root, cervical areas, and/or incisal/cusp tips [58]
  - In addition to caries, other adverse effects include plaque accumulation, gingivitis, periodontitis, other oral infections, difficulty wearing a prosthesis, and/or difficulty and discomfort talking/chewing/tasting [58].
- Try to identify the cause of xerostomia, which may be multifactorial.
- Provide recommendations
  - Drink more water, chew sugar-free gum or suck sugar-free candy, suck on ice chips, use a humidifier, avoid using alcohol-containing mouthwash, and avoid alcohol, caffeine, tobacco, spicy food [58] and marijuana [48].
  - Patients can use OTC products including patches, lozenges, sprays, gel, mouthrinses (e.g. Biotene).
  - The dentist can prescribe saliva substitutes.
- The dentist (if comfortable) or the physician can prescribe saliva stimulants (systemic medications) including pilocarpine hydrochloride and cevimeline [59] (beware the many contraindications).

Thumb-sucking and Pacifiers

- Can lead to an anterior open bite, increased overjet, and maxillary constriction.
- Dental changes depend on the amount of force applied, duration, and position of the digits in the mouth.
- Often children discontinue with peer pressure at school. Eliminate the habit before permanent incisors fully erupt.

Preventive Dentistry

- Treatment includes counseling, reminder therapy, reward system, and adjunctive therapy [20].
- According to the AAPD, if thumb- or finger-sucking continues past the age of three years a mouth appliance may be recommended [60].
- "Pacifiers can affect the teeth essentially the same way as sucking fingers and thumbs, but is often an easier habit to break" [61].

Sports Injuries

See Chapter 15.

Clinical Pearls

Tips

- Prophy polish: smear the polish with a gloved finger onto the teeth surfaces and then use the prophy angle to polish (vs. multiple times attempting to scoop the polish into the prophy angle and then polishing).
- Be cautious with the USS tip as it can lead to a needlestick injury! Anytime the USS it is not in use lay it flat on the tray table (Figure 5.11). Similarly, anytime a bur is not in use, remove it from the high- or slow-speed handpiece and lay it flat on the tray table.
- The dental assistant can assist you when using hand instruments by placing the surgical suction nearby to remove plaque and calculus from the instrument (Figure 5.12).
- Educating patients with poor oral hygiene:
  - Have the patient hold the mirror and scrape off plaque with the explorer to show the areas being missed when he or she is brushing and flossing.
  - Take before and after intraoral photos when performing a prophylaxis (Figure 5.13).
  - During a prophylaxis, clean half the arch and show the patient in the mirror the difference between the cleaned half and the half that has not been cleaned.
  - Use disclosing tablets or solutions.
- Customer service tips during the prophylaxis appointment:
  - Apply moisturizer (e.g. Vaseline) to the patient's lips before initiating the prophylaxis.
  - Adjust the head rest so that the patient is comfortable.
  - Place a bite block so that the patient does not get tired holding their mouth open throughout the procedure.
  - Offer different prophy paste flavors and let the patient choose.
  - Let the patient swish mouthrinse (e.g. Listerine) at the end of the prophylaxis appointment so that they don't leave the office tasting blood.
- When using the USS on the lower anteriors, pull the lower lip out to catch the water (Figure 5.14).
- When making custom fluoride trays, be sure the tray covers the entire clinical crown (i.e. including the root surfaces). This is different from bleaching trays (which should only cover the enamel) and occlusal guards (which cover about half of the clinical crown).

Figure 5.11 Be cautious with the USS and any burs on the handpieces. Prevent needlestick accidents by laying these sharps on the tray table when not in use. This is how the author had a needlestick accident.

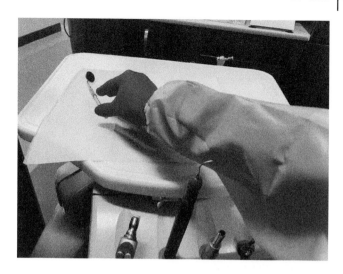

Figure 5.12 The dental assistant can use the surgical suction to remove plaque and calculus from the hand instrument to prevent a needlestick injury, which may occur when the dental assistant wipes the instrument each time with gauze.

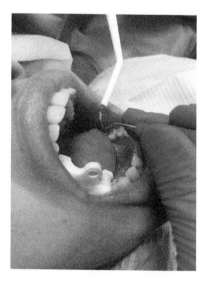

Figure 5.13 Take before and after photos with the intraoral camera for documentation and patient education.

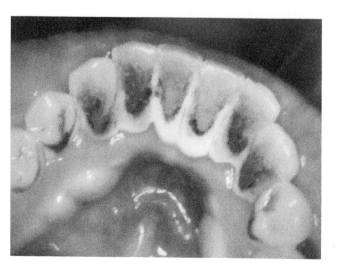

Preventive Dentistry

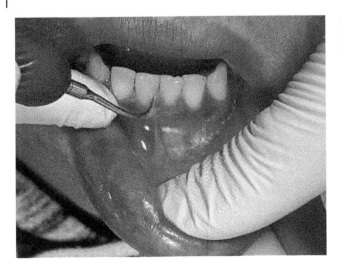

Figure 5.14 Pull the lower lip out to catch the water when using the USS on the lower anteriors.

Real-Life Clinical Questions Answered

Dental Hygienist's Question

- "When do we bill a child prophy versus an adult prophy?"
  - Prophylaxis codes are dentition specific (child = primary and transitional vs. adult = permanent and transitional). Some insurance companies have restrictions based on age [62].

Patients' Demands

- "I want a deep cleaning not a regular one."
  - Sounds like you want to make sure your cleaning is thorough, which I will make sure it is. We can only offer a deep cleaning if you have deep pockets between the gums and the teeth. Requesting a "deep cleaning" is not like requesting the gold versus the silver versus the basic carwash package to get your car cleaned. If there are no deep pockets we cannot go deep.
- "I don't want my daughter to have any fluoride."
  - I'm curious what your concerns are regarding the fluoride.
  - Seek to understand the reason. It could be as simple as the fee for fluoride varnish, concerns about fluorosis, or concerns about unfounded diseases associated with fluoride read on an internet blog.
  - If concerned about safety, remember the adage "the dose makes the poison" [63].
  - See section Fluoride Varnish.
  - Mention that almost every dental product used in the dental office contains fluoride; even the bonding agent for composite contains fluoride.

Patients' Comments

- "I brush every morning before breakfast."
  - While I'm glad to hear you are brushing, I recommend brushing after breakfast in order to remove the food particles from the teeth because the bacteria will feed on these food particles, secrete acid, and cause cavities.
- "I have arthritis so it is difficult for me to brush my teeth."
  - See section Oral Hygiene Instructions.

- "I don't floss because it makes my gums bleed."
  - Bleeding gums is a sign of gingivitis. Gingivitis is caused by plaque. Flossing removes plaque. The more you floss the less the gums will bleed.
- "I only floss if there is a piece of meat stuck between my teeth."
  - The ADA recommends daily flossing to prevent cavities and gum disease between all teeth [16] not just the ones with meat stuck between.
- "I use hard bristles because the soft don't clean my teeth as well."
  - The ADA recommends only using soft-bristled toothbrushes, as medium and hard can cause gingival abrasion [7].
- "I use an all-natural toothpaste so its fluoride-free."
  - Fluoride is also a naturally occurring element.
  - I'm glad to hear you are brushing as it mechanically removes plaque and food. My only concern is you are not getting the cavity-protecting benefits from fluoride.
  - See section Fluoride Varnish.
- "I always rinse with hydrogen peroxide."
  - Hydrogen peroxide is an antiseptic mouthwash. It can cause chemical burns in the mouth, usually associated with concentrations of 3% or higher [57].
  - I'd recommend using a different mouthrinse.

Patients' Questions

- "Is fluoride safe for my baby?"
  - Yes, fluoridated toothpaste is recommended as soon as teeth begin to come into the mouth [36].
- "I don't know how to brush my child's teeth because she's three years old, she is my first kid and when I try she runs out of the room with the toothbrush."
  - See Chapter 17.
- "Why do I have so many cavities? I don't eat sweets and I drink diet soda."
  - Bacteria feed on the food you eat, especially sugars and starches. The bacteria produce acid as a by-product of their digestion of the food, and this dissolves the tooth causing cavities. So even a diet that doesn't consist of sweets but consists of starches such as pasta, bread, cereal, pretzels, and/or crackers leads to cavities.
  - In addition, diet soda is very acidic, which causes erosion and weakens teeth [64]. When the teeth are weakened, they are at higher risk of becoming decayed.
  - Frequency is a big factor. How often do you snack and drink soda? And how often do you brush and floss?
- "I'll do whatever you say doctor. How can I lower my risk of getting cavities?"
  - See section Caries Management by Risk Assessment.
- "What can I do to get rid of bad breath?"
  - Bad breath in the morning is common. At night there is reduced saliva production, and if you are a mouth breather, the mouth will become even more dry. When saliva is not present to wash away the food particles and the bacteria from the mouth, the bacteria produce odors [65].
  - I recommend first identifying the culprit. Halitosis can have several causes, including poor oral hygiene, dry mouth, tooth decay, gum disease, surgical wounds, diet (e.g. garlic and onion, the odors of which are absorbed into the bloodstream and exhaled), postnasal drip, chronic sinusitis, throat infections, digestive system disturbances (e.g. GERD), and tobacco [66, 67].
  - Once the cause is identified, managing the halitosis will be easier.

Preventive Dentistry

- "What mouthwash do you recommend?"
  - It depends on your needs (see section Oral Hygiene Instructions).
- "Should I buy a Waterpik?"
  - The ADA recommends brushing twice a day and flossing once a day.
  - Waterpik is a brand of oral irrigators. I recommend these for patients with braces, bridges, implants, and/or isolated deep pockets as an adjunct to brushing and flossing.
- "I read that oil pulling is really healthy for your teeth and that charcoal toothpaste will whiten your teeth."
  - There is no scientific evidence that oil pulling reduces cavities, whitens teeth, or improves oral health and well-being. The ADA does not recommend oil pulling [68].
  - For charcoal toothpaste, see section Oral Hygiene Instructions.
- "I read that there is no benefit to flossing."
  - The ADA recommends daily flossing to reduce the likelihood of gum disease and tooth decay. Toothbrush bristles cannot clean efficiently between tight spaces [16].
- "Do I really have to brush for two minutes?"
  - Yes, in order to achieve clinically significant plaque removal [9].
- "I want a refill of that mouthwash in the brown bottle."
  - Is the chlorhexidine being used for gingivitis or for caries management?
  - If for gingivitis, it is not for long-term use due to side effects (see Chapter 16).
  - If for caries management, you may be due for a refill (see Chapter 16).
- "I need a mouthguard for football, what do you recommend?"
  - See Chapter 15.

References

1 US history.org (2020). The Electric Ben Franklin. https://www.ushistory.org/franklin/philadelphia/fire.htm (accessed 20 August 2020).

2 Centers for Disease Control and Prevention (CDC) (2020). Basics of oral health. https://www.cdc.gov/oralhealth/basics/index.html (accessed 20 August 2020).

3 Johnson, N.W., Glick, M., and Mbuguye, T.N. (2006). Oral health and general health. *Adv. Dent. Res.* 19: 118–121.

4 Featherstone, J.D.B., Crystal, Y.O., Chaffee, B.W. et al. (2019). An updated CAMBRA Caries Risk Assessment Tool for ages 0 to 5 years. *J. Calif. Dent. Assoc.* 47 (1): 37–47.

5 Featherstone, J.D.B., Alston, P., Chaffee, B.W., and Rechmann, P. (2019). Caries Management by Risk Assessment (CAMBRA): an update for use in clinical practice for patients aged 6 through adult. *J. Calif. Dent. Assoc.* 47 (1): 25–34.

6 Weinstein, P., Harrison, R., and Benton, T. (2004). Motivating parents to prevent caries in their young children. One-year findings. *J. Am. Dent. Assoc.* 135: 731–738.

7 American Dental Association (ADA) (2020). Oral health topics. Toothpastes. https://www.ada.org/en/member-center/oral-health-topics/toothpastes (accessed 19 August 2020).

8 American Dental Association (ADA) (2020). Accepted over-the-counter products. https://www.ada.org/en/science-research/ada-seal-of-acceptance/ada-seal-shopping-list (accessed 19 August 2020).

9 American Dental Association (ADA) (2020). Oral health topics. Toothbrushes. https://www.ada.org/en/member-center/oral-health-topics/toothbrushes (accessed 19 August 2020).

10 Beneduce, C., Baxter, K.A., Bowman, J. et al. (2009). Germicidal activity of antimicrobials and VIOlight Personal Travel Toothbrush sanitizer: an in vitro study. *J. Dent.* 38 (8): 621–625.

11 Ciancio, S.G. (2017). Baking soda dentifrices and oral health. *J. Am. Dent. Assoc.* 148 (11 Suppl): S1–S3. https://jada.ada.org/article/ S0002-8177(17)30822-X/fulltext (accessed 19 August 2020).

12 American Dental Association. Mouth Healthy. Natural teeth whitening: fact vs. fiction. https://www.mouthhealthy.org/en/ az-topics/w/natural-teeth-whitening (accessed 19 August 2020).

13 Anon (2003). Sensitive teeth: causes and treatment. *J. Am. Dent. Assoc.* 134: 1691.

14 The Kois Center: Advancing Dentistry Through Science. How much toothpaste should I use? https://www.koiscenter.com/patient-education/ smile/how-much-toothpaste-should-i-use (accessed 19 August 2020).

15 American Academy of Pediatric Dentistry (2020). Fluoride therapy. In: *The Reference Manual of Pediatric Dentistry*, 288–291. Chicago: AAPD.

16 American Dental Association (2020). Floss/ interdental cleaners. https://www.ada.org/ en/member-center/oral-health-topics/floss (accessed 19 August 2020).

17 Rose, L.F. and Mealy, B.L. (2004). *Periodontics: Medicine, Surgery, and Implants*. St. Louis, MO: Elsevier Mosby.

18 American Dental Association. Patient Smart Patient Education Center (2013). Flossing. https://www.ada.org/~/media/ADA/ Publications/Files/ADA_PatientSmart_ Flossing.pdf?la=en (accessed 19 August 2020).

19 American Academy of Periodontology (2018). Should you brush or floss first? New study suggests the ideal sequence for removing plaque. https://www.perio.org/ node/878?_ga=2.11497974.37167829 4.1585161364-1313695504.1539053453 (accessed 19 August 2020).

20 Casamassimo, P.S., Fields, H.W., McTigue, D.J., and Nowak, A.J. (2013). *Pediatric*

Dentistry: Infancy through Adolescence, 5e. St. Louis, MO: Elsevier Saunders.

21 Centers for Disease Control and Prevention (CDC) (2019). Pregnancy and oral health. https://www.cdc.gov/oralhealth/ publications/features/pregnancy-and-oral-health.html (Accessed 19 August 2020).

22 American Academy of Periodontology (2013). Expectant mothers' periodontal health vital to health of her baby. https:// www.perio.org/consumer/AAP_EFP_ Pregnancy (accessed 19 August 2020).

23 American Dental Association (2020). Mouth Healthy. Breastfeeding: 6 things nursing moms should know about dental health. https://www.mouthhealthy.org/en/az-topics/b/breastfeeding (accessed 19 August 2020).

24 Mark, A.M. (2019). Oral health care tips for caregivers. *J. Am. Dent. Assoc.* 150 (5): 480.

25 Misch, C.E. (2008). *Contemporary Implant Dentistry*, 3e. St. Louis, MO: Mosby.

26 GUM Red-Cote tablets. https://www. sunstargum.com/products/category-tablets/ gum-red-cote-tablets.html (accessed 19 August 2020).

27 Hingham, S., Hope, C., Valappil, S. and Smith, P. (2020). Caries process and prevention strategies: the environment. The Stephen curve. https://www.dentalcare.com/ en-us/professional-education/ce-courses/ ce371 (accessed 19 August 2020).

28 Hingham, S., Hope, C., Valappil, S. and Smith, P. (2020) Caries process and prevention strategies: the environment. Critical pH. https://www.dentalcare.com/ en-us/professional-education/ce-courses/ ce371 (accessed 19 August 2020).

29 Dawes, C. (2003). What is the critical pH and why does a tooth dissolve in acid? *J. Can. Dent. Assoc.* 69 (11): 722–724. https://www. cda-adc.ca/jcda/vol-69/issue-11/722.pdf (accessed 27 August 2020).

30 American Dental Association (2020). Mouth Healthy. 8 Bad brushing habits to break in 2020. https://www.mouthhealthy.org/en/ brushing-mistakes-slideshow (accessed 27 August 2020).

31 Kracher, C.M. (2020). Current concepts in preventive dentistry. Non- or low-acidogenic foods. https://www.dentalcare.com/en-us/professional-education/ce-courses/ce334/non-or-low-acidogenic-foods (accessed 19 August 2020).

32 Pavia, M., Pileggi, C., Nobile, C.G., and Angelillo, I.F. (2006). Association between fruit and vegetable consumption and oral cancer: a meta-analysis of observational studies. *Am. J. Clin. Nutr.* 83 (5): 1126–1134.

33 Colgate Professional. Mouth-healthy eating. (2002–2005). https://www.colgateprofessional.com/education/patient-education/topics/caries/mouth-healthy-eating (accessed 19 August 2020).

34 American Dental Association (2020). Mouth Healthy. Erosion: what you eat and drink can impact your teeth. https://www.mouthhealthy.org/en/az-topics/e/dietary-acids-and-your-teeth (accessed 19 August 2020).

35 American Academy of Pediatric Dentistry (AAPD) (2020). Healthy beverage consumption in early childhood: recommendations from key national health and nutrition organizations: Summary of oral health considerations. In: *The Reference Manual of Pediatric Dentistry*, 547–550. Chicago: AAPD.

36 American Dental Association (2018). *Fluoridation Facts*. https://www.ada.org/en/public-programs/advocating-for-the-public/fluoride-and-fluoridation/fluoridation-facts (accessed 20 August 2020).

37 Wright, K.F. (2015). Is your drinking water acidic? The comparison of the varied pH of popular bottled waters. *J. Dent. Hyg.* 89 (Suppl 2): 6–12.

38 BRITA (2014). Additional frequently asked questions. https://brita.ca/en/water-filtration-process/frequently-asked-questions (accessed 20 August 2020).

39 American Dental Association (2020). Mouth Healthy. Nutrition. https://www.mouthhealthy.org/en/adults-over-60/nutrition (accessed 19 August 2020).

40 American Academy of Pediatric Dentistry (AAPD) (2020). Policy on dietary recommendations for infants, children, and adolescents. In: *The Reference Manual of Pediatric Dentistry*, 84–86. Chicago: AAPD.

41 American Academy of Pediatric Dentistry (AAPD) (2020). Policy on early childhood caries (ECC): classifications, consequences, and preventive strategies. In: *The Reference Manual of Pediatric Dentistry*, 79–81. Chicago: AAPD.

42 American Dental Association (2020). Mouth Healthy. Nutrition. https://www.mouthhealthy.org/en/babies-and-kids/nutrition (accessed 11 May 2021).

43 Zarb, G. and Bolender, C. (ed.) (2004). *Prosthodontic Treatment for Edentulous Patients: Complete Dentures and Implant-Supported Prostheses*, 12e. St. Louis, MO: Elsevier Mosby.

44 U.S. Department of Agriculture. ChooseMyPlate. https://www.choosemyplate.gov (accessed 20 August 2020).

45 Hinode, D., Tanabe, S., Yokoyama, M. et al. (2006). Influence of smoking on osseointegrated implant failure. A meta-analysis. *Clin. Oral Implants Res.* 17 (4): 473–478.

46 Centers for Disease Control and Prevention (CDC) (2020). Frequently asked questions (FAQ) about 1-800-QUIT-NOW and the National Network of Tobacco Cessation Quitlines. https://www.cdc.gov/tobacco/quit_smoking/cessation/faq-about-1-800-quit-now/index.html (accessed 19 August 2020).

47 US Department of Health and Human Services (2008), Public Health Service. *Treating Tobacco Use and Dependence: 2008 Update*. https://www.ahrq.gov/sites/default/files/wysiwyg/professionals/clinicians-providers/guidelines-recommendations/tobacco/clinicians/references/quickref/tobaqrg.pdf (accessed 19 August 2020).

48 O'Neil, M. (ed.) (2015). *The ADA Practical Guide to Substance Use Disorders and Safe Prescribing*. Hoboken, NJ: Wiley Blackwell.

49 California Dental Association (2020). Treating young kids every day: 6-step infant oral care visit. Self-management goals for the parent/caregiver. https://www.cda.org/Portals/0/pdfs/tyke_self_mgmt_goals_for_parent.pdf (accessed 19 August 2020).

50 Wright, J., Tampi, M., Graham, L. et al. (2016). Sealants for preventing and arresting pit-and-fissure occlusal caries in primary and permanent molars. *Pediatr. Dent.* 38 (4): 282–294.

51 Soxman, J.A. (ed.) (2015). *Handbook of Clinical Techniques in Pediatric Dentistry*. Hoboken, NJ: Wiley Blackwell.

52 American Association of Pediatric Dentistry (AAPD) (2016). Evidence-based clinical practice guideline for the use of pit-and-fissure sealants. https://www.aapd.org/assets/1/7/G_EBD-Sealants1.PDF (accessed 23 April 2021).

53 Jenson, L., Budenz, A., Featherstone, J. et al. (2007). Clinical protocols for caries management by risk assessment. *J. Calif. Dent. Assoc.* 35 (10): 714–723.

54 Kanellis, M.J., Owais, A.I., Warren, J.J. et al. (2018). Managing caries in the primary dentition with silver nitrate: lessons learned from a clinical trial. *J. Calif. Dent. Assoc.* 46: 37–44.

55 Horst, J.A., Ellenikiotis, H., UCSF Silver Caries Arrest Committee, and Milgrom, P.M. (2016). UCSF protocol for caries arrest using silver diamine fluoride: rationale, indications, and consent. *J. Calif. Dent. Assoc.* 44 (1): 16–28.

56 Academy of General Dentistry (2015). Erosion and your teeth: a patient's guide to protecting tooth enamel. Brochure.

57 Neville, B.W., Damm, D.D., Allen, C.M., and Chi, A.C. (2016). *Oral and Maxillofacial Pathology*, 4e. St. Louis, MO: Elsevier Saunders.

58 American Dental Association (2019). Oral health topics. Xerostomia (dry mouth). https://www.ada.org/en/member-center/oral-health-topics/xerostomia (accessed 24 August 2020).

59 Jacobsen, P.L. (2013). *The Little Dental Drug Booklet: Handbook of Commonly Used Dental Medications*, 21e. Hudson, OH: Lexicomp.

60 American Academy of Pediatric Dentistry (2020). Frequently asked questions (FAQs). https://www.aapd.org/resources/parent/faq (accessed 6 May 2021).

61 American Dental Association (2020). Mouth Healthy. Thumbsucking and pacifier use. https://www.mouthhealthy.org/en/az-topics/t/thumbsucking (accessed 11 May 2021).

62 American Dental Association (ADA) (2020). *CDT 2020 Coding Companion: Training Guide for the Dental Team*. Chicago: ADA.

63 Toxipedia: Connecting Science and People. Paracelsus (1493–1534). https://www.asmalldoseoftoxicology.org/paracelsus (accessed 19 August 2020).

64 Colgate (2020). Sugar-free drinks: are they safe for teeth? https://www.colgate.com/en-us/oral-health/basics/nutrition-and-oral-health/sugar-free-drinks-are-they-safe-for-teeth-0115 (accessed 27 August 2020).

65 Colgate (2020). Bad breath from dry mouth and how to treat it. https://www.colgate.com/en-us/oral-health/conditions/bad-breath/bad-breath-from-dry-mouth-and-how-to-treat-it-0316 (accessed 19 August 2020).

66 Anon (2012). Bad breath: causes and tips for controlling it. *J. Am. Dent. Assoc* 143 (9): 1053.

67 American Dental Association (2020). Mouth Healthy. Bad breath: 6 causes (and 6 solutions). https://www.mouthhealthy.org/en/az-topics/b/bad-breath (accessed 19 August 2020).

68 American Dental Association (2020). Mouth Healthy. Oil pulling. https://www.mouthhealthy.org/en/az-topics/o/oil-pulling (accessed 19 August 2020).

Preventive Dentistry

6

Periodontics

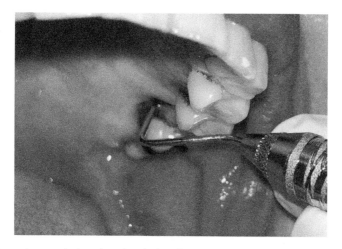

Figure 6.1   Finding a deep periodontal pocket during the comprehensive periodontal evalution.

Chapter Outline

- Real-Life Clinical Questions
- Relevance
- What is Periodontal Disease?
- Diagnosis: New Classification of Periodontitis
  - Chairside Guide to Periodontitis Staging and Grading
  - Periodontal Diagnosis Flowchart
  - Clinical Attachment Level
  - Furcation
  - Mobility
  - Occlusal Trauma
  - Fremitus

Clinical Dentistry Daily Reference Guide, First Edition. William A. Jacobson.
© 2022 John Wiley & Sons, Inc. Published 2022 by John Wiley & Sons, Inc.

Real-Life Clinical Questions

Dental Students' Questions

- "My patient is just here for a prophy. In the past he's had deep cleanings. Can I get a start check?"
- "The patient only needs SRP on a few teeth in the upper left. Do I bill SRP upper left 1 to 3 teeth and also a prophy?"
- "If the patient has severe bone loss but no deep pockets, should I do a prophy or SRP?"
- "Why do I have to remove the stains on the teeth?"
- "How do I know if I should put the patient on a three-, four-, or six-month periodontal maintenance schedule?"
- "The patient has an abscess but the tooth tests as vital. What could this be?"

Patients' Questions

- "What is periodontal disease?"
- "I was never told by my last dentist that I have gum disease. Why didn't he tell me?"
- "I brush and floss, I don't smoke, and I don't have diabetes so why do I have loose teeth?"
- "I don't smoke cigarettes, I just smoke pot which is natural. That shouldn't affect my teeth, right?"
- "Is periodontal disease contagious if I kiss someone?"
- "I heard your oral health is related to the rest of your body. Is that true?"
- "Will a deep cleaning help?"

- "What do you think about lasers for gum disease?"
- "What can I do to prevent more bone loss?"
- "Doc, how long will my teeth last?"

Patients' Demands

- "I only want a regular cleaning."
- "I need this form signed as clearance to begin orthodontic treatment."

Relevance

As a dentist you primarily treat two diseases, dental caries and periodontal disease. Almost half (47.2%) of adults aged 30 and older have some form of periodontal disease [1], and the American Academy of Periodontology (AAP) recommends that all adults receive an annual comprehensive periodontal evaluation to assess their periodontal health status and identify conditions that require additional treatment [2].

It is your responsibility to diagnose periodontal disease, understand the periodontal–systemic relationship, treat periodontal disease, and know when to refer to a periodontist.

What is Periodontal Disease?

Rose and Mealy [3] describe dental plaque [biofilm] as "complex microbial communities that form on virtually all surfaces of the teeth exposed to the bacteria-laden fluids of the mouth. Dental plaques are of considerable clinical importance because they are the primary etiologic agents in the development of dental caries and periodontal disease"

The AAP [4] defines periodontal disease as:

> an inflammatory disease that affects the soft and hard structures that support the teeth. In its early stage, called gingivitis, the gums become swollen and red due to inflammation, which is the body's natural response to the presence of harmful bacteria. In the more serious form of periodontal disease called periodontitis, the gums pull away from the tooth and supporting gum tissues are destroyed. Bone can be lost, and the teeth may loosen or eventually fall out. . . . Important risk factors include inherited or genetic susceptibility, smoking, lack of adequate home care, age, diet, health history, and medications.

Various forms of periodontal disease exist.

Diagnosis: New Classification of Periodontitis

- The new classification of periodontitis is from the 2017 World Workshop on the Classification of Periodontal and Peri-Implant Diseases and Conditions.
- Many forms of periodontal diseases exist within the following categories:
  - Periodontal health, gingival diseases and conditions
  - Periodontitis
  - Periodontal manifestations of systemic diseases
  - Peri-implant diseases and conditions [5] (see Chapter 14).

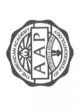

Staging and Grading Periodontitis

The 2017 World Workshop on the Classification of Periodontal and Peri-Implant Diseases and Conditions resulted in a new classification of periodontitis characterized by a multidimensional staging and grading system. The charts below provide an overview. Please visit **perio.org/2017wwdc** for the complete suite of reviews, case definition papers, and consensus reports.

PERIODONTITIS: STAGING

Staging intends to classify the severity and extent of a patient's disease based on the measurable amount of destroyed and/or damaged tissue as a result of periodontitis and to assess the specific factors that may attribute to the complexity of long-term case management.

Initial stage should be determined using clinical attachment loss (CAL). If CAL is not available, radiographic bone loss (RBL) should be used. Tooth loss due to periodontitis may modify stage definition. One or more complexity factors may shift the stage to a higher level. See **perio.org/2017wwdc** for additional information.

Periodontitis		Stage I	Stage II	Stage III	Stage IV
Severity	Interdental CAL *(at site of greatest loss)*	1 – 2 mm	3 – 4 mm	≥5 mm	≥5 mm
	RBL	Coronal third (<15%)	Coronal third (15% – 33%)	Extending to middle third of root and beyond	Extending to middle third of root and beyond
	Tooth loss *(due to periodontitis)*	No tooth loss		≤4 teeth	≥5 teeth

Complexity	Local	• Max. probing depth ≤4 mm
		• Mostly horizontal bone loss
			• Max. probing depth ≤5 mm
			• Mostly horizontal bone loss
				In addition to Stage II complexity:
				• Probing depths ≥6 mm
				• Vertical bone loss ≥3 mm
				• Furcation involvement Class II or III
				• Moderate ridge defects
					In addition to Stage III complexity:
					• Need for complex rehabilitation due to:
					  – Masticatory dysfunction
					  – Secondary occlusal trauma (tooth mobility degree ≥2)
					  – Severe ridge defects
					  – Bite collapse, drifting, flaring
					  – <20 remaining teeth (10 opposing pairs)

Extent and distribution	Add to stage as descriptor	For each stage, describe extent as: • Localized (<30% of teeth involved); • Generalized; or • Molar/incisor pattern			

Figure 6.2 Staging and grading of periodontitis. *Source:* courtesy of the AAP.

PERIODONTITIS: GRADING

Grading aims to indicate the rate of periodontitis progression, responsiveness to standard therapy, and potential impact on systemic health.

Clinicians should initially assume grade B disease and seek specific evidence to shift to grade A or C.
See **perio.org/2017wwdc** for additional information.

			Grade A: Slow rate	Grade B: Moderate rate	Grade C: Rapid rate
Primary criteria	Direct evidence of progression	Radiographic bone loss or CAL	No loss over 5 years	<2 mm over 5 years	≥2 mm over 5 years
Whenever available, direct evidence should be used.	Indirect evidence of progression	% bone loss / age	<0.25	0.25 to 1.0	>1.0
		Case phenotype	Heavy biofilm deposits with low levels of destruction	Destruction commensurate with biofilm deposits	Destruction exceeds expectations given biofilm deposits; specific clinical patterns suggestive of periods of rapid progression and/or early onset disease
Grade modifiers	Risk factors	Smoking	Non-smoker	<10 cigarettes/day	≥10 cigarettes/day
		Diabetes	Normoglycemic/no diagnosis of diabetes	HbA1c <7.0% in patients with diabetes	HbA1c ≥7.0% in patients with diabetes

The 2017 World Workshop on the Classification of Periodontal and Peri-Implant Diseases and Conditions was co-presented by the American Academy of Periodontology (AAP) and the European Federation of Periodontology (EFP).

Tables from Tonetti, Greenwell, Kornman. *J Periodontol* 2018;89 (Suppl 1): S159-S172.

Figure 6.2 (Continued)

Periodontal Diagnosis Flowchart

The flowchart in Figure 6.3 is helpful for formulating a periodontal diagnosis.

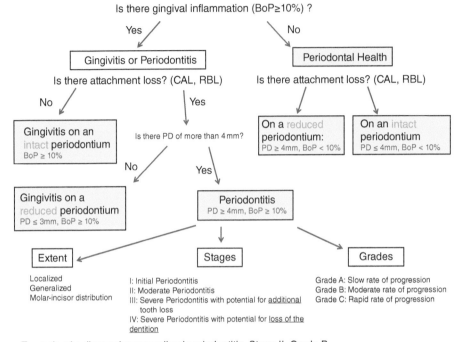

Example of a diagnosis: generalized periodontitis, Stage II, Grade B

Figure 6.3 Periodontal diagnosis flowchart. BOP, bleeding on probing; CAL, clinical attachment loss; PD, probing depths; RBL, radiographic bone loss; localized, <30% of teeth involved. *Source:* courtesy of Clara Kim, DMD, MS.

Clinical Attachment Level

- Using only probing depths is not accurate for diagnosing periodontal status, as the gingival margin is subject to change with inflammation/recession. The CEJ is a fixed reference point.
- Clinical attachment level (CAL) = [Pocket depths] + [Distance of gingival margin to CEJ].
  - Distance of gingival margin to CEJ is positive if the margin is apical to the CEJ or negative if the margin is coronal to the CEJ.
  - It is easy to determine distance of gingival margin to CEJ in recession, but is a challenge with the margin coronal to CEJ. Estimated by feeling CEJ with tip of probe [3].
- The term is amended to "clinical attachment *loss*" if there has been destruction to the periodontium.

Furcation (Glickman)

- Grade I: incipient lesion (feel a depression).
- Grade II: loss of interradicular bone and pocket formation but a portion of the alveolar bone and PDL remain intact (think a cul-de-sac).

- Grade III: through-and-through.
- Grade IV: through-and-through with gingival recession (clearly visible furcation) [7].
- Use a Nabers probe to assess, on lower molars B/L, on upper molars B/DP/MP.

Mobility (Miller Index of 1938)

1) First distinguishable sign of movement greater than normal (greater than physiologic movement).
2) 1 mm in any direction. (combined facial-lingual 2 mm).
3) >1 mm in any direction including teeth can be rotated or depressed into socket [8].

Occlusal Trauma

- Primary occlusal trauma: in a healthy mouth.
- Secondary occlusal trauma: associated with bone loss.
- Posterior bite collapse: loss of one or more posterior teeth which forces occlusion on the anterior teeth [3].

Fremitus

Movement of teeth created by patient's own occlusal forces. Have the patient tap their teeth together and move into excursions with your finger over buccal surfaces to feel fore movement.

- Class I: mild vibration detected.
- Class II: easily palpable vibration.
- Class III: visible movement of teeth [3].

What Is a Periodontal Abscess?

- There are two types of periodontal abscess:
  - Acute: very destructive process in the periodontium, not of pulpal origin, in a short period [3] (e.g. foreign body/food impaction such as popcorn husk).
  - Chronic: often associated with a preexisting periodontal pocket in which the orifice of the pocket becomes occluded by impaction of a foreign object (e.g. popcorn husk) or by healing and the purulent material cannot drain.
- Relevance: in the dental clinic 85% of toothaches will be of pulpal origin, and 15% will be of periodontal origin [3].
- Clinical signs: deep periodontal pocket, tooth mobility, signs range from localized swelling to face and neck swelling, sinus tract, lymphadenopathy, and/or normal pulp vitality testing [3].
- Radiographic signs: radiolucency lateral to root [3] (does not show if buccal or lingual).
- Symptoms:
  - Pain, tooth may feel high (extruded) [3].
  - May experience a bad taste (purulence).
  - May present as a fistula (closed or open).
- Potential complications: cellulitis which can occlude airway or cavernous sinus infection, serious systemic complications [3].
- For treatment, see Section Procedural Steps.

The Periodontal–Systemic Connection

- *Obesity and oral health*
  - Obesity is an inflammatory condition that can exacerbate the local inflammatory response in the periodontium.
  - Dental treatment: diet can be improved by treating dental disease (e.g. pain, establishing function), allowing the ability to eat a healthier range of foods, not limited to soft carbohydrates [9].
- *Diabetes and oral health*
  - Bidirectional relationship.
  - Hyperglycemia increases the risk of periodontal disease, and leads to hyposalivation and burning mouth and increased susceptibility to fungal infections. Hyperglycemia, not just a diagnosis of diabetes.
  - Periodontal disease, especially if severe, is a risk factor for developing type 2 diabetes and for progression of type 2 diabetes.
  - Dental treatment: nonsurgical periodontal treatment and extraction of hopeless periodontally compromised teeth decreases hemoglobin A1c and improves glycemic control [9].
- *Cardiovascular disease and oral health*
  - Strong association between both. May be due to unhealthy lifestyle (e.g. smoking, poor nutrition, lack of exercise).
  - "Cannot claim oral infections contribute to development or progression of cardiovascular events."
  - Dental treatment: no studies show improved cardiovascular health. However, oral microbes enter the bloodstream [9].
- *Renal disease and oral health*
  - Association: as renal disease progresses, the prevalence of periodontal disease increases.
  - Dental treatment: lack of evidence to support periodontal treatment improving renal health [9].
- *Pulmonary disease and oral health*
  - Association.
  - Periodontitis is a risk factor for pulmonary disease.
  - Plausible mechanism includes aspiration of periodontal pathogens during intubation, increasing the risk for aspiration pneumonia and ventilator-associated pneumonia.
  - Smoking most likely links the increased risk for chronic obstructive pulmonary disease and periodontitis.
  - Dental treatment: better outcomes in pulmonary disease treatment when free of periodontitis. Lack of evidence showing periodontal treatment reduces pneumonia-associated mortality [9].
- *Pregnancy and oral health*
  - During pregnancy there is an increase in prevalence, extent, and severity of gingivitis. Infrequently associated with clinical attachment loss.
  - Association between poor periodontal health and adverse pregnancy outcomes including preterm birth, low birthweight, and preeclampsia.
  - Dental treatment: lack of evidence to support periodontal treatment improving adverse pregnancy outcomes [9].
- *Cancer and oral health*
  - Association, and plausible that periodontal disease increases risk of cancer including oral, lung, colorectal, and pancreatic.
  - Dental treatment: lack of evidence to support periodontal treatment reducing risk of these cancers [9].

Radiographic Findings (see also Chapter 3)

Additional considerations include the following.
- Look for local irritating factors:
  - Calculus (around the CEJ or roots).
  - Poorly contoured restorations (e.g. open proximal contacts, overhangs) [10].
- Look for signs of early bone changes:
  - Anterior teeth: interproximal crestal bone blunting (no longer pointed/peak), loss of height [10].
  - Posterior teeth: interproximal crestal bone loss of density and rounding (no longer well defined and/or corticated), loss of height [10].
- Vertical osseous defects:
  - Single tooth versus multiple vertical osseous defects.
  - Early on may be seen as widening PDL at the crestal bone.
  - May not be visible when superimposed bone [10].
- Interdental craters:
  - Trough-like depression in crest of the interdental bone (may be seen at different levels buccally and lingually).
  - Appear as a band-like region of less dense bone at crest [10].
- Buccal or lingual cortical plate loss:
  - Root appears more radiolucent at crest.
  - Loss of cortical plate usually semicircular shape (often described as "trough" or "moat-like" appearance) [10].

Treatment Planning

Table 6.1 Treatment planning phases related to periodontal treatment.

Treatment phase	Description (may or may not apply)
Emergency phase	• Urgent treatment of pain, infection, trauma, and/or esthetic emergency
Data gathering phase	• Comprehensive periodontal evaluation • Full-mouth debridement (if necessary for diagnosing) • Periodontal risk assessment
Stabilization phase (to control disease)	• Extraction of hopeless teeth • SRP • One-month reevaluation • Replacement of defective restorations
Definitive phase	• Not applicable
Maintenance phase	• Periodontal maintenance (every 3, 4, or 6 months) • Comprehensive periodontal evaluation (annually)

For more detailed information, see Chapter 4. For treatment planning related to periodontal disease, see Table 6.1.

Assignment of Periodontal Maintenance Recall Schedule

Table 6.2 Indications and periodontal maintenance recall frequency.

Indications (if any of the following)	Periodontal maintenance recall frequency
Stage III/IV: severe periodontitis Extent: generalized Grade C: rapid rate of progression Poor oral hygiene	3 months
Stage II: moderate periodontitis Extent: localized Grade B: moderate rate of progression Fair oral hygiene	4 months
Stage I: initial periodontitis Extent: localized Grade A: slow rate of progression Excellent hygiene Healthy patients	6 months

Table 6.2 lists some indications to consider when determining the periodontal maintenance recall frequency for patients at the one-month reevaluation after SRP. The first periodontal maintenance is three, four, or six months from the most recent SRP, although this frequency can change for a patient over time.

When to Refer to a Periodontist

- Perquisite: when the patient is motivated to maintain a healthy periodontium.
- If any of the following, refer:
    - No improvement in CAL or worsening of condition.
    - Probing depths are 5 mm or greater.
    - Pseudopockets.
    - The patient is interested in a gum graft to cover recession (keep in mind that this will approach the level of interproximal bone, but will not cover 100% of a black triangle).
    - Furcations.
    - Aggressive periodontitis.
    - Mucogingival defects (when the width of keratinized tissue is <2 mm, it may be painful to brush) [3].
- A periodontist may be able to offer:
    - Comprehensive periodontal evaluation.
    - SRP and periodontal maintenance.
    - Flap surgery (debridement).
    - Osseous surgery (pocket depth reduction, recontouring the bone and gums making the teeth more accessible for daily hygiene).
    - Guided tissue regeneration/bone graft (regenerating bone and tissue to repair damage).
    - Gingivectomy.
    - Gum grafts.

- Crown lengthening.
- Sinus augmentation.
- Dental implants.
- Laser treatment.
- Periodontal plastic surgery.

Armamentarium

Table 6.3 lists some common instruments used for diagnosing periodontal disease, detecting calculus, and for the removal of biofilm and calculus.

Table 6.3 Armamentarium for periodontal treatment.

Instrument	Specifics	Indication
Periodontal probe: used for measuring pocket depths and the distance from the CEJ to the gingival margin		
Explorers Explorer provides superior tactile information. Use feather-light pressure to detect calculus with the 1–2 mm of the side of the tip with many close overlapping multidirectional strokes	Orban	Anteriors, F/L posteriors (not M/D)
	Pigtail	Normal to shallow pockets (care not to injure soft tissue)
	11/12	Normal to deep pockets
	TU17 Wilkins/ Tufts	Long shape to walk down tooth surface without potentially injuring soft tissue
Sickle scalers Only for enamel surfaces. Working-end has two cutting edges, therefore angle 70–80° toward tooth to prevent soft tissue trauma		
Universal curettes Supragingival and subgingival on any tooth in the mouth. Working-end has two cutting edges, therefore angle 70–80° toward tooth to prevent soft tissue trauma		
Gracey curettes Area-specific curettes for removal of supragingival and subgingival calculus and biofilm. Tilted (uneven) cutting edges at 70°, automatically at the proper angle. Lower cutting edge is the working cutting edge, instrument face tilt toward tooth	1/2, 3/4	Anterior
	5/6	Anterior/premolar
	7/8	Posterior: buccal/lingual
	11/12	Posterior: mesial
	13/14	Posterior: distal
Ultrasonic scaler (USS) Converts electrical energy into high-frequency sound waves that produce rapid vibrations to dislodge calculus, disrupt plaque biofilm, and flush out bacteria	Standard, broad	Supragingival heavy/medium calculus
	Standard, medium	Supragingival: medium/light calculus
	Slim perio, straight	Supragingival/subgingival
	Slim perio, curved paired	Deep pockets
Airflow technology		For biofilm removal after removal of calculus with a USS and/or hand instruments

Hand Instrument Advice

- Roll the handle of the instrument to achieve adaptation by wrapping the tip around tooth.
- Cover every square millimeter with multidirectional strokes: vertical strokes → oblique strokes → horizontal strokes [11].

Prophy Angle and Polishing Paste

- Objective: removal of extrinsic stains and supragingival plaque, improving the appearance of the dentition, and to demonstrate the standard of oral cleanliness.
- Various grits available (fine to extra coarse). Fine particle size removes the least amount of tooth structure.
- How to use:
  - Set to <20000 revolutions per minute (rpm) to decrease abrasion and decrease heat, which can damage the pulp.
  - Caution: do not abrade gingiva. The movement of the rubber cup is away from the gingiva.
- Contraindicated if there are decalcified enamel/carious lesions, or exposed root surfaces.
- A microscopic amount of tooth structure is lost [3].

Ultrasonic Scaler

- Converts electrical energy into high-frequency sound waves that produce rapid vibrations at 18000–50000 Hz (18–50 kHz) to dislodge calculus, disrupt plaque biofilm, and flush out bacteria.
- Piezoelectric ("piezo") devices are a type of USS.
- How to use:
  - Determine the setting:
    - High: don't use as it causes discomfort and can damage the tooth.
    - Medium: for removing calculus with fine mist of water.
    - Low: for deplaquing with halo/dripping water.
  - If the handpiece is warm you must use more water.
  - Adapt the 2–3 mm of the lateral surface to the tooth with feather-light lateral pressure.
    - Firm pressure decreases effectiveness.
    - Do not use the point (tip) against the tooth surface as this can damage the tooth.
    - Keep moving at all times along tooth surface.
    - Cover every square millimeter with multidirectional strokes: vertical strokes → oblique strokes → horizontal strokes.
- For implants: recommend using a protective tip on the USS (Figure 6.4).
- Contraindications:
  - Communicable diseases: due to aerosols (debris, microorganisms, and blood).
  - Cardiac implantable devices (consult with patient's cardiologist).
  - Young age: large pulp chamber, with risk of nerve damage.
  - Restorations/implants: chips/scratches/nicks amalgam, composite, and porcelain [11].
- Caution:
  - Do not contact the USS with any white spots (incipient lesions) on the tooth or you will create a cavitation (plaque trap).
  - Recommend placing the USS on a flat surface when not in use, to reduce the chance of a needlestick accident (see Figure 5.11).

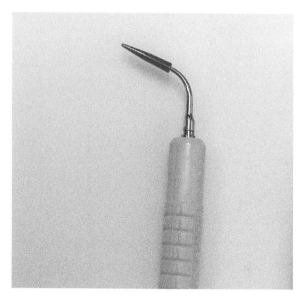

Figure 6.4 Dentsply Cavitron SofTip Ultrasonic Implant Insert to prevent scratching around titanium implants.

Procedural Steps

Comprehensive Periodontal Evaluation

Completed as part of the comprehensive oral evaluation (new patient exam) and annually.

- Radiographic findings (see Section Radiographic Findings).
- Full-mouth debridement (if necessary, for accurate diagnosis) (Figures 6.5 and 6.6).
- Inform the patient you are "doing a periodontal assessment."
- Comprehensive periodontal charting
  - Plaque score (a percentage calculated by the number of surfaces with plaque divided by total surfaces evaluated multiplied by 100).
  - Gingival margin (may identify recession or inflammation).
  - Probing depth (PD): six sites per tooth (See Figure 6.1).
  - Bleeding on probing (BOP): clinical sign of inflammation [3].
  - Suppuration on probing (clinical sign of inflammation) [3].
  - Mucogingival line (identifies mucogingival defects: pocket base at or beyond mucogingival junction).
  - CAL.
  - Furcations (Glickman system).
  - Mobilities (Miller system).
  - Occlusal trauma (primary or secondary).
  - Fremitus (functional mobility).
  - Teeth crowding.
  - Formulate and inform the patient of the diagnosis, prognosis, and treatment recommendations.
  - Document.

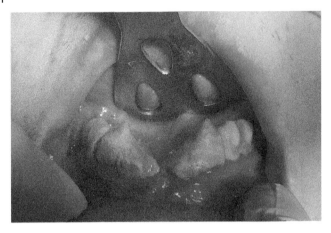

Figure 6.5 Due to the heavy amounts of calculus, a full-mouth debridement is necessary to obtain an accurate diagnosis of the periodontal condition.

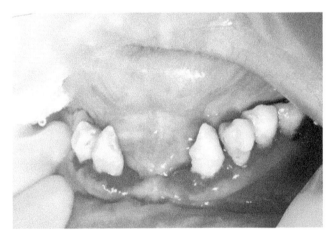

Figure 6.6 Image taken immediately following a full-mouth debridement.

Scaling and Root Planing

A nonsurgical periodontal treatment involving "careful cleaning of the root surfaces to remove plaque and calculus from deep periodontal pockets and to smooth the tooth root to remove bacterial toxins" [12]. One to four appointments are needed in total, depending on the distribution and severity of the calculus, and the time allotted.

- Preprocedural rinse (e.g. 1.5% diluted hydrogen peroxide or 0.12% chlorhexidine).
- Local anesthesia.
- USS (to remove calculus).
- Hand instrumentation (to remove calculus).
- Airflow (to remove the biofilm).
- Do not polish: if abrasive particles enter the gingival tissue without an intact epithelial barrier from instrumentation, delayed healing or a foreign body reaction may result [3].
- Floss.

- Review oral hygiene instructions.
- Smoking cessation (if applicable).
- Application of topical fluoride varnish low (sensitivity and root exposure), moderate, high, or extreme caries risk (see Chapter 5).
- Provide a personalized dental goody bag.
- Postoperative instructions:
  - Caution when eating not to bite lip/cheek/tongue.
  - Take ibuprofen before anesthetic wears off.
  - Warm saline rinses (½ teaspoon of salt per glass of lukewarm water) several times daily to reduce gingival inflammation.
  - May notice gum recession as swelling decreases.
  - May have tooth sensitivity to hot/cold for a few weeks, recommend desensitizing toothpaste.
  - If symptoms worsen or do not improve, return to the office.
- Document.

One-Month Reevaluation

Healing is assessed at four to six months after the last SRP. Identify problems that still persist.

- Comprehensive periodontal evaluation.
- Evaluation of patient's oral hygiene and recommendations.
- Determine if any plaque-retentive restorations contributing to the periodontal disease need to be replaced.
- Possible referral to periodontist if no improvement or worsening in periodontal condition.
- Assignment of periodontal maintenance recall schedule for long-term control of periodontal disease (three-, four-, or six-month frequency since the date of the most recent SRP).
- Document.

Periodontal Maintenance

Goal is "to prevent or minimize the reoccurrence and progression of periodontal disease in periodontally treated patients" [3]. This may alternate between the general dentist and the periodontist.

- Same as SRP, except one appointment for the full mouth.
- Preprocedural rinse (e.g. 1.5% diluted hydrogen peroxide or 0.12% chlorhexidine or Listerine).
- *Site-specific* SRP where indicated for removing calculus:
  - USS (to remove calculus).
  - Hand instruments (to remove calculus).
  - If no calculus, just remove the supragingival and subgingival biofilm and stains with airflow (e.g. Airflow by HuFriedy).
- Polish (if no airflow).
- Floss.
- Review oral hygiene instructions.
- Possible referral to periodontist if no improvement or decline in periodontal condition.
- Smoking cessation (if applicable).
- Application of topical fluoride varnish if low (sensitivity and root exposure), moderate, high, or extreme caries risk (see Chapter 5).

- Provide a personalized dental goody bag.
- Postoperative instructions:
  - Caution when eating not to bite lip/cheek/tongue.
  - Take ibuprofen before anesthetic wears off.
  - Warm saline rinses (½ teaspoon of salt per glass of lukewarm water) several times daily to reduce gingival inflammation.
  - May notice gum recession as swelling decreases.
  - May have tooth sensitivity to hot/cold for a few weeks, recommend desensitizing toothpaste.
  - If symptoms worsen or do not improve, return to the office.
- Document.

Periodontal Abscess Treatment

- Confirm the diagnosis (see Section What is a Periodontal Abscess?). Rule out pulpal involvement with a pulp vitality test.
- Local anesthesia.
- Localized SRP.
- Irrigate with sterile saline, 0.1% povidone-iodine, or 3% hydrogen peroxide.
  - Alternatively, make an incision to obtain full access to the root surfaces for debridement.
- Debride, suture, and prescribe twice daily chlorhexidine for one week.
- Prescribe antibiotics if systemic involvement (lymphadenopathy, swelling, fever, and/or malaise).
- Follow up one to two days after, weekly if necessary, until resolved [3].
- Document.

Prognosis

Table 6.4 Periodontal prognosis.

Favorable	The periodontal status of the tooth can be stabilized with comprehensive periodontal treatment and periodontal maintenance. Future loss of the periodontal supporting tissues is unlikely if these conditions are met
Questionable	The periodontal status of the tooth is influenced by local and/or systemic factors that may or may not be able to be controlled. The periodontium can be stabilized with comprehensive periodontal treatment and periodontal maintenance if these factors are controlled; otherwise, future periodontal breakdown may occur
Unfavorable	The periodontal status of the tooth is influenced by local and/or systemic factors that cannot be controlled. Periodontal breakdown is likely to occur even with comprehensive periodontal treatment and maintenance
Hopeless	The tooth must be extracted

Source: Kwok and Caton [13].

Prognosis is a somewhat subjective prediction of the probable course and final outcome of a disease (Table 6.4). It can be defined for different levels, such as of a tooth, of an arch, or of the entire dentition, and can differ at different times (before, middle, and after treatment). The "grading" described in the diagnosis of periodontal disease is related to the prognosis.

Charting Template

Recommend documenting the details of the procedure including the clinical findings:

- Hygiene (good/moderate/poor)
- Plaque (heavy/moderate/low)
- Calculus (heavy/moderate/low)
- Stain (heavy/moderate/low)
- Heme (heavy/moderate/low)

and that patient understands:

- Periodontal disease is a chronic progressive irreversible disease that leads to loss of teeth.
- Periodontal disease is treatable but not curable.
- SRP, regular periodontal maintenance, and patient's compliance with proper oral hygiene (along with not smoking and controlling A1c if diabetic) are all attempts to maintain the bone level to preserve the dentition and to help prevent further bone loss.
- At the one-month reevaluation after the last SRP, a periodontal evaluation will be completed. If no improvement is noted, a recommendation will be made to refer to a periodontist for additional treatment options.
- Failure to complete SRP, one-month reevaluation, periodontal maintenance long term, and follow through with the referral to the periodontist may result in tooth loss, pain, and infection.

Clinical Pearls

Troubleshooting

- Difficulty detecting calculus
  - Check the radiographs and make a mental note of the sites with calculus.
  - Detect with an explorer using a feather-light grip, exploring all the surfaces of each tooth.
    - You may hear a clicking sound, or it may feel like a speed bump if a ledge or ring of calculus is encountered, or it may feel gritty if there are spicules of calculus.
    - You can dry the teeth with the air syringe to help detect supragingival calculus, which appears chalky white, unlike the shiny tooth enamel [11].
  - Use the USS or hand instruments to remove calculus.
  - After removal, check for any remaining calculus with the explorer:
    - The tooth surface should feel as smooth as possible.
    - Every individual has different degrees of roughness/smoothness of their roots.
    - Do not over-instrument healthy areas.
  - Calculus harbors plaque.

Tips

- Periodontal charting
  - Maintain the periodontal probe in the sulcus for all three readings (on the buccal or lingual surface), i.e. "walk" the probe around the tooth.
  - Round numbers up.

- To avoid confusion as to which tooth you are working on when the dental assistant is recording the findings, recommend
  o Reading the pocket depths in threes (e.g. "3-2-3").
  o Informing the assistant that you are "crossing the midline" and occasionally confirming the tooth being probed (e.g. "now probing tooth the molar").
- For good customer service, if there is a lot of BOP, provide the patient with a cup of mouthwash to swish and expectorate so that they don't leave the office tasting blood.
- When working with your dental assistant, allow the assistant to go in first to position the high volume evacuator (HVE).
- When using hand instruments your assistant can suction the debris with a surgical suction.
- Recommend patients rinse with a mouthrinse (e.g. Listerine) at the end of the procedure so that individuals do not leave the office tasting blood in their mouth. If placing topical fluoride varnish, rinse prior to the varnish.
- Be sure to warn the patient prior to nonsurgical periodontal treatment (and full-mouth debridement) of the potential for gaps between the teeth, black triangles, and tooth sensitivity following treatment. Inform the patient the gums will get healthier but one of the side effects is the gums will shrink. Tooth sensitivity should dissipate over time, but enquire if any areas are already sensitive.
  - After the cleaning the patient may complain:
    o "Now I have gaps between my teeth" (after removal of calculus which filled the diastemas).
    o Of increased interproximal space due to soft tissue recession of the papilla (black triangles).
    o Of tooth sensitivity from recession.
- Oral hygiene instructions
  - I use a model showing the progression of periodontal disease as a patient education tool along with a periodontal probe, pointing out that gingivitis is reversible but the bone loss is not and discussing factors which increase the rate of progression ("grading" in the diagnosis; see Figure 6.2).
  - I recommend a Waterpik if pocket depths are 5 mm or greater while reminding patient's they still have to floss.
- SRP sequencing: recommend two or four visits:
  - Two visits
    o First visit: UR/LR
    o Second visit: UL/LL
    o Anesthetize only one side of the face per visit to reduce the risk of soft tissue trauma.
  - Four visits
    o LR → UR → UL → LL (following the same sequence to help you stay organized).
- Be sure to sharpen the hand instruments as a dull curette can burnish the calculus onto the roots making it harder to remove.

Miscellaneous

- Tray drug delivery systems: the AAP states that there is "no strong evidence that show adjunctive use of tray delivery systems is more effective than traditional non-surgical periodontal therapy alone" [12].

Real-Life Clinical Questions Answered

Dental Students' Questions

- "My patient is just here for a prophy. In the past he's had deep cleanings. Can I get a start check?"
  - If your patient has a history of surgical or nonsurgical periodontal treatment (SRP), then he is to be on a periodontal maintenance schedule, as he is always at risk for further periodontal destruction. With periodontal maintenance you clean the entire mouth in one visit and perform site-specific SRP. This is different from a prophy.
- "The patient only needs SRP on a few teeth in the upper left. Do I bill SRP upper left 1 to 3 teeth and also a prophy?"
  - Only bill SRP one to three teeth upper left quad and clean the rest of the mouth. We cannot bill both SRP and prophy. Be sure to document the remaining dentition was cleaned.
- "If the patient has severe bone loss but no deep pockets, should I do a prophy or SRP?"
  - It sounds like the patient's diagnosis is "periodontal health on a reduced periodontium." In this case if the pockets are shallow we treat with a prophy (or airflow technology after removal of calculus), closely monitor, and inform the patient of their condition and provide the option to refer to a periodontist.
- "Why do I have to remove the stains on the teeth?"
  - For esthetic reasons if extrinsic stains, and oftentimes it's a stained thin layer of calculus, which harbors bacteria, or stained biofilm.
- "How do I know if I should put the patient on a three-, four-, or six-month periodontal maintenance schedule?"
  - See Section Assignment of Periodontal Maintenance Recall Schedule.
- "The patient has an abscess but the tooth tests as vital. What could this be?"
  - See Section What is a Periodontal Abscess?

Patients' Questions

- "What is periodontal disease?"
  - See Section What is Periodontal Disease?
- "I was never told by my last dentist that I have gum disease. Why didn't he tell me?"
  - "I can't tell you precisely how long you have had the gum disease. What I can tell you is what I see today. Gum disease progresses at different rates in different people – and at different rates in the same person at different stages in life" [14].
- "I brush and floss, I don't smoke, and I don't have diabetes so why do I have loose teeth?"
  - There are many risk factors including inherited or genetic susceptibility, health history, and medications [4].
- "I don't smoke cigarettes, I just smoke pot which is natural. That shouldn't affect my teeth, right?"
  - See Chapter 1, *Marijuana*.
- "Is periodontal disease contagious if I kiss someone?"
  - Periodontal disease is an inflammatory host response to bacteria under the gums. The disease is not contagious; however, the bacteria can be spread through saliva [15].
- "I heard your oral health is related to the rest of your body. Is that true?"
  - See Section The Periodontal–Systemic Connection.
- "Will a deep cleaning help?"
  - The deep cleaning in combination with consistent good home care will help.

- The goal is to alter or eliminate the periodontal pathogens and reduce inflammation, improving periodontal health and decreasing the likelihood of disease progression. What can be expected as a successful outcome, combined with good home care, is decreased bleeding of the gums, reduction of inflamed gums, and gain in clinical attachment (Table 6.5). The healing results in the formation of a long junctional epithelium [3].

Table 6.5 Healing results after SRP.

Initial pocket depths (mm)	Pocket depth reduction (mm)	Clinical attachment level (mm)
1–3	0.03	0.34 (loss)
4–6	1.29	0.55 (gain)
7+	2.16	1.19 (gain)

- "What do you think about lasers for gum disease?"
  - According to the ADA at this time expert opinion is against recommending the use of photodynamic therapy with a diode laser for nonsurgical use as an adjunct to scaling and root planing because of the uncertainty over the clinical benefits and the evidence is lacking [16]. However, a recent systematic review found lasers have an adjunctive role in initial nonsurgical periodontal therapy [17].
- "What can I do to prevent more bone loss?"
  - The best way to prevent further bone loss is to brush your teeth after every meal, and floss and brush before going to sleep. Visit your dentist or periodontist at least twice a year [15]. If you smoke, quit; if you are diabetic, work with your medical provider to lower your blood sugar levels.
- "Doc, how long will my teeth last?"
  - See Section Prognosis.

Patients' Demands

- "I only want a regular cleaning."
  - "Due to your periodontal disease I am recommending (SRP or periodontal maintenance) in order to remove the bacteria from the roots of your teeth to help prevent further destruction, infection, pain, bone loss, loosening of teeth and eventual loss of teeth."
    - *If patient still refuses and only wants a prophy*: provide a periodontal treatment refusal form, which discusses recommended treatment, benefits of treatment, and the risk of no treatment, and have the patient sign it and retain in the records. The dentist is still legally and ethically liable for practicing within the standards of care and a patient cannot consent to substandard care. Recommend contacting your dental liability insurance company and/or consult with an attorney to discuss the medicolegal risk of "supervised neglect."
    - *If the patient is unable to afford treatment*: refer patient to a local community health clinic for treatment and document.
    - *If the patient refuses referral to a periodontist*: discuss the limitations of nonsurgical periodontal treatment (SRP and periodontal maintenance). Studies show the deeper the pockets, the less effective is nonsurgical periodontal treatment. Recommend contacting your dental liability insurance company and/or consult with an attorney to discuss medicolegal risk of "supervised neglect."

Periodontics

- "I need this form signed as clearance to begin orthodontic treatment."
  – If signs of periodontal disease (deep pockets, mobilities, furcations, RBL, recession, etc.) inform the patient.
    o "Due to your periodontal condition I will have to refer you to a periodontist to further evaluate the status of your gums and jawbones. I will not be able to sign off on your clearance for orthodontic treatment as the condition could worsen with braces causing loosening of teeth. A periodontist is better equipped to evaluate your condition."

References

1 Centers for Disease Control and Prevention (2013). Periodontal disease. http://www.cdc.gov/oralhealth/conditions/periodontal-disease.html#Risk (accessed 25 March 2020).

2 American Academy of Periodontology (2020). Comprehensive periodontal evaluation (CPE). http://www.perio.org/consumer/perio-evaluation.htm (accessed 25 March 2020).

3 Rose, L.F. and Mealy, B.L. (2004). *Periodontics: Medicine, Surgery, and Implants*. St. Louis, MO: Elsevier Mosby.

4 American Academy of Periodontology (2020). Periodontal Disease Fact Sheet. http://www.perio.org/newsroom/periodontal-disease-fact-sheet (accessed 3/27/2020.)

5 American Academy of Periodontology (2018). Classification of periodontal and peri-implant diseases and conditions. http://www.perio.org/sites/default/files/files/Classification%20at%20a%20glance.pdf (accessed 28 March 2020).

6 American Academy of Periodontology (2017). Staging and grading periodontitis. https://www.perio.org/sites/default/files/files/Staging%20and%20Grading%20Periodontitis.pdf (accessed 25 April 2021).

7 Glickman, I. (1972). *Clinical Periodontology: Prevention, Diagnosis, and Treatment of Periodontal Disease in the Practice of General Dentistry*, 4e, 242–245. Philadelphia, PA: Saunders.

8 Miller, S.C. (1938). *Textbook of Periodontia*, 1e. Philadelphia: Blakiston.

9 Glick, M. (2019). *The Oral–Systemic Health Connection. A Guide to Patient Care*, 2e. Chicago: Quintessence Publishing.

10 White, S.C. and Pharoah, M.J. (2008). *Oral Radiology: Principles and Interpretation*, 6e. St. Louis, MO: Mosby Elsevier.

11 Gehrig, J., Sroda, R., and Saccuzzo, D. (2019). *Fundamentals of Periodontal Instrumentation and Advanced Root Instrumentation*, 8e. Burlington, MA: Jones & Bartlett Learning.

12 American Academy of Periodontology (2020). Non-surgical periodontal treatment. http://www.perio.org/consumer/non-surgical-periodontal-treatment (accessed 28 March 2020).

13 Kwok, V. and Caton, J.G. (2007). Commentary: prognosis revisited: a system for assigning periodontal prognosis. *J. Periodontol.* 78 (11): 2063–2071.

14 Wright, R. *Tough Questions, Great Answers. Responding to Patient Concerns about Today's Dentistry*. Chicago: Quintessence Publishing.

15 American Academy of Periodontology (2020). Ask a periodontist. http://www.perio.org/?q=faq-page#n224 (accessed 27 March 2020).

16 Smiley, C.J., Tracy, S.L., Abt, E. et al. (2015). Evidence-based clinical practice guideline on the nonsurgical treatment of chronic periodontitis by means of scaling and root planing with or without adjuncts. *J. Am. Dent. Assoc.* 146 (7): 525–535.

17 Coluzzi, D., Anagnostaki, E., Mylona, V. et al. (2020). Do lasers have an adjunctive role in initial non-surgical periodontal therapy? A systematic review. *Dent. J. (Basel)* 8 (3): 93. https://doi.org/10.3390/dj8030093.

7

Operative Dentistry

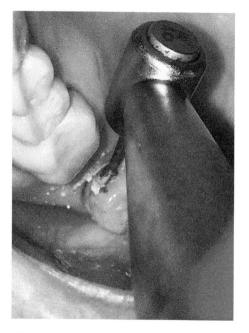

Figure 7.1 Removing decay with the slow-speed round bur until no more debris (which resemble eraser crumbs) are visible and the bur rattles off the hard healthy tooth structure.

Chapter Outline

- Real-Life Clinical Questions
- Relevance
- Clinical and Radiographic Exam
- Treatment Planning
- Informed Consent
- Armamentarium
- Procedural Steps
  - Cavity Preparation: External and Internal Outline Forms
  - Cavity Preparation: Principles and Tips

Clinical Dentistry Daily Reference Guide, First Edition. William A. Jacobson.
© 2022 John Wiley & Sons, Inc. Published 2022 by John Wiley & Sons, Inc.

Real-Life Clinical Questions

Dental Students' Questions and Comment

- "How can you tell there is still decay in the cavity prep?"
- "Where should the dots go on the composite when checking occlusion? Should there not be any dots on the filling?"
- "How would I know if I had a pulpal exposure? And what do I do?"
- "I didn't floss after because it was just an occlusal composite."
- "Sandwich technique?"
- "How do I know if we should do a large filling or a crown?"
- "What is the difference between a base and a liner?"

Dental Assistants' Questions

- "How long do I light cure this for?"
- "What instrument do you need doc?"

Patients' Concerns, Requests, Questions, and Comment

- "Is that a UV light?"
- "If you hit the nerve and place a protective layer, what is the chance I will need to get a root canal treatment?"
- "I'm here because I just had a filling and the tooth is hurting me."
- "I don't want my daughter to have any mercury fillings, so you need to use something else."
- "I want all these mercury fillings removed."
- "Can you make the water warm instead of cold?"
- "I just want caps on these teeth not fillings."
- "Why do I have so many cavities? I don't eat sweets and I drink diet soda."
- "Can I eat after this filling?"
- "Once my cavity is filled, I won't have to brush that tooth anymore?"
- "Does this have fluoride? Is this gluten free?"
- "Can you tell from the X-ray if I'm going to need a root canal?"
- "How long will a composite filling last me?"
- "Should I get veneers or composites to close these gaps?"
- "Will these fillings whiten once I bleach my teeth?"
- "If you told me I'd be sore I wouldn't have come in."

Relevance

"Operative dentistry is the area of general dentistry concerned with the treatment of diseases and/ or defects of the hard tissues of teeth, specifically the restoration of form, function and aesthetics of those hard tissues" [1]. Operative dentistry is a huge part of general dentistry and this chapter addresses basic principles along with providing numerous clinical pearls.

Clinical and Radiographic Exam

- Clinical exam
  - Evaluate *every* surface of *every* tooth: visual, tactile, and auditory assessment.
  - Check the condition of every existing restoration (i.e. crowns, amalgams, composites, etc.) with the tip of the explorer.
- Radiographic exam
  - Determine the type and number of radiographs necessary and interpret the findings (see Chapter 3).
  - For operative treatment, the PA should be current (taken within one year) to rule out any peri-apical pathosis.
- The author's sequence:
  - Review CC and pain level.
  - Review health history (see Chapter 1).
  - Conduct an EOE, IOE, and OCS and check occlusion (see Chapter 2).
  - Determine type and number of radiographs necessary (see Chapter 3).
  - Interpret and document all the radiographic findings on the odontogram (see Chapter 3).
  - Inform the patient "I will conduct the clinical exam. Some findings are only visible radiographically while other findings are only visible clinically, so we have to combine the two to come up with a treatment plan."
  - Confirm the radiographic findings and add additional clinical findings to the odontogram.
  - Take intraoral photos to document any clinical findings not visible radiographically (e.g. occlusal decay, crown open margin) in order to:
    - ○ Prevent being accused of overtreating by the dental insurance company if audited.
    - ○ Educate the patient of their conditions.
    - ○ Justify the proposed treatment plan when discussing with the patient, which helps develop trust.
  - If any cavity appears deep:
    - ○ Conduct endodontic diagnostic testing for pulpal and periapical diagnosis (see Chapter 8).
    - ○ Inform the patient the decay is always deeper than it appears radiographically. Warn the patient of possible outcomes:
      - ■ Large restoration.
      - ■ Possible need for a crown later on.
      - ■ Need for RCT, crown lengthening, buildup or a post and core, and a crown.
      - ■ Need for extraction and tooth replacement: discuss tooth replacement options (see Chapter 4).
  - Provide a comprehensive periodontal examination, as this can deem a tooth nonrestorable no matter how small the cavity is (see Chapter 6).
  - Combine all the findings and present the treatment plan (see Chapter 4).

Operative Dentistry

Treatment Planning

Table 7.1 Treatment planning phases related to operative dentistry.

Treatment phase	Description (may or may not apply)
Emergency phase	• NA
Data gathering phase	• Comprehensive oral evaluation • Medical history: medical consultation • EOE, IOE, and OCS • Full-mouth debridement (if necessary for diagnosing) • Radiographs and interpretation • Clinical findings • Periodontal evaluation • Intraoral photographs • Endodontic diagnostic testing • Caries and periodontal risk assessment • Parafunction and/or habits • Patient expectations • Referrals to specialists • Treatment plan discussion

Stabilization phase (to control disease)	• Caries control (bleaching if desired prior)
	  – Silver diamine fluoride
	  – Symptomatic teeth > larger cavities > smaller cavities
	• Replacement of defective restorations

Definitive phase	• NA
Maintenance phase	• Annual exam/periodic oral evaluation including reevaluation of "monitors" (e.g. incipient caries)

Informed Consent

- Discuss (and document) with the patient the risks, benefits and alternatives of treatment, including the risks of no treatment.
- As part of the verbal informed consent let the patient know the following.
  - For shallow cavities: tooth sensitivity after dental treatment is to be expected and should decrease over time. If the sensitivity remains or increases, the tooth may require further treatment (e.g. RCT and crown or extraction).
  - For deep cavities: the cavity appears deep so the plan is to remove the decay and evaluate how much tooth structure is remaining. The plan is to place a restoration; however, the tooth may require more treatment such as RCT, crown lengthening, buildup (or post and core) and a crown, or extraction. Additional treatment involves additional fees which may not be covered by the patient's insurance.

Armamentarium

- **Composite**
  - Resin composites contain four structural components: a polymer matrix, filler particles, a coupling agent, and an initiator system [2].
  - Indications: restorative dentistry, esthetic cases, minimally invasive dentistry.
  - Composite disadvantage: cost, isolation, leaking open margins, longevity, high caries risk, sensitivity, wear.
  - Packable composite: indicated for stress-bearing restorations.
  - Flowable composite: indicated for small low stress-bearing restorations (not as much filler and wear resistance as packable), cervical lesions, pediatric restoration, sealant substitute, age crack on anterior, repair defective margin.
- **Etch**: typically 35–37% phosphoric acid. Composed of acidic molecules that alter or remove the smear layer and demineralize the enamel and dentin and prepare it for bonding [2].
- **Prime**: helps make the hydrophilic dentin hydrophobic to accept the hydrophobic bonding agent [2].
- **Bond**: also known as bonding resin or adhesive resin. Becomes incorporated with the primed dentin and once cured forms the structural support of the bonded interface between the tooth and the restoration [2].
- **Amalgam ("silver fillings")**
  - Amalgam is an alloy of mercury with another metal or metals [3].
  - High-copper amalgams contain 12–30% copper and 40% silver by weight [4].
  - Indications: moisture contamination/hard to isolate areas, high caries risk, nonesthetic zone, bruxer (wears like enamel).
  - Contraindications: if allergic or sensitive to any metals in amalgam (e.g. silver, tin, copper) or mercury [5].
  - Disadvantage: esthetics, cannot polish for 24 hours.
  - Controversy: due to mercury content of amalgam.
    - The ADA supports amalgam as safe, affordable, and durable [6].
    - The FDA in "clinical studies in adults and children ages 6 and above have found no link between dental amalgam fillings and health problems" [5].
    - The World Health Organization (WHO) consensus statement states amalgam is considered safe, but in rare instances causes local side effects or allergic reaction. No evidence has been shown of adverse health effects due to mercury released from placement and removal of amalgam. No evidence supporting removal of amalgam relieved general symptoms. Patients reporting symptoms should be referred to "other health care professionals for diagnosis and treatment if symptoms persist" [7].
- **Glass ionomer (GI)**
  - GI: chemically bound to tooth structure (dentin) and releases fluoride [2].
  - Resin-modified glass ionomer (RMGI): contains elements of conventional GIs and light-cured resins but most similar to conventional GIs. They are fluoride releasing and are not indicated for use in occlusal load-bearing areas in permanent teeth [2].
  - GI/RMGI chemically bonds to dentin, not enamel [2].
    - Do not dry GI/RMGI.
    - Requires use of cavity conditioner.

Operative Dentistry

- ○ Advantages: moisture contamination, fluoride releasing.
- ○ Disadvantages: not as strong, not for class I/II/IV on permanent teeth.
- – Examples of products
  - ○ GC Cavity Conditioner: 20% polyacrylic conditioner removes smear layer and conditions the tooth for optimal chemical adhesion. Apply for 10 seconds, rinse with water, and dry without desiccating. Apply GI [8].
  - ○ Fuji II LC: light cured (LC) RMGI. Must layer and light cure if >2 mm [9].
  - ○ Fuji IX: self-cured GI.
  - ○ Fuji Triage: as sealant for partially erupted molars, floor of endo access after obturation, stepwise cavity excavation.
  - ○ Fuji Lining LC: liner.
- **Calcium hydroxide** (e.g. Dycal): acts as a mechanical barrier for a pinpoint exposure.
  - – Stimulates reparative dentin formation with direct pulpal contact [10].
  - – Has antimicrobial activity as a result of its alkaline pH [11].
- **MTA** (mineral trioxide aggregate)
  - – Indications: include pulp capping, pulpotomies, treatment of root perforations.
  - – In one study, dentinal bridges were observed in 100% of MTA cases and only 60% of calcium hydroxide cases [12].

Procedural Steps

Cavity Preparation: External and Internal Outline Forms

Class II Cavity Prep for Amalgam or Composite (Conventional Design) (Figure 7.2)

For composite it is permissible to have enamel on the pulpal floor. Note for amalgam preparations the proximal walls converge occlusally (see Figures 7.3 and 7.4).

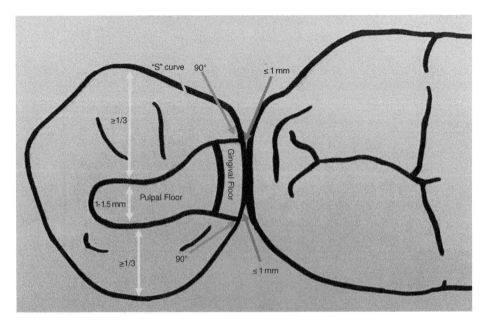

Figure 7.2 An occlusal view of an ideal Class II prep with labels.

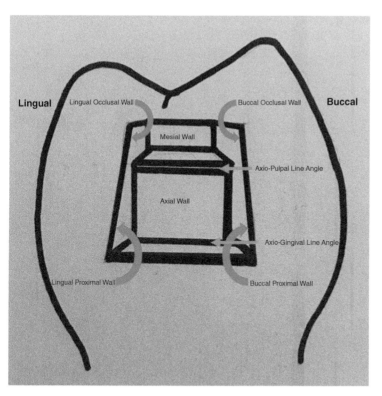

Figure 7.3   An interproximal view of an ideal Class II prep with labels.

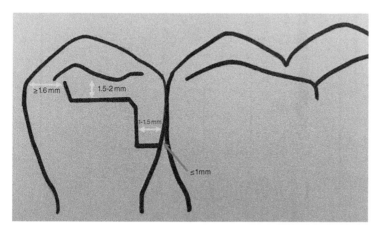

Figure 7.4   A lingual view of an ideal Class II prep with labels.

Class III Cavity Prep for Composite.

Determine if facial or lingual access is required based on the location of decay in order to keep an intact lingual or facial wall. Note the incisal wall is not broken (the incisal wall is located at the midpoint of the proximal contact). Note convex axial wall parallel to tooth surface. Minimal lingual (or facial, depending on access) extension of ≤0.05 mm so contact broken. Stay within the marginal ridge (MR). See Figures 7.5 and 7.6.

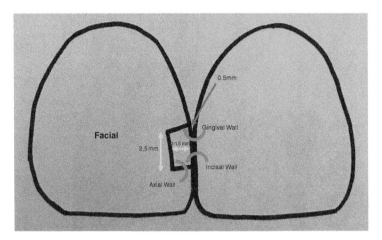

Figure 7.5 Facial view of an ideal Class III prep with labels.

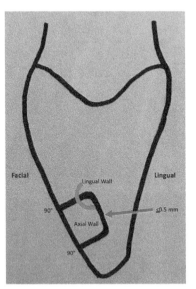

Figure 7.6 Interproximal view of an ideal Class III prep with labels.

Class IV Prep

The secondary bevel on a Class IV prep (Figure 7.7) is shaped like a sunburst (Figure 7.8).

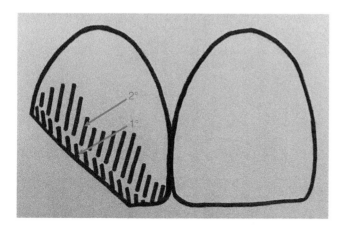

Figure 7.7   Facial view of an ideal Class IV prep with labels.

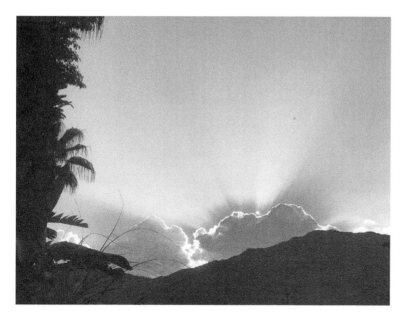

Figure 7.8   Sunburst.

Class V prep for Composite and Amalgam (Figures 7.9 and 7.10)

Note that the pulpal wall is convex and parallel to the tooth surface. The composite prep is divergent and beveled, whereas the amalgam prep has retention groves.

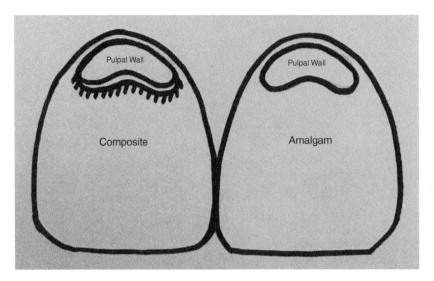

Figure 7.9 Facial view of an ideal Class V prep with labels.

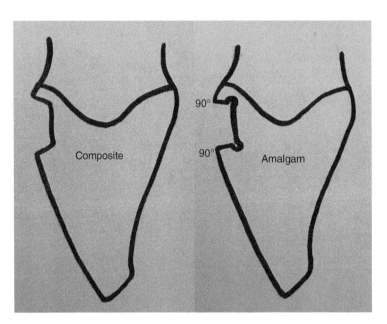

Figure 7.10 Interproximal view of an ideal Class V prep with labels.

Creating a Trough

Create a trough along the incisal edge to remove the decay while preserving tooth structure around the trough. Bevel the enamel along the incisal edge (Figure 7.11).

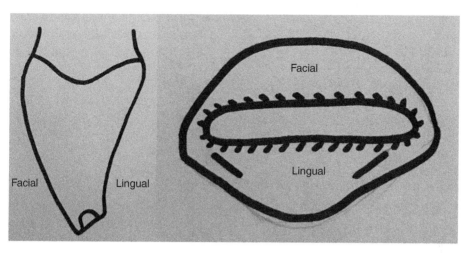

Figure 7.11   Creating a trough.

Cavity Preparation: Principles and Tips

Amalgam Cavity Preparation
- Requires mechanical retention: the cavity prep requires converging walls. One can add retention grooves.

Composite Cavity Preparation
- Both mechanical and chemical retention:
  - Composite bonds to enamel.
  - Bevel enamel for improved retention.

- Converging walls are not required: the walls can be parallel or diverging.
- A goal of "adhesive dentistry" is to remove the decay and conserve as much tooth structure as possible. It is not necessary to connect the decay in a pit to the decay on another part of the tooth.

Removing Caries
- First double check the radiograph and *all surfaces* of the tooth clinically to prevent:
  - treating the wrong tooth
  - overtreating (when caries is limited to enamel)
  - treating a part of the tooth and missing another surface which was also decayed.
- Remove the gross decay with the high-speed bur.
- If interproximal caries (i.e. Class II, III):
  - Protect the adjacent tooth from being nicked.
    - ○ Use a proximal protector (e.g. FenderWedge, Wedgeguard) (Figure 7.12). Caution: it is still possible to drill into the adjacent tooth.
    - ○ Or can pre-wedge with a wooden wedge (also prevents nicking the papilla).
    - ○ Or can leave a shell of enamel and remove with hand instruments (e.g. hatchet, hoe) (Figure 7.13).
      - ■ One study determined that 40–60% of Class II preps resulted in iatrogenic damage of the adjacent tooth [13], while another study resulted in 100% damage of the adjacent tooth [14].

- ▪ If you cut the adjacent tooth, there is an increased risk of decay due to loss of the outer layer of enamel. A plaque trap can form, and even if there is no decay the damage may be misdiagnosed on a BW as decay by another provider and prepped later on, removing healthy tooth structure.
- Remove the remaining decay with the slow-speed round bur (Figure 7.1).
  - Use the largest sharp round bur that fits. If the bur is too small, it can perforate.
  - Make sure the handpiece is set to F (i.e. forward) not R (i.e. reverse) which would burnish the decay instead of remove it.
  - Avoid hand instruments near the pulpal wall (e.g. spoon excavator) as pressure can lead to pulpal exposure [11].
  - One can use caries-indicating dye to verify that all caries has been removed prior to restoring.
- Check all surfaces of the cavity prep for any remaining decay prior to restoring.
- *Class III*:
  - Determine if facial or lingual access is needed.
  - Place the bur perpendicular to tooth structure and begin to prep.

- *Class IV*:
  - Check occlusion prior to restoring to determine the interincisal space to determine length of tooth.
  - Have patient bite edge-to-edge ("like a bulldog" or "as if biting your nails").
  - Select the shade: prior to prepping the tooth, place a small amount of packable composite on the tooth and light cure to check shade (no etching/bonding) as a mock-up. Obtain the patient's verbal approval of the shade; once checked, remove by flicking off the composite with the explorer.
  - Long-term precautions:
    - ○ Inform the patient that restoration may have to be replaced multiple times over a lifetime.
    - ○ If there are multiple large class IV buildups of teeth, an occlusal guard may be required.
    - ○ Nail biting and other chewing habits can compromise the restoration over the long term.
    - ○ Warn the patient that the restoration can, and probably will, become stained over time.
  - Prep design: the primary bevel is short and hides the fracture at 45°; the secondary bevel is shallow and scalloped at 60° for esthetic blending and retention. Is the fractured piece available to bond to tooth? See Chapter 10.
- *Class V*:
  - If caries, restore. Warn patient that it is not possible to determine depth of caries using radiography because it produces a two-dimensional image. Tooth may require additional treatment (e.g. RCT, crown lengthening) or may not be restorable.
  - If abfraction:
    - ○ If the patient has esthetic concerns, restore.
    - ○ If there is sensitivity, try a conservative treatment first (e.g. desensitizer, OTC desensitizing toothpaste, topical fluoride). If inadequate relief, restore.
    - ○ If there is a plaque trap, restore.
    - ○ If compromised tooth structure is present, restore.
    - ○ If preventing further abrasion, restore and recommend soft toothbrush.
    - ○ Repair may not be retentive if the patient is clenching/grinding or occlusion is not treated.
    - ○ Recommend beveling the enamel with a diamond bur.

Figure 7.12   One method of protecting the adjacent tooth when prepping.

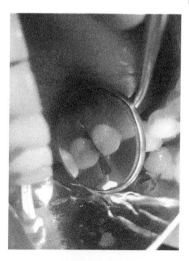

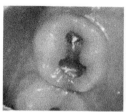 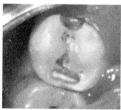 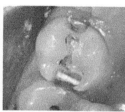 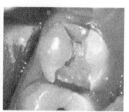

Figure 7.13   Another method of protecting the adjacent tooth when prepping.

Cavity Restoration: Principles and Tips

General Restoration Principles

- Class II/III:
  - After placing the matrix and wedge, check for a good seal between the matrix band and the tooth (i.e. no gap for the tip of an explorer to fit into to prevent overhang). Make sure there is no saliva seepage and rinse any blood and debris before restoring.
  - After restoring, if a wooden wedge was used verify that the tip did not break and become dislodged in the gingiva.
  - Check contact with floss that shreds easily (e.g. Floss Singles). Do not use dental tape, which is too forgiving and never shreds and can therefore mask a rough or sharp contact or an overhang. This will give the patient a false impression that the contour is smooth, who then returns home and complains of difficulty flossing.
- Always floss after every restoration to remove excess bonding agent. Also, with the explorer check the sulcus for excess bonding agent. Figure 7.14 shows #20 O composite being flossed to remove the bonding agent trapped interproximally.

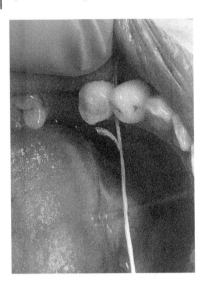

Figure 7.14 Always floss after placing a restoration to remove excess bonding agent.

- Be sure to adjust and polish the margins until they become undetectable to prevent a plaque (and stain) trap (Figure 7.15).

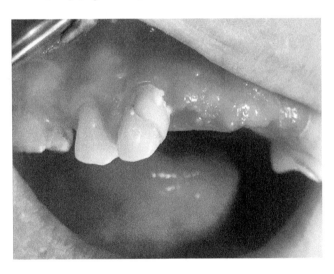

Figure 7.15 A composite restoration without flush margins has become a stained plaque trap.

Composite Restorations

- Disinfect the cavity prep. Three disinfectants have been recommended in various continuing education courses: chlorhexidine, Gluma, and isopropyl alcohol.
- In order to ensure that excess composite beyond the cavosurface bonds to the enamel:
  - Selectively etch the enamel beyond the cavosurface, rinse, and dry.
  - Place self-etching adhesive in the cavity prep and beyond the cavosurface. Scrub and dry until no longer moving but shiny (following the manufacturer's guidelines). Verify that the bonding agent is adequately mixed before applying (i.e. a homogeneous consistency).

- Restore:
  - Dispense flowable composite into the deepest portions of the prep to fill all the nooks and crannies.
  - Tease out the bubbles with the perio probe and then light cure.
  - Dispense packable composite:
    - Lightly tap into place (don't condense as with amalgam).
    - Light cure every 2-mm layer.
  - Check if the margins are detectable. If detectable, adjust with the finishing bur until undetectable. Can use the tip of the flame bur for tactile sensation.
- Check occlusion and adjust as needed (before polishing). Ask the patient "Does the bite feel even? Can you feel the teeth contacting normally on the side that isn't numb?" Adjust as needed.
- Polish. Ask the patient "Does the filling feel smooth? Any rough or sharp spots?" Polish as needed. See Section Postoperative Instructions.
- *Class II*:
  - Place the sectional matrix, ring, and wedge (or Tofflemire if no adjacent tooth). Wedge placed from the lingual (larger embrasure).
  - Rinse the cavity prep with water and dry.
  - Etch and bond following manufacturer's instructions.
  - Four options to restore:
  1) Place packable composite and create wall with the ball burnisher or the microbrush, light cure and pack composite using layering technique.
  2) Place flowable composite on the gingival floor and along the cavosurface and light cure followed by layers of packable composite.
  3) Place packable composite in layering technique.
  4) Bulk fill composite material (following manufacturer's instructions).
  - Remove the ring and bend the matrix against the adjacent tooth.
  - Light cure the B and L (prior to removing wedge and matrix to prevent blood from contaminating the uncured composite).
  - Check for contact with floss. Floss should "snap" and not shred or snag/catch.
- *Class III*:
  - Place a curved Mylar strip and wooden wedge. The wedge should be snug enough to separate the teeth and below the cavosurface of the gingival wall and inserted from the lingual (larger embrasure).
  - Restore:
    - by creating small balls of packable composite; or
    - by creating a proximal wall first; or
    - with flowable composite; or
    - flowable composite along the cavosurface, then light cured, followed by packable composite.
  - If the cavity prep is a "tunnel" place the Mylar strip and apply pressure with one's finger to support the matrix. Place the first layer, light cure, remove finger and use this to lightly pack more layers of composite. If too much pressure is applied, the composite may be dislodged.
  - Create properly shaped MR.
- *Class IV*:
  - Creating the lingual wall (Figure 7.16).

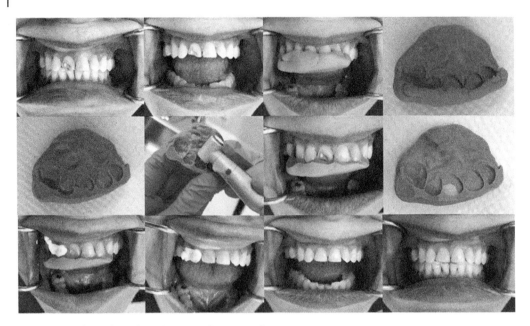

Figure 7.16 Steps for a Class IV composite restoration.

- o Mix putty matrix and place on the lingual to create a lingual index. Once the putty is set, remove. With a high-speed bur trim the desired shape of the tooth. Then wrap Teflon adjacent to the tooth. Etch/bond following manufacturer's instructions. Place composite on the lingual index, seat the matrix, lightly tap against the tooth, light cure, remove lingual index, and now there is a lingual wall to which layers of composite can be added.
  - ■ Is the fractured piece available to use for the lingual index? Hold in place with packable composite on facial and light cure, obtain a putty matrix of lingual, slice putty as lingual index (template).
  - ■ Is the fractured piece available to re-attach? See Chapter 10 Real-Life Questions, Concerns, and Demands Answered.
  - o Another approach involves placing a Mylar strip and a wooden wedge beneath the contact. Etch/bond (following the manufacturer's instructions). Hold the Mylar strip with finger pressure on the lingual as packable composite is dispensed to build a lingual wall. Light cure. Continue to add layers of composite.
  - o To create an esthetic restoration, use enamel and dentin shades for layering.
- • *Class V:*
  - – Pack a dry cord. Use lidocaine plus 1:100 000 epinephrine for hemostasis.
  - – If the cavity prep is entirely on a root surface, restore with RMGI.
    - o Use cavity conditioner (following manufacturer's instructions).
    - o Place RMGI (start at the most apical portion to avoid creating a void). If self-curing wait for the materials to set.
    - o Adjust with burs until the sulcus is free of restorative material and margins are not detectable.
    - o Do not dry the RMGI.
      - ■ Clinical pearl: After placing the RMGI/GI, insert the periodontal probe into the sulcus in the middle of the tooth and drag it to one side of the tooth to remove the excess, then place the probe in the center and drag to the other side to remove the excess (like the action of windshield wipers) (Figure 7.17).

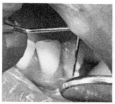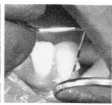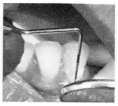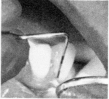

Figure 7.17 A clinical pearl for shaping and removing excess material when restoring a Class V with RMGI/GI.

- If a portion of the cavity prep is on the root surface and a portion is on enamel.
  - Restore the root surface first:
    - Cavity conditioner.
    - RMGI.
  - Restore the portion on the enamel:
    - Etch and bond the enamel (following the manufacturer's instructions).
    - Place composite.
  - Adjust with burs until the sulcus is free of restorative material and margins are not detectable.
  - Do not dry the RMGI.
- If the entire cavity prep is surrounded by enamel restore with composite.

Amalgam Restorations
- Mix the amalgam in the amalgamator.
  - If undermixed: crumbly consistency.
  - If overmixed: soupy consistency.

- Quickly condense small amounts of amalgam, reaching the deepest portion first.
- Overpack the cavity prep by ≥1 mm.
- Burnish the anatomy (football burnisher, ball burnisher, acorn burnisher).
- Carve to remove excess amalgam: pressure should be on tooth not amalgam. Carvers rest half on enamel, half on amalgam, with the tip at the central groove, not on the opposing incline plane.
- Wipe with wet or dry cotton roll.
- To check occlusion, ask patient "Bring your teeth together lightly. Don't bite hard."
- Adjust occlusion as needed with the spoon or Cleoid-Discoid carver.
- Check if the margins are detectable; if detectable, carve until undetectable.
- Wait 24 hours to polish with a brownie then a greenie; can also adjust with football finishing bur.
- See Section Postoperative Instructions.
- *Class II*:
  - Caution: amalgam may show in the esthetic zone (e.g. #12 MO).
  - Place the Tofflemire matrix band (from the buccal) and wedge (from lingual, larger embrasure).
  - Burnish the matrix band below the MR against the adjacent tooth to establish contact while maintaining tight seal of box.
  - Condense layers of amalgam into the gingival floor before pulpal floor.
  - Condense, burnish, carve.
  - Remove the wedge, followed by the Tofflemire matrix once the amalgam is set by wrapping it against the adjacent tooth and sliding it out in the buccal or lingual direction. If using wooden wedges, verify that no tips break and remain in the gingiva.
  - Check contact by flossing apically and pulling out the side.

– When flossing, slide apically and up toward the contact, hugging the tooth to remove excess amalgam (don't slide through contact which may break the contact).
– Hug the tooth with carver from cervical occlusally to remove any overhangs.
– To check occlusion, ask patient "Bring your teeth together lightly. Don't bite hard."

Other Restorative Scenarios

Sandwich Techniques

GI is used as an intermediate layer between the dentin and resin composite (e.g. Class II and V).

Open Sandwich Technique

- With this technique the GI is at the gingival margin of the cavity preparation and is exposed.
- Indications: when there is no remaining enamel at the most apical portion of the cavity preparation (e.g. subgingival Class II and V).
- Steps: cavity conditioner step, place GI or RMGI on dentin, etch the enamel, bond the enamel and dentin, and place composite.

Closed Sandwich Technique

- With this technique the GI is completely covered by the resin composite.
- Indications:
  - Class V: when there is no enamel to bond to and the shade of GI does not match the tooth. GI or RMGI can be placed with a layer of composite covering it.
  - Deep extensive Class I: RMGI can be placed for the bulk of the restoration with composite on the top layer bonded to enamel; this is more wear resistant.
- Steps: cavity conditioner step, place GI or RMGI on dentin, etch the enamel, bond the enamel and dentin, and place composite.

Indirect Pulp Capping and Stepwise Excavation

- Indications (all conditions must be present): permanent teeth with immature apices, deep carious lesions considered likely to result in pulp exposure during excavation, no history of subjective pretreatment symptoms, pretreatment radiographs should exclude periradicular pathosis, and patient fully informed that endodontic treatment may be indicated in the future [15].
- First visit: "caries is excavated leaving affected dentin adjacent to the pulp. Calcium hydroxide or other biologically compatible material is placed over the dentin followed by a base, and the tooth is soundly restored" [15].
- Second visit, six to eight months later: "the restorative material and residual caries mass is removed, and the tooth is restored" [15].
- Recommend using Fuji Triage as it is colored pink and alerts dentist, hygienist, or dentist at other office that the final caries excavation and restoration has not yet been completed.

Indirect Pulp Cap

- "Procedure in which the nearly exposed pulp is covered with a protective dressing to protect the pulp from additional injury and to promote healing and repair via formation of secondary dentin. This code is not to be used for bases or liners when all caries has been removed" [16].
- The protective material could be MTA, or GI, in close proximity to the pulp (e.g. the axial wall and/or pulpal floor).

- Do not extend the material to the cavosurface.
- Etch/bond following manufacturer's guidelines and restore with composite.
- See Section Postoperative Instructions.

Direct Pulp Cap

- "Procedure in which the exposed pulp is covered with a dressing or cement that protects the pulp and promotes healing and repair" [16].
- If caries appears deep and there is potential for mechanical pulpal exposure:
  - Endo test prior to anesthetizing for preoperative diagnosis.
  - Prep the tooth with rubber dam isolation.
  - If pulpal exposure, and the tooth is vital, blood will be seen. If unsure, place cotton pellet into the cavity prep, remove and observe for presence of blood (check that blood is not from the gingiva).
  - Disinfect the cavity prep by swabbing the dentin with a cotton pellet dampened in sodium hypochlorite.
  - Irrigate the cavity prep with sterile saline (not with the water from the unit as it is not sterile).
  - Dry.
  - Place direct pulp capping material. Various materials are available, such as calcium hydroxide (e.g. Dycal), bioceramics such as MTA and Endosequence BC RRM-Fast Set Putty. A study found that MTA has a higher success rate with less pulpal inflammatory response and more predictable hard dentin bridge formation than calcium hydroxide [17].
  - Cavity conditioner.
  - Cover direct pulp capping material with a GI in order to tack the pulp capping material into place.
  - Etch/bond following manufacturer's instructions.
  - Restore with composite.
  - See Section Postoperative Instructions.

Class II/III with Large Gingival Embrasures

- Inform the patient that due to bone loss/recession (clinical attachment loss) this will continue to be a food trap. If the patient complains of continued food trapping, provide samples or recommend purchase of interdental brushes.
- Consider stacking wedges in the same direction, or opposite directions, or wrapping a wedge in Teflon in order for the wedge to fit snugly between the teeth.

Deep Decay and Questionable Prognosis

- Inform the patient that the plan is to "remove decay and reevaluate" before deciding to extract the tooth, as extraction is irreversible. The patient may understand language such as "It's 50/50 whether or not the tooth can be saved."
- Warn patient tooth may require RCT/crown lengthening/buildup/post and core/crown or extraction.
- Remove decay and asses the tooth's restorability (see Figure 11.4): remaining tooth structure, ferrule, crown/root ratio, mobility, proximity to pulp.

Operative Dentistry

Class II Composite with an Anatomic Concavity on the Proximal Surface

- Tooth anatomy may be concave at the neck of the tooth.
- Figure 7.18 shows a well-sealed, but problematic, matrix placement against the concavity of the tooth with multiple stacked wedges. This leads to a poorly contoured tooth with an open proximal contact, which will lead to food impaction.
- Consider deep margin elevation technique.

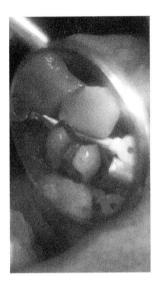

Figure 7.18 Challenges faced with restoring a Class II on a tooth with a concavity (a sealed margin at the expense of an open proximal contact). This is not recommended.

Deep Margin Elevation for Subgingival Class II Composite

- If deep subgingival caries, use an endodontic bur to access and remove the deep decay. If regular burs are used, the head of the handpiece may hit the tooth preventing the bur from reaching the decay.
- For procedure, see Figure 7.19.

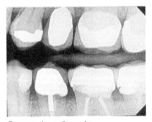

Preoperative radiograph:
#21 DO with D subgingival recurrent
decay and an open margin

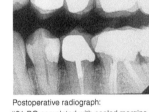

Postoperative radiograph:
#21 DO completed with sealed margins

Margin elevation
matrix band

Place the band
subgingivally

Confirm band
placement

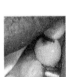

Fuji II to
equigingival height
keeping the contact
"broken"

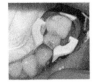

V3 Sectional
Matrix System
placed for
composite

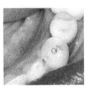

Checked
occlusion and
contours,
adjusted, and
polished

Figure 7.19 The deep margin elevation technique used to restore tooth #21 DO.

Diastema Closure

- Evaluation:
  - Inform the patient of the alternatives to composite: veneers, orthodontic treatment, and no treatment.
  - Preoperative evaluation: will closing the diastemas result in unesthetic disproportionally wide teeth unless in combination with esthetic crown lengthening?
  - Measure the mesial–distal width of the teeth. If one tooth is smaller, add more composite to that one.
- Steps:
  - (Optional) impressions: pour-up models, mount, diagnostic wax-up, fabricate putty lingual index from wax-up.
  - Bevel enamel with a diamond bur.
  - Etch/bond following manufacturer's instructions.
  - With a Mylar matrix placed in the sulcus, place packable composite and tap into place with a microbrush, light cure, and add more layers.
  - Remove the Mylar strip and evaluate the contours; adjust as needed.
  - Check with floss to verify no shredding.
  - Restore the adjacent tooth. Alternatively, make impressions, pour the models, mount, create a diagnostic wax-up, fabricate a putty index, and use the putty index to build the lingual walls.

Tips for Getting Good Anatomy

- Review dental anatomy (beyond the scope of this book), including embrasures, contact areas, height of contours, and line angles.
- Use the contralateral tooth as a reference for the tooth's anatomy.
- Class I/II on mandibular first premolars: use the acorn burnisher to create the pits ("snake eyes").
- Class I/II on maxillary molars: think "MOB, DOL." Slide the acorn burnisher across the tooth in these directions to re-create the grooves.
- Class I/II on mandibular first molars: think "MOL, BOB." Slide the acorn burnisher across the tooth in these directions to re-create the grooves with the L coming from the center of the tooth.
- Class I/II on mandibular second molars: think "positive" sign. Slide the acorn burnisher across the tooth in these directions to re-create the grooves.
- Class II MRs: to create round MRs, slice the excess composite off with an angled plastic instrument at a 45° angle. The MR should be the same height as the adjacent MR. A rounded MR (vs. flat) will help guide the floss between the teeth.
- Class IV: use a flat diamond bur that looks like "thick crust pizza" without water to adjust the incisal edge until it is level with the adjacent (if a central) or contralateral (if a lateral) tooth. Teeth #8 and #9 should be mirror images of each other. Be sure to include the facial line angles.
- Class V: rest the plastic instrument on the tooth structure beyond the composite (apically) and slide across the tooth to re-create the tooth contour.

Operative Dentistry

Postoperative Instructions

- General
  - Continue with oral hygiene to prevent recurrent decay.
  - Any exposed surfaces of teeth are still at risk of decay.
  - If the bite feels "off," return to the office for a bite adjustment.
  - Tooth sensitivity is to be expected and should decrease over time; OTC pain medication is recommended. If tooth sensitivity remains or increases, you experience spontaneous pain, and/or there is lingering pain to cold, return to the office. The tooth may require further treatment including RCT or extraction. This treatment may be referred to a specialist, and may not be covered by dental insurance.
  - If the cavity was at or below the gumline, the gum tissue may be sore. Rinse with warm salt-water several times a day and take OTC pain medication as needed.
  - Beware not to bite your cheek, lip, or tongue until the anesthetic wears off. If you are hungry, recommend eating soft foods until the anesthetic wears off. If you bite yourself by accident (e.g. cheek, lip), apply vitamin E oil.

- Composite
  - The restoration is set and you may eat.
  - The restoration will stain over time from highly staining foods, drinks, tobacco, and mouthwashes.
  - If the filling was placed on the edge of a front tooth (e.g. class IV) do not bite into anything hard like apples and don't chew your nails, as this will fracture the filling. With these types of fillings you will likely require replacement in future.

- Amalgam
  - Not fully set until 24 hours have elapsed.
  - No hard or crunchy foods for the first 24 hours until the filling is fully set. Eat soft foods only, as the restoration may crack, fall out, or develop a void.
  - You may experience sensitivity as metal conducts hot and cold faster than tooth structure.
  - You can return to polish the restoration after 24 hours.

- Indirect pulp cap
The cavity was deep and a protective layer was placed beneath the restoration. The tooth may require RCT in the future. We will monitor the tooth at future visits for any new signs and symptoms. Call if the tooth causes any pain.
- Direct pulp cap
  - The cavity was deep and reached the pulp tissues. The tooth will require RCT and possibly a crown.
  - Or the cavity was deep and while cleaning out the tooth there was a very small mechanical exposure of the pulp tissues. A protective material was placed to cover the exposure and then the restoration was placed. The tooth may require RCT in the future. The status of the tooth will be assessed at future visits for any new signs and symptoms [15]. Call if the tooth causes any pain.
- Stepwise caries excavation
  - For the permanent tooth with immature apices, please return in six to eight months for removal of the "temporary" filling and residual decay for placement of a permanent restoration [15]. The status of the tooth will be assessed at future visits for any new signs and symptoms. RCT may be indicated in the future.

Clinical Pearls

Troubleshooting

Unsatisfactory Restorations

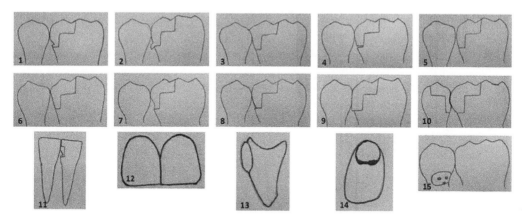

Figure 7.20 Radiographs taken at the recall exam may reveal unsatisfactory restorations. Problems and solutions are provided in the text.

The numbers on Figure 7.20 refer to the problems and solutions listed below.

1) *Problem*: Class II wedge silhouette.
   Solution: wedge placement was too far occlusal. Redo. Place the wedge apical to the gingival floor.
2) *Problem*: Class II overhang.
   Solution: Redo. The matrix was not flush against the tooth. Also, the matrix may have initially been flush against the tooth but if the tooth was burnished heavily or in an occlusal–apical direction, the matrix may have moved away from the tooth. Verify a tight seal between the tooth and matrix band prior to restoring.
3) *Problem*: Class II MR overlapping appearance on bitewing at recall.
   Solution: To repair adjust with high-speed bur. In the future when placing composite at the MR, "slice" the composite with the plastic instrument at a 45° angle to create a rounded MR prior to light curing.
4) *Problem*: Class II open margin.
   Solution: Redo. Make sure plastic instrument does not pull composite away from the gingival floor. Dab instrument in composite wetting resin to prevent pulling. Consider placing flowable composite into the box, teasing out the bubbles with the periodontal probe, and light curing, followed by layers of packable composite. This will prevent the opportunity for the packable composite to "pull away" from the gingival floor.
5) *Problem*: Class II open contact.
   Solution: Redo. The matrix was not burnished against the adjacent tooth, and/or the matrix was too thick, and/or the wedge was too small and did not provide adequate pressure to separate from neighboring teeth, and/or sectional ring was not tight enough to adequately separate the teeth, and/or the Tofflemire matrix band was overly tightened.
6) *Problem*: Class II pinpoint contact, in which the contact is too far occlusal. The poor proximal contour resulted in a large embrasure, creating a food trap.

Solution: Redo. Use a sectional matrix band, not a Tofflemire matrix band for more natural contours and contact. If the contact is too far occlusal and the restoration requires adjusting, the contact may be lost when adjusting creating an open contact.

7) *Problem*: Class II undercontoured due to Teflon placement with wedge when attempting to create a marginal seal with the matrix.

Solution: Redo. Consider margin elevation technique to avoid this.

8) *Problem*: Class II undercontoured (also referred to as "sub") due to Tofflemire matrix band overly tightened and placed occlusal to the gingival floor.

Solution: The matrix band must be flush against the tooth apical to the cavosurface.

9) *Problem*: Class II overcontoured (also referred to as "plus") due to not placing a wedge. This "step" of composite can also occur if the matrix band is burnished in a cervical-occlusal direction, when the matrix should be burnished in a buccal-lingual direction.

Solution: Redo. Be sure to place a wedge for Class II restorations.

10) *Problem*: adjacent Class IIs "spooning." The molar Class II is overcontoured, and the premolar Class II is undercontoured.

Solution: When restoring adjacent Class IIs, or "kissing caries," place adjacent sectional matrices (1, 2), wedge (3), and ring (4). Restore one tooth, then remove the matrix of the restored tooth (e.g. 1) and lightly burnish the remaining matrix (2). Having both matrices placed at the beginning allows for optimal contours of both teeth, preventing one from being overcontoured and impinging on the space for the adjacent tooth's contour. See Figure 7.21.

11) *Problem*: Class III wedge silhouette. The wedge placement was too far incisal.

Solution: Redo. Place the wedge apical to the cavosurface. Sometimes the interdental papilla will have to be traumatized in order to place the wedge in the appropriate location. The gingiva will heal, so warn patient it may be sore.

12) *Problem*: diastema closure, or Class IV. Teeth appear splinted and difficult to insert floss (seen clinically).

Solution: Create an incisal embrasure when adapting the composite prior to light curing. If already cured, adjust with the high-speed bur. The incisal embrasure will also help guide the floss in when flossing.

13) *Problem*: Class V overcontoured (clinically).

Solution: when placing restorative material, adapt the plastic instrument to the tooth to match the contour of the tooth. If already cured/set, adjust with the high-speed diamond bur.

14) *Problem*: Class V marginal stains due to overhangs (clinically).

Solution: Prior to restoring, etch and bond *beyond* the cavosurface (not just in the cavity prep) as it is difficult to see the edge of the composite placement in the cavity prep and if composite goes beyond the cavity prep will still be bonded to enamel. If not etched/bonded beyond the cavosurface, the composite will be cured but not bonded to the enamel, creating an overhang resulting in stains and possible recurrent decay.

15) *Problem*: Class V voids.

Solution: if using flowable composite, tease out the bubbles with a periodontal probe prior to curing.

Figure 7.21 Follow this sequence for restoring "kissing caries."

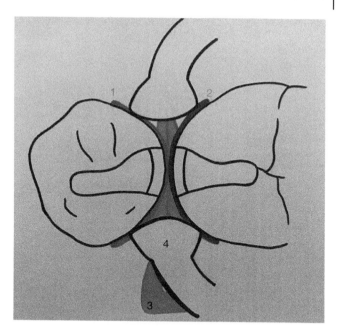

Other Problems

- Determining which direction to place the wedge for Class IIs and IIIs. The embrasure size dictates the direction of wedge placement. Place the wedge from the side with the larger embrasure, often the lingual.
- Excess gingival tissue blocking cavity preparation and restoration. This requires gingivectomy and there are various options with advantages and disadvantages, including electrosurgery, laser, scalpel, or a coarse or medium diamond bur to remove some gingiva followed by a hemostatic agent. Various specific gingivectomy burs on the market (e.g. CeraTip, GingiBur kit, and Preppi, a small round fine finishing diamond).
- Hemostasis control with Class II/III/IV/V: this is a good opportunity to emphasize oral health instructions. Can anesthetize with lidocaine, can use hemostatic agents (e.g. Viscostat, Hemodent).
- Composite Class II: alternative technique for obtaining contact when using a Tofflemire. If the Tofflemire is thick and you're concerned you will not obtain adequate proximal contact, place flowable at the base of the gingival floor and light cure. Then after placing a layer of packable composite, insert a cured piece of composite with cotton pliers (Figure 7.22). Remove the cotton pliers and use a burnisher to apply pressure on the cured piece of composite against the adjacent tooth and light cure for half the time. Remove the burnisher, and complete light curing to obtain proximal contact. Finish restoring the tooth with more layers of composite.

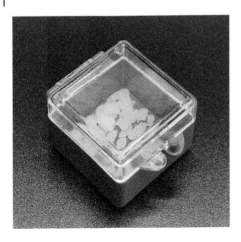

Figure 7.22   Pre-cured pieces of packable composite.

- Be prepared for surprises. A Class I may turn into a Class II when more caries are discovered while prepping the pulpal floor. Occlusal decay can spread to the interproximal without the typical triangular shape seen interproximally on the radiograph. See Figure 7.23.

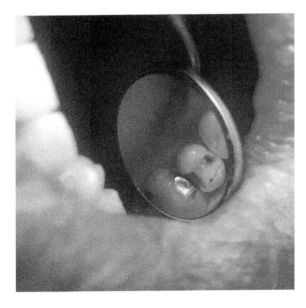

Figure 7.23   A DO cavity preparation. While prepping the pulpal floor, decay was noted on the M which was not apparent radiographically, turning the DO into an MOD.

- Class II slot design versus conventional: not been as retentive for amalgams/composites as conventional preps. Especially for composite there is more enamel to bond to with the conventional cavity prep design.
- If composite becomes contaminated during placement, re-etch/bond following manufacturer's instructions and add composite.
- If the patient does not want a bite block, explain why this helps you.
  - Stabilizes the jaw so not working on a moving target! Having a moving target introduces risk of trauma to teeth/soft tissue. If the patient bites down, the bur can drill deeper into the tooth leading to damage or a pulpal exposure.
  - Patient is able to rest their jaw during the procedure.
  - More working space for the dentist and assistant.

- Bonding agent stuck interproximally and unable to floss. Try to remove with explorer tip or use floss threader or Superfloss to floss beneath the contact and pull occlusally/incisally to dislodge the excess bonding material.
- Heavy contact (Class II/III): discomfort due to pressure and inaccessible for flossing.
  - Class II/III: wedge to separate teeth if unable to slide the interproximal polishing strip, polish, remove the wedge, and check the contact. Repeat as necessary.
- No contact (Class II/III/IV): leads to food impaction, localized bone loss, and recurrent decay. Redo the restoration.
- Unsure if cavitated/decayed interproximally on an adjacent proximal surface? When prepping the cavitated tooth you will gain direct visual/tactile access to the adjacent surface in question to evaluate.
- Partial denture wearer:
  - Check the fit of the partial prior to avoid being accused of a loose fitting partial once the restoration is completed.
  - Verify the partial still seats completely with the new restoration and adjust as needed.
- Patient unsure if bite is correct because of anesthetic. Check occlusion on the side of the mouth that is not anesthetized with articulating paper and tug (paper should tear). Inform the patient that he or she can return if the bite feels odd.
- Shade selection: see Chapter 11.
- Hypocalcification/(chalky) white lesions:
  - This is active caries if dull and white versus shiny and white.
  - If cavitated in the center and white lesions wrap around entire surface of tooth, do not remove entire white lesion. Restore only where the tooth is cavitated (plaque trap) and treat the white spot with fluoride applications.
- Patient reports "In order for my teeth to come together properly, I have to bite and slide my jaw slightly." This means the teeth are contacting on the incline plane, so adjust incline plane.
- Cavity preparation so small that instruments or restorative material cannot be introduced. You cannot work in a cave, so the cavity prep must be enlarged. If the condenser instrument is too large, composite can be condensed with a microbrush.
- Patient says she was told her filling "is leaking" and wants this filling removed. Leaking refers to an open margin in which oral fluids are leaking into the tooth between the restoration and tooth. Leaking does not refer to the restoration dissolving and leaking into the mouth.
- Nearby teeth sensitive to air/cold water when using the high-speed handpiece. Dispense bite registration to cover the sensitive teeth from the cold water/air and continue treatment (Figure 7.24).

Figure 7.24 One approach to protecting cold-sensitive teeth during a cavity preparation.

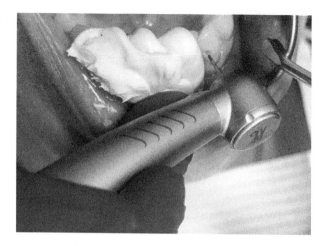

- Unsure if the dark pit on a tooth is a stain or cavity? Consider the patient's caries risk. Monitor, or if high risk may be able to assume it is decay.
- Shredding/catching floss on the restoration but cannot tell where to adjust? Insert the floss and pull it out slowly; the instant the floss catches, carefully inspect the position of the floss in order to determine the location of the overhang that requires adjusting.

Tips

- To minimize the discomfort when administering local anesthesia (except for inferior alveolar nerve block) warn the patient that they will feel a pinch and dispense only a small amount of anesthetic. Wait one minute and go back into the same spot to dispense the rest of the local anesthetic. Patients will appreciate this.
- Hold the mouth mirror further away from the mouth to reduce splatter and fog. Have your assistant blow air on the mirror to "defog" and to remove water and occasionally rinse off debris. Have your assistant wipe the mirror with alcohol if the reflection is blurry (e.g. from topical anesthetic).
- When placing a matrix band, use the following analogy for patients: it is similar to placing masking tape around a window or door frame prior to painting, which is tedious but necessary to prevent paint from marking those surfaces that are to remain unpainted.
- To produce a lifelike appearance when restoring a maxillary central incisor, rub articulating paper on the facial to see the anatomy, including the location of the lobes and developmental grooves in order to replicate this in the adjacent tooth with diamond burs (Figure 7.25).

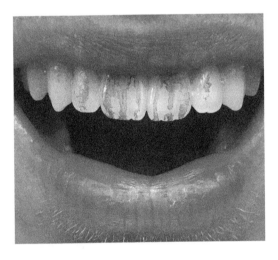

Figure 7.25 Articulating paper revealing the subtle anatomy on the maxillary central incisors.

- If the hand instrument does not fit in the cavity prep to tap the composite into place, try using a microbrush instead.
- Wooden wedges: place with cotton pliers and use the opposite end to push the wedge forcefully between teeth.
- A blue Mylar strip is easier to see on the tray table and for placement on the tooth than the clear Mylar strips.
- Erosion:
  - Wear appears as flat surfaces on teeth, while erosion can appear as cupping, dimpling, and troughing on incisal edges, and has a melted candle appearance.

- – If cupping/dimpling on occlusal surfaces are restored with composite, you may have to remove the entire restoration if the opposing cusp occludes with the base of the dimple. Always check occlusion beforehand.
  - – Maxillary anterior lingual surfaces with erosion: check occlusion beforehand when evaluating restorability. The opposing teeth may have supraerupted to contact the maxillary anterior lingual surfaces. When prepping anterior teeth with erosion on the lingual, place grooves and notches for retention, roughen with football bur, etch, bond, place flowable, light cure, and place packable which bonds to flowable to restore.
- If severely worn incisal edges or occlusal surfaces are present, create trough and fill with composite and packable will bond to flowable.
- Interproximal decay adjacent to a tooth planned for extraction. Extract the tooth first; once it heals you will have direct access to the interproximal caries. The preparation can be more conservative (e.g. M vs. MO) and easier to restore. See Figure 7.1.
- Etching:
  - – Do not get any etch on the soft tissue as it will cause a chemical burn on the mucosa (e.g. patient's lower lip).
  - – After etching tooth, have the assistant encompass the tooth with the HVE to suction the etching material prior to rinsing with water to prevent spreading the etch onto the soft tissue.
- Time efficiency: for cavity preps and crown preps, minimize the number of bur changes during the procedure.
- Limited interocclusal space to build up tooth. Options include:
  - – Intrude the opposing tooth with orthodontic treatment.
  - – Enameloplasty "lightly dusting portion of superficial enamel layer." Obtain and document the patient's verbal consent to do this.
  - – Opening the bite by increasing VDO (beyond the scope of this book).
- Converging versus diverging walls in cavity prep? Picture this from the perspective of the bacteria in the cavity. Need converging walls for mechanical retention when placing amalgam; need diverging walls for inlays and onlays.
- Radiographic void/bubbles in composite:
  - – If you placed it, then monitor. If someone else placed it, redo.
  - – This may have been flowable composite in which the operator did not tease out the bubbles with a periodontal probe prior to light curing.
- Improving skill set for esthetic cases: take photos before and after procedure to analyze contours of teeth; you may see more when analyzing the photos than looking in the mouth. Learn from every experience.
- Uses of Teflon tape in dentistry
  - – Class II: to obtain a better adapted matrix which seals the cavosurface place a ball of Teflon between the matrix and wedge.
  - – Class II/III with recession: instead of double wedging, wrap a wooden wedge in several layers of Teflon tape for better anatomy.
  - – Class III/IV: wrap around adjacent tooth to obtain contact when restoring without use of a matrix and wedge. The thickness of Teflon is negligible.
    - ○ Caution: if wrapping around adjacent tooth for a Class III, without using a wedge and matrix, you may end up with an overcontoured restoration with a flat interproximal surface.
  - – Veneer cementation: wrap around the adjacent tooth to prevent splinting teeth with veneer cement.
  - – Implant crowns: placed beneath composite layer on screw-retained implant crowns.
  - – Protect adjacent tooth from etch by wrapping proximal wall with Teflon.
  - – Train dental assistants to refer to it as "Teflon tape" not "plumbers tape."

- Goal with adhesive dentistry is to conserve tooth structure; however, if amalgam restoration is butting up against the composite you plan to place, then remove the entire amalgam restoration. The composite will not bond to the amalgam and the composite may fall out.
- Drying the bonding agent
  - Do not remove the entire bonding agent by applying too much air; start from afar and slowly approach tooth. Lightly dry until the bonding agent is no longer moving but still appears shiny.
  - Make sure there is no moisture contamination by blowing air on the back of your gloved hand with the air/water syringe. If droplets of water are seen on the glove, then there will be moisture contamination. Instead use the HVE for the stream of air.
- Composite wetting resin is used to moisten dry composite and improve glide of instrument.
- Optiguard is used to fill the marginal gaps. After adjusting the occlusion and polishing, etch the composite, rinse, dry, apply Optiguard and light cure following manufacturer's instructions.
- Pumice occlusal surface (clean tooth) before caries removal.
- Patient management: inform patients during the procedure that things are going well and as planned to calm them.
- Rubber dam:
  - Recommended for composite restorations. When the patient breathes the mouth mirror becomes foggy. Similarly, this moisture contaminates the composite.
  - Quadrant isolation allows more room for the assistant to suction; in addition, a Class I restoration may turn into a Class II restoration if more decay is found.
  - Inverting the dam: can use a plastic instrument or wrap floss around a tooth and have floss cross over and pull outward so as to tighten the floss.
  - Class II/III:
    - Must isolate more than one tooth, and include adjacent.
    - Place a wooden wedge when prepping interproximally to avoid tearing rubber dam with bur.

Real-Life Clinical Questions Answered

Dental Students' Questions and Comments

- "How can you tell there is still decay in the cavity prep?"
  - See Figure 7.26 for some of the colors found on and in teeth.
  - Use your three senses:
    - *Look* at the color (Figure 7.27).
    - *Feel* the dentin (by scratching not poking) in the questionable area and compare it to the dentin in the part of the cavity prep you are confident is not decayed. May feel soft, sticky, leathery, or rubbery.
    - *Listen* to the explorer against the dentin (turn the HVE off). Does it sound hard?
  - Active caries may have a red brick color, not to be confused with blood from the pulp. Evaluate the distance from the pulp horn radiographically.
  - Caries begins as a white-spot lesion which is porous, but over time takes up stains and may become brown or black [18].
  - Try to achieve a uniform color, but remember:
    - Could be uniform color and still contain caries.
    - Do not chase the stain to achieve a desired color of dentin as this removes more tooth structure and leads to pulpal exposure.
  - Consider using a caries-indicating dye to verify that all caries has been removed.

- ○ Gentle probing does not disrupt surface, whereas forceful pressure causes irreversible damage [18] and cavitation [19].
- ○ Scratch, don't poke.
- When diagnosing caries may see shadowing in the enamel (Figure 7.28).
- When removing decay with the slow-speed round bur it often appears as a powder or eraser crumbs (Figure 7.1).
- Once reaching hard healthy tooth structure, the round bur will rattle off the tooth.
- When determining if composite still remains inside the cavity prep when replacing a restoration, the composite is usually opaque, monochromatic compared to tooth structure, and feels like plastic.
- Active caries means there is ongoing mineral loss due to metabolic activity in the biofilm. If active and cavitated, treat; if active and not cavitated, use nonoperative treatment (e.g. fluoride). Active noncavitated lesions may be turned into arrested/inactive noncavitated carious lesions.
- Treat cavitated caries as it is difficult to control the biofilm by oral hygiene when the lesion is cavitated. Treatment involves restoration [18].

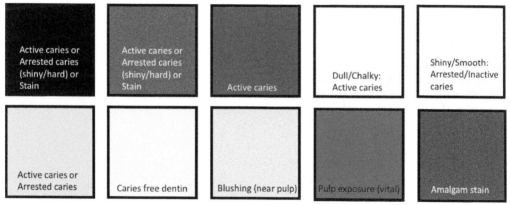

Figure 7.26   Diagram of colors found on and inside teeth.

Figure 7.27   Note the difference between the color of the dentin on the pulpal floor and that of the gingival floor and axial wall.

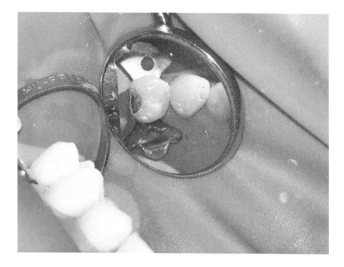

Operative Dentistry

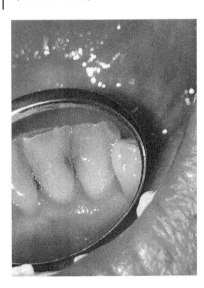

Figure 7.28 Note the shadowing through the enamel at the proximal contact.

- "Where should the dots go on the composite when checking occlusion? Should there not be any dots on the filling?"
  - Do not take the tooth out of occlusion as the opposing tooth or the tooth being restored may supraerupt (also the patient may bite their tongue or cheek if there is space).
  - The dots may or may not be on the filling depending on the location and the bite.
  - Recommended before cavity preparation: check occlusion with the articulating paper. Try to remember the location of the "dots" or take an intraoral photo.
  - After restoring: dry the occlusal surfaces of the restored tooth and opposing tooth by having patient bite on a stack of gauze.
  - Coat the articulating paper with petroleum jelly to reduce the false-positive marks.
  - Use red/blue articulating paper (black can be used instead of blue). Sequence of use as follows:
    - Red paper for dynamic occlusal marks: ask patient to "Bite and slide teeth left, right, forward, back."
    - Blue paper for static occlusal marks: ask patient to "Tap tap."
    - Evaluate red and blue marks:
      - Posterior teeth:
        (a) Every tooth must have at least one blue mark (don't take the tooth out of occlusion).
        (b) No blue on incline planes (or patient will have to bite and slide teeth into place).
        (c) No red without blue.
      - Anterior teeth:
        (a) Only have red [20] (exception: edge-to-edge anterior occlusal relationship).
- "How would I know if I had a pulpal exposure? And what do I do?"
  - One way to determine if there is a pulpal exposure is to look for bleeding. If the pulp is necrotic there will not be any bleeding, but hopefully you determined this in advance by endo testing the tooth. If it is difficult to see, place a cotton pellet using cotton pliers into the cavity prep; after a few seconds remove the cotton pellet and inspect for any blood. A false positive can occur if blood from the gingiva was contacted or blood from the gingiva entered the cavity prep. For treatment, see Section Direct Pulp Cap.
- "I didn't floss after because it was just an occlusal composite."

- When you dry the bonding agent it often spreads to the interproximal surface and splints the teeth together. Sometimes the bonding agent also spreads into the sulcus. You must always floss after every restoration and check the sulcus for excess bonding agent. See Figure 7.14.
- "Sandwich technique?"
  - Open sandwich technique: Class II when the cavity prep is subgingival. Hold the matrix, place Fuji, light cure, remove the matrix, remove overhangs, or contour with plastic instrument, then use a sectional matrix (better contour/contact).
  - Closed sandwich technique: since the composite bonds to enamel and RMGI bonds to dentin, use RMGI in the deep portions contacting dentin and composite for the remaining restoration.
- "How do I know if we should do a large filling or a crown?"
  - Sometimes an indirect restoration is better for creating ideal contours, as it is made outside the mouth.
  - Onlay/inlay procedures beyond scope of this book.
  - Indications for crown, see Chapter 11.
- "What is the difference between a base and a liner?"
  - Liner: also referred to as "pulp-capping agents" [21]. Relatively thin layer [22].
  - Base: thermal protection for the pulp and mechanical support for a restoration [21]. Implies a degree of strength to restore part of the missing tooth structure [22].

Dental Assistants' Questions

- "How long do I light cure this for?"
  - Never guess. Go to the primary source. Empower and train your assistants. Look up the manufacturer's guidelines and learn these setting times for the materials used in your office. Consider creating an easily accessible card with these setting times in the operatory.
- "What instrument do you need doc?"
  - Learn the names (e.g. condenser, ball burnisher, football burnisher, plastic instrument, acorn).

Patients' Concerns, Requests, Questions, and Comments

- "Is that a UV light?"
  - Light-cured resin composites require a photoinitiator to activate the polymerization reaction (so that the material sets). Visible light is required and the most energy is delivered in the range 460–480 nm (blue light). Offices may possess light-emitting diode (LED) or quartz–tungsten–halogen (QTH) lights. It is not a UV light [2].
- "If you hit the nerve and place a protective layer, what is the chance I will need to get a root canal treatment?"
  - If there is a mechanical exposure, there is a fairly high success rate (studies vary: 92.2% [23] or 80% [11]), so it is not likely you will require RCT. If it is an exposure due to the caries, there is only a 33.3% success rate, so it is much more likely you will require RCT [23]. Teeth with carious exposure should be root canal treated [11].
- "I'm here because I just had a filling and the tooth is hurting me."

- How many days has it been since the restoration was placed (could be postoperative sensitivity)? What is your pain level on a scale of 0–10? What are your symptoms? Tender on biting? Likely in hyperocclusion, adjust bite. Sensitive to cold? Possibly reversible pulpitis or irreversible pulpitis. See Chapter 10.

- "I don't want my daughter to have any mercury fillings, so you need to use something else."
  - Seek to understand why the parent is opposed to amalgam restorations.
  - As the healthcare professional, provide your treatment plan recommendations, including the risks, benefits, advantages, disadvantages, and alternatives, including second opinion. If you believe amalgam restorations are in the best interest of the patient's oral health, you can always suggest the parent have a second opinion. Determine how much you are willing to compromise, if at all.

- "I want all these mercury fillings removed."
  - Seek to understand why the patient is requesting this procedure. Is it due to esthetics? Claimed mercury poisoning?
  - Consider the risks involved:
    o The FDA does not recommend removing amalgam restorations if in satisfactory condition (not fractured, no recurrent decay) as removing amalgam will result in "unnecessary loss of healthy tooth structure, and exposes you to additional mercury vapor released during the removal process" [5].
    o Any time a tooth is drilled there is a risk of pulpal inflammation and the tooth requiring further treatment such as RCT and crown.
  - If amalgam is removed, use rubber dam isolation to reduce mercury vapor exposure and to prevent large pieces of amalgam from being swallowed or aspirated. Can remove with a 330, or consider using the amalgam buster diamond bur (geometric hourglass shape).

- "Can you make the water warm instead of cold?"
  - Unfortunately, I can't control the temperature of the water. Which teeth are sensitive? What I can offer is placing some bite registration material over these sensitive teeth during the procedure. This typically helps. The alternative would be to anesthetize other areas of your mouth (see Figure 7.24).

- "I just want caps on these teeth not fillings."
  - Let me evaluate these teeth first and provide my recommendations. In most cases it is better to conserve tooth structure. Capping teeth may be doing a disservice to you, especially if you have a high caries risk. Capping the teeth simply moves the location of your future cavities to the gumline, which makes it harder to save your teeth later down the line if decay forms. A composite restoration can save more tooth structure. Veneers are another option which are much more conservative than caps.

- "Why do I have so many cavities? I don't eat sweets and I drink diet soda."
  - See Chapter 5.

- "Can I eat after this filling?"
  - See Section Postoperative Instructions.

- "Once my cavity is filled, I won't have to brush that tooth anymore!"
  - You only have to brush and floss the teeth you want to keep.

- "Does this have fluoride? Is this gluten free?"

- Refer to the primary source (the manufacturer's guidelines) for accuracy when answering a patient's question. You may be surprised to discover that fluoride is in the bonding agent you use for your composites. Recommend having a binder in the office containing all the manufacturer's guidelines.
- "Can you tell from the X-ray if I'm going to need a root canal?"
  - I would have to test the tooth to determine if it needs a root canal. The radiograph shows how deep a cavity is on the chewing surface or in between the teeth, but it is not possible to determine the depth on the front or back of the tooth since it is a two-dimensional image. Anytime a tooth is worked on the pulp may become inflamed and require RCT.
- "How long will a composite filling last me?"
  - According to Delta Dental (dental insurance company) amalgam lasts 10–15 years and composites five to seven years [24].
  - According to the position statement by the American College of Prosthodontists:
    - o No true direct filling "substitute" yet exists for amalgam.
    - o A five-year study demonstrated that multisurface composites were replaced and repaired at nearly twice the rate of amalgam restorations.
    - o Another study reported twice the failure rate for composites versus amalgam by the eighth year, and by 10–11 years 40–50% of the composites had failed [25].
- "Should I get veneers or composites to close these gaps?"
  - There are advantages and disadvantages to each.
    - o Veneer (beyond scope of this book):
      - ▪ Advantages: longer lasting, does not stain.
      - ▪ Disadvantages: irreversible, harder to repair (must replace), time-consuming, cost, may require an occlusal guard.
  - Composite:
    - o Advantages: reversible, conservative, less expensive, easier to repair, cost.
    - o Disadvantage: stains.
- "Will these fillings whiten once I bleach my teeth?"
  - No. Fillings, crowns, and any exposed root surfaces (cementum) will not bleach. In addition, teeth with silver fillings can appear darker due to the translucency of teeth.
- "If you told me I'd be sore I wouldn't have come in."
  - This is a reminder to always review postoperative instructions so the patient knows what to expect. See Section Postoperative Instructions.

References

1 American Dental Association (2016). Operative dentistry becomes first interest area in general dentistry to receive recognition. https://www.ada.org/en/publications/ada-news/2016-archive/november/operative-dentistry-becomes-first-interest-area-in-general-dentistry-to-receive-recognition (accessed 15 May 2021).

2 Hilton, T.J., Ferracane, J.L., and Broome, J.C. (ed.) (2013). *Summit's Fundamentals of Operative Dentistry. A Contemporary Approach*, 2e. Chicago: Quintessence Books.

3 (1989). *Webster's Unabridged Dictionary of the English Language*. New York: Portland House.

4 Craig, R.G. (ed.) (1993). *Restorative Dental Materials*, 9e. St. Louis, MO: Mosby.

5 U.S. Food and Drug Administration (2021). Dental amalgam fillings. https://www.fda.gov/medical-devices/dental-devices/dental-amalgam-fillings (accessed 15 May 2021).

6 American Dental Association. Statement on dental amalgam. https://www.ada.org/en/about-the-ada/

ada-positions-policies-and-statements/
statement-on-dental-amalgam (accessed
15 May 2021).

7 FDI World Dental Foundation (1997). WHO
consensus statement on dental amalgam.
https://www.fdiworlddental.org/who-
consensus-statement-dental-amalgam
(accessed 15 May 2021).

8 GC America Inc. Product Catalog (2019).
http://www.gcamerica.com/
catalog2019/08-06-2019/GCA-
Catalog-08-06-2019.pdf (accessed
15 May 2021).

9 GC America Inc (2020). GC Fuji II LC. http://
www.gcamerica.com/products/operatory/
GC_Fuji_II_LC (accessed 15 May 2021).

10 Stanley, H.R. (1981). *Human Pulp Response to
Restorative Dental Procedures*. Storter:
Gainesville, FL.

11 Torabinejad, M. and Walton, R.E. (2009).
Endodontics: Principles and Practice, 4e. St.
Louis, MO: Saunders Elsevier.

12 Min, K.S., Park, H.J., Le, S.J. et al. (2008).
Effect of mineral trioxide aggregate on dentin
bridge formation and expression of dentin
sialoprotein and heme oxygenase-1 in human
dental pulp. *J. Endod.* 34: 666–670.

13 Medeiros, V.A. and Seddon, R.P. (2000).
Iatrogenic damage to approximal surfaces in
contact with class II restorations. *J. Dent.*
28 (2): 103–110.

14 Lussi, A. and Gygax, M. (1998). Iatrogenic
damage to adjacent teeth during classical
approximal box preparation. *J. Dent.* 26 (5–6):
435–441.

15 American Association of Endodontists (2013).
Guide to Clinical Endodontics, 6e. Chicago:
AAE https://www.aae.org/specialty/clinical-
resources/guide-clinical-endodontics.

16 American Dental Association (2016). CDT
Code Check phone app.

17 Li, Z., Cao, L., Fan, M., and Xu, Q. (2015).
Direct pulp capping with calcium hydroxide or
mineral trioxide aggregate: a meta-analysis.
J. Endod 41 (9): 1412–1417.

18 Fejerskov, O. and Kidd, E. (ed.) (2003). *Dental
Caries. The Disease and its Clinical
Management*, 2e. Copenhagen: Blackwell
Munksgaard.

19 Casamassimo, P., Fields, H., McTigue, D., and
Nowak, A. (2013). *Pediatric Dentistry: Infancy
Through Adolescence*, 5e. St. Louis, MO: Elsevier.

20 Patel, V. (2018). Where is the bite? Everyday
occlusion. *The Nugget*. Sacramento Dental
District Society.

21 Powers, J.M. and Sakaguchi, R.L. (ed.) (2006).
Craig's Restorative Dental Materials, 12e. St.
Louis, MO: Mosby Elsevier.

22 Gladwin, M. and Bagby, M. (2013). *Clinical
Aspects of Dental Materials: Theory, Practice
and Cases*, 4e. Philadelphia, PA: Lippincott
Williams & Wilkins.

23 Al-Hiyasat, A.S., Barrieshi-Nusair, K.M., and
Al-Omari, M.A. (2006). The radiographic
outcomes of direct pulp-capping procedures
performed by dental students: a retrospective
study. *J. Am. Dent. Assoc.* 137 (12): 1699–1705.

24 Delta Dental (2018). The facts on fillings:
amalgam vs. resin composite. https://www.
deltadentalins.com/oral_health/amalgam.
html (accessed 15 May 2021).

25 American College of Prosthodontists (2018).
Position statement: dental amalgam. https://
www.prosthodontics.org/about-acp/position-
statement-dental-amalgam/ (accessed
15 May 2021).

8

Endodontics

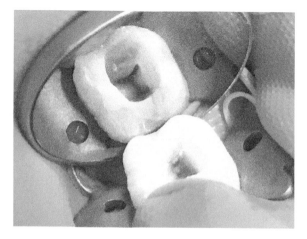

Figure 8.1 Color changes found on the pulp-chamber floor of tooth #18 acting as a "roadmap" for locating canals. Note the size of this access is larger than ideal due to the removal of caries prior.

Chapter Outline

- Real-Life Clinical Scenarios
- Relevance
- Clinical and Radiographic Exam
- Diagnostic Testing
  - Pulp Sensitivity Testing
  - Periapical Testing
  - Biting Test
  - Mobility
  - Anesthetic Test
- Diagnostic Terminology
- Formulation of Pulpal and Periradicular Diagnoses
- Types of Tooth Fractures
- Treatment Type and Indications
- AAE Endodontic Case Difficulty Assessment Form and Guidelines
- Treatment Planning

Clinical Dentistry Daily Reference Guide, First Edition. William A. Jacobson.
© 2022 John Wiley & Sons, Inc. Published 2022 by John Wiley & Sons, Inc.

Real-Life Clinical Scenarios

Dental Students' Questions

- "How do I pulp test a tooth?"
- "I'm not going to be an endodontist so why do I need to know the endo access shape for every tooth?"
- "How do I know if the patient needs a pulpotomy or a pulpectomy?"
- "How can I tell if it's a cracked tooth?"
- "How do I know if this is a periodontal abscess or endodontic abscess?"
- "I'm trying to drill out this temporary material to do the core buildup and it feels really hard and I'm afraid of damaging the floor of the pulp chamber."
- "When should we get a CBCT of the tooth?"
- "How long will it take for the PARL to heal?"
- "How do I know if the tooth needs a retreatment or endodontic surgery?"

Dental Assistant's Comment

- "I don't like using the rubber dam and you don't need it for this buildup."

Patients' Comments

- "Ever since I fell down this tooth has been dark"
- "Doc, the tooth doesn't hurt so I'll let you know when it hurts, then we can schedule the root canal."
- "I know which tooth it is that needs the root canal. You don't have to test it."
- "No. You are not going to put something cold on my teeth."
- "I had the root canal done one week ago [with the endodontist] and it still hurts."
- "I went to the endodontist and he said the tooth is fractured so it cannot be saved."

Patients' Requests

- "The temporary fell out a few weeks ago but it doesn't hurt." (Figure 8.2)
- "I had my root canal done and need you to do the crown." (Figure 8.3)

Patients' Questions

- "What is a root canal?"
- "What is better? Extracting the tooth and getting an implant or a root canal and a crown?"
- "How do you clean out the infection if it is in the bone?" (Figure 8.4)
- "How much pain should I expect to be in after?"
- "Did the specialist do a bad job on my root canal?"
- "Doc I cannot afford a crown right now for the tooth I had a root canal done on and the specialist said I need a crown. How long can I wait?"

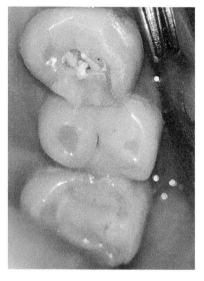

Figure 8.2 Food debris (along with saliva and bacteria) packed into the endodontic access of a recently root canal-treated tooth contaminating the canals.

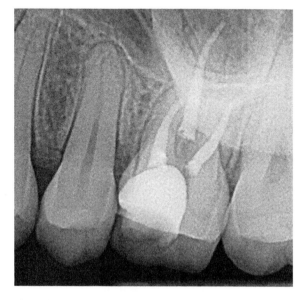

Figure 8.3 Periapical radiograph of tooth #14 which was recently root canal treated.

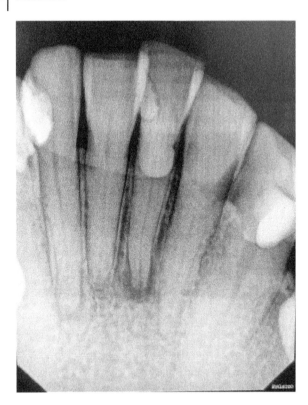

Figure 8.4 Tooth #24 has a PARL.

Relevance

Every tooth in the mouth has a pulp, and every pulp is at risk of becoming injured and diseased. Even if you intend to refer all of your root canal treatments to an endodontist, you should still be able to provide emergency treatment to alleviate your patient's pain (i.e. ability to provide pulpotomy, pulpectomy, or pulpal debridement). This chapter provides practical endodontic material to help guide you.

Clinical and Radiographic Exam

- Review the medical and dental history (see Chapter 1).
- Vitals: does the patient have a fever? Need for antibiotics?
- Patient interview:
  - Chief complaint in the patient's own words.
  - Time of onset (enquire about any recent dental treatment).
  - Ask about provoking factors.
  - Palliation: what relieves the pain? Provides insight about the severity.
  - Progression: are symptoms worsening?

- Quality of pain: quick/sharp indicates reversible cause; dull/spontaneous, throbbing indicates irreversible pulpitis; dull/achy indicates referred muscle pain; electrical/jolt indicates neuralgia.
  - Radiation of pain?
  - Severity of pain (scored on a scale of 0–10):
    - Current pain level
    - At its worst
  - Timing (duration, frequency)? Useful tip: spontaneous is indicative of irreversible pulpitis.
  - Change in bite?
  - Pain on biting? Useful tip: may indicate periapical inflammation.
  - How are you sleeping? Provides insight about the severity if awakened from sleep or unable to sleep.
- Clinical exam
  - EOE, IOE, and OCS (see Chapter 2).
    - Facial swelling?
    - Tender and/or swollen lymph nodes?
    - Trismus?
    - Extraoral or intraoral sinus tract? See Figures 10.6a and 10.6b
    - Parulis?
    - Intraoral swelling?
    - Trouble breathing?
  - Trauma? See Appendix A.
  - Clinical findings
    - Caries? Fracture? Defective restoration?
    - Periodontal evaluation (see Chapter 6).
    - Cracked tooth? See Section Types of Tooth Fracture.
    - Occlusion
- Radiographic exam
  - Interpret the radiographs (see Chapter 3).
- Diagnostic tests
  - See Section Diagnostic Testing.
- Determine restorability
  - Is the tooth restorable? Be sure the tooth is restorable if planning RCT (e.g. before sending the patient to the endodontist) (see Figure 11.4).
    - If the tooth is crowned and it has recurrent decay or an open margin, make a preliminary impression for a temporary crown. Remove the crown and evaluate restorability before RCT.
    - If the tooth has a defective filling (i.e. fractured, open margin, recurrent decay), remove the restorative material and decay and evaluate restorability before RCT.
  - Determine treatment (see Section Treatment Type and Indications).
  - Determine who will treat (see Section AAE Endodontic Case Difficulty Assessment Form and Guidelines).

Diagnostic Testing

An example of diagnostic testing is shown in Table 8.1.

Endodontics

Table 8.1 An example of diagnostic testing results.

Tooth no.	Percussion (–, no response; +, pain)	Palpation (–, no response; +, pain)	Cold (–, no response; +, normal response; ++, lingering)	Electric pulp test (–, no response; +, normal response)	Probing depths (mm)	Mobility	Occlusion (hypo-occlusion normal; hyperocclusion)
18	–	–	+	+	324 323	0	WNL
19	+	+	–	–(>80)	434 434	1	Hyperocclusion
20	–	–	+	+	323 323	0	WNL
21	–	–	+	+	323 323	0	WNL
22	–	–	+	+	323 323	0	WNL
23	–	–	–	–(>80)	222 222	0	WNL
24	–	–	+	+	223 322	0	WNL
14	–	–	+	+	323 334	0	WNL
30	–	–	+	+	434 434	0	WNL

In this case, #19 was the tooth in question. The entire quadrant was tested, along with the opposing tooth #14 and the contralateral tooth #30. The diagnosis was pulpal necrosis and symptomatic apical periodontitis. Tooth #23 was previously root canal treated.
Note that if a patient takes an NSAID 35–40 minutes before assessment, this could impact the outcome of the diagnostic tests.

Pulp Sensitivity Testing

Determines the status of the pulpal tissues.

Cold Test

Tell the patient to raise their hand if they feel cold and to keep it raised for the period of time they feel the sensation, so that you know (i) if they feel the cold stimulus and (ii) its duration.

- Saturate a cotton pellet with refrigerant spray (e.g. Endo Ice, which contains 1,1,1,2-tetrafluoroethane and fragrance) until it is dripping. Shake off any excess. Touch the tooth without contacting any soft tissue and do not allow any spray to drip onto the soft tissue. Once the patient feels the cold stimulus (by raising their hand) remove the cotton pellet and observe the duration of the sensation (amount of time patient's hand is raised).
- Don't use a cotton tip applicator as the wood absorbs the cold.
- If the cotton pellet is frozen solid, reuse or replace.
- Test the tooth in question last. If it is a "hot tooth" the pain will linger and will supersede all other responses and will mask symptoms. You might also find pathosis on another tooth during endodontic testing.
- Test all the teeth in the quadrant, an opposing tooth, and a contralateral tooth.
- Do not inform the patient which tooth is being tested.
- If there are conflicting responses (e.g. response to cold when testing a root canal-treated tooth) perform a control test by secretly spraying next to but not onto the cotton pellet and apply it to the tooth, knowing that it should not elicit a response. If the patient responds, then the response is a false positive. Refer to the Endodontist if there are inconclusive or conflicting endodontic diagnostic test results. (Figure 8.5 and Table 8.2).
- In some cases cold can relieve the pain if there is advanced intrapulpal inflammation with formation of an intrapulpal abscess. A patient may complain of symptoms to heat relieved by cold. To reproduce the symptoms you can perform a heat test by rolling two to three gutta percha cones into a ball, heating the ball, and placing it on the tooth. Evaluate if the patient feels pain, and then place a cold cotton pellet to evaluate if the cold relieved the pain.

Figure 8.5   Determining if the patient responds to cold when the stimulus is room temperature. Note the cotton pellet is not being sprayed but the patient believes it is.

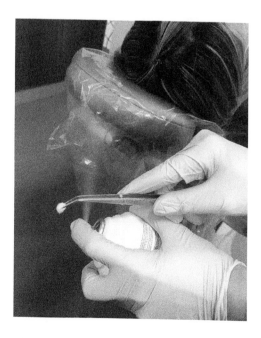

Endodontics

Table 8.2 Cold test false positives and false negatives.

False positive (a necrotic or RCT-treated tooth with a response)	• Cold contacting the gingiva or cold transferred to adjacent teeth [1]
False negative (a healthy tooth with no response)	• Calcified canals [1] • Metal, ceramic or ceramometal crowns have a delayed response to cold. May take up to 30 seconds until a response is felt

Electric Pulp Test

An adjunct to thermal tests to determine pulp vitality. Read the manufacturer's instructions of your device. For patients with a pacemaker, see Chapter 1.

- Set the wheel to 6 (rate at which intensity increases).
- Attach the lip clip to the patient's lips.
- Dry the teeth to be tested.
- Dip the probe in a small amount of fluoride gel. Topical fluoride gel (or a gel toothpaste) conducts electricity better than toothpaste and is recommended for the medium between the tooth and the electrode.
- Contact the tooth. The light will indicate that an electrical contact has been made.
- Remove from the tooth once the patient experiences a sensation (pulsating pressure, warmth, or tingling sensation). If no sensation is experienced, increase the intensity until the scale indicates 80, at which point the light starts flashing and the probe should be removed from the tooth. (Note that the numbered scale on the machine is arbitrary.) Wait 2 seconds between teeth being tested [2].
- Tell the patient "I will apply a small amount of current to the tooth and you will feel a little tingling sensation. You get to control it." Have the patient hold the end of the handpiece to ground it and once a sensation is felt the patient can release it and the circuit is broken (relieves some anxiety for the patient to be in control). With this approach you do not use the lip clip.
- Tables 8.3 and 8.4 show the range of normal responses and false-positive and false-negative responses.

Table 8.3 Electric pulp test: range of normal responses.

Teeth	Normal range
Anteriors	10–40
Premolars	20–50
Molars	30–70
Vital tooth	1–79
Nonvital tooth	80 +

Source: Based on Vitality Scanner Model 206. Instruction Guidelines [2].

Table 8.4   Electric pulp test: false positives and false negatives.

False positives (a necrotic or RCT-treated tooth with a response)	• A patient may sense stimulation in an adjacent tooth contacting the tooth being tested • A patient may sense a periodontal neural stimulus rather than pulpal nerve stimulus (recommend have the patient feel the difference between the tip contacting gingiva vs. tooth)
False negatives (a healthy tooth with no response)	• Moisture on the surface of the tooth making contact with gingiva • Metal restoration on the tooth making contact with gingiva • Severe calcifications • Conditions resulting in degradation of the neural response • Porcelain crowns (can use a Mini-Tip to contact tooth structure beneath the crown margin; the outside is insulated and can contact gingiva as long as the tip contacts tooth structure)

Source: Based on Vitality Scanner Model 206. Instruction Guidelines [2].

Periapical Testing

Determines the status of the periapical tissues.

- Percussion: tap the occlusal/incisal with the butt end of the mirror handle to determine periapical inflammation.
- Palpation: palpate with a finger around the apex of the tooth on the facial and on the lingual. In areas where root tips are close together use a cotton applicator (finger could overlap multiple roots). Pain indicates periapical inflammation.

Biting Test

- Perform when a vertical root fracture or cusp fracture is suspected. Inform the patient you want to know if there is discomfort on biting or upon release. You can use a Tooth Slooth on individual cusps, a cotton tip applicator, the rubber portion of a prophy angle, or the rubber portion of the saliva ejector.
- If there is pain on release, it is a classic sign of a cracked tooth or cuspal fracture. Could also have pain on biting, or both (likely a cracked tooth).

Mobility

With periapical inflammation there can be some mobility as the inflammation elevates the tooth in the socket. Alternatively, it could be due to periodontal disease.

Anesthetic Test

Performed when nonodontogenic pain is suspected. Anesthetize and if the pain is not relieved, then it is likely not of pulpal origin.

Endodontics

Diagnostic Terminology (Figure 8.6)

Recommended Terms

AAE Consensus Conference Recommended Diagnostic Terminology

Pulpal

Normal pulp	A clinical diagnostic category in which the pulp is symptom-free and normally responsive to pulp testing.
Reversible pulpitis	A clinical diagnosis based on subjective and objective findings indicating that the inflammation should resolve and the pulp return to normal.
Symptomatic irreversible pulpitis	A clinical diagnosis based on subjective and objective findings indicating that the vital inflamed pulp is incapable of healing. Additional descriptors: lingering thermal pain, spontaneous pain, referred pain.
Asymptomatic irreversible pulpitis	A clinical diagnosis based on subjective and objective findings indicating that the vital inflamed pulp is incapable of healing. Additional descriptors: no clinical symptoms but inflammation produced by caries, caries excavation, trauma.
Pulp necrosis	A clinical diagnostic category indicating death of the dental pulp. The pulp is usually nonresponsive to pulp testing.
Previously treated	A clinical diagnostic category indicating that the tooth has been endodontically treated and the canals are obturated with various filling materials other than intracanal medicaments.
Previously initiated therapy	A clinical diagnostic category indicating that the tooth has been previously treated by partial endodontic therapy (eg, pulpotomy, pulpectomy).

Apical

Normal apical tissues	Teeth with normal periradicular tissues that are not sensitive to percussion or palpation testing. The lamina dura surrounding the root is intact, and the periodontal ligament space is uniform.
Symptomatic apical periodontitis	Inflammation, usually of the apical periodontium, producing clinical symptoms including a painful response to biting and/or percussion or palpation. It might or might not be associated with an apical radiolucent area.
Asymptomatic apical periodontitis	Inflammation and destruction of apical periodontium that is of pulpal origin, appears as an apical radiolucent area, and does not produce clinical symptoms.
Acute apical abscess	An inflammatory reaction to pulpal infection and necrosis characterized by rapid onset, spontaneous pain, tenderness of the tooth to pressure, pus formation, and swelling of associated tissues.
Chronic apical abscess	An inflammatory reaction to pulpal infection and necrosis characterized by gradual onset, little or no discomfort, and the intermittent discharge of pus through an associated sinus tract.
Condensing osteitis	Diffuse radiopaque lesion representing a localized bony reaction to a low-grade inflammatory stimulus, usually seen at apex of tooth.

Figure 8.6   American Association of Endodontists Consensus Conference Recommended Diagnostic Terminology. *Source:* AAE Consensus Conference Recommended Diagnostic Terminology [3].

Formulation of Pulpal and Periradicular Diagnoses (Figure 8.7)

Remember that if test results are inconsistent and do not support a pulpal and apical diagnosis, then the toothache could be nonodontogenic (see Chapter 10). If you cannot diagnose it, don't treat it. Refer to a specialist to evaluate.

Diagnosis	Signs and Symptoms	Radiographic Appearance	Response to Pulp Tests[2]	Response to Periapical Tests[3]
Pulpal Diagnosis				
Normal Pulp (NP)[4]	None	No radiographic changes on radiographs	Response	No changes in responses to periapical tests
Reversible Pulpitis (RP)	May have Sharp Pain		Response	
Symptomatic Irreversible Pulpitis (SIP)[5]	Sharp Pain, but may have Deep, Dull, Gnawing Pain, Spontaneous Pain, Referred Pain, or a Past History of Pain		Response (may be extreme and/or lingering)	
Asymptomatic Irreversible Pulpitis (AIP)[5]	None, but may have a Past History of Pain		Response	
Pulp Necrosis (PN)	No Response		No Response	
Previously Treated (PT)[6]	No Response		No Response	
Previously Initiated Therapy (PIT)[6]	No Response		With or Without Response	
Periradicular (Periapical) Diagnosis?				
Normal Apical Tissues (NAT)[5]	None (WNL)[9]	No Periapical Changes	Not applicable	None (WNL)
Symptomatic Apical Periodontitis (SAP)[10]	Pain	1. No Significant Changes (may have widene pdl) or 2. Apical Radiolucency		Painful Response
Asymptomatic Apical Periodontitis (AAP)[11]	None (WNL)	Apical Radiolucency		None (WNL)
Acute Apical Abscess (AAA)[12]	Swelling With or Without Pain	With or Without Apical Radiolucency		With or Without Painful Response
Chronic Apical Abscess (CAA)[13]	Sinus Tract Without Pain (usually)	With or Without Apical Radiolucency		Usually No Response
Condensing Osteitis (CO)[14]	With or Without Pain	Radiopacity, may be framing a coexistent radiolucency		With or Without Response

Figure 8.7 Formulation of pulpal and periradicular diagnoses [4]. *Source:* Ørstavik, D. (2020). *Essential Endodontology: Prevention and Treatment of Apical Periodontitis.* Wiley-Blackwell.

Types of Tooth Fractures

Table 8.5 Types of tooth fractures.

Longitudinal tooth fracture	Description	Treatment	Prognosis	Additional information
Craze lines	• Limited to enamel • Asymptomatic	None	Very good	• Common in adults • Buccal, lingual, and marginal ridges of posteriors • Vertically on anteriors
Fractured cusp	Symptoms: not spontaneous, only when stimulated; brief sharp pain on masticatory release; may be cold sensitive	• Three-quarter or full coverage crown down to fracture • If cusp is not mobile, full coverage crown to hold the segments	Very good	• Usually associated with Class II restorations or caries • Tooth is usually vital
Cracked tooth	Symptoms: acute pain on mastication of grainy tough foods and sharp brief pain with cold. Other symptoms vary based on the pulpal and periapical status	Extraction (if crack extends to the pulp chamber floor)	Questionable to poor	• Usually mesiodistally crossing one or both marginal ridges and extends subgingivally • Radiographically not visible if mesiodistally • From most common to least common locations: mandibular second molar > mandibular first molar > maxillary second molar > maxillary premolar • May evolve into a split tooth or develop a periodontal defect • Percussion from one direction may induce pain by separating the crack while percussion from another direction may be painless
Split tooth	• Tooth segments are separable • Symptoms: pain on mastication, periodontal abscess	Varies: if severe requires extraction; may require RCT, crown lengthening, orthodontic extrusion, removal of segments, buildup, crown	Varies	• Radiographic: horizontal bone loss interproximally or at furcation • See Figures 10.10 and 10.11
Vertical root fracture	Involves the root only (from the apex up or begins midroot)	Varies: exploratory surgery (flab reflection), root amputation, hemisection, or extraction	Hopeless	Two major causes include post placement and obturation

Source: Based on Torabinejad and Walton [1].

Treatment Type and Indications

Table 8.6 Treatment type and indications.

Treatment type	Indications
Nonsurgical RCT	*Primary teeth* • Irreversible pulpitis or necrosis with no permanent successor • Pulpal necrosis with or without periradicular disease • Treatment will not jeopardize the permanent successor *Permanent teeth* • Symptomatic or asymptomatic irreversible pulpitis, with or without periapical disease • Necrotic pulp with or without periradicular disease • Teeth with a pulp that would be compromised during dental procedures • Restorative reason when placement of a core and possibly a post is necessary for retention of a fixed restoration • Cracked or fractured teeth with pulpal involvement • Teeth with thermal hypersensitivity that significantly interfere with normal function, when alternative methods have failed to reduce hypersensitivity • When teeth must be preserved over extraction in those receiving systemic treatment, including head and neck radiation treatment, bisphosphonates, chemotherapy, and/or corticosteroids [5]
Nonsurgical retreatment	• Continued periradicular pathosis, with symptoms • Radiographic evidence of a deficiency in the quality of root canal obturation when periradicular pathosis or symptoms continue after endodontic treatment • Persistent symptoms • Anticipated restorative or prosthetic procedures that could compromise any preexisting root canal obturations • Anticipated restorative or prosthetic procedures on a tooth where the previous treatment quality is questionable • Salivary contamination when bacterial leakage into the root canal system is suspected
Apicoectomy (endodontic surgery)	• Symptomatic periradicular pathosis following endodontic treatment • Periradicular lesion that enlarges after endodontic treatment • Marked overextension of obturating materials interfering with healing • Access for periradicular curettage, biopsy, or to an additional root • Access for root-end preparation and root-end filling • When the apical portion of the root canal system of a tooth with periradicular pathosis cannot be cleaned, shaped and obturated

Notes:
Table limited to only three types of endodontic procedures; more exist. Determine if in-house or referring (see Section Referral to an Endodontist).
Source: Based on American Association of Endodontists [6].

Endodontics

AAE Endodontic Case Difficulty Assessment Form and Guidelines (Figure 8.8)

american association of endodontists

AAE Endodontic Case Difficulty Assessment Form and Guidelines

Patient Information

Full Name

Street Address   Suite/Apt

City   State/Country   Zip

Phone

Email

Disposition

Treat in Office: ○ Yes ○ No

Refer Patient to:

Date

Guidelines for Using the AAE Endodontic Case Difficulty Assessment Form

The AAE designed the Endodontic Case Difficulty Assessment Form for use in endodontic curricula. The Assessment Form makes case selection more efficient, more consistent and easier to document. Dentists may also choose to use the Assessment Form to help with referral decision making and record keeping.

Conditions listed in this form should be considered potential risk factors that may complicate treatment and adversely affect the outcome. Levels of difficulty are sets of conditions that may not be controllable by the dentist. Risk factors can influence the ability to provide care at a consistently predictable level and impact the appropriate provision of care and quality assurance.

The Assessment Form enables a practitioner to assign a level of difficulty to a particular case.

Levels of Difficulty

MINIMAL DIFFICULTY
Preoperative condition indicates routine complexity (uncomplicated). These types of cases would exhibit only those factors listed in the MINIMAL DIFFICULTY category. Achieving a predictable treatment outcome should be attainable by a competent practitioner with limited experience.

MODERATE DIFFICULTY
Preoperative condition is complicated, exhibiting one or more patient or treatment factors listed in the MODERATE DIFFICULTY category. Achieving a predictable treatment outcome will be challenging for a competent, experienced practitioner.

HIGH DIFFICULTY
Preoperative condition is exceptionally complicated, exhibiting several factors listed in the MODERATE DIFFICULTY category or at least one in the HIGH DIFFICULTY category. Achieving a predictable treatment outcome will be challenging for even the most experienced practitioner with an extensive history of favorable outcomes.

Review your assessment of each case to determine the level of difficulty. If the level of difficulty exceeds your experience and comfort, you might consider referral to an endodontist.

Criteria and Subcriteria	MINIMAL DIFFICULTY	MODERATE DIFFICULTY	HIGH DIFFICULTY
A. PATIENT CONSIDERATIONS			
MEDICAL HISTORY	☐ No medical problem (ASA Class 1*)	☐ One or more medical problem (ASA Class 2*)	☐ Complex medical history/serious illness/disability (ASA Classes 3-5*)
ANESTHESIA	☐ No history of anesthesia problems	☐ Vasoconstrictor intolerance	☐ Difficulty achieving anesthesia
PATIENT DISPOSITION	☐ Cooperative and compliant	☐ Anxious but cooperative	☐ Uncooperative
ABILITY TO OPEN MOUTH	☐ No limitation	☐ Slight limitation in opening	☐ Significant limitation in opening
GAG REFLEX	☐ None	☐ Gags occasionally with radiographs/ treatment	☐ Extreme gag reflex which has compromised past dental care
EMERGENCY CONDITION	☐ Minimum pain or swelling	☐ Moderate pain or swelling	☐ Severe pain or swelling

The contribution of the Canadian Academy of Endodontics and others to the development of this form is gratefully acknowledged. The AAE Endodontic Case Difficulty Assessment Form is designed to aid the practitioner in determining appropriate case disposition. The American Association of Endodontists neither expressly nor implicitly warrants any positive results associated with the use of this form. This form may be reproduced but may not be amended or altered in any way. © American Association of Endodontists, 180 N. Stetson Ave., Suite 1500, Chicago, IL 60601; Phone: 800-872-3636 or 312-266-7255; Fax: 866-451-9020 or 312-266-9867; E-mail: info@aae.org; Website: aae.org

Access additional resources at aae.org

 american association of endodontists

Figure 8.8 AAE Endodontic Case Difficulty Assessment Form and Guidelines. *Source:* Courtesy of the American Association of Endodontists (AAE) [7].

Criteria and Subcriteria	MINIMAL DIFFICULTY	MODERATE DIFFICULTY	HIGH DIFFICULTY
B. DIAGNOSTIC AND TREATMENT CONSIDERATIONS			
DIAGNOSIS	☐ Signs and symptoms consistent with recognized pulpal and periapical conditions	☐ Extensive differential diagnosis of usual signs and symptoms required	☐ Confusing and complex signs and symptoms: difficult diagnosis ☐ History of chronic oral/facial pain
RADIOGRAPHIC DIFFICULTIES	☐ Minimal difficulty obtaining/interpreting radiographs	☐ Moderate difficulty obtaining/interpreting radiographs (e.g., high floor of mouth, narrow or low palatal vault, presence of tori)	☐ Extreme difficulty obtaining/interpreting radiographs (e.g., superimposed anatomical structures)
POSITION IN THE ARCH	☐ Anterior/premolar ☐ Slight inclination (<10°) ☐ Slight rotation (<10°)	☐ 1st molar ☐ Moderate inclination (10-30°) ☐ Moderate rotation (10-30°)	☐ 2nd or 3rd molar ☐ Extreme inclination (>30°) ☐ Extreme rotation (>30°)
TOOTH ISOLATION	☐ Routine rubber dam placement	☐ Simple pretreatment modification required for rubber dam isolation	☐ Extensive pretreatment modification required for rubber dam isolation
CROWN MORPHOLOGY	☐ Normal original crown morphology	☐ Full coverage restoration ☐ Porcelain restoration ☐ Bridge abutment ☐ Moderate deviation from normal tooth/root form (e.g., taurodontism microdens) ☐ Teeth with extensive coronal destruction	☐ Restoration does not reflect original anatomy/alignment ☐ Significant deviation from normal tooth/root form (e.g., fusion dens in dente)
CANAL AND ROOT MORPHOLOGY	☐ Slight or no curvature (<10°) ☐ Closed apex (<1 mm in diameter)	☐ Moderate curvature (10-30°) ☐ Crown axis differs moderatel from root axis. Apical opening 1-1.5 mm in diameter	☐ Extreme curvature (>30°) or S-shaped curve ☐ Mandibular premolar or anterior with 2 roots ☐ Maxillary premolar with 3 roots ☐ Canal divides in the middle or apical third ☐ Very long tooth (>25 mm) ☐ Open apex (>1.5 mm in diameter)
RADIOGRAPHIC APPEARANCE OF CANAL(S)	☐ Canal(s) visible and not reduced in size	☐ Canal(s) and chamber visible but reduced in size ☐ Pulp stones	☐ Indistinct canal path ☐ Canal(s) not visible
RESORPTION	☐ No resorption evident	☐ Minimal apical resorption	☐ Extensive apical resorption ☐ Internal resorption ☐ External resorption
C. ADDITIONAL CONSIDERATIONS			
TRAUMA HISTORY	☐ Uncomplicated crown fracture of mature or immature teeth	☐ Complicated crown fracture of mature teeth ☐ Subluxation	☐ Complicated crown fracture of immature teeth ☐ Horizontal root fracture ☐ Alveolar fracture ☐ Intrusive, extrusive or lateral luxation ☐ Avulsion
ENDODONTIC TREATMENT HISTORY	☐ No previous treatment	☐ Previous access without complications	☐ Previous access with complications (e.g., perforation, non-negotiated canal, ledge, separated instrument) ☐ Previous surgical or nonsurgical endodontic treatment completed
PERIODONTAL-ENDODONTIC CONDITION	☐ None or mild periodontal disease	☐ Concurrent moderate periodontal disease	☐ Concurrent severe periodontal disease ☐ Cracked teeth with periodontal complications ☐ Combined endodontic/periodontic lesion ☐ Root amputation prior to endodontic treatment

*American Society of Anesthesiologists (ASA) Classification System **Class 1:** No systemic illness. Patient healthy. **Class 2:** Patient with mild degree of systemic illness, but without functional restrictions, e.g., well-controlled hypertension. **Class 3:** Patient with severe degree of systemic illness which limits activities, but does not immobilize the patient. **Class 4:** Patient with severe systemic illness that immobilizes and is sometimes life threatening. **Class 5:** Patient will not survive more than 24 hours whether or not surgical intervention takes place. *www.asahq.org/clinical/physicalstatus.htm*

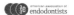

Figure 8.8 (Continued)

Treatment Planning (Table 8.7)

Table 8.7 Treatment planning phases related to endodontic treatment.

Treatment phase	Description (may or may not apply)
Emergency phase	Urgent treatment of pain, infection, trauma, and/or esthetic emergency
Data gathering phase	Endodontic diagnostic testing
Stabilization phase (to control disease)	Caries control (bleaching if desired prior) • Symptomatic teeth > larger cavities > smaller cavities
Definitive phase	Crowns
Maintenance phase	Follow-up of RCT tooth

- Discussion of additional fees: if additional treatment is necessary to save the tooth beyond RCT (e.g. crown lengthening, post and core, buildup, and/or a crown), discuss the fees *prior to* RCT. This is to prevent the patient from paying for RCT and then not being able to afford the additional treatment necessary to save the tooth, which may result in loss of the tooth.
- RCT and crown lengthening sequence:
  1) Determine if crown lengthening is required.
  2) Complete the RCT (in-house or refer to the endodontist).
  3) Prep the tooth and fabricate a temporary crown to the desired margins for the definitive crown.
  4) Refer to the periodontist for crown lengthening.
  5) Healing time: 8–12 weeks (restorative), four to six months (for esthetic cases).
  6) Refine the crown prep, make the final impression, and deliver the crown.
- Follow-up visits after RCT:
  - A one-month follow-up to verify a sinus tract has healed.
  - A six-month follow-up and additional follow-ups as necessary until healing is complete. This involves clinical and radiographic examination.
- Restore: once the tooth is asymptomatic.

Referral to an Endodontist

- Be sure the tooth is restorable before sending the patient to the endodontist for treatment.
- Be sure the patient can afford restorative treatment, including possible need for crown lengthening, post and core, core buildup, and a crown.
- If you suspect that crown lengthening is needed, or have determined this is needed, inform the endodontist the tooth is planned for RCT, then crown lengthening, then a definitive restoration.
- Emphasize to the patient being referred for RCT:
  - If postoperative complications occur, such as continued pain, return to the specialist for follow-up.
  - If the temporary filling falls out, you may need retreatment. Make sure they return soon for the definitive restoration (i.e. filling or crown) to prevent contamination (coronal leakage) into the root canal system and to prevent the tooth from fracturing off.
  - I need to see you back within one month to complete the crown. Timing is critical as the tooth can fracture and no longer be savable.

Sample Referral Form

History (including CC):
Tooth #:
Prognosis:
Diagnosis:

Pulpal:
- Normal pulp
- Reversible pulpitis
- Symptomatic irreversible pulpitis
- Asymptomatic irreversible pulpitis
- Pulp necrosis
- Previously initiated treatment
- Previously treated

Periapical Diagnosis:
- Normal apical tissues
- Symptomatic apical periodontitis
- Asymptomatic apical periodontitis
- Acute apical abscess
- Chronic apical abscess

- Inconclusive or conflicting diagnostic test results
- Other:

Treatment:
- Evaluation only
- Evaluation and appropriate treatment
- Nonsurgical root canal treatment or endodontic surgery
- Endodontic retreatment or endodontic surgery
- Post space preparation
- Prefabricated post and buildup
- Core buildup
- Orifice barrier and a temporary filling
- Other:

Additional remarks: (e.g. tooth planned for crown lengthening after RCT)
Please send endo report to: (email address/fax)

Informed Consent

- Informed consent is legally required for endodontic treatment.
- Be familiar with the informed consent forms in your office and be able to answer the patient's follow-up questions.
- Informed consent is governed by state law.
- There is no "one size fits all" consent form, due to the range of procedures and variances in state law.

Endodontics

- The AAE recommends that you consult with your professional liability carrier for specific guidance including sample forms.
- The informed consent must be in a face-to-face conversation that discloses the following:
  - The diagnosis
  - The nature of the proposed treatment or procedure
  - Risks reasonably associated with the proposed treatment or procedure
  - Prognosis after the proposed treatment or procedure
  - Feasible alternatives to the proposed treatment or procedure
  - Risks associated with declining treatment, and that "no treatment" is an alternative.
- There must be an opportunity for the patient and/or guardian to ask questions.
- The patient must sign the form, and may require the provider's signature, and/or a witness to sign.
- In some states, a notation that consent was obtained may be required in the medical/dental record [8].
- Sample of an informed consent form is shown below:

Sample Informed Consent Form

I hereby authorize _____ to perform root canal treatment on tooth number: _____.

I understand that a root canal treatment is a procedure to retain a tooth, which may otherwise require extraction. Although root canal treatment has a very high degree of clinical success, it is still a biological procedure, so its success cannot be guaranteed.

I (or my child/ward), _____, have been informed that I (or my child/ward) require an endodontic procedure (root canal treatment) to retain this tooth and that I fully understand the following:

1) Failure to follow this recommendation will most likely result in:
   a) The loss of the tooth.
   b) Bone destruction due to an abscess.
   c) Possible systemic (affecting the whole body) infection.
2) 5–10% of root canal treatments fail and many require retreatment, periapical surgery, or even extraction.
3) During cleaning of the tooth, tools may break and lodge permanently in the tooth. Also, an instrument may perforate the root wall. Although this occurs rarely, broken tools or perforations can cause root canal treatments to fail. This may lead to the need for further more complex treatment or referral to a root canal specialist (endodontist) or loss of the tooth.
4) Possible complications associated with root canal treatments are cracked teeth, blocked canals, curved roots, and gum disease. These are rare complications that can make the treatment impossible.
5) During or after the root canal treatment, there are some complications that could arise. These possible complications include swelling, bleeding, pain, infection, permanent or temporary numbness/tingling of the lip and/or tongue.
6) On occasion, while performing the root canal treatment, the cleaning solution used can cause sudden pain followed by rapid swelling that can last for a while. This pain and swelling will go away with time. Treatment involves waiting and taking pain medications if needed.

7) When making an access (opening) through an existing crown or by placing a rubber dam clamp, damage could occur to the existing crown and a new crown may be necessary following endodontic therapy.

8) Successful completion of the root canal treatment does not prevent future decay or fracture of the tooth.

9) Temporary fillings are usually placed in the tooth following root canal treatment. These endodontically treated teeth usually need a buildup and a crown will be required in order to restore the tooth to proper function and appearance. Failure to place the recommended final restoration, such as a crown, on a completed root canal treated tooth can result in tooth fracture or recurrent decay which in turn can result in failure of the root canal and eventual need for treatment or extraction.

There are risks involved in administration of anesthetics, analgesics (pain medication), and antibiotics.

I will inform the doctor of any previous side effects or allergies.

_____   _____

Date   Patient or Patient's Parent/Guardian Signature

_____   _____

Date   Witness to Signature

Armamentarium

- **Rubber dam/dental dam**: "Tooth isolation using the dental dam is the standard of care [and] is integral and essential for any non-surgical endodontic treatment." The rubber dam minimizes the risk of oral bacteria entering the root canal system, aids in visualization to maintain a clean operative field, and prevents ingestion or aspiration of dental materials, irrigants, and instruments [6]. On rare occasions with tooth alignment or rotations, a rubber dam may be placed after the access cavity preparation but no files or irrigation may be used without the rubber dam [5] (especially when crowned).
  - Rubber dam punch: used for punching a hole in the rubber dam for the clamp. The hole sizes, from largest to smallest, are for the clamp, molars, smaller molars, premolars, canines, upper anterior, and lower anterior.
  - Clamp anatomy: bow (faces distal), forceps holes, jaws (may be serrated) and four points, and wings (unless wingless). The advantage of a winged clamp is being able to place it into the mouth as one unit (Figure 8.9). Examples of clamp sizes are shown in Table 8.8.
  - If seepage, consider a smaller size dam punch or a liquid dam.
  - Sometimes with lack of tooth structure the gingiva must be clamped. Expect some postoperative discomfort.
  - Steps for placement: evaluate the mesial–distal width of the tooth being clamped. Select the appropriate winged clamp. Ligate the clamp with floss. Try the clamp for fit and stability. Remove the clamp and attach to the rubber dam with the frame and transfer to the mouth as one unit.
  - Liquid rubber dam: there are different products on the market, help seal areas of seepage between the tooth and rubber dam.

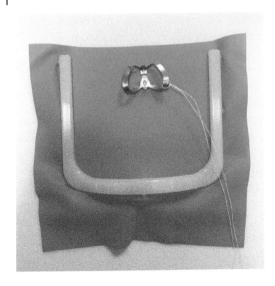

Figure 8.9 Winged #9 clamp should have the appearance of a butterfly flying into the patient's mouth.

Table 8.8 Clamp sizes for teeth.

Teeth	Clamp size
Anterior	9
Premolar and molar	2A
Small premolar	1
Large upper molar	14
Large lower molar	56

- **Files**: used for cleaning and shaping the canals. Files must contact and plane all walls to debride completely [1].
  - Length: typically 21, 25, and 31 mm long.
  - Size: refers to the diameter at the tip in hundredths of a millimeter, e.g. a #20 file is 0.20 mm in diameter at the tip. Sizes range from #6 to #140.
  - Taper: for example, 0.04 or 0.06 means that for every millimeter of length from the tip, the diameter increases by 0.04 or 0.06 mm.
  - Hand files: stainless steel and relatively inflexible [1]. See Figure 8.10.
  - Rotary files: nickel–titanium files. More flexible and adapt better to fine curved canals than stainless steel hand files. No cutting end and less likely to transport [1]. Do not pre-curve as this will weaken the file. A nickel allergy is not a contraindication as nickel–titanium is an alloy and not pure nickel. Even if the metals separate, this will not create a reaction. See Figure 8.11.

Figure 8.10 A hand file being inserted into the canal.

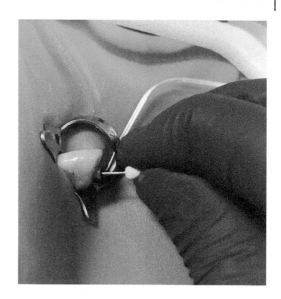

Figure 8.11 A rotary file being inserted into the canal.

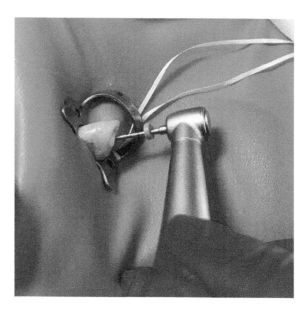

- **Endodontic microscope**: while loupes can magnify two and a half to six times, a microscope can magnify 4–25 times. Microscopes can improve ergonomics and visualization, and reduce eye muscle strain and fatigue (preventing eyes from rotating medially) [8].
- **Apex locator**: electronic device to help determine the length of the root canal (i.e. working length). Read the manufacturer's instructions. For patients with a pacemaker, see Chapter 1. Try to avoid causes of inaccurate measurements, which include:
  - An extremely dry canal
  - A large apical foramen (immature tooth or root resorption)
  - A large periapical lesion
  - A blocked canal

- – Contact of the file with:
  - o the gingiva (from a broken clinical crown)
  - o metal (e.g. PFM crown)
  - o caries in which the caries contacts the gingiva
  - o pulpal tissue or debris in the canal
- – Accessory canal
- – Root fracture
- – Gutta percha present in the canal
- – Blood, saliva, or chemical solutions overflowing from the canal to the gingiva [9].
- **Endo Ice**: a refrigerant spray used for vitality testing. See Section Pulp Sensitivity Testing for details of use.
- **Electric pulp test**: see Section Pulp Sensitivity Testing for detailed instructions of use.

Dental Materials

- **Sodium hypochlorite (NaOCl)**
  - – Purpose: also known as household bleach, it is used S36 to mechanically flush debris from the canal and dissolve vital and necrotic tissue. It has both antimicrobial and lubricating actions. Because of toxicity, extrusion must be avoided to prevent a "sodium hypochlorite accident" [1].
  - – Concentration ranges from 0.5 to 5.25%, but commonly used at 2.5% [1].
  - – Precautions
    - o *Do not* get in the patient's eyes (always use eye protection)
    - o *Do not* get on skin or soft tissue
    - o *Do not* get on clothes/shoes (will bleach)
    - o *Do not* extrude out the apex or a sodium hypochlorite accident may occur.
      - ▪ Extrude gently. The needle must be in the apical one-third for efficient irrigation; move up and down to produce agitation. Bend the needle or place a rubber stopper to control the depth of the needle.
      - ▪ Do not let the needle bind inside the tooth. It must be placed loosely in the canal. Use a side-venting needle.
      - ▪ Caution with an open apex.
    - o *Always* have the surgical suction on and resting on the tooth before delivering NaOCl to the tooth.
    - o Protocol for sodium hypochlorite accident:
      - ▪ Significance: can cause a life-threatening emergency (if swelling on the floor of the mouth compromises the airway) [1].
      - ▪ Signs and symptoms: sudden prolonged and sharp pain during irrigation followed by rapid diffuse swelling. This will subside spontaneously with time.
      - ▪ Treatment is palliative:
        - a) Analgesics and reassure the patient [1].
        - b) Irrigate with a lot of sterile saline.

     c) Inform the patient there may be bruising.

     d) If soft tissue was destroyed to the basement membrane, may require a tissue graft. If some tissue sloughing is present, a tissue graft may not be necessary if necrotic tissue is absent.

- Follow up with the patient to monitor progress [1].

- **Glycerin**
  - Purpose: a mild alcohol used as a lubricant placed on the shaft of files or deposited into the canal orifice to reduce the torsional forces on the instruments (i.e. hand and rotary files) and to decrease the potential for fracture.
    - Glycerin is recommended for hand files.
    - Lubricant is not needed for rotary files if sufficient sodium hypochlorite. Lubricant can create more friction and contribute to instrument fracture.

- **Ethylenediaminetetraacetic acid** (EDTA)
  - Purpose: used for removal of the smear layer (composed of organic pulpal materials and inorganic dentinal debris and may include bacteria and by-products). EDTA also deactivates sodium hypochlorite [1]. This allows gutta percha to adapt better, increases sealer adhesion, and decreases leakage.
  - Concentration: 17%.

- **Sodium perborate**
  - Purpose: the material of choice for internal bleaching. Once the powder is mixed with water it forms sodium metaborate, hydrogen peroxide, and nascent oxygen. More easily controlled and safer than hydrogen peroxide [1].
  - Concentration: powder form as 95% sodium perborate.

- **Calcium hydroxide**
  - Purpose: has antimicrobial activity due to the alkaline pH, and may dissolve necrotic tissue, bacteria, and their by-products [1]. Some brands (e.g. Ultradent's UltraCal) include a plastic canula; do not bind it in the canal and as you express the material back out to prevent extrusion.

- **Gutta percha**
  - Purpose: used for obturating the canals, it is composed of about 75% zinc oxide, 20% gutta percha, and binders, opaquers, and coloring agents [1]. Gutta percha is a rubber-like material from Brazilian trees.

- **Sealer**
  - Purpose: Provides a fluid-tight seal between the gutta percha and the canal walls. Variety of materials available, including zinc ocide–eugenol (ZOE), bioceramics, and epoxy resins. Zinc oxide–eugenol based sealers have a long history of success.

Endodontic Access

- You must have a knowledge of dental anatomy, including the likelihood of encountering multiple canals.
- Use the "rules of symmetry" to aid in locating the number and position of orifices in the pulp chamber floors, especially in teeth that are heavily restored, malpositioned, or calcified. This should aid in reducing the likelihood of perforating the tooth.

Endodontics

Rules of Symmetry

Table 8.9 Rules of symmetry.

Relationship of the pulp chamber to the clinical crown	
Law of centrality	The floor of the pulp chamber is always located in the center of the tooth at the level of the CEJ
Law of concentricity	The walls of the pulp chamber are always concentric to the external surface of the tooth at the level of the CEJ
Law of the CEJ	The CEJ is the most consistent, repeatable landmark for locating the position of the pulp chamber
Relationship of the pulp-chamber floor	
Law of symmetry 1	Except for maxillary molars, the orifices of the canals are equidistant from a line drawn in a mesial distal direction through the pulp-chamber floor
Law of symmetry 2	Except for maxillary molars, the orifices of the canals lie on a line perpendicular to a line drawn in a mesial distal direction across the center of the floor of the pulp chamber
Law of color change	The color of the pulp-chamber floor is always darker than the walls
Law of orifice location 1	The orifices of the root canals are always located at the junction of the walls and the floor
Law of orifice location 2	The orifices of the root canals are located at the angles in the floor–wall junction
Law of orifice location 3	The orifices of the root canals are located at the terminus of the root developmental fusion lines

Source: Based on Krasner and Ranjow [10].

The rules of symmetry are concerned with the relationship of the pulp chamber to the clinical crown, the relationship of the pulp chamber floor, and the color of the pulp-chamber floor, and provide a "roadmap." Note that it is more visible in larger chambers but not always visible (see Figure 8.1).

Teeth and Relevant Information (Table 8.10)

Table 8.10 Teeth and relevant information.

Teeth	Relevant information
Maxillary	
Central incisors	• Canals: 100% of the time have one canal
	• Tooth length/crown length/root length: 23.5 mm/10.5 mm/13 mm [11]
	• Outline form: triangular with apex at cingulum. As pulp recedes, more ovoid
	• Access steps: with a round bur perpendicular to the lingual surface, penetrate 2–3 mm, and then reorient the bur along the long axis
	• Dentin shelves: remove the lingual shelf
	• Midroot canal shape: round

(Continued)

Table 8.10 (Continued)

Teeth	Relevant information
Lateral incisors	• Canals: 100% of the time have one canal (unless dense en dente) • Tooth length/crown length/root length: 21 mm/9 mm/13 mm [11] • Outline form: triangular with apex at cingulum. As pulp recedes, more ovoid • Access steps: with round bur perpendicular to the lingual surface, penetrate 2–3 mm, and then reorient the bur along the long axis • Dentin shelves: remove the lingual shelf • Midroot canal shape: wider faciolingual • Precautions: root apex has a distal curve, don't transport. Tooth may have dens invaginatus with varying degrees of complexity
Canines	• Canals: 100% of the time have one canal • Tooth length/crown length/root length: 27 mm/10 mm/17 mm [11] • Outline form: ovoid. With attrition the access is closer to the incisal edge • Access steps: with a round bur perpendicular to the lingual surface, penetrate 2–3 mm, and then reorient the bur along the long axis • Dentin shelves: remove the lingual shelf • Midroot canal shape: wide faciolingual with slight hourglass shape
First premolars	• Canals: two, but could be one, and rarely three (two buccal and one palatal) • Tooth length/crown length/root length: 22.5 mm/8.5 mm/14 mm [11] • Outline form: ovoid in the faciolingual direction • Access steps: with round bur within the incline planes. If three canals, triangular with the apex at the palatal • Dentin shelves: remove the buccal and lingual dentin shelves • Midroot canal shape: if two separate canals, avoid. If one canal wide buccal–lingual • Precautions: mesial concavity. Do not perforate the mesial
Second premolars	Same as maxillary first premolar except: • Canals: two, but could be one, and rarely three (two buccal and one palatal) • Outline form: ovoid in the faciolingual direction. If three canals, triangular with the apex at the palatal
First molars	• Pulp chamber location: typically, cusp tip to pulp horn is 6 mm, pulp chamber height 1.5–2 mm, floor of pulp chamber to furcation 3 mm [12] • Canals: assume four canals (60% of the time). MB1, MB2, DB, P • Tooth length/crown length/root length: buccal 19.5 mm/7.5 mm/12 mm; palatal 20.5 mm/7.5 mm/13 mm [11] • Outline form: triangular with apex at the palatal. Oblique ridge left intact. DB canal in line with the buccal groove. Palatal canal largest, slightly distal to the ML cusp. MB1 canal slightly distal to the MB cusp. MB2 canal is 1–3 mm lingual to MB1 and slightly mesial to a line from MB1 to the palatal canal • Dentin shelves: remove the MB shelf for the MB1 and MB2, remove the DB shelf for the DB, remove the P shelf for the P • Midroot canal shape: P canal is wide mesiodistally. MB canal is wide buccolingually
Second molars	• Same as maxillary first molars except less common to have four canals but still plan for it and look for it
Third molars	• Varied, typically three canals with fused roots; consider extraction • Tooth length/crown length/root length: 17.5 mm/6.5 mm/11 mm [11]

Endodontics

(*Continued*)

Endodontics

Table 8.10 (Continued)

Teeth	Relevant information
Mandibular	
Central incisors	• Canals: 20–40% of the time have two canals. Careful examination with angled radiographs and exploration with a precurved hand file for the lingual canal • Tooth length/crown length/root length: 21.5 mm/9 mm/12.5 mm [11] • Outline form: triangular with apex at cingulum. As pulp recedes, more ovoid. With attrition, access is more incisal • Access steps: with round bur perpendicular to the lingual surface, penetrate 2–3 mm, and then reorient the bur along the long axis, straightening it up toward the incisal edge (not toward the cingulum) • Dentin shelves: remove the lingual shelf • Midroot canal shape: if one canal a ribbon-like shape broad faciolingually, or two canals • Miscellaneous: if crowding or receded canal, a facial approach may be used • Precautions: do not perforate the facial
Lateral incisors	Same as mandibular central incisors except: • Tooth length/crown length/root length: 23.5 mm/9.5 mm/14 mm [11]
Canines	Same as mandibular central incisors except: • Canals: may contain two • Tooth length/crown length/root length: 27 mm/11 mm/16 mm [11] • Access shape: ovoid
First premolars	• Canals: one (70%), two, or three and often divide deep within the root • Tooth length/crown length/root length: 22.5 mm/8.5 mm/14 mm [11] • Outline form: ovoid in the buccolingual dimension located buccal to the central groove • Dentin shelves: remove the lingual shelf • Midroot canal shape: round • Precautions: complex anatomy. May have a "fast break" (appears as one canal that disappears into multiple small canals)
Second premolars	Same as mandibular second premolars except: • 85% have one canal • Tooth length/crown length/root length: 22.5 mm/8.0 mm/14.5 mm [11]
First molars	• Pulp chamber location: typically, cusp tip to pulp horn is 6 mm, pulp chamber height 1.5–2 mm, floor of pulp chamber to furcation 3 mm [12] • Canals: MB, ML, DB, DL, and one D canal 70% of the time • Tooth length/crown length/root length: 21.5 mm/7.5 mm/14 mm [11] • Outline form: rectangular or trapezoidal. The MB canal is under the MB cusp and slightly distal to MB cusp, ML on central groove slightly distal to MB canal, D canal at the intersection of the buccal, lingual, and central grooves, DB canal buccal and mesial to the D canal • Dentin shelves: remove the MB shelf for the MB canal, the ML shelf for the ML canal, if one D canal the D shelf for the D canal, or the DB shelf for the DB canal and the DL shelf for the DL canal • Midroot canal shape: round for all canals, except if one D canal then ovoid in the faciolingual direction • Precaution: concavity in the furcation. Avoid perforation or stripping
Second molars	Same as mandibular first molars except: • Canals: MB, ML, DB, DL, and one D canal 92% of the time • Tooth length/crown length/root length: 20 mm/7 mm/13 mm [11]
Third molars	• Varied and consider extraction • Tooth length/crown length/root length: 18 mm/7 mm/11 mm [11]

Source: Based on Torabinejad and Walton [1].

Endodontic Access Tips

Figure 8.12 Endodontic access shapes.

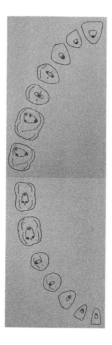

- Refer to Table 8.10 and Figure 8.12.
- The goal is to have straight-line access to the apical portion of the canal or to the first curvature.
- Before accessing, identify the shape of the CEJ by probing around the tooth. Important to note the shape, for example, of concavities to avoid perforating.
- Look at the bur from all angles with the mirror to avoid perforation.
- Bitewing radiographs give a more accurate anatomic position and information for posterior teeth than periapical radiographs.
- You may have to remove a Class V restoration because it can obstruct the view on the bitewing of the pulp-chamber shape and location for posteriors.
- The high-speed round bur may not "drop" into the chamber if it is narrow occluso-apically.
- Remove the pulp horns. If not removed, then bacteria will be left in the access and discoloration will follow. With a round bur engage the pulp-chamber walls laterally under the overhang and pull up (occlusally).
- Do not remove the marginal ridges in the access.
- Keep in mind the location of the dentin shelf to remove with the rotary files.
- Keep in mind the midroot shape when cleaning, shaping, and obturating.
- Keep in mind that anatomic variations exist with the number of roots, number of canals, canal morphology (e.g. round, hourglass, ovoid, bowling pin, kidney bean, C-shaped).

Procedural Steps

- Remember you are held to the same standards as endodontists if you provide RCT.
- Many different approaches, philosophies, techniques, materials, and systems for RCT.
- Be sure you have all the equipment necessary, including fully functioning units, charged batteries, and adequate supplies (e.g. sufficient small hand files, gutta percha points).
- Be familiar with procedural accidents, and how to prevent, recognize, and treat.

Endodontics

Pulpotomy

- Definition: removal of the inflamed tissue restricted to the pulp chamber [13]. Note: removing tissue from the radicular pulp only. This is typically only for molars as there must be a defined pulp chamber that is clearly differentiated from the radicular pulp.
- Indications: a vital pulp with symptomatic irreversible pulpitis with or without symptomatic apical periodontitis when time does not permit a pulpectomy [1].
- Obtain verbal/written consent.
- Eye protection for the patient.
- Local anesthesia.
- Cold test to verify profound anesthesia.
- Rubber dam isolation.
- Access the pulp chamber, flush with sodium hypochlorite, and place calcium hydroxide, cotton, or foam, and a temporary filling to seal the endodontic access.
- Occlusal adjustment taking the tooth out of occlusion.
- Initiate RCT within six months to avoid another painful episode [13].
- If swelling, consider incision and drainage: release fluid pressure, reduce microbial and inflammatory mediators, and prevent the spread of infection to deeper fascial tissues [13].
- If swelling, lymphadenopathy, fever, and/or malaise, prescribe antibiotics (see Chapter 16).
- See Section Postoperative Instructions.

Pulpectomy

- Definition: extirpation of the inflamed tissues in the root canal system. There is a 90% success rate in reducing postoperative pain, from moderate–severe to mild/no pain [13] (Figure 8.13). Referred to as a "pulpal debridement" if the pulp is necrotic.
- Indications:
  - For emergency cases to relieve pain.
  - Requires an adequate amount of time to clean and shape when there is pulpal necrosis without swelling, with localized swelling, or with diffuse swelling [13] (pulpal debridement).
  - Adequate amount of time required to clean and shape when vital (pulpectomy).
- A common mistake is partial removal of the pulp. Do not enter the pulp unless you are prepared to clean and shape all the canals. This can lead to greater postoperative pain [13].
- Obtain verbal/written consent.
- Eye protection for the patient.
- Local anesthesia.
- Cold test to verify profound anesthesia.
- Rubber dam isolation
- Clean and shape (see Sections Nonsurgical Root Canal Treatment and Follow-up).
- After cleaning and shaping, insert calcium hydroxide into the canals and place a cotton pellet and a temporary filling.
- Occlusal adjustment to take the tooth out of occlusion (to decrease discomfort).
- If swelling, consider incision and drainage to release fluid pressure, reduce microbial and inflammatory mediators, and prevent the spread of infection to deeper fascial tissues [13].
- If swelling, lymphadenopathy, fever, and/or malaise, prescribe antibiotics (see Chapter 16).
- See Section Postoperative Instructions.

Figure 8.13 Size 10 hand file with retained pulpal tissue during a pulpectomy.

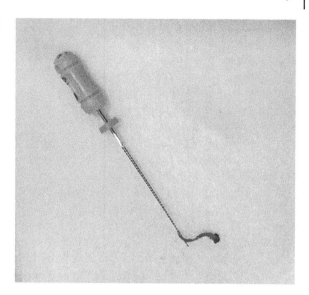

Table 8.11 Summary of emergency treatments for teeth.

Tooth status	Treatment if limited time	Treatment if adequate time
Vital	Pulpotomy	Pulpectomy (more effective at alleviating pain)
Necrotic	Recommend pulpal debridement	Pulpal debridement

Nonsurgical Root Canal Treatment

- Before the procedure evaluate the preoperative radiographs (Table 8.12).
  - BW and PA for posterior: evaluate the size, shape and location of the pulp chamber.
  - PA for anterior.
  - Measure the preoperative working length (WL) (Figure 8.14).
- Explain the procedure.
- Obtain written and verbal consent.
- Mirror check only if the patient is not convinced which tooth is showing a positive cold test.
- Provide eye protection (i.e. to prevent getting sodium hypochlorite in the eyes and to protect the eyes from sharp files).
- Local anesthesia.
- Obtain a preliminary impression (for a future temporary crown).
- Mark the tooth with a Thompson stick (to ensure the correct tooth is accessed once the rubber dam is placed).
- Cold test to verify profound anesthesia.
- Presence of sinus tract? Perforate and irrigate with saline.
- Place the rubber dam.
- Remove decay: "Complete removal of existing restorative materials in their entirety provide[s] a better coronal seal and allow[s] a more complete understanding of the remaining tooth structure and restorability of the tooth following treatment" [5].
- Deroof the pulp chamber.

- Document the intrapulpal status (e.g. bleeding, suppuration, necrotic): if suppuration, drain or suction it.
- Intrapulpal injection of local anesthetic:
  - Warn the patient "You will feel pressure."
  - Can cause tachycardia temporarily.
  - Not indicated if necrotic.
- Verify all canals are accessed:
  - Scout the canals with a small hand file (size 10, or 6 or 8).
  - If the file does not advance, bend the last 5 mm.
- Use the Apex locator with a #15 file (minimum size for radiograph) to determine the WL (Figure 8.15). Advance until it displays "apex" (you are at the tip of the tooth) and then withdraw slowly until halfway between "apex" and 1 (1 should be close to 1 mm). If a large PARL, recommend to be at 1.
- Working length PA: the file should be 0.5–1 mm from the radiographic apex [5].
- If the radiographic WL looks good, then set the rubber stopper on all the files to the WL.
- Refine the access with a non-end-cutting bur (keep pulp chamber floor anatomy intact).
- Clean and shape with hand files and rotary files (Figure 8.16).
  - How to use hand files and rotary files
    - Sequence: lubricate, clean and shape, irrigate, recapitulate, repeat.
    - Clean and shape:
      - Lubricate every hand file (e.g. with glycerin). For rotary files, use sodium hypochlorite as the lubricant.
      - With every file insert and when removing brush along the B, repeat along M, repeat along L, repeat along D and remove.
      - Clean the flutes of the file with an alcohol wipe.
      - Inspect the file for unwinding, overwinding, or breakage.
    - Irrigate with sodium hypochlorite.
    - Recapitulate using a #15 hand file to WL (to loosen debris and prevent blockage).
  - The goal is to keep the apical foramen as small as practical.
  - Remove the dentin shelves (go in direction of that canal, e.g. MB canal shape in the M and B direction).
  - Pre-flare with the hand files
    - Combine reaming and filing:
      - Reaming: clockwise and counterclockwise.
      - Filing: up and down motion.
    - Lubricate, insert the file, ream and file, wipe debris off with an alcohol wipe, irrigate, recapitulate, repeat.
    - Continue from size #10 up to #25. Files above #25 do not bend well, and can cause a ledge, perforation, or transportation.
- Pre-flare with Gates Glidden to two-thirds the WL (slow speed 800 rpm).
  - For removal of dentin shelves.
  - $WL \times \frac{2}{3} = x$ (size 2), then $x - 3$ mm is size 3, and $x - 6$ mm is size 4.
  - Gates Glidden creates a large amounts of debris, so requires copious irrigation.
  - Direct the cutting away from the furcations on multirooted teeth
- "Crown down" with rotary files to reduce the risk of fracture and to remove the most diseased portion before proceeding apically, reducing the likelihood of packing debris blocking canals, and allowing deeper irrigation.
  - Use 350 rpm (slow speed).

- Lateral brushing on the out movements.
- Begin with a large file and move sequentially down to a smaller file until you reach the WL.
  - ○ File sizes #30–35 in most canals reaches the WL.
  - ○ Smallest file size recommended to WL is #25 (if smaller the gutta percha may not reach and become crinkled).
  - ○ Largest file size may go to #40 in large canals (e.g. palatal root or mandibular molar).
- Select a master apical cone that coincides with the master apical file size.
  - Measure the WL on the cone and crimp it with the cotton pliers.
  - Place to the WL; should feel tug back.
- Master apical cone PA.
- For warm vertical obturation: (Figure 8.17)
  - Remove the master apical cone.
  - Pre-fit the plugger for the down-pack to see which is the largest that fits and goes down 4–5 mm shy of the WL. Place a rubber stopper on the plugger.
  - Place 17% EDTA for one minute (or citric acid 10%).
  - Dry the canals with paper points.
  - Coat the master apical cone with sealer: only coat the apical one-third for warm vertical obturation.
  - Place sealer in the canal walls with a size #15 hand file.
  - Slowly insert the master apical cone until it reaches WL (use the crimp as your reference guide).
  - Obturate one canal at a time.
  - Warn the patient "You will feel warm and pressure temporarily."
  - Down-pack: with a heated plugger insert into the canal in increments until 5 mm short of the WL. Wait 10 seconds, place a burst of heat and remove (twist and pull).
  - Down-pack PA (optional, to verify that the apical 5 mm are sealed).
  - If a post and core is planned, place the post (see Chapter 11).
  - Pack with a cold hand plugger.
  - Back fill
    - ○ Verify the back-fill tip reaches the gutta percha (5 mm from the WL). If not, go back to down-pack.
    - ○ Extrude the back-fill gutta percha on a gauze to confirm it is working.
    - ○ Dip the tip in sealer.
    - ○ Insert the back-fill tip and contact the gutta percha in the canal, wait for five seconds (to melt the most coronal portion of the gutta percha) and then extrude as the tip "pushes" you out.
  - Pack the gutta percha with a cold hand plugger so that it is below the CEJ: can remove the excess gutta percha with a high-speed bur.
- Coronal seal
  - Determine if placing a temporary or permanent restoration today.
  - For post and core and crowns, see Chapter 11.
  - Remove any sealer and gutta percha from the pulp chamber, which can make the tooth appear dark (clean with alcohol on a cotton pellet).
  - Temporary coronal seal:
    - ○ Dry the walls.
    - ○ Place glass ionomer over the gutta percha (e.g. Limelite, Vitrebond).
    - ○ Place a piece of foam or a cotton pellet.
    - ○ Pack Cavit against the walls in layers (requires 3–4 mm for strength/seal) or place Fuji Triage.

Endodontics

- Permanent coronal seal:
  - ○ Place glass ionomer over the gutta percha (e.g. Limelite, Vitrebond).
  - ○ Fill the chamber with Fuji IX.
- Remove the rubber dam/clamp, and adjust the occlusion.
- Postoperative PA:
  - Evaluate the PA.
  - Check for a homogeneous radiopaque appearance free of voids and filled to WL [5] with a continuous tapering conical form.
  - Is a puff of sealer present? May be well tolerated and absorbed by the periradicular tissue over time but should be prevented. Will be destructive if compacted into periradicular tissues, the maxillary sinus, or the mandibular canal [5] (Figure 8.18).
  - Overfills/extrusion: may prevent healing and could be associated with nerve damage and permanent injury (paresthesia and dysesthesia) [5].
- Administer a long-acting anesthetic.
- If symptomatic on biting, enameloplasty for a very light occlusion.
- See Section Postoperative Instructions.

Table 8.12   Radiographs for nonsurgical root canal treatment.

Preoperative radiographs

BW and PA* (if posterior)
PA* (if anterior)
*Angled PA if possibility of more than one canal

Working radiographs

1 PA (working length)
1 PA (master apical cone)
1 PA (optional, to see the down-pack)
1 PA (postoperative without rubber dam/clamp, with a filling)

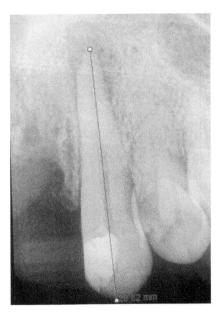

Figure 8.14   Preoperative radiographic working length measurement.

Figure 8.15 Using the Apex locator to determine the working length.

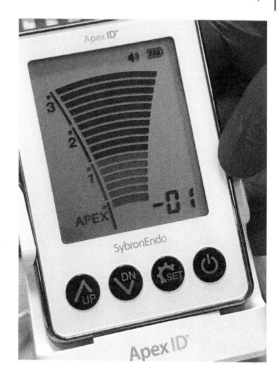

Figure 8.16 EndoRing used to hold and measure hand and rotary files.

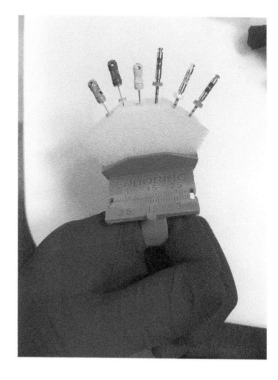

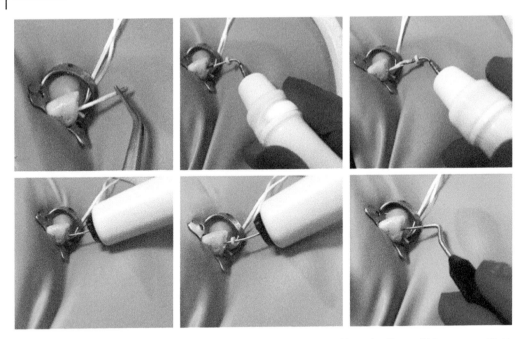

Figure 8.17 Warm vertical obturation. Placement of the master cone with sealer. Shear off the excess with the down-packing instrument to leave 5 mm of gutta percha for the apical seal. Use the backfill instrument to fill the remaining portion of the canal. Use a hand plugger instrument to pack the gutta percha apical to the CEJ.

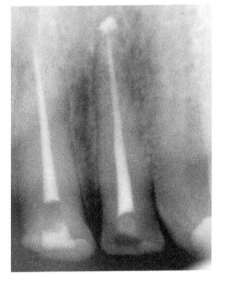

Figure 8.18 Postoperative PA. Note that the "puff" of sealer should be prevented.

Follow-up

- Timeline
  - At one month to evaluate if the sinus tract has healed (only if applicable). In an immunocompetent patient it should heal within two to three weeks; if a smoker/diabetic/immunocompromised, it can take longer. If a parulis, it can take time for the tissue to retract.

- – At six months.
- – Possibly at one year if still healing.
- Clinical exam
  - – Evaluate clinically for the absence of pain, swelling, sinus tract, and soft tissue destruction (e.g. probing depths) [1].
  - – Check pocket depths and mobility.
  - – Percuss and palpate.
  - – Cold test only if the tooth is still sensitive.
  - – Verify the restoration is still intact.
- Radiographic exam
  - – Evaluate the PA and check for any PARL.
  - – See Table 8.13 for the prognosis based on the PARL.

Table 8.13   Prognosis based on radiolucency.

Prognosis	Radiolucency?
Success	• Resolved • None developed
Questionable	• Remained the same size • Decreased in size but not significantly
Failure[a]	• Remained the same size • Enlarged • Developed

[a] Do not tell the patient the root canal "failed." Better to explain to the patient that "the bone didn't heal."
Source: Torabinejad and Walton [1].

- Internal bleaching
  - – Various internal (nonvital) bleaching techniques exist for root canal-treated teeth. The walking bleach technique is described here.
  - – Indications: discolorations of pulp chamber origin, dentin discolorations, and discolorations not amenable to external bleaching (Figure 8.19).
  - – Procedural steps:
    - o Verbal and written consent.
    - o Clinical and radiographic exam:
      - ▪ If retreatment necessary, complete prior to internal bleaching.
      - ▪ Evaluate the quality and shade of the existing restorations on the tooth for possible replacement.
    - o Determine the preoperative shade of the tooth with a shade guide.
    - o Take preoperative photographs (at the first and subsequent visits).
    - o Rubber dam isolation.
    - o Remove the restoration sealing the endodontic access.
    - o Remove any obturating material in the pulp chamber to the gingival margin.
    - o "Open" any pulp horns for access.
    - o Remove all composite, taking care not to perforate the tooth.

o If any discoloration from a metallic restoration, remove a thin layer of the stained dentin with a slow-speed bur.
o Mix sodium perborate with water, saline, or anesthetic material to the consistency of wet sand.
o Pack the material into the pulp chamber.
o Condense and remove excess liquid with a dry cotton pellet.
o Leave 3 mm of space for temporary material.
o Place temporary material (e.g. Cavit, IRM) to seal the access.
o Schedule next visit to repeat the procedure two to six weeks later [1].
o See Section Postoperative Instructions.

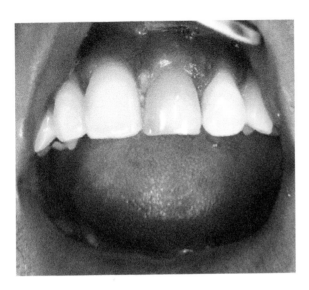

Figure 8.19 Note tooth #9 is discolored.

Postoperative Instructions

Nonsurgical Root Canal Treatment

- Day 1
  - Take care during the first several hours, especially when eating, not to bite your cheek, lip, or tongue until the numbness wears off.
  - Eat soft foods and be sure to stay hydrated with water.
  - Postoperative discomfort is expected and varies.
  - Take 600 mg of ibuprofen and alternate with 500 mg of acetaminophen every two hours (instead of taking the two medications together, in which case both can wear off at the same time) to prevent greater peaks and valleys of postoperative pain.
  - The gums may be sore from the rubber dam clamp. To reduce swelling swish warm salt water rinses 10–20 times a day.
- Week 1
  - It is normal to have some discomfort when chewing food.
  - Continue taking ibuprofen and acetaminophen as needed.
  - Discomfort can peak on day three, but is highly dependent on the amount of preoperative pain (especially if periradicular; if only pulpal pain is present, then RCT should relieve the pain).
  - Continue eating soft foods and progress to harder foods once comfortable to do so.

- If a temporary filling was placed:
  - ○ It is normal for a small amount to wear off.
  - ○ If the entire filling falls out, return to the office as soon as possible.
  - ○ If the temporary filling involves the surfaces between the teeth, be careful when flossing: pull out the side of the tooth to prevent dislodging the temporary filling.
- Crown appointments: if a crown was recommended, any delay can result in the tooth breaking and no longer being salvageable. In addition, any leakage of bacteria in the mouth into the root canal-treated tooth can also cause failure.
- Six-month follow-up: in order to track the healing process, return for a six-month follow-up appointment. More follow-up appointments may be necessary.

Pulpotomy, Pulpectomy, or Pulpal Debridement

- Same postoperative instructions as for nonsurgical root canal treatment.
- Be sure to return to the office (or to the endodontist) soon for RCT as delays can result in pain, systemic involvement, and other complications such as a fractured tooth.

Internal Bleaching

- The bleaching agent works slowly and any lightening may not show for two to six weeks.
- It may be necessary to perform the internal bleaching up to four separate times to achieve the desired results. After four times, further attempts may not improve the results.
- Be sure to return for replacement of the temporary filling with a permanent filling.

Procedural Accidents

You should be familiar with types of procedural accidents, including prevention, how to identify once they have occurred (radiographically, signs, symptoms), treatment, and prognosis.
Types of procedural accidents include:

- Perforation
- Ledge formation
- Creating an artificial canal (transportation)
- Root perforation
- Separated instrument
- Aspiration or ingestion
- Extrusion of irrigants ("sodium hypochlorite accident") (see Section Dental Materials)
- Overfilling (extrusion)
- Vertical root fracture [1].

Charting Template

Treatment records should include:

- Chief complaint(s) in the patient's own words
- Pain level (0–10)

Endodontics

- Current medical and dental history
- Radiographic findings
- Results of diagnostic tests and clinical examination
- Pulpal and periradicular diagnosis
- Treatment recommendations
- Informed consent (in some states, a notation that consent was obtained may be required in the medical/dental record) [14]
- Treatment rendered, including pulpal status on entry
- Prognosis
- Recommendations for tooth restoration
- Any prescriptions and consultations [6]

Clinical Pearls

Troubleshooting

- Unsure if the patient is numb before accessing the tooth? Cold test the tooth. If there is no response, proceed. If there is a response, add more anesthetic.
- Unsure if you have reached the pulp horns or the pulp chamber floor?
  - See Table 8.9.
  - The pulp chamber, if large enough, may have a "roadmap" on the pulp chamber floor connecting the orifices.
  - Take care not to perforate the floor. Recommend opening the canals carefully while determining if at the pulp horn or floor. This process may deroof the pulp chamber.
  - You could also take a radiograph to evaluate how far you have gone with your bur.
- File not reaching the WL? Never force a file; it can untwist, weaken, or break. Go back to the smaller previous file and enlarge the canal more.
- Premolar with two canals that converge?
  - Determine which canal is longer with the hand files.
  - Let's call one file A, the other B.
    - ○ Try in A then B, and try in B then A. If one file goes in further (A or B), that file is longer and is reaching the WL. Obturate the file that reaches WL first to prevent blockage of the canal.
- Difficulty differentiating multiple files on the radiograph? Can use different size files, different types of file (e.g. Hedstrom file and a K-file), or the SLOB rule.
- Master cone that appears crinkled in the apical third? Recommend cutting it shorter and reaching WL and feeling "tug back" and taking a new PA.
- Gutta percha not reaching WL? Either clean and shape more, or decrease the gutta percha size to reach WL and measure the length to prevent extruding out the apex.
- Hyperemic pulp? To control hemostasis:
  - Use a hemostatic agent (e.g. Viscostat) and compress with a cotton pellet, or
  - Administer intrapulpal anesthetic with epinephrine, or
  - Insert a paper point with a hemostatic solution for one minute, then rinse with sodium hypochlorite.
  - Difficulty obturating a C-shaped canal? These are complex. Refer to an endodontist. Prior to initiating RCT and finding a C-shaped canal, evaluate the radiograph. If a molar has a conical root, this may be indicative of a C-shaped canal.

Tips

- One versus two appointments for RCT:
  - One appointment for asymptomatic patients.
  - Two appointments: for complex or time-consuming cases, where exudate is present, the patient or dentist is tired or impatient, or when severe symptoms are present because if pain persists it is harder to manage once obturated.
- Billing advice: only bill the diagnostic radiograph (e.g. one PA) for diagnosis; all the other "working radiographs" during the treatment are included in the global RCT fee, including a postoperative radiograph within 30 days.
- Be careful when using the down-pack heated plugger not to apply pressure with your finger to push it apically as it is very hot (200°C or 400°F).
- When using hand or rotary files, occasionally measure the WL on the file as the rubber stopper can slide up the file.
- Don't rely on the WL from the last visit (that you or another dentist measured) as it may be inaccurate. Retake the WL.
- When removing Cavit from the pulp chamber placed by the endodontist, use an ultrasonic scaler.
- Select reverse on the rotary handpiece if you want to push material down apically (e.g. calcium hydroxide).
- For the percussion test, if a tooth is extremely sensitive try percussing with your finger. If no response, then use the end of the mouth mirror handle.
- Anesthetizing a mandibular molar when it is a "hot tooth":
  - Premedicate with ibuprofen.
  - Aim high for the inferior alveolar nerve block. Anesthetize with a plain anesthetic so it does not burn (i.e. mepivacaine) followed by two cartridges of lidocaine.
  - Long buccal with one cartridge of articaine.
  - Wait 10 minutes.
  - Cold test:
    - If still symptomatic, lingual infiltration to anesthetize the mylohyoid nerve.
    - Consider intraosseous injection.

Real-Life Clinical Scenarios Answered

Dental Students' Questions

- "How do I pulp test a tooth?"
  - See Section Diagnostic Testing
- "I'm not going to be an endodontist so why do I need to know the endo access shape for every tooth?"
  - Even if you plan to refer every root canal to an endodontist, you still need to be able to offer palliative treatment to help relieve your patients of intense pain. For this reason, you need to know how to access any tooth in the mouth, even a third molar.
- "How do I know if the patient needs a pulpotomy or a pulpectomy?"
  - See Table 8.11.
- "How can I tell if it's a cracked tooth?"
  - See Table 8.5.

Endodontics

- "How do I know if this is a periodontal abscess or endodontic abscess?"
  - See Section Diagnostic Terminology.
  - See Section Formulation of Pulpal and Periradicular Diagnoses.
  - See Chapter 6, section What is a Periodontal Abscess?
- "I'm trying to drill out this temporary material to do the core buildup and it feels really hard and I'm afraid of damaging the floor of the pulp chamber."
  - Did you obtain the endodontic report? Always be sure to obtain and read the report prior to proceeding with treatment (e.g. core buildup, crown prep). The report will provide information regarding the treatment completed, the prognosis, and recommendations. See Figure 8.20 for examples of critical information found in endodontic reports. Obtain the report from the specialist and do not take the patient's word for what happened.

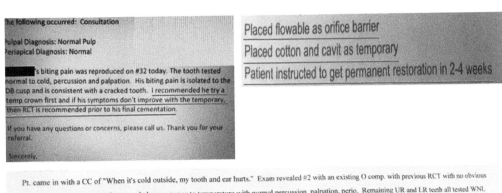

The following occurred: Consultation

Pulpal Diagnosis: Normal Pulp
Periapical Diagnosis: Normal

_____'s biting pain was reproduced on #32 today. The tooth tested normal to cold, percussion and palpation. His biting pain is isolated to the DB cusp and is consistent with a cracked tooth. I recommended he try a temp crown first and if his symptoms don't improve with the temporary, then RCT is recommended prior to his final cementation.

If you have any questions or concerns, please call us. Thank you for your referral.

Sincerely,

Placed flowable as orifice barrier

Placed cotton and cavit as temporary

Patient instructed to get permanent restoration in 2-4 weeks

Pt. came in with a CC of "When it's cold outside, my tooth and ear hurts." Exam revealed #2 with an existing O comp. with previous RCT with no obvious PA pathology. Vitality testing revealed no response to temperature with normal percussion, palpation, perio. Remaining UR and LR teeth all tested WNL without lingering pain.

Dx. #2- previously treated with normal apical tissue. RCT re-tx. was not recommended. Informed pt. of normal findings. Told pt. pain to cold involving her ear is likely non-odontogenic. Pt. will consult with an ENT physician for evaluation. Please let me know if I can be of further assistance.

Figure 8.20 Examples of portions of endodontic reports with critical information for the general dentist regarding the patient's treatment plans.

- "When should we get a CBCT of the tooth?"
  - CBCT (Figure 8.21) should not be used routinely for endodontics. Indications include:
    - When the patient's history and clinical exam demonstrate that the benefits outweigh the potential risks.
    - When the imaging cannot be met by lower-dose two-dimensional radiography [15].
    - May be necessary to evaluate the existence of extra canals, complex morphology, curvatures and/or dental developmental anomalies [5].

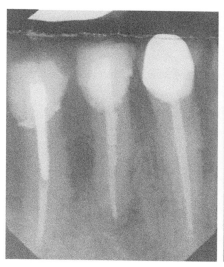
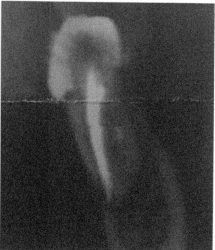

Figure 8.21 CBCT image on an endo report of a missed lingual canal.

- "How long will it take for the PARL to heal?"
  - This depends on the size of the lesion, severity of the disease, and the host response.
  - See Section Procedural Steps: Follow-up.
- "How do I know if the tooth needs a retreatment or endodontic surgery?"
  - See Table 8.6.

Dental Assistant's Comment

- "I don't like using the rubber dam and you don't need it for this buildup."
  - This decision is not up to your dental assistant. Rubber dam isolation is considered the standard of care for endodontic treatment [6]. When removing the temporary filling to place a permanent buildup, the gutta percha will be exposed. Bacteria in the mouth can reenter the endodontic access and recontaminate the canals. Always use the rubber dam (Figure 8.22).
  - Remove Cavit with slow speed and irrigate with sterile saline because the water lines are not sterile if using the high speed with water.

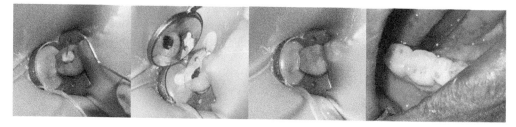

Figure 8.22 Always use rubber dam isolation for nonsurgical endodontic treatment, including removal of temporary filling and placement of a core buildup.

Endodontics

Patients' Comments

- "Ever since I fell down this tooth has been dark"
  - There are many reasons for teeth discolorations; however, with a history of trauma it may cause intrapulpal hemorrhage that results in disrupted blood vessels, hemorrhage, and lysis of erythrocytes. It is theorized that the by-products of tissue disintegration enter the dentinal tubules causing discoloration [1]. The discolored tooth may be necrotic. Recommend clinical/radiographic exam and endodontic testing. Tooth may require RCT and the patient may be interested in internal bleaching.
- "Doc, the tooth doesn't hurt so I'll let you know when it hurts then we can schedule the root canal."
  - If you recommend RCT and the patient declines, the patient needs to be aware of the risks involved with no treatment. This includes loss of tooth, bone destruction which can lead to loss of the tooth and other teeth, and systemic infection.
  - A patient cannot consent to substandard treatment. Contact your malpractice carrier and/or lawyer for guidance.
- "I know which tooth it is that needs the root canal. You don't have to test it."
  - Inform the patient that referred pain is a real phenomenon and you want to confirm the diagnosis as this will dictate the treatment. Do not take the patient's word. Imagine believing the patient, then completing the RCT only to find that the painful symptoms continue because it was a different tooth that needed RCT. Pain can be referred from the upper arch to the lower arch, from a distal tooth to a more mesial tooth, but rarely crosses the midline.
- "No. You are not going to put something cold on my teeth."
  - Explain to the patient why it is necessary to diagnose the tooth before initiating RCT.
  - Inform the patient that you only intend to hold the cold against the tooth until the first sign is felt and then the cold will be removed.
  - If the cold test is refused, inform the patient that you cannot provide RCT as you would be guessing which tooth needs treatment and the patient could end up with two or three teeth requiring RCT.
- "I had the root canal done one week ago [with the endodontist] and it still hurts."
  - Is the pain decreasing, the same, or increasing?
  - If the tooth still hurts, recommend the patient return to the endodontist for evaluation. Similarly, with third molar postoperative pain after treatment by an oral surgeon, recommend the patient return to the specialist.
- "I went to the endodontist and he said the tooth is fractured so it cannot be saved."
  - Do not proceed based on what the patient says. You must obtain the endodontic reports to receive the communication directly from the endodontist. Imagine taking the patient's word and extracting the tooth when the patient only said this because he or she did not want to pay for RCT.

Patients' Requests

- "The temporary fell out a few weeks ago but it doesn't hurt." (See Figure 8.2)
  - Evaluate if the gutta percha is exposed. If the gutta percha is exposed with an orifice barrier or is covered in a worn-down temporary filling, then the prognosis is better.
  - If the gutta percha is exposed it has been contaminated.

- If the gutta percha is exposed and there is still caries on the tooth, then there is even more bacterial contamination.
- Recommend the patient return to the endodontist.
- If the patient does not want to return, warn the patient the tooth may require retreatment, endodontic surgery, or extraction in the future. Will monitor the tooth for signs and symptoms.
- Place rubber dam isolation, irrigate with sodium hypochlorite, and place a definitive restoration.
- "I had my root canal done and need you to do the crown." (See Figure 8.3)
  - Be sure to obtain the endodontics report.
  - Take an updated radiograph.
  - If the endodontic treatment appears satisfactory:
    o Rubber dam isolation.
    o Replace the temporary with a permanent material and crown if indicated.
  - If you are concerned about how the endodontic treatment appears on the radiograph (e.g. extrusion of gutta percha in the palatal canal; see Figure 8.3):
    o Contact the endodontist and have the patient return for a follow-up.
    o If the tooth is symptomatic or asymptomatic.
    o Replace the temporary filling with Fuji IX as an orifice barrier.
    o Contact the endodontist and have the patient return for a follow-up.
    o Do not permanently cement a crown until the tooth is asymptomatic and the concerns are resolved.

Patients' Questions

- "What is a root canal?"
  - When a cavity reaches the pulp in a tooth, the pulp becomes contaminated and inflamed. This can cause a toothache and an abscess and systemic problems. RCT is a process in which we access the tooth, disinfect the roots, and seal it so that it does not become recontaminated and allows the bone to heal. If you picture a candle in which the wax is the tooth and the wick is the pulp, we remove the wick and replace it with a different material.
- "What is better? Extracting the tooth and getting an implant or a root canal and a crown?"
  - Not everyone is a candidate for implants and both implants and root canals can fail. No guarantees in dentistry.
  - Many studies out there and you need to look at the criteria for what is considered a "success."
  - The results are comparable.
  - Better to maintain the natural tooth if possible as the biologic interface is natural and the tooth is resilient because the PDL absorbs the shock.
- "How do you clean out the infection if it is in the bone?" (See Figure 8.4)
  - We cannot directly clean the portion beyond the apex with nonsurgical RCT (vs. endodontic surgery). However by cleaning, shaping, and obturating the canals and removing the source of the infection, the host response (immune system) should clear up the remaining infection in the bone over time. We will follow up after the RCT to make sure the bone is healing properly.

Endodontics

- "How much pain should I expect to be in after?"
  - If you have preoperative pain you can expect to have more pain after RCT compared with someone who had no preoperative pain. With any dental procedure there can be some discomfort afterwards and this varies from tooth to tooth within the same individual.
  - A study found that calling the patient to follow-up the day after the dental appointment reduced pain perception and analgesic needs [16]. Be sure to document the telephone encounter.
- "Did the specialist do a bad job on my root canal?"
  - Try to determine on what basis this question is being asked.
    - Is the tooth symptomatic?
    - Is the patient fishing for ammunition for a lawsuit?
  - Do not speak poorly of other dentists or their work. What you say could be used in court against another dentist and creates distrust among other problems. Be objective: you can only report based on what you see today. You do not know the circumstances under which the endodontist was working (e.g. uncooperative patient, limited mouth opening, bleeding, a hot tooth).
  - In addition, outside the USA treatment techniques are different. Knowing in which country the RCT was completed can give a clue to the techniques and materials used. It comes down to the presence of pathosis, the presence of symptoms, and restorative considerations.
- "Doc I cannot afford a crown right now for the tooth I had a root canal done on and the specialist said I need a crown. How long can I wait?"
  - While I cannot provide you with a specific length of time you can wait (could fracture within days), I can tell you that the longer you go without the crown the greater the risk is that this tooth will fracture and we will have to extract it. There are many factors, including how much tooth structure is remaining, the opposing teeth, and the amount of wear and tear the teeth suffer (e.g. diet, grinding, or clenching). Studies show that for premolars and molars full-coverage crowns are recommended and as time passes the risk of failure increases [17].
  - See Section Treatment Planning.

References

1 Torabinejad, M. and Walton, R.E. (2009). *Endodontics: Principles and Practice*, 4e. St. Louis, MO: Saunders Elsevier.

2 Vitality Scanner Model 206. Instruction Guidelines. SybronEndo. https://www.kerrdental.com/kerr-endodontics/vitality-scanner-2006-electronic-pulp-tester-diagnose#docs (accessed 10 February 2021).

3 American Association of Endodontists (AAE) (2009). AAE Consensus Conference Recommended Diagnostic Terminology. *J. Endod.* 35 (12): 1634. https://www.aae.org/specialty/wp-content/uploads/sites/2/2017/07/aaeconsensusconferencerecommendeddiagnosticterminology.pdf.

4 Michell, J.K. Sorting out endodontic symptoms. http://www.augusta.edu/dentaltable/pdfs/goals/relievepain/sortingOut6.pdf (accessed 10 February 2021).

5 American Association of Endodontists (2020). *Treatment Standards*. Chicago: AAE. https://www.aae.org/specialty/wp-content/uploads/sites/2/2018/04/TreatmentStandards_Whitepaper.pdf (accessed 1 May 2021).

6 American Association of Endodontists *Guide to Clinical Endodontics*, 6e. Chicago: AAE https://www.aae.org/specialty/clinical-resources/guide-clinical-endodontics.

7 American Association of Endodontists (2019). AAE endodontic case difficulty assessment form and guidelines. https:// f3f142zs0k2w1kg84k5p9i1o-wpengine. netdna-ssl.com/specialty/wp-content/ uploads/sites/2/2019/02/19AAE_ CaseDifficultyAssessmentForm.pdf (accessed 10 February 2021).

8 American Association of Endodontists (2016). The dental operating microscope in endodontics. *Winter 2016 Endodontics: Colleagues for Excellence.* Available at https:// www.aae.org/specialty/newsletter/dental-operating-microscope-endodontics (accessed 10 February 2021).

9 Apex Locator Root ZX II Canal Measurement Module (2007). Operations Instructions. https://www.dentsply.com/content/dam/ dentsply/web/en_US/Govt_School/ SterilizationProcedures/DENTSPLY-Maillefer-Root-ZXII-Apex-Locator-2vm3owk-en-1308. pdf (accessed 10 February 2021).

10 Krasner, P. and Ranjow, H.J. (2004). Anatomy of the pulp-chamber floor. *J. Endod.* 30 (1): 5–16.

11 Nelson, S.J. (2009). *Wheeler's Dental Anatomy, Physiology and Occlusion*, 9e. St. Louis, MO: Saunders Elsevier.

12 Deutsch, A.S. and Musikant, B.L. (2004). Morphological measurements of anatomic landmarks in human maxillary and mandibular molar pulp chambers. *J. Endod.* 30 (6): 388–390.

13 American Association of Endodontists (2017). Management of endodontic emergencies: pulpotomy vs. pulpectomy. *Fall 2017 Endodontics: Colleagues for Excellence.* https:// www.aae.org/specialty/wp-content/uploads/ sites/2/2017/10/COL041Fall2017EndodonticE mergencies.pdf (accessed 1 May 2021).

14 American Association of Endodontists (2020). Informed consent. https://www.aae.org/ specialty/clinical-resources/treatment-planning/informed-consent (accessed 10 February 2021).

15 American Association of Endodontists (2016). AAE and AAOMR Joint Position Statement. Use of cone beam computed tomography in endodontics: 2015/2016 Update. https:// f3f142zs0k2w1kg84k5p9i1o-wpengine. netdna-ssl.com/specialty/wp-content/ uploads/sites/2/2017/06/conebeamstatement. pdf (accessed 1 May 2021).

16 Touyz, L.Z. and Marchand, S. (1998). The influence of postoperative telephone calls on pain perception: a study of 118 periodontal surgical procedures. *J. Orofac. Pain* 12: 219–225.

17 Nagasiri, R. and Chitmongkolsuk, S. (2005). Long-term survival of endodontically treated molars without crown coverage: a retrospective cohort study. *J. Prosthet. Dent.* 93 (2): 164–170.

18 Ørstavik, D. (2020). *Essential Endodontology: Prevention and Treatment of Apical Periodontitis.* Wiley-Blackwell

Endodontics

9

Oral Surgery

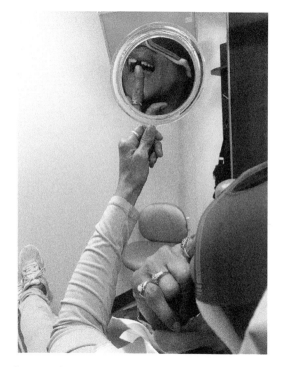

Figure 9.1 Before extracting a tooth a mirror check is completed. This is analogous to a "time out" in the operating room. The patient is asked to point to the tooth/teeth planned for extraction(s) that day. Alternatively, the patient could point using a cotton tip applicator.

Chapter Outline

- Real-Life Clinical Questions
- Relevance
- Clinical and Radiographic Exam

Clinical Dentistry Daily Reference Guide, First Edition. William A. Jacobson.
© 2022 John Wiley & Sons, Inc. Published 2022 by John Wiley & Sons, Inc.

Real-Life Clinical Questions

Dental Students' Comments

- "I told my patient we can pull her tooth today."
- "When do I need to suture?"
- "How should the extraction site look after one week? Is this normal or infected?"

Dental Assistant's Question

- "Which forceps do you want me to pass you?"

Patients' Concerns

- "What is the likelihood I'll end up with permanent numbness like you mentioned on the consent form?"
- "As a Muslim I cannot have any animal products."
- "I don't think I'm numb, I feel you touching the gum."
- "Every time I scratch this area, I feel my skull bone."
- "I think I now have an infection where the tooth was pulled, it looks yellow."
- "I think I have a dry socket."
- "You left a piece of tooth, see it sticking out?"
- "I saw the oral surgeon last week and my mouth really hurts and there is a tooth fragment"

Patients' Requests

- "Come on doc, just pull the tooth, try your best, I believe in you, I can't afford the oral surgeon."
- "You yanked the tooth out of my skull and you're not going to give me any strong pain medications?"

Patients' Questions

- "Should I get my third molars taken out?"
- "Can I take my tooth home after you extract it?"
- "Are you going to give me antibiotics after pulling my tooth for the infection?"
- "What can I eat after my tooth is pulled?"
- "Should I use Listerine to gargle with after my tooth is pulled?"
- "How long will I be sore?"
- "How will I know if I get a dry socket?"
- "What is in the dry socket medicine?"

Relevance

As a dentist you should be able to provide simple tooth extractions. This is a skill sought after by your patients. Equally important is the ability to interpret the radiographs and clinical findings to assess the level of case difficulty so that you know when to refer out to a specialist.

Clinical and Radiographic Exam

- Determine if the tooth is restorable or nonrestorable (see Figure 11.4).
- If the tooth is deemed nonrestorable and planned for extraction:
  - Determine if the extraction is of minimal, moderate, or high difficulty (Table 9.1).
  - If high difficulty, consider referring to an OMFS.

Table 9.1 Extraction case difficulty assessment.

	Minimal difficulty	Moderate difficulty	High difficulty
Patient considerations			
Health history	• ASA 1 (see Chapter 1) [1]	• ASA 2 (see Chapter 1) [1]	• ASA 3–5 (see Chapter 1) [1] • Blood thinners without lab values • History of oral/IV bisphosphonates or antiresorptive therapy • History of radiation to head and neck • History of chemotherapy • Poor historian • Under the influence of drugs/alcohol • Questionable mental state (ex/ dementia)

Oral Surgery

(Continued)

Table 9.1 (Continued)

	Minimal difficulty	Moderate difficulty	High difficulty
Behavior	• Cooperative and compliant [1]	• Anxious but cooperative [1]	• Uncooperative [1] • Severe anxiety • Severe psychological disorder • Requesting sedation • Bad attitude • Drug-seeking behavior • Speaks poorly of previous dentist • Litigious history • Patient pressuring you to work outside of your scope • If you are uncomfortable
Pain/swelling	• Minimum pain or swelling [1]	• Moderate pain or swelling [1]	• Severe pain or swelling [1] • Difficulty breathing. Refer to the ER
Anesthesia	• No history of anesthesia problems [1]		• Difficulty achieving anesthesia [1]
Ability to open	• No limitation [1]	• Slight limitation in opening [1]	• Significant limitation in opening [1]
Gag reflex	• None [1]	• Gags occasionally with radiography or treatment [1]	• Extreme gag reflex which has compromised past dental care [1]
Diagnosis	• Simple		• Confusing, complex, lacks certainty
Clinical findings			
Eruption status	• Erupted		• Partially erupted • Unerupted • Supraerupted (requires alveoplasty)
Clinical crown condition	• No restoration • No decay		• Large restoration/crown • Severely decayed
Mobility	• Mobility 3[a]	• Mobility 0, 1, 2	• Ankylosed (tooth makes a metal sound when percussed)
Adjacent teeth (risk of damage/further mobility)	• No decay or restorations • No bone loss/no mobility		• Large restorations • Mobile
Radiographic findings			
Image quality	• Diagnostic image		• Unclear image (unable to confirm outline of roots), superimposed structures

Table 9.1 (Continued)

	Minimal difficulty	Moderate difficulty	High difficulty
Location of decay	• Supragingival decay	• Equi-gingival decay • Subgingival decay	• Subcrestal decay
Bone loss	• Severe bone loss		• No bone loss + deeply decayed • Dense bone
Periodontal ligament	• Visible PDL		• No visible PDL
Periapical radiolucency	• PARL (less bone)		• No PARL • Large PARL (risk of damaging adjacent structures including sinus and inferior alveolar nerve)
Root canal treated	• Not root canal treated		• Previously root canal treated (weaker)
Root form	• Conical single root • No/slight curvature	• Thin roots • Multiple roots • Long root trunk and bifurcated	• Flared roots • Roots that diverge and converge at apex locking in bone • "Banana"-shaped roots • Bulbous roots • Dilaceration • Primary molar roots encircle a tooth bud
Proximity to the floor of the maxillary sinus	• Not close to maxillary sinus	• Root tips at maxillary sinus	• Significant portion of the root surface along the maxillary sinus • A pneumatized sinus
Adjacent roots	• Wide root proximity		• Close root proximity
Proximity to the inferior alveolar nerve	• Not close to inferior alveolar nerve		• Intimate relationship with inferior alveolar nerve
Risk of maxillary tuberosity fracture	• Minimal risk		• Max molar with pneumatized sinus • Isolated maxillary molar
Risk of mandibular fracture	• Minimal risk		• Thin atrophied mandible with long tooth root and/or large PARL, deeply impacted teeth

Type of extraction	• Simple		• Surgical:
			  – Troughing buccal bone
			  – Sectioning roots

[a] A tooth may appear very mobile but have a root fracture located far apically, allowing a portion of the tooth to move while the apical portion of the root is well anchored into the socket.
Always verify the entire tooth has been removed (Figure 9.2).
Source: American Association of Endodontists [1].

Oral Surgery

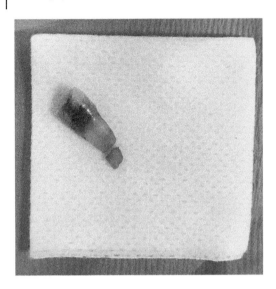

Figure 9.2 Always verify the entire tooth is out. One way is by holding the fragments together like puzzle pieces to verify.

Examples of Minimally Difficult Extractions

See Figure 9.3.

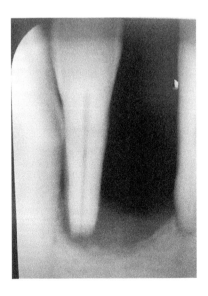

Figure 9.3 Tooth #26 with severe bone loss (and external resorption of the apex).

Examples of Moderately Difficult Extractions

See Figure 9.4.

Figure 9.4 Root tip #8 with equigingival and subgingival decay.

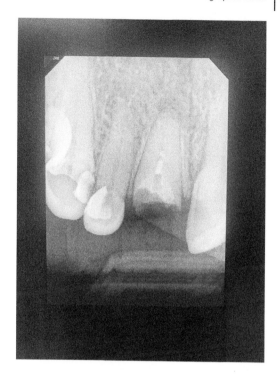

Examples of Highly Difficult Extractions

See Figures 9.5–9.11.

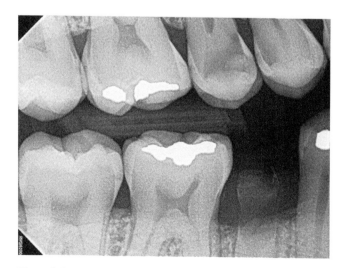

Figure 9.5 Tooth #29 with subcrestal decay that required a surgical extraction: bitewing radiograph.

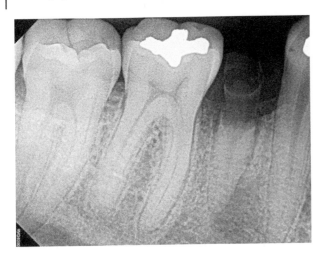

Figure 9.6 Tooth #29 with subcrestal decay that required a surgical extraction: periapical readiograph.

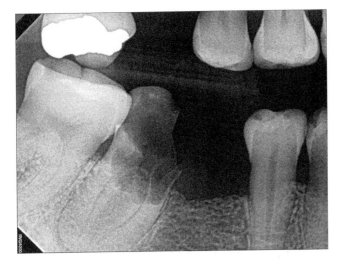

Figure 9.7 Tooth #31 with subcrestal decay that required a surgical extraction.

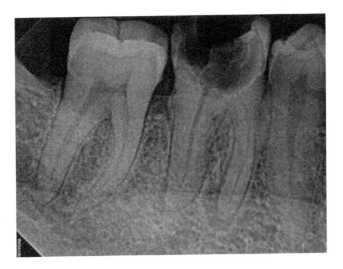

Figure 9.8 Tooth #31 "banana"-shaped mesial root that required sectioning.

(a)

(b)

(c)

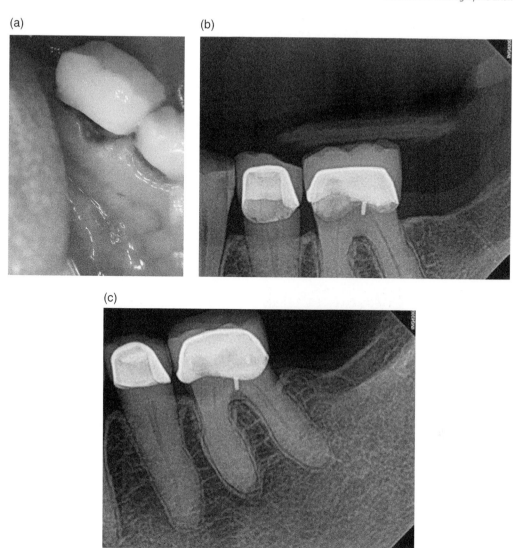

Figure 9.9 (a–c) Tooth #19 has a PFM crown, subgingival root caries on the lingual, and bulbous roots. The crown fractured off and the tooth required sectioning.

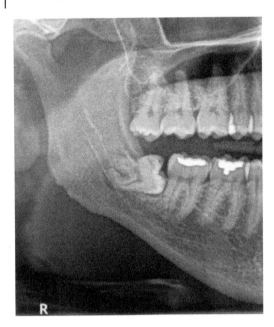

Figure 9.10 Tooth #32 on the panoramic radiograph appears to have an intimate relationship with the inferior alveolar nerve. Refer to an OMFS. In this case, the patient ended up with permanent paresthesia after the extraction.

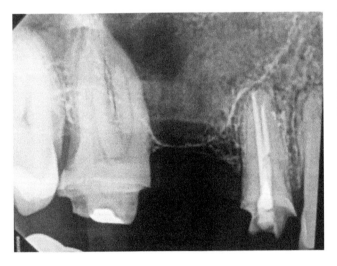

Figure 9.11 If tooth #2 were to require an extraction, refer to an OMFS due to the significant portion of the mesiobuccal root surface along the maxillary sinus. This could lead to a large opening between the mouth and the maxillary sinus (i.e. oral–antral communication).

Treatment Planning (Table 9.2)

Table 9.2 Treatment planning phases related to extractions.

Treatment phase	Description (may or may not apply)
Emergency phase	• Urgent treatment of pain, infection, trauma, and/or esthetic emergency
Data gathering phase	• Referrals to specialists (e.g. oral maxillofacial surgeon)

Stabilization phase (to control disease)	• Extraction of hopeless teeth
	• Caries control (bleaching if desired prior)
	  – Silver diamine fluoride
	  – Symptomatic teeth > larger cavities > smaller cavities (may involve extractions if a tooth is deemed nonrestorable)

Definitive phase	• Orthodontics (may request extractions)
	• Tooth replacement (may recommend extractions for prosthodontic purposes):
	  – Fixed partial denture (bridge)
	  – Implant
	  – RPD
	  – Complete denture

Maintenance phase	• Possible

Figure 9.12 Treatment planning for extractions.

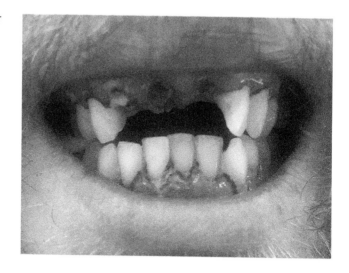

Additional Tips

• When treatment planning for extractions (Figure 9.12), plan for the "surgical extraction" fee so the patient is prepared to pay the higher fee. If the extraction ends up being a "simple extraction" then the fee will be lower for the patient.

• In cases involving many extractions, explain to the patient that "It is in your best interest to see an oral maxillofacial surgeon as you may be able to have all the extractions completed in one visit (after a consultation visit), with one recovery, and less chances of postoperative complications versus multiple extraction visits here."

Referral to Oral Maxillofacial Surgeon

- Refer patient for evaluation and treatment noting tooth/teeth to be extracted, the nonrestorable diagnosis, and alveoplasty as needed.
- Document if the referral is urgent, noting the patient's pain level.
- Document the plan, for example: "Plan is to have the patient heal for six to eight weeks followed by impressions for maxillary and mandibular complete dentures."
- If many teeth are planned for extraction, clearly document which teeth are to be "saved" and not extracted.

Informed Consent

- Informed consent is governed by state law.
- Contact your professional liability carrier and/or attorney for specific guidance and forms.
- A sample consent form is shown below.

Information and Consent for Oral Surgery

[Provider's name] has reviewed my case and determined that my dental condition is best treated by an extraction of tooth/teeth number(s): _____

This procedure is normally performed in the dental office using local anesthesia, sometimes supplemented with other medications.

The expected benefit from this procedure is: _____

There may be alternatives to the removal of this tooth/teeth. These alternatives include:

- Removal of decay
- Root canal treatment
- Periodontal treatment

As with any dental treatment, there could be complications. While these complications are rare, they do occasionally occur. They include, but are not limited to, the following:

- Dry socket
- Unusual pain, swelling, and/or discomfort after treatment
- Infection which may require medications, follow-up treatment or additional care
- Temporary pain, tingling or altered sensation of the lip, face, chin, gums and/or tongue. Numbness may become permanent
- Damage to adjacent teeth, restorations or gums
- Possible deterioration of my condition which may result in additional tooth loss
- The need for replacement of restorations or other appliances in the future
- An altered bite, which may require adjustment
- If upper teeth are removed, there is a chance of a sinus infection or opening between the mouth and the sinus cavity. This could result in an infection or the need for further treatment. A root tip, bone fragment or piece of a dental instrument may be left in my body and need to be removed. Treatment by an oral surgeon will result in fees for which the patient (or guardian) is responsible.

I have read and understand all of the information contained in this form and the dentist has discussed the risks, benefits and alternatives to this treatment. I have informed [Provider's name] of all medical and/or dental conditions or other circumstances that may affect the success of this procedure. I have had all of my questions answered and understand that, if I wish, I may have a second opinion before this procedure is performed. I accept the risks described on this form and give [Provider's name] permission to proceed with the removal of my tooth/teeth, or oral surgery as explained.

Printed Patient Name_____

Signature and Date_____

MRN Date of Birth_____

Signature of Guardian for Minors_____

Printed Provider Name_____

Provider Signature and Date_____

Armamentarium (Table 9.3)

Table 9.3 Extraction armamentarium.

Tooth #	Forceps	Extraction movements	Caution
8/9	150/1	Facial/lingual clockwise/ counterclockwise, end facial	• Don't nick the nasopalatine nerve/artery • See Figure 9.13
7/10	150/1	Facial/lingual	• Caution distal root curve
6/11	150/1	Facial/lingual	• Caution thin buccal plate
5/12	150/151 A	Buccal/lingual	• Caution fragile slender root tips • Don't perforate the sinus or lose a root tip in the sinus
4/13	150/151 A	Buccal/lingual	• Don't perforate the sinus or lose a root tip in the sinus
2/3/14/15	150/88L/88R	Buccal/lingual	• 88L/88R (left or right side) use action shown in Figure 9.8 • Don't perforate the sinus or lose a root tip in the sinus • Don't nick the greater palatine (GP)/lesser palatine (LP) artery • See Figure 9.14

(Continued)

Oral Surgery

Table 9.3 (Continued)

Tooth #	Forceps	Extraction movements	Caution
1/16	210 Forceps	Buccal	• Palatal bone thin, max. tuberosity thin; if sinus pneumatization and excess pressure can fracture the tuberosity • Don't perforate sinus or lose root tip in sinus Don't nick GP/LP artery – Have patient almost biting to maximize working room in the posterior – Tooth should "roll" out distally – Alternate positions from parallel to long axis of the tooth to perpendicular [2]
23/24/25/26	151, Ash/Bird Beak	Facial/lingual, rotate slightly	• Rotate only slightly, D curved tip
22/27	151, Ash/Bird Beak	Facial/lingual, rotate slightly	• 20% D curved tip
20/21/28/29	151, Ash/Bird Beak	Buccal/lingual, rotate	• Don't nick mental nerve/artery
18/19/30/31	151/23 Cowhorn	Buccal/lingual	• Cowhorn: make sure beaks are seated subgingivally and use a "pumping" action • Don't cause nerve trauma to inferior alveolar/lingual nerve • See Figures 9.15 and 9.16
17/32	222 Forceps		• Don't cause nerve trauma to inferior alveolar/lingual nerve
1–32	Rongeurs (side-cutting and end-cutting)		• Alveoplasty • Grabbing lose root tip, removing bone spicules
A-J	150S		• Caution with the succedaneous tooth bud
K-T	151S		• Caution with the succedaneous tooth bud
Root tips	65/Cryer elevator (east/west)/root tip picks		

Other Equipment and Materials

• Forceps:
   – Maxillary forceps: from the side have an "S" shape.
   – Mandibular forceps: from the side have an arched shape.

- Extracting maxillary teeth: deliver in facial/buccal direction and upward (away from lower arch to avoid traumatizing those teeth).
- Extracting mandibular teeth: deliver in facial/buccal direction and downward (away from upper arch to avoid traumatizing those teeth) [3].
- Elevators:
  - #9 Molt periosteal elevator: pointed end to elevate interdental papilla and broad end to elevate mucoperiosteum from the bone [3].
  - Straight elevator: for all upper/lower teeth. Concave side toward tooth perpendicularly or at angle to tooth, seated on buccal of tooth between tooth and socket [3]. Looks like a shoe-horn. A luxator looks similar except more of a wedge (no concavity).
- Retractors:
  - Weider retractor: retracts the tongue.
  - Minnesota retractor.
- Curette: periapical curette is spoon-shaped to remove granulation tissue, cysts, bone chips, and foreign bodies [3].
- Other equipment:
  - Ashe forceps.
  - Scalpel.
  - Bone file: serrated file cuts only in pull direction; crosshatched file cuts in push and pull direction.
  - Mirror/explorer/probe.
  - Rubber bite block.
  - Cotton pliers.
  - Needle holder: crosshatched to stabilize the needle (not parallel).
  - Scissors.
  - Local anesthetic, syringe, needle, topical anesthetic.
  - Sterile surgical gloves for oral surgery. Provide a higher level of infection control for surgery and are thicker, minimizing the risk of tears/punctures.
- Sutures
  - Various materials and diameters, cross-sectional needle shape/size.
  - Absorbable: made of gut or vital tissues from various animals
    - Plain gut suture: easier to tie knots, resorbs sooner (eight days [3]).
    - Chromic gut suture: harder to tie knots, lasts longer and resorbs (12–15 days [3]).
  - Nonabsorbable: requires patient to return for removal seven days later.
    - Silk suture: easy to use.
    - Nylon: alternative if religious contraindication to animal products (e.g. Muslim).
- Surgical handpiece:
  - Use only rear-venting surgical handpieces when performing oral surgery to avoid subcutaneous or submucosal emphysema [3] (Figure 9.17).
  - Different from regular dental handpieces which force air toward the bur.
- Miscellaneous products:
  - Sterile saline and monoject syringe: irrigate debris/foreign bodies to avoid post-extraction granuloma [3].
  - Dry socket paste [4]
    - Iodoform: antiseptic (kills microorganisms).
    - Butamben: analgesic.
    - Eugenol (from clove oil): analgesic.

Oral Surgery

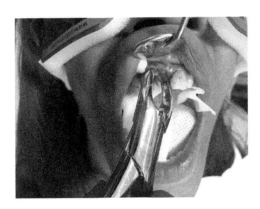

Figure 9.13 #150 Forceps used in a counterclockwise motion in this instance.

(a)

(b)

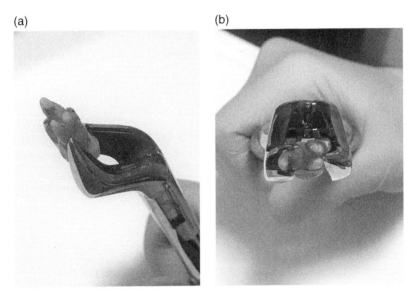

Figure 9.14 (a, b) #88R engaging all three furcations of the upper right maxillary molar.

(a)

(b)

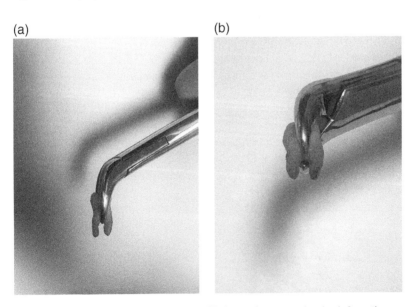

Figure 9.15 (a, b) #23 Cowhorn for mandibular molars engaging both furcations.

(a) (b)

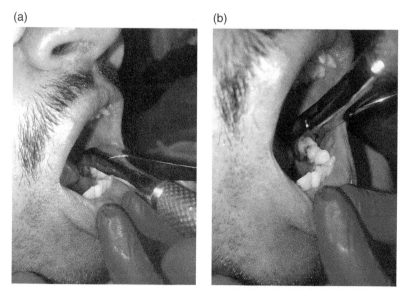

Figure 9.16 (a, b) #23 Cowhorn beaks are seated subgingivally on tooth #19 and are being used with a "pumping" action.

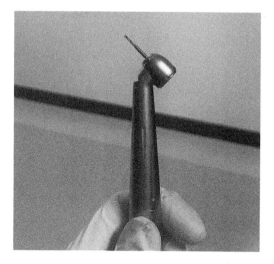

Figure 9.17 A rear-venting surgical handpiece.

Extraction Steps

- Chief complaint.
- Review medical history.
- Clinical and radiographic evaluation.
- Clinical and radiographic diagnosis.
- Determine difficulty level and decide if referring to an OMFS (see Table 9.1).

- Discuss risks, benefits and alternatives, answer questions, and obtain verbal and written informed consent. Address postoperative pain plan (i.e. medications) as part of the informed consent (do not move forward if there is disagreement) (see Chapter 16).
- Mirror check with a witness present. Have the patient hold the mirror and point to the tooth planned for extraction in front of the dental assistant and the dentist (see Figure 9.1).
- Local anesthesia.
- Check if area adequately anesthetized. Inform the patient: "I'm going to check if you are numb by first checking a part of your mouth that is not numb for comparison. [Press gingiva with periotome in an area that is not numb.] Can you feel this? [Then press around the tooth planned for extraction.] What about this area?" (See Figures 9.18 and 9.19).
- Inform the patient "You will feel a lot of pressure during the procedure, pushing and pulling. We cannot get rid of that sensation. If you feel sharp pain, raise your left hand because I'm on your right side with sharp instruments. If you feel any discomfort, we can numb you up some more. You may hear some cracking sounds, but don't be alarmed, oftentimes the tooth is brittle and pieces break off."
- Place throat pack (Figure 9.20). Be very careful if the patient has a cough, as the gauze can be aspirated when the individual inhales immediately before a cough.
- Use the periotome to sever the PDL around the entire tooth (if not done, you can tear tissue) (Figure 9.21).
- Use the straight elevators (small, medium, or large) to expand the socket by placing the small elevator between the tooth root and socket (not between teeth) as far apical as possible with the concave side facing the tooth root. Turn clockwise and hold. Turn counterclockwise and hold until the elevator can completely twist within the space between the tooth and socket. Then go up in size and repeat. Use the alveolar ridge as a fulcrum, not the adjacent tooth (risk of fracture and PDL damage) (Figures 9.22 and 9.23). Note, the straight elevator is usually perpendicular to the long axis of the tooth. Twist the elevator in the direction as if "scooping" the tooth out of the socket.
- Select proper forceps (see Section Armamentarium), and do not use until the tooth has mobility score of 3. Apply pressure apically. Hold facial/buccal for 10 seconds, then hold lingual for 10 seconds. Be patient, and use slow controlled movement.
  - Patient may worry if the procedure is taking a while.
  - Reassure the patient: "Don't be concerned if this seems to be taking a long time. I prefer to take my time and remove the tooth in one piece, if possible. I do not want to rush the procedure." (See Figures 9.24 and 9.25).
- Deliver the tooth (Figure 9.26).
- Inspect the tooth to verify root is intact (Figure 9.27). Apex should be round and dull (unless root resorption), not sharp/flat/shiny.
- Inspect the socket for debris, bone fragments or tooth fragments.
- Curette the socket. Enucleate any cysts or granulation tissue and remove any foreign debris (Figure 9.28).
  - Curette laterally (not apically) if near the maxillary sinus, nasal floor, or inferior alveolar or mental nerve.
  - Granulation tissue may develop into a cyst.
- Irrigate the socket with sterile saline only (not water from unit, which is not sterile) (Figure 9.29).
- Compress the ridge. Rationale: the socket has been expanded, so compress to prevent bulbous/irregular/undercut ridge or bony protuberance (Figure 9.30).
- Palpate the ridge for any sharp edges; if present, smooth with bone file/rongeurs and irrigate again with sterile saline
- Optional:

- Hemostatic material placement (Figure 9.31).
- Bone socket preservation.
- Suture (may be indicated).
- Fold and wedge gauze and have patient bite for 30 minutes so there is pressure over the socket (Figures 9.32 and 9.33). Tell the patient to not simply bite the gauze as this does not provide pressure (Figure 9.34).
- Consider a long-acting anesthetic (e.g. bupivacaine).
- Provide verbal and written postoperative instructions
- Provide a bag with extra gauze, ice pack, and the written postoperative instructions (Figure 9.35).
- Verify that hemostasis has been achieved prior to dismissal.
- Documentation.
- Optional: follow-up phone call to patient that evening and document the telephone encounter.

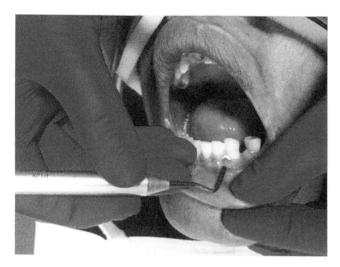

Figure 9.18 Comparing an area that is not anesthetized to an area that is anesthetized.

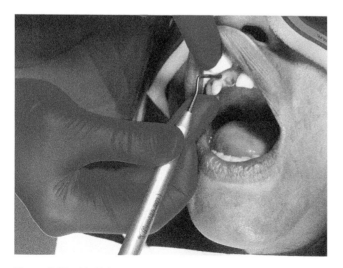

Figure 9.19 Verifying the tissue is anesthetized around the tooth planned for extraction.

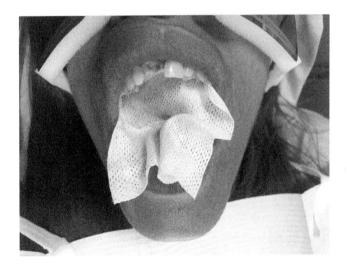

Figure 9.20 Gauze throat pack to prevent the patient from swallowing or aspirating tooth fragments.

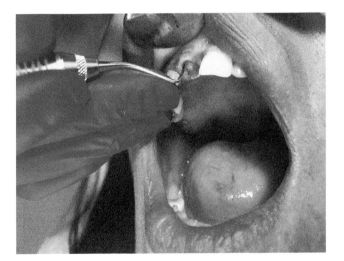

Figure 9.21 A periotome used to sever the PDL.

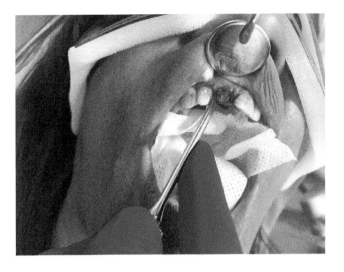

Figure 9.22 A straight elevator placed as far apical as possible. In this image the straight elevator is parallel to the long axis of the tooth. Of note, the straight elevator is usually perpendicular to the long axis of the tooth and used in a twisting motion as if "scooping" the tooth out of the socket.

Figure 9.23 Rotating the straight elevator and holding it in place for 10 seconds.

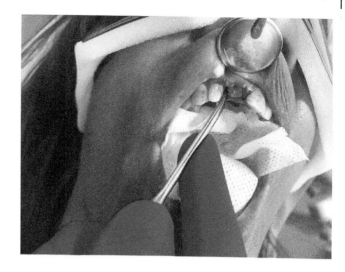

Figure 9.24 Placing the 150 forceps as far apical as possible.

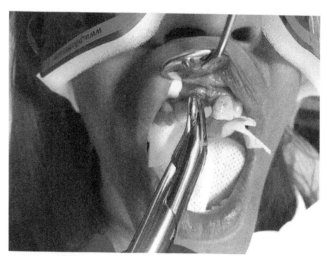

Figure 9.25 Rotating the 150 forceps clockwise and counterclockwise (not recommended if more than one root). Hold in one direction and count 10 seconds and then hold in the other direction and count 10 seconds.

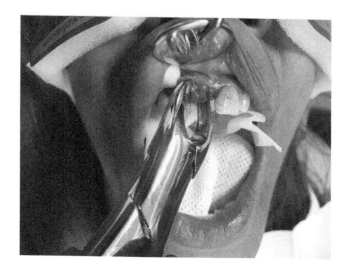

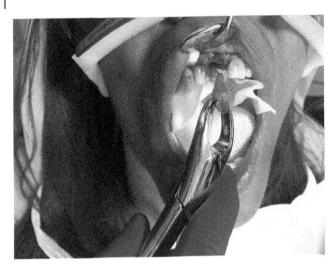

Figure 9.26   Delivering tooth #8.

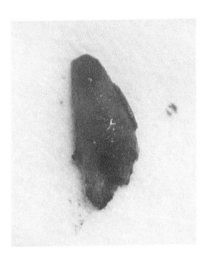

Figure 9.27   Carefully inspecting tooth #8 for any missing fragments. When in doubt take a postoperative PA radiograph to verify.

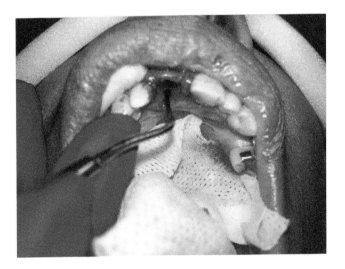

Figure 9.28   Curetting the extraction site.

Figure 9.29 Irrigating the debris with sterile saline. Warn the patient may taste salt water.

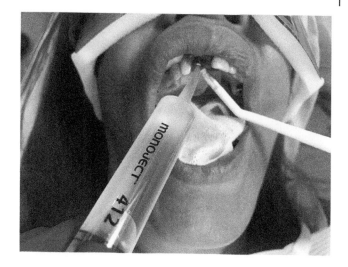

Figure 9.30 Ridge compression following expansion at the extraction site. This helps to avoid a patient returning to the office stating "Now I have a bump on my gums."

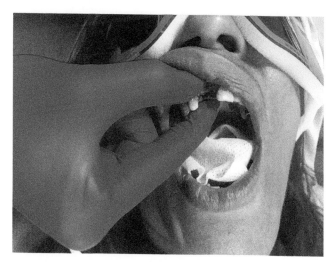

Figure 9.31 Placement of a hemostatic agent, in this case Surgifoam (consider any religious contraindications to using animal products).

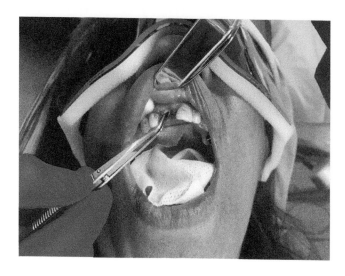

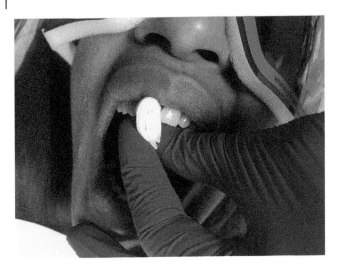

Figure 9.32 Folding the gauze.

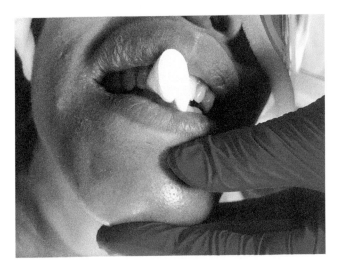

Figure 9.33 Have the patient bite to create firm pressure on the extraction site for 30 minutes. Show the patient in the mirror the proper placement of the folded gauze.

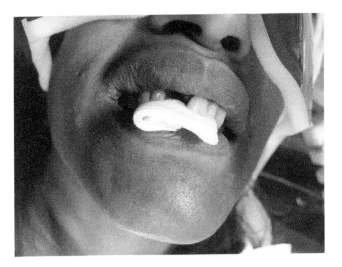

Figure 9.34 Tell the patient to not simply bite the gauze as this does not provide pressure. Also show the patient the improper way of placing the gauze so that they understand that pressure is needed.

Figure 9.35 Written postoperative instructions, ice pack, and gauze.

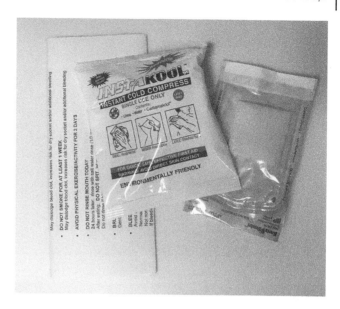

Related Surgical Procedures

Primary Teeth Extractions
See Chapter 17.

Surgical Extraction
"Surgical removal of erupted tooth requiring removal of bone and/or sectioning of tooth, and including elevation of mucoperiosteal flap if indicated" [5]. You can "divide and conquer" by converting multirooted teeth into multiple single-rooted teeth. When the roots are curved on a molar, recommend sectioning the tooth. At times a premolar with multiple roots may also require sectioning (e.g. sectioning a maxillary premolar mesiodistally).

Maxillary Molar Surgical Extraction
- Tooth #3 deeply decayed with flared roots which have a wider height of contour compared to the CEJ of the tooth (Figure 9.36, 9.37).
- If attempting to use forceps this tooth will be "locked" into the bone.
- Tooth must be sectioned.
- Section the molar by drilling a "Y" shape (Figure 9.38) (similar to the "Mercedes Benz" symbol) reaching the furcations to separate all three roots and use straight elevators to loosen and remove with root tip forceps. Place the elevator between the tooth root and the socket and push into the space created by previously removed root.
- Always inspect the root tips to verify removal of the entire tooth (Figure 9.39).

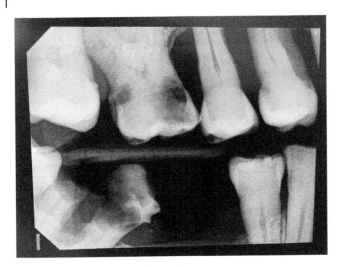

Figure 9.36 Preoperative bitewing of #3. Note the flared roots.

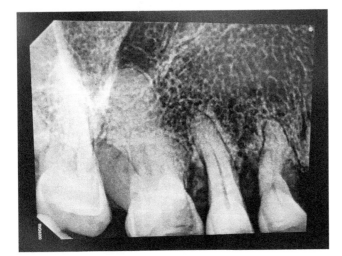

Figure 9.37 Preoperative periapical of #3.

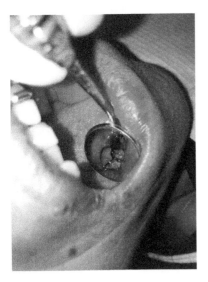

Figure 9.38 Sectioned molar #3 (similar to the "Mercedes Benz" symbol).

Figure 9.39 Inspecting tooth #3 fragments.

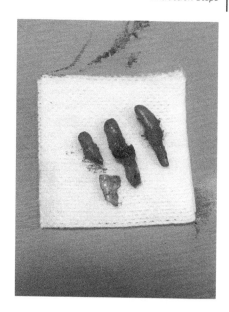

Mandibular Molar Surgical Extraction

- Tooth #18 is a deeply decayed/brittle tooth with no bone loss, zero mobility (Figure 9.40, 9.41, 9.42).
- If attempting to use forceps, this tooth will crumble.
- Tooth must be sectioned.
- Section the molar by drilling buccal to lingual (Figure 9.43) reaching the furcation to separate the two roots and use straight elevators to loosen and remove with root tip forceps.
- Always inspect the root tips to verify removal of the entire tooth (Figure 9.44).

Figure 9.40 Preoperative bitewing of #18 with deep decay to the pulp and subcrestal decay.

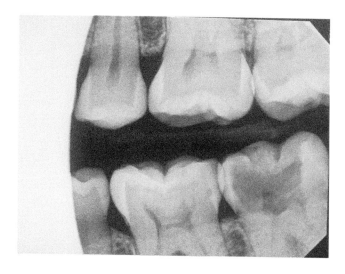

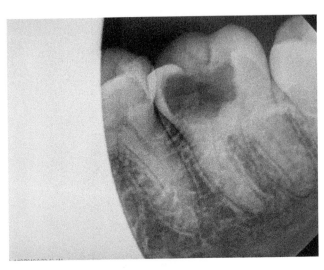

Figure 9.41 Preoperative periapical of #18.

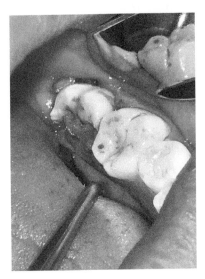

Figure 9.42 Inspecting tooth #18 before sectioning.

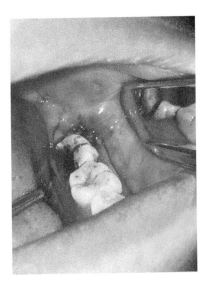

Figure 9.43 Tooth #18 immediately after sectioning the tooth to separate the two roots.

Figure 9.44 Inspecting tooth #18 fragments.

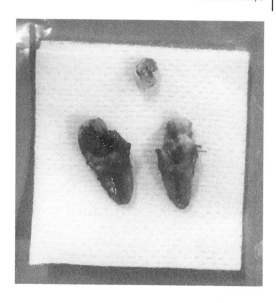

Reflecting a Flap and Troughing Bone

- At times a tooth will be broken and/or decayed below the crestal bone and require reflecting a flap and troughing bone in order to access the tooth for removal (Figure 9.45).
- First make an incision and reflect the tissue for visibility (Figure 9.46).
- Drilling bone requires a lot of irrigation.
- When troughing the bone, "hug the tooth" (Figure 9.47); err on the side closer toward the tooth being extracted not toward the adjacent tooth.
- Irrigate with sterile saline to avoid contaminating the bone/subcutaneous tissue/bloodstream with microorganisms from the water line tubing. The water line tubing cannot be reliably sterilized in dental units. For this reason, sterile saline as a coolant/irrigator must be used when performing oral surgery.
- Irrigation helps cool the bone when drilling. The high temperature of the bur (>106°F, 41°C) causes necrosis of bone cells, leading to poor healing.
- If troughing bone and you are unable to remove the root tip and there is compromised visibility, take a radiograph to reorient.

Figure 9.45 Unable to extract tooth #31 as the remaining tooth structure is all below the crestal bone.

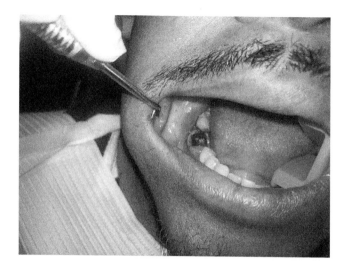

Oral Surgery

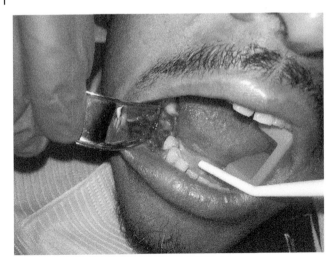

Figure 9.46 An incision was made with the base of the flap wider for better access and visibility prior to using the surgical handpiece to remove bone.

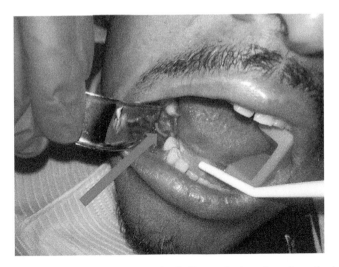

Figure 9.47 The blue curved line indicates the location where the bone was removed with the surgical handpiece ("troughing the bone") in order to gain better access for the straight elevators.

Incision

- Try to avoid making flaps, as it is traumatic and takes longer to heal. If you can see the tooth or the root, the extraction can be flapless most of the time.
- Best to incise if the tooth is "spongy" (soft due to decay) to access stronger healthier tooth structure.
- Vertical releasing incisions should start at the buccal vestibule and end at the interdental papillae [3].

- Use a scalpel in one continues movement contacting bone. Repeated strokes at the same place can often impair wound healing [3].
- Ensure the base of the flap is wider apically to ensure blood circulation to prevent necrosis.

Sutures

- Indicated to hold a flap over a wound, reapproximating the wound edges [3]. If the flap is not sutured but the wound margins approximate themselves, it will likely heal in the right position, but to ensure precise approximation of the papilla suturing is recommended.
- Multiple interrupted sutures: if one loosens or falls out, it will not influence the other sutures [3].
- Steps for suturing
  - Take healthy "bites" with the needle to avoid tearing the flap with the suture (Figure 9.48).
    - "Two forward, one back, one forward"
      - Wrap the end with needle around the needle holder twice ("two forward") creating the surgeon's knot/double-wrapped knot, placing the flap into position. (Helpful hint: "I'm being too forward.")
      - Single-wrap knot ("one back") creates the safety knot.
      - Tighten.
      - Single-wrap knot ("one forward").
      - Rationale: knots in different directions square the knot to reduce the likelihood of unwinding.
    - Make sure knot is on the side and not over the actual incision: it tightens easier, there is less irritation, and is easier to cut/remove [3].
    - Tip: wet the suture with sterile saline as you tighten down the first throw, as the sutures dry out and don't cinch down well.
- Have the dental assistant dab the bleeding site with gauze for better visualization (Figure 9.49).

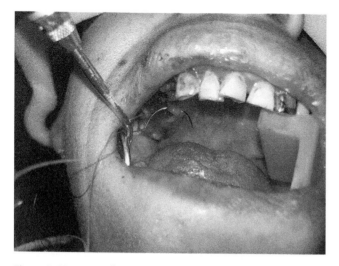

Figure 9.48 Taking "healthy bites" (adequate amount of soft tissue) to prevent tearing the soft tissue with the suture.

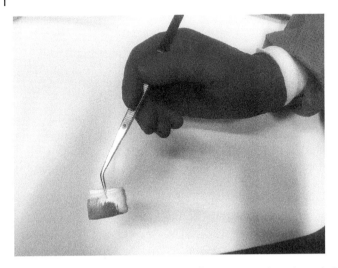

Figure 9.49 Have the dental assistant "dab" the bleeding site to help with visualization.

Alveoplasty

- To smooth or recontour the alveolar bone to facilitate the healing procedure and successful placement of future prosthetic restorations. In addition, uneven bone injures soft tissue causing severe pain/inflammation.
- Injury, stability, retention problems.
- After extracting a tooth/teeth, palpate the soft tissue for any sharp or rough areas. If a sharp area is detected, use rongeurs and warn the patient "You will hear a snap/loud sound as I remove and smooth some sharp edges" as the sound may startle the patient (Figures 9.50 and 9.51).
- Full denture: can create a surgical stent, after all extractions, seat and check for blanching. With #15 scalpel contact bone and make incision along crestal bone, reflect flap with periosteal elevator, use rongeurs to cut jagged parts, smooth with bur or bone file, remove excess gingiva, irrigate with sterile saline and suction. Try on surgical stent. If blanching is present, more alveoplasty required; if not, suture with interrupted sutures.

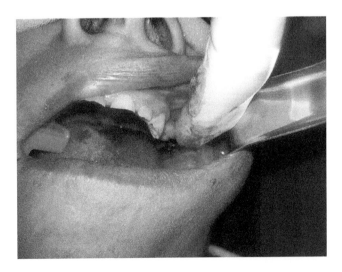

Figure 9.50 After extraction of tooth #14, the soft tissue was plapated to check for any sharp edges.

Figure 9.51 A sharp edge was noted, so the soft tissue was reflected and a razor-sharp edge of the inter-radicular septum was found. Area was smoothed with the bone file, irrigated with sterile saline to remove debris, and the flap repositioned and palpated to check for any remaining sharp edges.

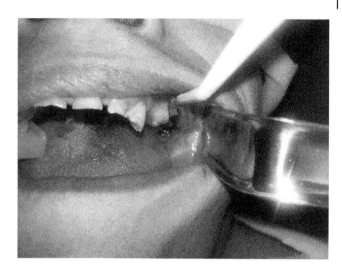

Intraoral Incision and Drainage

- There can be swelling without pus (Figure 9.52). If there is no pus, the abscess has not matured.
- You can empty out half of the cartridge of local anesthetic (e.g. lidocaine) and then place the needle in the abscess and aspirate. If blood is present don't incise; if pus, then incise and drain.
- If pus, anesthetize. Don't reuse the needle in healthy part of the mouth.
- Incise the height of contour of swelling with scalpel, open with hemostat, drain, suction, irrigate with sterile saline, place the rubber drain for three to five days and stabilize it with a suture. Provide patient with a monoject syringe and prescription bottle of sterile saline to irrigate. Patient must return for follow-up visits each day to irrigate and monitor progress (swelling should decrease each day). Once swelling subsides, remove drain/sutures and allow incision to heal itself (do not suture).
  - Use a Penrose drain with a silk suture, or a piece of rubber dam material with a silk suture. Purpose of the rubber is to prevent the incision from closing.
  - Palatal abscess: just barely pierce the mucosa with scalpel to prevent nicking artery.
- For extraoral incision and drainage, refer to ER or to an OMFS.

Figure 9.52 An incision made at the height of contour of an abscess on the hard palate. No pus only blood as the abscess had not matured.

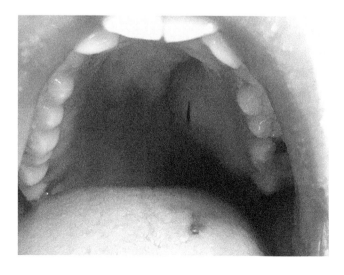

Oral Surgery

Danger Zones with Oral Surgery
- Maxillary:
  - Incisive palatine nerve: caution with incision or reflecting tissue.
  - Greater palatine nerve: caution with incision or reflecting tissue.
- Mandibular:
  - Mental nerve: caution curetting apically or with incision.
  - Inferior alveolar nerve: caution curetting apically if near or with incision.
  - Long buccal nerve: caution with incision.
  - Lingual nerve: caution with incision or sectioning a molar

Extraction Postoperative Instructions

Provide both verbal and written instructions (Figure 9.35).

- *Bleeding*
  - Bite on gauze as a pressure bandage for 30 minutes.
    - If replacing, moisten the gauze in your mouth with cold water prior to removal to prevent pulling off the clot.
    - Discontinue biting on gauze once the bleeding has slowed sufficiently or stopped.
  - Normal to have blood-tinged saliva for a 24–48 hours.
  - Not normal for the mouth to fill with bright red blood. If bleeding starts apply pressure by biting on gauze for two hours. You can also use a moistened tea bag (tannic acid promotes formation of a blood clot). Continuous hard pressure is needed to stop bleeding.
  - Place a towel over the pillow at night to prevent blood staining. Sleep with your head slightly elevated and avoid bending over.
- *Pain*
  - Normal and should decrease each day. Take medications as instructed and stay hydrated.
- *Avoid trauma*
  - You will be numb for several hours. Try to avoid scratching or biting your cheek, tongue, or lips.
- *Diet*
  - Not a time for dieting as proper nutrition (especially proteins) is necessary for wound healing.
  - Not eating can lead to nausea and vomiting.
  - Stay hydrated, especially when taking ibuprofen.
  - First day recommend cold soft foods. Some suggestions include fish (salmon, tuna), mashed potatoes, hummus, cottage cheese, scrambled eggs, macaroni and cheese, avocado, smoothie/milkshake without a straw, high calorie drinks (e.g. Ensure, Boost).
  - Avoid hot beverages (e.g. coffee) or soup, as this can dissolve the clot.
  - Avoid seeds/rice/popcorn for the first few days as these can become lodged in the extraction site.
- *Avoid dry socket*
  - Avoid getting a dry socket, which can occur up to five days postoperatively. If it occurs return to the office for the dentist to irrigate the socket and place a dressing.
  - Do not disturb the clot. Keep tongue/fingers away from the surgical site.
  - Do not spit. This can dislodge the blood clot.
  - Do not drink from a straw for five days. This can dislodge the blood clot.
  - Do not smoke for at least one week. Smoking increases risk of dry socket and delays healing. The longer you refrain, the less chance of postoperative problems.

- Avoid alcohol. This can dissolve the clot.
- Avoid carbonated beverages for several days. This can dissolve the clot.
- *Rinsing*
  - Do not rinse your mouth for 24 hours.
  - After 24 hours you can rinse with salt water (half teaspoon of salt per glass of lukewarm water) 10–20 times a day after eating.
  - Do not spit; instead let the water dribble out the mouth.
  - Do not rinse vigorously for the next five days.
  - Do not rinse if bleeding occurs.
- *Brushing*
  - Resume brushing and flossing of teeth beginning the day after extraction. Avoid the healing clot site, but floss the adjacent teeth.
- *Avoid physical exercise/activity*
  - For two days.
- *Swelling*
  - Normal, can last up to 10 days. Maximum swelling on day 3 and should decrease.
  - Cold versus warm compress
    - Extraction day 1, 2, 3 (peak): apply cold compress for 10–15 minutes, repeated every 30 minutes for four to six hours [3]. Keep your head elevated when sleeping by using a few pillows.
    - Days 4–7: apply warm compress for 20 minutes on and off.
    - Exception: do not use cold if there is swelling from infection; this will constrict vessels and blood flow leading to suboptimal delivery of antibiotics due to reduced circulatory perfusion.
- *Trismus*
  - Muscle stiffness causing difficulty opening the mouth can occur and can last one to three weeks.
  - Recommend warm compress.
- *Bruising*
  - Can occur and may last one to two weeks (especially if older age group, stiches placed, or diabetic). No treatment required.
- *Sores/abrasions*
  - May occur on the lips and/or corners of mouth due to stretching. Use Vaseline to keep moist.
- *Canker sores*
  - Occasionally occur after surgery and disappear after one week. No treatment.
- *Sutures*
  - If placed in your mouth will dissolve over time. It is OK if you swallow the sutures.
  - Do not play with the sutures.
  - Sutures may have a bad taste or odor.
- *Sharp edges or pieces of socket bone*
  - Bone spicules are common and disappear within 8–10 weeks, or may have to be removed.
  - A sharp edge may have to be smoothed down at a future appointment.
- *Sinus precautions*
  - If the tooth was in close proximity to the sinuses:
    - No sneezing with your mouth closed for one week.
    - No blowing your nose for one week.
    - No snorting for one week.
    - If you have a stuffy nose, use an OTC decongestant for one week.

If the patient has any questions or concerns, tell them to call the office number or, in case of emergency, the EMS.

Oral Surgery

Charting Template

Tooth Extraction # ___
  CC (free text)
  Preoperative BP/pulse:
  Discussion with the patient regarding the risks, benefits, and alternatives of the extraction, answered questions, and both written and verbal consent were obtained
  Mirror check (the patient held the mirror and when asked to point to the tooth/teeth planned for extraction the patient pointed to the correct tooth/teeth planned for extraction with the dentist and the dental assistant as a witness)
  Extraoral/intraoral exam (free text)
  Clinical findings (free text)
  Radiographic findings (free text)
  Diagnosis (*select one or more of the following*):
    Perio nonrestorable
    Caries nonrestorable
    Fractured nonrestorable
    Root tip
    Removal for prosthodontic purposes
  20% Benzocaine topical anesthetic placed
    (1/2/3/4/5/6/7/8/9/10) cartridges
  (*Select all that apply*)
  2% Lidocaine with epinephrine 1:100 000
  4% Septocaine with epinephrine 1:100 000
  3% Carbocaine without epinephrine
  0.5% Marcaine with epinephrine 1:200 000
  (*Select location*)
  IA, L, LB
  Local infiltration
  GP
  NP
  M
  PSA
  MSA
  ASA
  Gauze throat pack placed
  Periotome, straight elevators, delivered tooth with forceps
  Curetted socket laterally, rinsed with sterile saline
  Simple noncomplicated extraction (Yes/No)
  Surgical extraction (Yes/No) (*Select all that apply*: tooth sectioned/bone removed with surgical handpiece while assistant irrigated with sterile saline)
  Surgifoam placed (Yes/No)
  3-0 Chromic gut suture (Yes/No; if yes how many sutures placed?)
  Gauze placed over extraction site with patient biting/applying pressure

POIG written/verbal (Copy of postoperative instructions in chart)
Verified hemostasis was achieved
RX (free text)
Postoperative BP/pulse
NV (free text)

Clinical Pearls

Troubleshooting

- Unsure if your instrument is contacting the maxillary sinus membrane (or nasal floor) or granulation tissue?
  - Use a 27-gauge needle and insert it into the socket. If needle contacts bone it is safe to curette the granulation tissue. If needle does not contact bone and enters sinus/nasal floor, then do not curette apically. Do not try this on mandibular molars as it can traumatize the inferior alveolar nerve (Figure 9.53).
  - Alternatively, ask the patient to perform the Valsalva technique and look for bubbles (there must be blood or sterile saline in the socket to see bubbles). Be sure patient blows nose very gently to avoid creating a perforation.
  - Optional: take a radiograph to reorient yourself and locate sinus.
  - Sometimes the granulation tissue or radicular cyst comes out attached to the tooth (Figures 9.54 and 9.55).
- Buccal plate fracture: if the buccal plate is mobile but adheres to the periosteum (soft tissue) suture after extracting the tooth, let it heal. If the buccal plate is mobile and loose, then remove. If the buccal plate is on the root of the tooth that was extracted, the patient may experience more postoperative pain. Risk with upper/lower canines (Figure 9.56).
- Evaluating third molar position: even the OMFS may not know the exact position without a CBCT or by actually performing surgery. Tooth could be overlapping second molar or causing root resorption of second molar. Options: take occlusal radiograph, SLOB rule (see Chapter 3) or refer to the OMFS for evaluation.
- Dry socket
  - Clinically, look for a missing clot or partially missing clot (Figure 9.57). It will appear dark/black/empty inside. Check from all angles; could be adjacent to a bone spicule. There may be food debris.
  - Could be missing the clot beneath the surface further down in the socket. If the periodontal probe drops right into an empty socket, the clot is missing and there should be some resistance. There should be no suppuration (pus), facial swelling, fever, or malaise, which are signs of infection that may require antibiotics (see Chapter 16).
  - Radiographically, verify that no foreign body is in the socket such as a root or bone fragment which will need to be removed.
  - Anesthetize (optional).
  - Irrigate with sterile saline to flush out debris.

- Place dry socket paste into socket with monoject syringe (Figure 9.58). Inform patient pain relief will occur within five minutes, then leave room and return five minutes later to check on patient. May have to repeat 24 hours later to relieve pain for longer duration.
  o Two alternatives as follows:
    ■ Anesthetize. Then irrigate with 50/50 mix of hydrogen peroxide (antibacterial and effervescent to move debris to surface) and sterile saline. Place dry socket paste, place Surgifoam, and suture.
    ■ Place dry socket paste over ¼ inch-wide iodoform gauze strip, warn patient of some initial discomfort followed by relief within five minutes. Patient should return after three to five days for removal and replacement if still symptomatic.
- Trouble removing a fractured root tip after extracting the tooth? If you adequately loosened the tooth by elevating it and you are trying to reach the loose root tip at the base of the socket, use an endodontic hand file to retrieve it (Figure 9.59).
- Avoid being accused of extracting the wrong tooth: an essential part of the consent procedure is to perform a mirror check with your dental assistant paying attention (not setting up the room). Insist that this dental assistant stays as a witness until the end of the procedure (which avoids the situation where it is your word against the patient's). Patient must hold mirror and point to the tooth planned for extraction; it is helpful to describe the teeth around the one planned for extraction, for example "not the tooth with the chip behind it, not the tooth with the silver filling in front of it." A mirror check is similar to a "time-out" in the operating room for surgeries. Be sure to inform the patient that after the extraction there may be other teeth with problems contributing to the pain.
- Bleeding
  - If concerned you have nicked an artery such as the greater palatine, apply pressure with gauze and hold and wait for 10 minutes. Verify that hemostasis has been achieved before alowing the patient to leave. It can be alarming to ask the patient to bite for 10 minutes and return only to see fresh blood dripping with a pulse. This is due to the patient not biting hard enough/lack of adequate pressure to create hemostasis.
  - Purchase tissue gel (PeriAcryl) to minimize bleeding after extraction, especially if concerned about bleeding (medication/condition). The violet-colored option is more visible than the clear option and helps indicate where you placed the material.

- Unable to see due to the bleeding
  - Have your dental assistant irrigate the surgical site with sterile saline and suction with the surgical suction to improve visualization.
  - Note that if a root tip is almost out of the socket, make sure the assistant does not push the root tip back into the socket with the surgical suction.
- Considering leaving a root tip behind? If retrieval of a small root tip (<5 mm) is too risky and the root tip is not loose and not infected, leaving it in the socket is an option. Be sure to take a postoperative PA and inform the patient of the risks of removal and of leaving the root tip, and schedule a six-month follow-up visit.

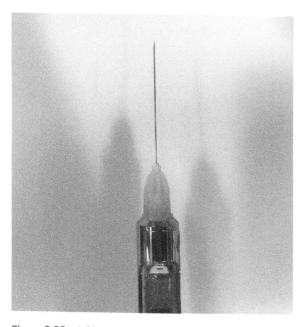

Figure 9.53 A 27-gauge needle is used to check if it is safe to curette granulation tissue in close proximity to the sinus or nasal floor.

Figure 9.54 Preoperative PA of tooth #10 with a large PARL.

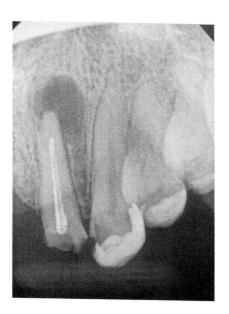

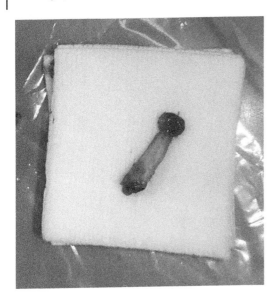

Figure 9.55 Granulation tissue or radicular cyst attached to the apex of tooth #10.

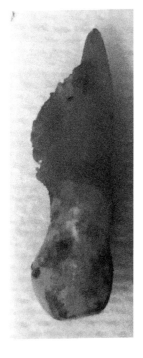

Figure 9.56 Extracted tooth #6 with attached buccal plate. Expect more postoperative pain and an osseous defect, and try to avoid this from occurring in future.

Figure 9.57   The patient reported she was sucking on a hard candy and then experienced severe pain at the recent extraction site of tooth #7. Upon inspection, only part of the clot remained. Diagnosis: dry socket.

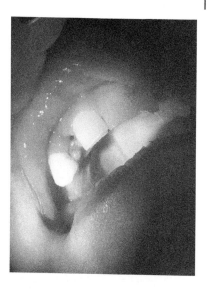

Figure 9.58   Dry socket paste placed into the extraction site with a monoject syringe.

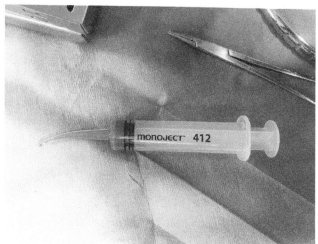

Figure 9.59   An endodontic hand file (size 08) was used to retrieve a loose fracture root tip remaining in the extraction site.

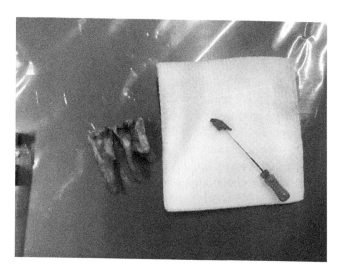

Tips

- Ergonomics: position patient in the chair so that his or her mouth is at/below the surgeon's elbow. Position patient for upper extractions with the maxillary arch at 90° to the floor (tilt head back with chin up) in the supine position and for lower extractions with mandibular arch parallel to floor to 30° in the semi-supine position.
- Extractions
  - When using the elevator during luxation, place gauze on palatal/lingual side to avoid injuring your finger or the patient's tongue/floor of mouth if elevator slips [3].
  - Always use a bite block for mandibular extractions to prevent injuring the TMJ from excessive force.
  - Don't let the dental assistant throw away the fractured tooth pieces. Keep these on gauze to piece together like a puzzle to verify the entire tooth was extracted.
    - If unsure, take a PA to verify that no fragments remain.
    - Similarly, don't allow your dental assistant to dispose of the cartridges of local anesthetic during the procedure as it is easy to lose count of the quantity. You must document the exact amount of anesthetic used.
  - Place forceps beaks as apically as possible and be sure beaks are between root and bone, not over bone.
  - Prevent trauma to the opposing tooth once the forceps pulls the tooth out as follows:
    - Lower teeth: using nondominant hand, place thumb under patient's chin, retract with index finger, and place middle finger over beaks of forceps.
    - Upper teeth: "L" shape with nondominant thumb and index finger, thumb under the beaks of the forceps.
  - If you extract the tooth and there is bleeding in the gums but not in the socket, scratch the inside of the socket with a small elevator to cause bleeding to form a clot and prevent a dry socket. Don't send patient home with a dry socket.
  - Multiple extractions sequence: maxillary before mandibular (longer for anesthesia to take effect on lower and prevent debris from falling into lower sockets) and posterior before anterior.
  - Removing maxillary third molars: extracting #1/16, have patient close mouth almost completely in order to reach.
  - Removing maxillary canine root: prepare a flap, reflect flap, and use surgical drill with #8 round bur and remove bone on buccal plate to expose more root structure prior to placing elevator [2].
  - Removing lone standing maxillary molar:
    - To avoid fracturing the maxillary tuberosity, sectioning the molar is indicated and tooth should not be removed in one piece.
    - Creating a mucoperiosteal flap, removing buccal bone and sectioning the molar will eliminate pressure which could fracture the tuberosity and expose the sinus [2].
  - Tooth not moving with elevators? Don't panic, be patient, and go around the tooth 360°. An OMFS at a continuing education course noted that "every tooth has a magic spot" (or the "purchase point") at which the tooth will move.
  - Going surgical. If after 10 minutes you are still unable to get the tooth mobile, consider going "surgical." This may require sectioning the tooth, reflecting a mucoperiosteal flap, and troughing the bone. Sectioning the tooth first is the most conservative route, as an incision delays healing and removing any bone creates a bony defect. However, proper flap reflection and

conservative bone removal if necessary will heal better than traumatized tissue from excessive forces.

- Avoid extractions in the afternoon on Friday; if there are complications and/or you need to refer to an OMFS, finding an office that is open and available will be a challenge.
- An OMFS at a continuing education course recommended that after extraction, scrape out granulation tissue, rinse the socket with hydrogen peroxide to decontaminate (bacteria cause dry socket), then saline (do not rinse with chlorhexidine as it kills cells), then Gelfoam, and suture.

- Always have a justification for the extraction and document this. If not visible radiographically (e.g. decay, partial eruption) take intraoral photos for the patient's record.
- Understanding the consent form
  - Necessary to answer patient's questions and for you to know what risks to look out for.
  - Inform patient that this is not meant to frighten or alarm but helps him or her make an informed decision.
  - Do not allow your assistant to simply hand the consent form to the patient and say "sign here" as the patient must understand the form.
  - "Possible deterioration of my condition which may result in additional tooth loss" can be misinterpreted when a patient has periodontal disease and adjacent teeth have slight mobility, which after the extraction may have even more mobility due to the bone loss.
  - Also note that it is not uncommon for the teeth adjacent to an extraction site to later develop sensitivity due to recession. Recommend placing desensitizing medicament (e.g. Seal and Protect) once the patient complains of sensitivity.
  - Damage to adjacent teeth can occur, such as cavitating an incipient lesion on an adjacent tooth, fracturing porcelain on an adjacent crown.
  - Bone fractures can occur on an angular mandibular third molar or an isolated distal maxillary molar.
- Understanding the postoperative instructions
  - Emphasize to patients the postoperative instructions. The goal is for the clot to survive two weeks. Do not allow the dental assistant to simply hand the instructions to the patients; similarly, you would not simply hand the consent form to the patient. You must read this to the patient and make sure they understand.
  - Dental assistant can begin to explain the postoperative instructions while the dentist is seeing another patient or while waiting for patient to become numb.
  - Swelling peaks at day 3, and thus a cold compress is recommended as it causes vasoconstriction, decreasing leakage of fluid from the vessels to the extraction site. Patient should sleep elevated to decrease swelling.
  - Warm compress causes vasodilation and helps the blood vessels to carry away fluids. It is recommended starting at day 4.
  - Swelling after day 4, or if swelling subsides and develops again, may be a sign of infection.
  - Mouth is not sterile and occasionally an infection can occur after extraction, with signs including malaise, fever, and swelling that increases after the third day.
  - Dry gauze could potentially remove clot and sutures, so recommend wetting the gauze.
  - Recommend warm wet black tea (caffeinated) bag for hemostasis, as it contains tannic acid which promotes blood clot. Do not use herbal or green tea.
  - Rest to reduce bleeding and help healing. Keep head elevated.
  - Trismus is due to inflammation and/or swelling in the muscles and can last for days to longer than two weeks. Recommend warm moist wash cloth at 15-minute intervals, soft diet, NSAIDs, and mouth opening exercises 10 times daily.

- Facial and neck swelling can be serious and life-threatening and these patients should be referred to the ER.
  - Submental: may obstruct breathing.
  - Pharyngeal: may obstruct breathing (tonsil region).
  - Sublingual: may obstruct breathing (floor of mouth).
  - Unable to open mouth to access tooth due to severe swelling/trismus.
  - Severe facial swelling in which patient no longer looks human.
  - Any patient having trouble breathing: in the ER, intravenous antibiotics may be given. IV antibiotics are analogous to using a fire hydrant compared with a hose (oral antibiotics).
- Easy way to place needle into the sharps container: hold the suture in the hand and the needle with the needle-holder making the suture taut and have the dental assistant cut the suture right above the needle. With the needle-holder, drop the needle into the sharps container. If the suture is not cut, it is a challenge to get the entire suture and needle into the small opening of the sharps container.
- Effects of a follow-up phone call to the patient: a study has revealed that calling the patient to follow up on their recovery "significantly reduces pain perception and number of analgesics used for relief." The callers were "reassuring and positive about surgical outcomes" [6]. So, call your patient that evening or the next day to follow up on them!
- Analgesics: refer to Chapter 16.
- If a patient requests sedation for extractions due to anxiety, do not try to convince this individual to undergo extraction without sedation, simply refer. Trying to extract a tooth in a highly phobic patient who screams when you apply the slightest amount of pressure can turn into a nightmare. A patient who runs out the door during the extraction attempt, or one where you are unable to extract the entire tooth, requires referral to an oral surgeon. Be sure to save the signed consent form for your records – do not allow your dental assistant to shred the form.
- Local anesthesia
  - While local anesthesia before consent saves time, it is better to avoid this as the patient could claim they were too impaired after local anesthesia to give full consent.
  - Lower molar: two cartridges for inferior alveolar/lingual nerve block, one to two for long buccal nerve block. Upper molar: two cartridges.
  - It is hard to obtain profound anesthesia for a "hot tooth." Add PDL injections all around tooth in the sulcus, and intrapulpal if the nerve is exposed, or intraosseous. Consider mylohyoid injection too. Studies have shown that preemptive administration of an NSAID increases the success rate of inferior alveolar nerve block.
  - To find the greater palatine, 90% of the time it is between the second and third molar, so if teeth #1 and #16 are missing go distal to the second molar.
  - If a yellow color appears when aspirating during inferior alveolar nerve block, it is buccal fat/adipose tissue.
- Child or elderly patient: ligate the gauze with floss so that child's parent or elderly patient's caregiver can remember there is gauze inside the patient's mouth and to help prevent aspiration.
- Extraction site healing stages:
  - Tooth extraction (day 1): hemorrhage and blood clot (red/white blood cells).
  - Initial angiogenesis (day 1 to week 3): new blood vessels form from the broken ends of blood vessels in the PDL. The blood clot begins to shrink, granulation tissue (from new capillaries and fibroblasts) forms at the apex and spreads upward. New bone trabeculae form at the apex.

- New bone formation (three to four weeks): entire socket filled with granulation tissue. Bone growth forms a lattice of woven bone while crestal bone, especially interproximally and on thinner facial plate, continues to resorb (complete epithelial closure of the socket occurs at three to six weeks).
- Bone growth (four to six weeks): new bone trabeculae have thickened and filled the apical two-thirds of the socket.
- Bone reorganization (six weeks to four months): the primary bone trabeculae remodel to form thicker secondary spongiosa (more mature bone) while cortical lining of the socket is still resorbing.
- Radiographic sign of healing: when lamina dura (which represents the cribriform plate) is no longer present. Typically occurs after three to six months, depending on tooth size, number of roots, and amount of trauma [7].
- Sinus perforation
  - Apices of maxillary posterior teeth may be coronal to the sinus floor or part of the sinus floor, or pathosis may reach the sinus floor.
  - Everyone's anatomy is different, but in general teeth in closest proximity to the maxillary sinus, in descending order, are the maxillary first molar 1, maxillary second molar, and maxillary second premolar.
  - If a large oral–antral communication is diagnosed, refer to an OMFS.
  - If a 1–2 mm oral–antral communication is found, recommend placing an absorbable gelatin sponge (e.g. Surgifoam), suturing, and prescribing antibiotics and OTC decongestants.

Real-Life Clinical Questions Answered

Dental Students' Comments

- "I told my patient we can pull her tooth today."
  - Student did not know how to assess the tooth for the level of extraction difficulty. The tooth was of high difficulty level, not an appropriate level for a dental student (see Section Extraction Case Difficulty Assessment).
- "When do I need to suture?"
  - Recommend suturing any time you make an incision in order for the mucos to be reapproximated (brought together) [3].
- "How should the extraction site look after one week? Is this normal or infected?"
  - It is a good idea for you to know what "normal healing" looks like and in order to inform patients what to expect.
  - I tell my patients "At first the extraction site will be bright red, the next day it will appear dark red, over the next two weeks you will have a clot that appears yellow. About one month into healing the gum will close over the extraction site and match the color of your gums." It takes several months for the bone to heal.
  - How does it look and are there any symptoms? Any suppuration, swelling, fever, malaise (signs of infection)? Tender on palpation?
  - See Figures 9.60–9.63.

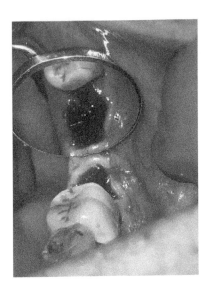

Figure 9.60 Extraction site immediately after tooth extraction. Note the bright red color of blood.

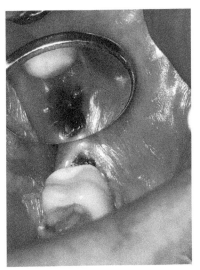

Figure 9.61 Extraction site 24 hours later. Note the dark red color of clot.

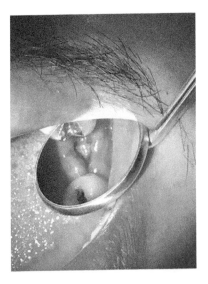

Figure 9.62 Extraction site two weeks postoperatively. Note the yellow color of the healing clot.

Figure 9.63 Extraction site one month postoperatively. Note the pink appearance of the gum.

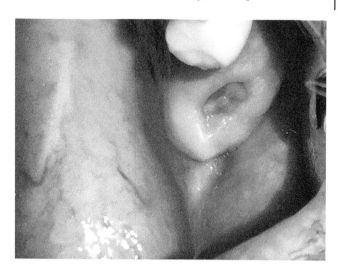

Dental Assistant Questions

- "Which forceps do you want me to pass you?"
  - Learn the names of instruments in order to communicate with your dental assistant like a professional (see Section Armamentarium).

Patients' Concerns

- "What is the likelihood I'll end up with permanent numbness like you mentioned on the consent form?"
  - Great question. I want you to know the risks so that you feel more comfortable about deciding whether or not you want this tooth extracted. There is no surgery without risk. One must also weight these risks to the risks of not providing treatment. This risk is more associated with extraction of lower wisdom teeth. The risk of permanent paresthesia is less than 1%. The risk of paresthesia in general is 0.35–8.4%. Usually this is not permanent and regenerates over time. Risk factors include patients over age 24, horizontally impacted third molars, close radiographic proximity to mandibular canal, and treatment by inexperienced surgeons [8].
    - Incidence of persistent inferior alveolar nerve involvement present after six months varies from 0.9% to zero [9–12].
    - Incidence of persistent lingual nerve damage varies from 0.5% to zero [13].
    - Effects of long buccal nerve damage are generally not noted [14].
    - Incidence of mylohyoid nerve damage up to 1.5% [15].
- "What is the chance of me getting a dry socket?"
  - For routine extractions the incidence of dry socket, or alveolar osteitis, is 0.5–5%. With mandibular third molars the incidence ranges from 1 to 37.5%. Risk factors for dry socket include surgical trauma/difficulty of surgery, extraction of mandibular third molars, oral contraceptives (estrogen), smoking (dose dependent: 20% for pack per day smokers, 40% if smoking same day; unclear if systemic or local effect such as heat or suction is the culprit), preexisting local bacterial infection, and increased risk with age [16].
- "As a Muslim I cannot have any animal products."

   – "I appreciate you communicating this with me. I will be sure that we don't use any animal products in your mouth today."
   - o Ask about preferences against animal or human products.
   - o Avoid animal products which are in plain gut suture, chromic gut suture, silk sutures, anything with gelatin such as Gelfoam (gelatin hemostatic agent), prescribing medications in gel capsules, and certain bone grafts.
   - o Instead use nylon suture and Surgicel for hemostasis (cellulose derived from plants) and prescribe medications in liquid or tablet form.
   - o Ask for permission to touch the patient's face.
   - o *Know your dental materials!*
   - o Potential religious contraindications:
     - ▪ Jewish: pig (porcine), includes gelatin and certain bone graft materials.
     - ▪ Muslim: pig (porcine), includes gelatin and certain bone graft materials.
     - ▪ Hindu: cow (bovine), includes gelatin and certain bone graft materials.
- "I don't think I'm numb, I feel you touching the gum."
   – You will feel pressure but you shouldn't feel pain. If it's painful raise your left hand and I will anesthetize you more.
- "Every time I scratch this area, I feel my skull bone."
   – Do not scratch the extraction site as this will disturb and remove the clot leading to a painful dry socket.
- "I think I now have an infection where the tooth was pulled, it looks yellow."
   – Refer to the third Dental Students' Comments.
- "I think I have a dry socket."
   – "What makes you think you do?" Listen carefully and perform a clinical and possibly radiographic exam.
   – Is it within five days of the extraction?
- "You left a piece of tooth, see it sticking out?"
   – "Let me take a look. Sometimes we remove the entire tooth but there can be a fragment of a tooth or bone that remains which the body tries to push out."
     - o Take radiograph; if extracting a bone spicule, obtain verbal/written consent for oral surgery.
     - o A bone spicule may self-exfoliate, resorb, or require extraction (Figure 9.64).

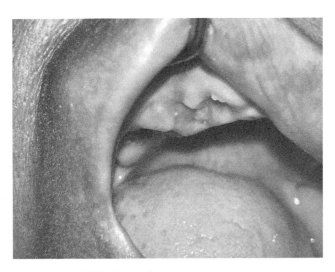

Figure 9.64   Visible bone spicule.

- "I saw the oral surgeon last week and my mouth really hurts and there is a tooth fragment"
  - "You will have to return to the oral surgeon as she is responsible as your treating specialist." (You are liable if you intervene in any complication yourself.)

Patients' Requests

- "Come on doc, just pull the tooth, try your best, I believe in you, I can't afford the oral surgeon."
  - Listen to your gut. Do not let a patient pressure you into providing treatment you are not comfortable performing, because if it goes wrong you will be blamed by the patient. It is dangerous to let a patient persuade you, as there can be irreversible damage and malpractice. Tell the patient "This is out of my scope, it is beyond my comfort level, and it is best you see a specialist." You are not a failure because you don't have the training and experience to treat every situation.
- "You yanked the tooth out of my skull and you're not going to give me any strong pain medications?"
  - Discuss postoperative pain management during the informed consent process so that the patient knows what to expect in order to make an informed decision.
  - Refer to Chapter 16.

Patients' Questions

- "Should I get my third molars taken out?"
  - "Let me evaluate the tooth and the radiographs to determine if removal is indicated."
    - According to the American Association of Oral and Maxillofacial Surgeons White Paper Position statement, evaluate patient's medical and dental history, symptoms, eruption status, position of tooth, functionality, periodontal and caries status, imaging for disease status and adjacent anatomy, and risk associated with removal or retention. Increased difficulty and risk of complication with age. A decision should be made before mid-thirties. If third molars are "associated with disease or at high risk of developing disease, should be surgically managed. In absence of disease or significant risk of disease, active clinical and radiographic surveillance is indicated" [17].
    - Typically, extraction is recommended in the following circumstances: partially erupted, causing adjacent tooth root resorption, preventing eruption of second molar, pain, decay, recurrent decay, high caries risk, periodontally involved or high periodontal risk, under age 25 with three-quarter root formed.
    - If unsure, refer to an OMFS to evaluate and to determine if surgery indicated.
- "Can I take my tooth home after you extract it?"
  - According to the CDC you may keep your tooth: "Once an extracted tooth is returned to a patient, it is no longer considered a potential risk to dental health care personnel and is no longer subject to the provisions of the Occupational Safety and Health Administration (OSHA) Bloodborne Pathogens Standard" [18].
- "Are you going to give me antibiotics after pulling my tooth for the infection?"
  - Usually no (unless indicated) as once the tooth has been extracted the source of infection has been removed.
- "What can I eat after my tooth is pulled?"
  - I recommend eating cold soft food. Avoid anything very hot like soup or coffee which could dissolve the blood clot and avoid anything small that could get into the socket and interfere with healing, such as seeds, rice or popcorn.

Oral Surgery

  o Let comfort be your guide.
  o Protein is important for wound healing. Some foods you may want to consider are fish (salmon, tuna), mashed potatoes, hummus, cottage cheese, scrambled eggs, macaroni and cheese, avocado, smoothie/milkshake without a straw, high calorie drinks (e.g. Ensure, Boost).
  o Don't forget to stay hydrated, especially when taking high doses of ibuprofen.
- "Should I use Listerine to gargle with after my tooth is pulled?"
  – No. Listerine contains alcohol which can dissolve the clot and lead to a painful dry socket. Instead we recommend you avoid rinsing your mouth for the first 24 hours. After that you can rinse gently with warm salt water (half teaspoon of salt per glass of water) 10–20 times daily. Be sure to avoid vigorous swishing and forceful spitting by letting the salt water dribble out your mouth.
- "How long will I be sore?"
  – Everyone and every tooth extraction heals differently. A patient may tell me they were only sore for one evening, and then the same patient may tell me on another tooth we extracted that they were sore for two weeks. There are various factors involved, but the pain should be less severe with each passing postoperative day and last up to two weeks. If the pain persists or gets worse, return to the office. We will prescribe you analgesics to relieve the pain; however, the pain may not be completely relieved but only partially relieved.
    o Pain immediately after the extraction in most cases can be managed with analgesics.
    o Pain can peak around 12 hours after extraction and then diminishes rapidly.
    o Significant pain rarely persists longer than two days after surgery.
- "How will I know if I get a dry socket?"
  – Typically, the pain will be subsiding the day of the extraction, and then between the first and third day (or first five days) *after* the extraction you will have an increase in pain. You may experience throbbing radiating pain (such as to the ear) which may be hard to localize. This is from the disintegrated dislodged blood clot leading to delayed healing and necrosis of the bone surface [3]. If this occurs come back into the office for treatment. If you are unable to come in, purchase OTC 20% benzocaine and place it in the extraction site.
- "What is in the dry socket medicine?"
  – It is a prescription paste mixture of iodoform, which kills microorganisms, butamben, an analgesic, and eugenol, from clove oil [16]. Eugenol acts as an anesthetic and has anti-inflammatory and antibacterial properties [19].

References

1 American Association of Endodontists. AAE endodontic case difficulty assessment form and guidelines. https:// f3f142zs0k2w1kg84k5p9i1o-wpengine. netdna-ssl.com/specialty/wp-content/ uploads/sites/2/2019/02/19AAE_ CaseDifficultyAssessmentForm.pdf (accessed 10 February 2021).

2 Gaum, L.I. (2011). *Oral Surgery for the General Dentist*, 2e. Hudson, OH: Lexicomp.

3 Fragiskos, F.D (2010). *Oral Surgery*. Springer.

4 Septodont. Alvogyl, paste for dental use. www.septodont.co.uk/sites/default/files/ Alvogyl%20Patient%20information%20 leaflet%20S%2005%2006%20047%2011%2000. pdf (accessed 13 March 2020).

5 American Dental Association (2016). CDT Code Check phone app

6 Touyz, L.Z. and Marchand, S. (1998). The influence of postoperative telephone calls on pain perception: a study of 118 periodontal

surgical procedures. *J. Orofac. Pain* 12 (3): 219–225.

7 Misch, C.E. (2008). *Contemporary Implant Dentistry*, 3e. St. Louis, MO: Mosby Elsevier.

8 Sarikov, R. and Juodzbalys, G. (2014). Inferior alveolar nerve injury after mandibular third molar extraction: a literature review. *J. Oral Maxillofac. Res.* 5 (4): e1.

9 Chaparro-Avendano, A.V., Perez-Garcia, S., Valmaseda-Castellon, E. et al. (2005). Morbidity of third molar extraction in patients between 12 and 18 years of age. *Med. Oral Pathol. Oral Cir. Bucal* 10 (5): 422–431.

10 Schultze-Mosgau, S. and Reich, R.H. (1993). Assessment of inferior alveolar and lingual nerve disturbances after dentoalveolar surgery, and of recovery of sensitivity. *Int. J. Oral Maxillofac. Surg.* 22 (4): 214–217.

11 Gulicher, D. and Gerlach, K.L. (2001). Sensory impairment of the lingual and inferior alveolar nerves following removal of impacted mandibular third molars. *Int. J. Oral Maxillofac. Surg.* 30 (4): 306–312.

12 Queral-Godoy, E., Valmaseda-Castellon, E., Berini-Aytes, L., and Gay-Escoda, C. (2005). Incidence and evolution of inferior alveolar nerve lesions following lower third molar extraction. *Oral Surg. Oral Med. Oral Pathol. Oral Radiol. Endod.* 99 (3): 259–264.

13 Blackburn, C.W. and Bramley, P.A. (1989). Lingual nerve damage associated with the removal of lower third molars. *Br. Dent. J.* 167 (3): 103–107.

14 Merrill, R.G. (1979). Prevention, treatment, and prognosis for nerve injury related to the difficult impaction. *Dent. Clin. North Am.* 23 (3): 471–488.

15 Carmichael, F.A. and McGowan, D.A. (1992). Incidence of nerve damage following third molar removal: a West of Scotland Surgery Research Group Study. *Br. J. Oral Maxillofac. Surg.* 30 (2): 78–82.

16 Kolokythas, A., Olech, E., and Miloro, M. (2010, 2010). Alveolar osteitis: a comprehensive review of concepts and controversies. *Int. J. Dent.* 249073.

17 American Association of Oral and Maxillofacial Surgeons (2016). White Paper. Management of third molar teeth. https:// www.aaoms.org/docs/govt_affairs/ advocacy_white_papers/management_ third_molar_white_paper.pdf (accessed 13 March 2020).

18 Centers for Disease Control and Prevention (CDC). Extracted teeth. https://www.cdc.gov/ oralhealth/infectioncontrol/faqs/extracted-teeth.html (accessed 13 March 2020).

19 Colgate. Dry socket paste: is it worth trying? https://www.colgate.com/en-us/oral-health/ conditions/wisdom-teeth/dry-socket-paste-is-it-worth-trying-0117 (accessed 13 March 2020).

Oral Surgery

10

Toothaches

"Listen to the patient, he is telling you the diagnosis."

Sir William Osler [1]

Figure 10.1 The patient after being asked to point to the location where she is experiencing pain.

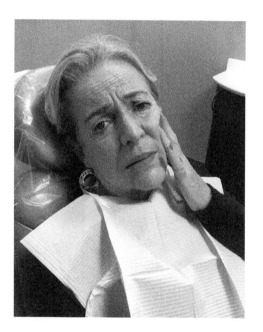

Chapter Outline

- Real-Life Questions, Concerns, and Comments
- Relevance
- Treatment Planning
- Dental Trauma Armamentarium
- Nonodontogenic Toothaches (Referred Pain)
- Teledentistry and Toothaches
- Clinical Pearls

Clinical Dentistry Daily Reference Guide, First Edition. William A. Jacobson.
© 2022 John Wiley & Sons, Inc. Published 2022 by John Wiley & Sons, Inc.

- Troubleshooting
- Tips
- Real-Life Questions, Concerns, and Demands Answered
- References

Real-Life Questions, Concerns, and Comments

Dental Students' Questions

- "I don't know what to do if a patient walks in with a toothache?"

Dental Assistant's Question

- "The patient has several teeth bothering her today. How many X-rays should I take?"

Office Manager's Question

- "What is considered a true emergency or an urgent appointment?"

Patients' Concerns

- "The tooth you did the filling on hurts when I bite or chew food."
- "Can this tooth be saved?"
- "Gum hurts under my denture."
- "I have a bump or pimple on my gums."
- "This broken tooth is cutting my tongue."

Patients' Questions

- "Does the X-ray show the tooth fracture?"
- "I don't know if this is a toothache or if it is related to my sinus problems?" (Figure 10.1)
- "Here is my son's broken tooth. Can you attach it back on?" (Figure 10.2)

Figure 10.2   A tooth fragment.

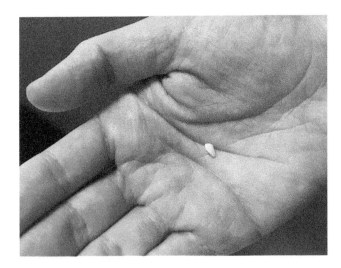

Patients' Demands

- "My crown fell off and I just need you to glue it back on."
- "You need to pull this tooth out. This one hurts."
- "I need antibiotics for this."
- "I need something stronger than ibuprofen, like Norco."

Relevance

As a general dentist, you are the go-to person for toothaches. Each case is unique and involves problem-solving. Having a systematic approach with checklists will help you determine the diagnosis, and reduce the likelihood of oversights.

Treatment Planning

The first phase of a treatment plan is the emergency phase, i.e. the urgent treatment of pain, infection, trauma, and/or esthetic emergency. A toothache checklist is shown in Table 10.1 and a dental trauma checklist in Table 10.2.

Table 10.1   Toothache checklist.

Dental history	☐ Recent dental treatment ☐ Pending dental treatment	
Vitals	☐ BP and pulse ☐ Temperature >38°C (100.4°F)	
Chief complaint	• Tooth/area: • Onset: • Provocation: • Palliation: • Progression:	• Quality: • Radiation: • Severity (0–10): currently and at its worse • Timing (duration, frequency): • Interferes with sleep:
Extraoral exam	☐ Facial swelling ☐ Lymphadenopathy ☐ Trauma ☐ Trismus ☐ Sinus tract	
Intraoral exam	☐ Palatal/mandibular tori ☐ Bilateral linea alba ☐ Scalloped tongue ☐ Ulceration ☐ Swelling ☐ Parulis/sinus tract	

(Continued)

Table 10.1 (Continued)

Oral cancer screening	☐ No abnormalities detected ☐ Other:
Radiographic findings	☐ Caries or fracture to enamel/dentin/pulp/subgingival/root/recurrent on surfaces: M/O/I/D/B/L/F ☐ Calcified ☐ Resorption (internal/external) ☐ Root tip ☐ PARL ☐ RCT ☐ Open apex ☐ Bone loss: horizontal/vertical ☐ Crown/root ratio: <1 : 1, 1 : 1, >1 : 1 ☐ Violation of biologic width (or will be) ☐ Widened PDL ☐ Restoration ☐ Post and core/crown
Clinical findings	☐ Caries or fracture: to enamel/dentin/pulp/subgingival/root/recurrent on surfaces: M/O/I/D/B/L/F ☐ Root tip ☐ Unsatisfactory restoration: fractured/missing/open margin ☐ Sensitive to air ☐ Erosion/attrition/abrasion ☐ Food impaction ☐ Partially erupted
Periodontal evaluation	☐ Pocket depths B _____ L _____ ☐ Recession B _____ L _____ ☐ BOP ☐ Suppuration ☐ Mobility: 1/2/3 ☐ Fremitus ☐ Furcation involvement: Grade 1/2/3/4 ☐ Hygiene: good/moderate/poor
Endodontic diagnostic tests	☐ Tooth in question: _____ ☐ Control teeth: _____ ☐ Cold test: WNL/transient pain/lingering/no response ☐ Electric pulp test: <80/= 80 ☐ Percussion: + (tender)/− (WNL) ☐ Palpation: + (tender)/− (WNL) ☐ Biting: painful/pain upon release
Occlusion	☐ Heavy ☐ Light ☐ Not in occlusion ☐ Supraerupted ☐ Intruded ☐ Crossbite ☐ Open bite ☐ Edge-to-edge
Parafunction	☐ Bruxer/clencher ☐ Recent stress ☐ History of/wears occlusal guard ☐ Other habits:
Restorability	☐ Restorable ☐ Nonrestorable ☐ Questionable ☐ Adequate ferrule: 360° of both 1.5–2 mm dentin height and 1–1.5 dentin thickness ☐ Requires ortho extrusion ☐ Inadequate ferrule (need for crown lengthening. Consider crown/root ratio, furcation, esthetics)
Origin of dental pain	☐ Odontogenic ☐ Nonodontogenic
Diagnosis	
Prognosis	☐ Good ☐ Fair ☐ Poor ☐ Questionable ☐ Hopeless

Source: William Jacobson, DMD, MPH.

Table 10.2 Dental trauma checklist.

Date and time of trauma?

Suspect abuse?	☐ Dentists are mandated to report abuse of children (<18 years old) and the elderly (≥65 years old).

Head trauma?	☐ Rule out concussion or hemorrhage
	    ☐ Symptoms include loss of consciousness, amnesia, nausea/vomiting, confusion, blurred vision, uneven pupils, slurred speech
	    ☐ If positive findings immediately refer to a medical doctor [2]

Lacerations or bruises	☐ Take extraoral/intraoral photos for documentation (e.g. may be used for a future police report)
Missing tooth fragment and a lip laceration?	☐ Take a radiograph of the lacerated soft tissue (Figure 10.3)
Gingival contours	☐ Evaluate for bone displacement.
Tooth positioning	☐ Evaluate the tooth position in the arch from various angles (e.g. facial and incisal) (Figure 10.4) ☐ Does the patient feel a change in their bite?
Tooth color	☐ Evaluate the tooth color compared to the adjacent teeth. Is it discolored (yellow, gray, pink, brown)?
Radiographs	☐ Panoramic or CBCT if suspect jaw fracture ☐ Two PAs from different angles ☐ BW
Radiographic findings	☐ Permanent tooth? ☐ Open or closed apex? ☐ Primary tooth? ☐ Evaluate the distance between the root and the socket (Figure 10.5) ☐ Root fracture? ☐ Root resorption?
Refer to the Trauma Guidelines	☐ See Appendix A

Figure 10.3 Taking a radiograph of the lower lip to rule out any embedded tooth fragments.

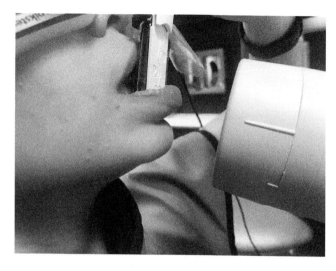

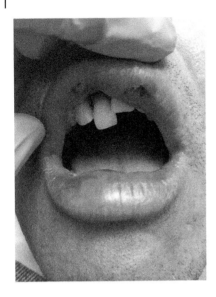

Figure 10.4   Evaluate the position of the tooth in the arch.

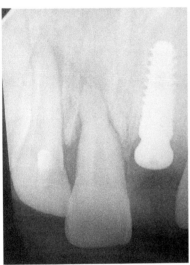

Figure 10.5   Evaluate the distance from the root to the socket.

Dental Trauma Armamentarium

- Storage media in descending order of preference: milk, Hanks' balanced salt solution (HBSS), saliva, saline, water [3].
- MTA or calcium hydroxide.
- Flexible splint material 0.016 inch or 0.4 mm, or nylon fishing line (0.13–0.25 mm).
- 0.12% alcohol-free chlorhexidine bottles.
- Root canal treatment supplies, extraction supplies, and cold compress.

Nonodontogenic Toothaches (Referred Pain)

If the diagnosis is confusing, consider nonodontogenic pain as part of your differential diagnosis (Table 10.3). Do not perform any irreversible dental treatment if the diagnosis is not clear.

Table 10.3   Nonodontogenic toothache (referred pain).

Nonodontogenic toothache	Description	Treatment
Myofascial toothache	• Origin: skeletal muscles • Unique features: determine if the pain is reproducible with palpation of trigger points for about 6–10 seconds. Have patient point to where pain is occurring and trace it to where pain refers. **Trigger point** — **Referred pain to** Temporalis — Maxillary Masseter — Maxillary/mandibular posterior/TMJ Lateral pterygoid — Maxillary sinus/TMJ Anterior digastric — Mandibular incisors Sternocleidomastoid — Oral structures and forehead Trapezius — Mandible/temporalis	• Local anesthetic of strained muscle, warm or cold compress, muscle stretching, massage, restful sleep [4] • Refer to an orofacial pain doctor, oral surgeon, ENT, or medical provider. Think muscle pain before nonodontogenic nerve pain (author recommended)
Cardiac toothache	• Origin: cardiac ischemia • Unique features: local anesthetics and analgesics fail to alleviate dental pain, worsened with exceptional activities and alleviated with rest, feel pressure	• Immediate referral to medical provider [4]
Sinus toothache (sinusitis)	• Origin: inflammation or infection in maxillary sinus • Unique features: pain on palpation of infraorbital region, or pain by bending over with head below the knees; radiograph may show radiopaque sinus or thickened lining (roots may protrude into sinus with only Schneiderian membrane between roots and sinus) • Also note: tooth infection can lead to sinus infection	• Possibly nasal decongestants, possible antibiotics, refer to ENT or medical provider [4]
Neurovascular toothache	• Origin: also known as headaches such as migraines and trigeminal autonomic cephalalgia	• Refer to medical provider [4]
Neuropathic toothache	• Origin: neural structures, conditions such as trigeminal neuralgia • Unique feature: "electrical" pain for a few seconds, most severe pain ever experienced. (Anecdotal report from author's relative: "sharp constant pain all day long and worse when stimulated")	• Refer to medical provider [4]
Neoplastic toothache	• Origin: oral cancer or systemic cancers	• Refer to oral surgeon or medical provider [4]
Psychogenic toothache	• Origin: psychological • Unique feature: variable	• Refer to psychiatrist or psychologist [4]
Temporomandibular joint disorders, cervical pain disorders, and systemic diseases [5]	• Varies	• Refer to an orofacial pain doctor, oral surgeon, or medical provider

Teledentistry and Toothaches

- **Prior to calling the patient**
  - Determine if the patient is of record. If so, is there any pending treatment (e.g. a tooth that is already planned for extraction)?

- **Phone visit**
  - Block your personal number or use the office phone.
  - First introduce yourself: "This is Dr. _____ from _____. May I speak to _____."
  - Ask the patient to confirm their date of birth and to consent to a telephone visit
  - Consider asking the patient to send a photo to help your assessment and for the patient's record. If a virtual visit, ask the patient if he or she consents to taking a screenshot to upload into the records (e.g. swollen face, broken tooth).
  - Document the time of the call and the duration.
  - If no answer, attempt three times and document times of calls.

- **Ask the patient**
  - How can I help you today?
  - Pain level from 0 to 10 ("10 being the worst pain imaginable and 0 being no pain").
  - Pain level currently and at its worst.
  - Description of the pain.
  - What makes it feel better? What makes it feel worse?
  - Is the gum sore?
  - Sharp edge?
  - Swelling? Visible on outside of face if looking in mirror?
  - Any trouble breathing? (Compromised airway)
  - Fever (>38°C, 100.4°F)?
  - Tender lymph nodes or neck muscles?
  - Difficulty opening the mouth wide?
  - Bleeding gums?
  - Recent trauma?
  - Taking medication to manage the pain or the infection?
  - What medication, dosage, and frequency?
  - Rate pain level on scale of 0–10 when taking medication. Is it tolerable?
  - Recent dental work?
  - Last dental visit.
  - Medical conditions? Medications? Allergies? Surgeries? Hospitalizations?

- **Consider the arsenal of supplies outside your office for the patient to use** (if unable to be seen by you soon enough)
  - Prescriptions: antibiotics, analgesics, viscous lidocaine.
  - OTC: ibuprofen, acetaminophen, 20% benzocaine, desensitizing toothpaste, ortho wax, mouthguards, temporary filling and cement, denture adhesive, oral hygiene products, mouthrinses.
  - Home: warm salt-water rinses, teabag (tannic acid for hemostasis).

- **Warn the patient**
  - If between now and the in-person visit the patient develops any facial swelling, malaise, fever, or tender lymph nodes, tell them to call back, as they may need antibiotics.
  - If any trouble breathing tell them to call EMS and to go to the ER.

- **Determine how soon to schedule the patient's visit (urgency level)**
  - See Table 10.4
  - Set the patient's expectations ahead of time.
  - Inform the patient an in-person visit is needed. This will involve a clinical and radiographic exam to determine what treatment is recommended. The treatment may be completed in the office or may be referred to a specialist.

Clinical Pearls

Troubleshooting

- Trouble determining which tooth is causing pain in a mouth full of broken teeth or root tips? Percuss each tooth and observe which elicits the most painful response to determine which tooth to prioritize for extraction.
- Trouble determining the offending tooth when a parulis is present?
  - A parulis (i.e. gumboil or stoma) may appear on the gingiva and you may be uncertain as to the source. The parulis could be adjacent to the infected tooth, between two teeth (and both may have PARLs), or several teeth away from the infected tooth. When a parulis is present it means the infection has burrowed its way through the bone and soft tissue in order to drain.
  - To trace the sinus tract, dry the soft tissue, place topical anesthetic, inform the patient that they will feel some pressure, and insert a medium-size gutta percha point into the sinus tract. If you feel resistance, change the angulation until the gutta percha goes in freely. Add rope wax to hold the gutta percha in place against a tooth and take a PA. This will indicate the source and confirm your diagnosis (Figure 10.6).

(a)

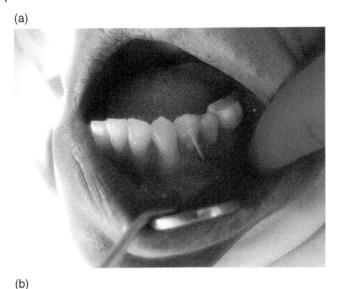

(b)

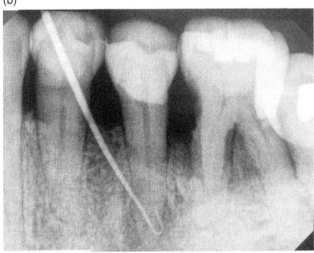

Figure 10.6 (a, b) Tracing a sinus tract to determine or confirm the offending tooth.

- Trouble determining if the patient is grinding or clenching their teeth or a patient who is unaware of their parafunctional habits? Ask the patient about their stress levels and look for signs including a bilateral linea alba, a scalloped tongue, abfractions, worn dentition, and tender masseter and temporalis.
- Trouble diagnosing the pulpal condition with the cold test on a patient with questionable responses? If the responses from the cold test do not make sense, such as responses to cold on a root canal-treated tooth (a "false positive"), then out of the patient's vision pretend to spray the cotton pellet (i.e. spray right next to, but not on, the pellet so that the patient hears the sound of the spray) and then place the pellet on a vital tooth. If the patient responds to cold, then it is another "false positive" and you should refer to an endodontist. Do not initiate treatment where the diagnosis is inconclusive.
- Potential dilemma with restorability (and sequencing): a patient attends with a severe toothache on a tooth with an existing crown and you want to refer the patient to the endodontist immediately for RCT. How do you know if the tooth is restorable? See Chapter 4, section Real-Life Questions Answered.

Tips

- "Listen to the patient, he is telling you the diagnosis" said Sir William Osler [1].
  - Listen more than talk. Do not rush. Do not make hasty decisions. Do not make assumptions. When in doubt, refer out.
- Diagnosis:
  - Check all surfaces of a tooth, including:
    - ○ The gumline (Figure 10.7).
    - ○ The pits and fissures with an explorer. The tooth may appear intact and then the explorer drops into a crack, wedging the tooth apart and revealing a split tooth (Figure 10.8).
  - To determine if percussion sensitive, be sure to percuss at various surfaces of a tooth.
  - Typically, if the patient complains that the toothache interferes with their sleep, then the tooth requires more than a filling – it requires RCT or extraction.
  - Ask open-ended questions and do not give patients the words you are looking for, such as "electric" or "burning."
  - Remember that it is not always "toothache" but can be "gumache." For example, a 50 year old with erupted third molars, no caries, and pain 10/10 on #32 was anesthetized, followed by SRP of the 6-mm pockets around tooth #32. Patient was contacted the next day and the pain was gone.
  - A recent composite you completed broke and the patient comes in for replacement. Don't assume it simply needs the filling redone. Take a BW and PA; you may find a PARL and the tooth may require RCT, buildup, and a crown instead.
- Trust no one:
  - Always be sure to obtain your own diagnosis. If the patient has seen another dentist and that dentist diagnosed and treatment planned for RCT and the patient is on your schedule for RCT, do not begin RCT! Do not rely on the diagnosis from your colleague. Obtain your own diagnosis. It could be a misdiagnosis and only require a composite restoration, or pain could be casued by food impaction.
  - Similarly, do not take the patient's word for what the specialist recommended. Always obtain the report from the specialist.
- If the patient is in your office due to discomfort after treatment by a specialist (e.g. an endodontist or an OMFS) be sure to send the patient back to the specialist. It is the responsibility of the specialist, so do not get involved.
- A sharp broken tooth is irritating a patient's tongue or cheek and you are unable to offer a same-day extraction or restoration. Smooth the sharp edge with a white diamond bur (high speed with water) until the patient is satisfied. This does not require local anesthetic.
- Documentation:
  - If prescribing antibiotics, document why it was indicated.
  - If the patient refuses treatment options, make sure you document what you offered and what was refused (such as "Offered to write a prescription for ibuprofen and acetaminophen," "Offered to administer a long-acting local anesthetic," "Offered same-day extraction, and the patient refused"). Also document that you warned the patient of the consequences of no treatment and/or delayed treatment and that the patient understood.

Toothaches

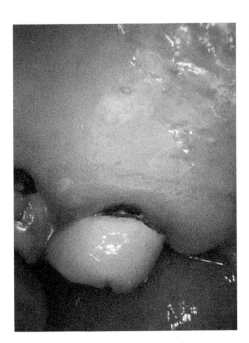

Figure 10.7 Check all surfaces of the tooth, including the gumline. A #2 PFM crown had recurrent decay which was missed by the dental provider.

(a)

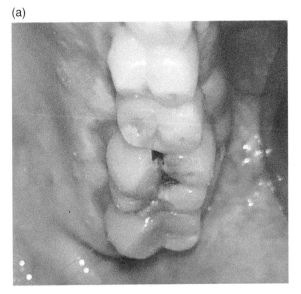

Figure 10.8 (a, b) A tooth causing pain appeared intact but on further investigation with an explorer revealed a split tooth. The tooth was deemed nonrestorable and extracted.

(b)

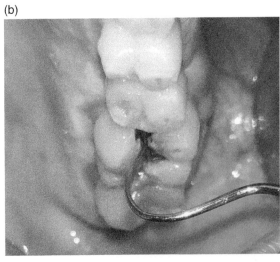

Real-Life Questions, Concerns, and Demands Answered

Dental Students' Questions

- "I don't know what to do if a patient walks in with a toothache?"
  - Approach each case systematically to discover an accurate diagnosis. The diagnosis dictates the treatment plan. It is easy to overlook checking the pocket depths or occlusion during the visit and once the patient leaves you are unable to go back in time and check these things. For this reason, using a toothache checklist (see Table 10.1) is useful. It also helps you later on in the day when you are charting rather than relying on your memory.

Dental Assistant's Questions

- "The patient has several teeth bothering her today. How many X-rays should I take?"
  - Inform the patient that due to limited time he or she should indicate which tooth is causing the most pain and take a radiograph of that tooth. We can address the other teeth at the next visit (the new patient exam).

Office Manager's Question

- "What is considered a true emergency or an urgent appointment?"
  - If a patient calls the office, use Table 10.4 to help you screen the patient to determine the level of urgency and determine how soon they should be seen. If the patient is having trouble breathing tell them to call EMS and go to the ER.

Table 10.4   Prioritization for scheduling dental emergencies.

Emergency type	Description	When to schedule
True dental emergencies	• According to the ADA "are potentially life threatening and require immediate treatment to stop ongoing tissue bleeding [or to] alleviate severe pain or infection." Examples are uncontrolled bleeding, bacterial infection with intraoral or extraoral swelling that may compromise the patient's airway, or trauma involving the facial bones potentially compromising the patient's airway [6] • True emergencies disrupt the patient's sleep/ability to eat, has bothered the patient a few hours to two days, and pain medications are ineffective [7]	Same day
Urgent	• Tooth sensitivity, sore spot, pain managed by OTC medications, broken filling, broken denture/partial, temporary/permanent crown fell off	Within seven days
Nonurgent	• Dental exams, cleanings, fillings, removable procedures, anything elective, etc.	Next available opening

Toothaches

Patients' Concerns

- "The tooth you did the filling on hurts when I bite or chew food."
  - Determine if the occlusion on the restoration is heavy as this can make the tooth sore to biting and chewing. The patient may have been too numb at the filling appointment to determine if the bite felt normal. Adjust the occlusion and see if the patient reports immediate relief. If the occlusion was not heavy, recommend endodontic diagnostic testing. It is common to have some soreness after recent dental work.
- "Can this tooth be saved?"
  - Saving the tooth is always my goal; however, I need to complete a clinical and radiographic evaluation to determine if it is savable.
- "Gum hurts under my denture."
  - Useful tip: If there is a traumatic ulceration on the gums, mark it with the Thompson stick and seat the denture to transfer the mark so you know exactly where to adjust the denture. Remove the denture from the mouth, adjust it with an acrylic bur, and seat back in the mouth. Ask the patient by how much (as a percentage) it has improved. Also have the patient bite on two cotton rolls (one on each side) and to imagine chewing food to see if it still hurts. May require more adjusting and a follow-up visit.
- "I have a bump or pimple on my gums."
  - Likely a parulis/gumboil. May require tracing the sinus tract if uncertain as to which is the offending tooth, or to confirm the offending tooth (see Figure 10.6 and Section Troubleshooting).
- "This broken tooth is cutting my tongue."
  - For palliative treatment, if limited time and unable to provide definitive treatment (such as an extraction or a restoration), adjust with a white stone bur (high speed) until the patient is satisfied.

Patients' Questions

- "Does the X-ray show the tooth fracture?"
  - "Signs and symptoms often are not present early but manifest months, years, or decades after fracture initiation" [7].
  - Fractures can be a diagnostic challenge and oftentimes are not visible on radiographs. Depending on location and severity, diagnosis may require other forms of radiographs, exploratory periodontal surgery, or endodontically accessing the tooth for further evaluation.
  - See Chapter 8 for types of tooth fractures.

- "I don't know if this is a toothache or if it is related to my sinus problems?"
  - See Section Nonodontogenic Toothaches (Referred Pain).
- "Here is my son's broken tooth, can you attach it back on?" (see Figure 10.2)
  - Inform the parent that sometimes it works, sometimes it doesn't. Advantage: looks more esthetic than composite.
  - Steps: place tooth fragment in sterile saline for 30 minutes to hydrate. Evaluate if there is pulpal involvement of the tooth and treat as necessary. It is best not to adjust the tooth and the fragment to ensure the best fit. If an indirect or direct pulp cap is necessary, you may have to gain some space on the tooth fragment for the material. Bevel the facial and lingual of the tooth and the fragment. Etch the beveled portions, rinse, and dry. Use a bonding agent with a thin film thickness. Place bonding agent on the tooth and the fragment. Hold the fragment tightly against the tooth and light cure. Place a thin layer of flowable composite along the facial and lingual of the tooth and light cure. Check occlusion, adjust as necessary, and polish.

Patients' Demands

- "My crown fell off and I just need you to glue it back on."
  - Oftentimes it is not as simple as just cementing the crown back on the tooth. We need to figure out the cause for the loss of retention. Typically, it is a bad sign if a permanent crown has fallen off. Loss of retention could be due to recurrent decay, a tooth/buildup fracture (if the tooth is attached to the intaglio of the crown), or an overly tapered crown prep. Do not re-cement the crown if there is a risk of swallowing and aspirating the crown. If the fit of the crown is very snug, you could permanently re-cement it and treatment plan a new crown as it is unlikely to remain cemented.
- "You need to pull this tooth out. This one hurts."
  - "Thanks for pointing to the tooth that is bothering you. I don't want to make any hasty decisions so I need to take a closer look. I've had patient's in the past with referred pain so I want to be 100% certain that this is the tooth causing the pain." Even if the patient is demanding you pull a specific tooth, you are the doctor and you must complete a thorough clinical and radiographic exam and there must be an indication for the extraction. With referred pain, you could extract a tooth and not resolve the toothache. I have had patient's in the chair crying and requesting that a specific tooth be pulled that had no indication for extraction.
    - Example 1: patient crying and pointing to #20 requesting extraction. Upon further evaluation, it was determined that #18 was causing referred pain. Referred pain can be from:
      - an upper tooth to a lower tooth
      - from a posterior tooth to a more mesial tooth
      - does not cross the midline.
    - Example 2: patient crying and pointing to #3 with no indication for extraction. Upon further evaluation, the patient was referred to her medical provider and diagnosed with migraines. Once she began taking medication for her migraines, the toothache went away.
    - In both cases imagine if the tooth the patient wanted out was extracted. This irreversible treatment would not have resolved the toothache and the patient would not be happy.
    - Also, when in doubt, refer out.
- "I need antibiotics for this."
  - See Chapter 16, section Real-Life Questions Answered.
- "I need something stronger than ibuprofen, like Norco."
  - See Chapter 16, section Real-Life Questions Answered.

References

1 Jane Sarasohn-Kahn, MA, MHSA. Listening to Osler Listening to the Patient: How to Liberate Health Care at Liberation (2019). https://liberatehealth.medecision.com/listening-to-osler-listening-to-the-patient (accessed 22 March 2020).

2 McCrory, P., Meeuwisse, W.H., Aubry, M. et al. (2013). Consensus statement on concussion in sport: the 4th International Conference on Concussion in Sport, Zurich, November 2012. *J. Athl. Train.* 48: 554–575.

3 DiAngelis, A.J., Andreasen, J.O., Ebeleseder, K.A. et al. (2012). International Association of Dental Traumatology guidelines for the management of traumatic dental injuries: 1. Fractures and luxations of permanent teeth. *Dent. Traumatol.* 28: 2–12.

4 Balasubramanian, R., Turner, L.N., Fischer, D. et al. (2011). Non-odontogenic toothache revisited. *Open J. Stomatol.* 1: 92–102.

Toothaches

5 Neville, B.W., Damm, D.D., Allen, C.M., and Chi, A.C. (ed.) (2016). *Oral and Maxillofacial Pathology*, 4e. St. Louis, MO: Elsevier.

6 American Dental Association (2020). ADA develops guidance on dental emergency, nonemergency care. http://www.ada.org/en/publications/ada-news/2020-archive/march/ada-develops-guidance-on-dental-emergency-nonemergency-care (accessed 22 March 2020).

7 Torabinejad, M. and Walton, R.E. (2009). *Endodontics: Principles and Practice*, 4e. St. Louis, MO: Saunders Elsevier.

11

Crown and Bridge

Kind of Esthetic

Porcelain Fused Metal

○ Non Precious ○ High Precious (white)
○ Semi Precious ○ High Precious (yellow)

Full Metal Crown

○ Non Precious ○ Semi Precious (white)
○ Gold milled (58%, 2%)
○ Gold casted (call us for %)

All Ceramic

○ Full Contour Zirconia
○ Porcelain Fused to Zirconia
○ E-max Staining Tech.
○ E-max Layering Tech.

Margin Design

Facial

○ M/P Junction
○ Porcelain Margin

Lingual

○ M/P Junction
○ Metal Margin

All Around

○ 360° Porcelain Margin
○ 360° Metal Margin
○ 360° M/P Junction

Metal Design

○ Metal Lingual
○ Metal Occlusal *Excluding* Buccal Cusp
○ Metal Occlusal *Including* Buccal Cusp
○ Cingulum Rest
○ Occlusal Rest (Mesial/Distal)
○ Fit to Partial

Pontic Design

If Insufficient Room

○ Please Call
○ Reduce Die
○ Reduction Coping
○ Spot on Opposing
○ Metal Island

Return For

○ Die Trim   ○ Frame Work
○ Diagnostic Wax View ○ Bisque Bake

Sex: ○ Male ○ Female Age: _____

CONTACTS
Light ○
Regular ○
Tight ○

OCCLUSION
Light ○
Regular ○
Tight ○

SURFACE FINISH
☐ High Glaze
☐ Polished Gloss
☐ Satin Finish
☐ Low Gloss

OCCLUSAL STAIN
☐ None
☐ Light
☐ Medium
☐ Dark

A: ☐ Sanitary Spaced
B: ☐ Sanitary Contact
C: ☐ Buccal Lap
D: ☐ Full Lap
E: ☐ Ovate _____ mm

A B C D E

STUMP: _____

SHADE: _____

○ Check Here For Custom Shade

Collage of lab prescriptions.

Chapter Outline

- Real-Life Clinical Scenarios
- Relevance
- Clinical and Radiographic Exam
- Treatment Planning Considerations
  - Terms Used in this Chapter
  - Ferrule
  - Biologic Width
  - Indications and Considerations for Crowns
  - Indications and Considerations for Bridges

Clinical Dentistry Daily Reference Guide, First Edition. William A. Jacobson.
© 2022 John Wiley & Sons, Inc. Published 2022 by John Wiley & Sons, Inc.

Real-Life Clinical Scenarios

Dental Students' Questions

- "How do we know if the tooth needs a filling, or a buildup, or a crown?"
- "I'm not good at shade selection. Any advice?"
- "Doctor, did I invade the biologic width?"
- "Do I send the patient for crown lengthening before I prep the crown?"
- "What is flash?"
- "Do I take a bitewing before and after cementing the crown?"
- "How do I check for interferences?"

Dental Students' Comments

- "I'm doing a crown because it was treatment planned by the last student."

- "For crowns, I always treatment plan PFMs."
- "I've never cut off a crown before, I hope the tooth is OK underneath."
- "Today I am prepping a survey crown."

Dental Assistant's Questions

- "Doc, every time I make the temporary it breaks and sticks on the tooth."
- "At the crown delivery appointment, I just took the temporary crown off and the buildup broke. What should I do?"

Patients' Questions

- You section off an existing crown and determine the tooth is not restorable. The patient yells "You're telling me now I have to get the tooth pulled when I thought I was just getting my crown replaced?"
- "Doc I cannot afford a crown right now but I just had a root canal done and the specialist said I need a crown. How long can I wait?"
- "Which type of crown will last the longest?"
- "The temporary broke again, should I sleep with my partials in until I get the permanent crowns?"
- "How do you know if I have a cavity under the crown? Can you pull the crown off to see and then put it back on?"
- "Do you recommend a bridge or an implant?"

Patient's Comments

- Crown not seating at the delivery appointment and patient said "The temporary crown fell off the next day but I figured I'd see you in a week for the permanent crown and it wasn't bothering me so I didn't call."
- At the crown delivery appointment, patient said "Doc, this tooth is so sensitive to cold."

Patient's Demand

- "My crown fell off and I just need you to glue it back on."

Colleague's Question

- "When are we supposed to worry about incisal guidance?"

Scenarios

- A dental student tries on a crown and no open margins are detected. Once the student cements the crown, the crown now has an open margin on the buccal.
- A dental student permanently cemented a crown on the patient without showing the patient how it looks in the mirror for shade selection approval.
- A dental assistant loads the permanent crown with Fuji IX instead of Fuji CEM.
- A dental student makes a full arch final impression and it becomes locked in beneath a bridge.

Relevance

Crown and bridge falls within the scope of general dentistry. A crown protects a tooth from fracturing and a bridge replaces missing teeth. This chapter provides only clinically relevant material, photos, and illustrations to help guide you.

Clinical and Radiographic Exam

Carefully evaluate the condition of every existing crown/bridge and the teeth considered for crown/bridge
- Clinical exam
    - Decay (initial or recurrent)? (Figure 11.2)
    - Fractured?
    - Ferrule? (See Section Treatment Planning and Figure 11.6)
    - Virgin tooth?
    - Existing restoration satisfactory?
        - Open margins on existing crowns? (Check with the explorer/floss/radiograph) (Figure 11.3)
        - Contours? (Esthetic? Food trap?)
        - Shade?
        - Proximal contacts?
        - Occlusion?
    - Periodontal status? See Chapter 6
    - Pulpal/periapical status? See Chapter 7
    - Occlusion
        - Posterior stops? If not, will you have to fabricate wax occlusal rims and full arch impressions so that the lab technician can properly articulate the models?
        - Crossbite? Open bite?
            - Determine which are the functional and nonfunctional cusps
        - Tipped tooth or adjacent teeth?
        - Is the tooth so severely supraerupted it will require endodontic treatment to permit shortening the crown to correct the occlusal plane or extraction? (Figure 11.4)
    - Shade match? See Section Treatment Planning
- Radiographic exam
    - All teeth being prepared for a crown/bridge need a recent (less than one year old) PA to rule out any periapical pathosis.
    - Interpret radiographs (see Chapter 3)
    - Carefully evaluate the distance of the restorative material (e.g. core buildup, composite) relative to the crestal bone to assess the likelihood that the tooth will require crown lengthening (Figure 11.5).

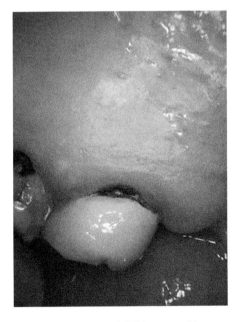

Figure 11.2 Tooth #2 PFM crown with recurrent decay on the palatal root surface.

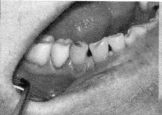
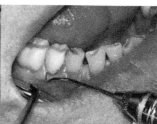

Bitewing: #29 existing
Zirconia crown has closed margins

#29 Zirconia crown appears to have closed margins

#29 Zirconia crown has an open margin in which the tip of the explorer fits inside about 3 min.
Always check the margins of existing crowns with the explorer.

Figure 11.3   Tooth #29 open margin on clinical evaluation.

Figure 11.4   A patient lost her #2 temporary crown provided by another dental office. Her chief complaint was "I'd like a crown put in here." Tooth #2 has supraerupted and is now occluding with #31.

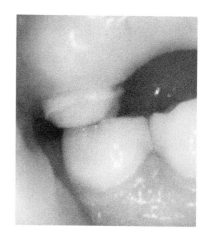

Figure 11.5   Tooth #14 D was not examined carefully enough preoperatively and the patient was told she needed crown lengthening mid-treatment (while attempting a final impression). This should be avoided. Best to carefully evaluate and warn the patient of any possible additional treatment ahead of time.

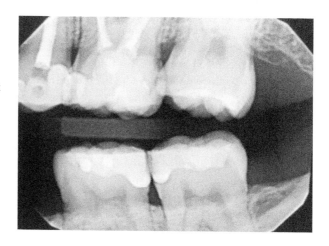

Treatment Planning Considerations

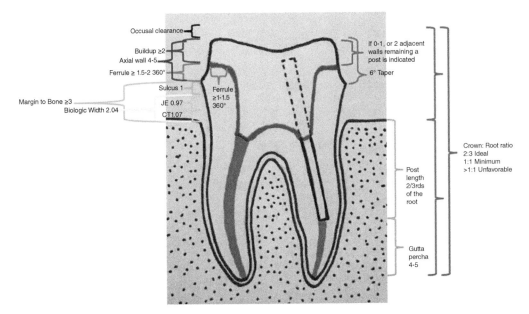

Figure 11.6 Dimensions to consider when evaluating a tooth. The units for all the numbers are in millimeters (mm). JE, junctional epithelium; CT, connective tissue.

Terms Used in this Chapter

- **Crown**: full coverage.
- **PFM**: porcelain fused to metal crown. Porcelain for esthetics, and metal coping for strength. The metal coping covers and protects the tooth.
- **Bridge**: also known as a fixed partial denture (FPD). Replaces missing teeth.
- **Prep**: preparation, i.e. the tooth that has been reduced to a smaller version of itself to allow space for the crown or bridge material.
- **Abutment**: the tooth structure supporting the crown or retainer (FPD).
- **Retainer**: the tooth (crown) on the bridge.
- **Pontic**: the tooth being replaced on the bridge.
- **Connector**: located between the retainer and pontic of a bridge. The connector may be **rigid** (soldered) or **nonrigid** (similar to a lock and key, to transfer stress to the bone rather than the connector) [1]. Nonrigid connectors are also used when a single path of insertion cannot be achieved with nonparallel abutments (e.g. tiled molar and an upright premolar).
- **Provisional**: temporary (e.g. provisional crown).
- **Definitive**: permanent (e.g. definitive crown).
- **Matrix**: the preliminary impression of the abutment tooth before being prepared for fabricating the provisional crown.
- **PVS**: polyvinyl siloxane, the impression material used for crown and bridge. Also referred to as VPS (vinyl polysiloxane).
- **Stump**: the prepared tooth for a crown/bridge (i.e. the dentin) typically used to describe the "stump shade."

Ferrule

- "A band or ring used to encompass the root or crown of a tooth" [2].
- Refers to the amount of solid tooth structure above the bone level needed to retain a crown.
- Analogies for describing ferrules to patients to explain why adequate tooth structure is necessary:
  - Like trying to get a baseball cap to fit on a person's shoulder, instead of a person's head.
  - Like hair extensions, you need enough hair to attach the extensions to.
- This term is used when assessing restorability (must also take into consideration other factors).
- Requirements:
  - Ferrule height: 1.5–2 mm of sound dentin.
  - Ferrule width: 360° of 1–1.5 mm of sound dentin.
  - Axial wall height for retention: 4–5 mm (ferrule + core buildup).
    - Post and core: if coronal to the minimum ferrule (2 mm) and only none or one wall of dentin remains, or two adjacent walls of dentin remain, then endodontic treatment and a post and core is needed to retain a crown.

Biologic Width

- "The combined width of connective tissue and junctional epithelial attachment formed adjacent to a tooth and superior to the crestal bone."
- Biologic width = junctional epithelium (0.97 mm average) + connective tissue (1.07 mm average) = 2.04 mm [2].
- To measure the biologic width on a tooth:
  - Estimate from the bitewing (only interproximals) (see Figure 11.5).
  - Hygiene should be under control without any signs of inflammation for accuracy.
  - Measure the pocket depths around the tooth: requires a minimum 1 mm sulcus depth.
  - Anesthetize.
  - "Sound the bone" with the periodontal probe around the tooth (place the probe deep enough until crestal bone is contacted).
  - Do not place the crown margin <3 mm from the crestal bone [3]: 2 mm from the crestal bone is the closest; <2 mm violates the biologic width.
  - When prepping, especially anterior, be sure to follow the rise and fall of the CEJ interproximally.
  - Tooth may require crown lengthening or orthodontic extrusion to avoid violating the biologic width.
- Violation of biologic width
  - Signs and symptoms:
    - The patient may complain of discomfort when measuring pocket depths.
    - Gingival inflammation, bleeding on probing, bone loss, recession.
  - Estimate from the bitewing (only interproximals).
  - Measure the pocket depths around the tooth.
  - Anesthetize.
  - "Sound the bone" with the periodontal probe around the tooth contacting the crestal bone.
  - Subtract the pocket depth from the "sounding bone" depth. If <2 mm anywhere, the biologic width has been violated.
  - Treatment: crown lengthening or orthodontic extrusion
    - With crown lengthening you must consider:
      - Esthetics (anterior gingival margin).
      - Furcation involvement (posterior).

- Crown/root ratio (minimum 1 : 1).
- Root sensitivity of adjacent teeth with exposed cementum.
- With orthodontic extrusion: maintains the gingival level but decreases the crown/root ratio.
- For sequencing crown lengthening
  - Prep the tooth and fabricate a temporary crown prior to crown lengthening to aid the periodontist in determining the bone level and for easier access and visibility.
  - If RCT is needed, complete RCT prior to crown lengthening as the RCT could deem the tooth nonrestorable (e.g. fractured root, endodontic complication).
  - Sequence: assess restorability, RCT (if indicated), core buildup and temporary crown, crown lengthening, healing time, refine the prep and final impression, definitive crown.
- Taper (Figure 11.7): the more nearly parallel the opposing walls are, the greater the retention. However, parallel walls in the mouth produce undercuts which must be avoided. Opinions differ regarding exact amount of taper:
  - 6° (ideally) to 10° is typically taught in dental schools.
  - As low as 10° for anteriors and as high as 22° for molars [1].

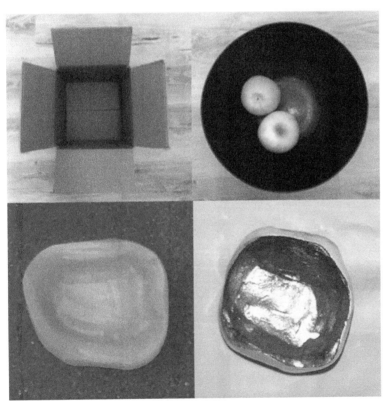

Figure 11.7   An analogy when looking at the intaglio (i.e. internal surface) of a crown. On a retentive crown, the intaglio should appear similar to the inside of a cardboard box (but with a slight taper and no sharp internal line angles). On a poorly retentive crown, the intaglio will appear similar to the inside of a bowl.

Indications

Factors to consider when deciding between a direct restoration (e.g. composite, amalgam) versus an indirect restoration (e.g. crown).

- Replacing a crown:
  - Existing post and core? Likely inadequate tooth structure beneath.
  - Subgingival margins and/or recurrent decay? More of a challenge to obtain a final impression and restore. May violate the biologic width (see Section Biologic Width).
- Amount of remaining tooth structure: need a crown for strength and protection?
- Loss of incisal edge
  - Anteriors: "traumatic or pathological destruction of the crown of the tooth which involves four or more tooth surfaces including at least the loss of one incisal angle" and "the facial or lingual surface shall not be considered involved for a mesial or proximal restoration unless the proximal restoration wraps around the tooth to at least the midline."
  - "loss of an incisal angle which involves a minimum area of both half the incisal width and half the height of the anatomical crown."
  - "incisal angle is not involved but more than 50% of the anatomical crown is involved" [4].
- Loss of a cusp
  - Is it a functional cusp (more stress, recommend crown)? Or a nonfunctional cusp (less stress bearing)?
  - Premolars: "Traumatic or pathological destruction of the crown which involves three or more tooth surfaces including at least one cusp."
  - Molars: "Traumatic or pathological destruction of the crown which involves three or more tooth surfaces including at least two cusps" [4].
    - For patients. with insurance coverage, it is important to be aware of insurance guidelines. Please note that insurance guidelines are fickle and that insurers don't always follow their own guidelines. Best to always preauthorize so that there are no surprises (i.e. unexpected bill in the mail).
- Posterior root canal treated tooth
  - "While cuspal coverage is typically recommended in the posterior dentition following root canal procedures, this may not be necessary in some instances" such as "teeth with minimal structural loss, intact marginal ridges, a conservative access preparation, and no pre-existing cracks, the clinician may consider a direct intracoronal bonded restoration as a valid option" [5].
  - Recommend full coverage crown. Not necessary for anterior unless severely weakened. Check if well obturated and no periapical pathology or symptoms before placing a crown.
- Cracked tooth syndrome.
- Esthetics:
  - Changing the shape of a tooth.
  - Changing the shade of a tooth that cannot be altered by bleaching (e.g. tetracycline stains).
  - Highly visible tooth in a highly discriminating patient.

Considerations

- Plaque control and caries risk: if high caries risk (high caries risk (HCR) and/or extensive plaque, weigh the pros and cons of placing a crown. You may simply be moving the location for caries to develop (the gumline). Consider a direct restoration until plaque control is improved for a direct restoration.

- Retention: is there a short tooth and/or limited interocclusal space?
- Adequate tooth structure for ferrule: minimum 1.5–2 mm ferrule necessary (with 1–1.5 mm thick dentin). Additional buildup material used to provide a total of 4–5 mm axial height for retention. If inadequate ferrule and axial height, expect the patient to return with the crown in their hand and the abutment cemented inside from the tooth sheering off.
- Periodontal health: check mobility, bone loss, gingival health (see Chapter 3).
- Biologic width violated? (see Section Biologic Width and Figure 11.6).
- Is a post indicated? (see Section Post and Core and Figure 11.6).
- Crown/root ratio for abutment tooth (see Figure 11.6).
  - <1 : 1 (favorable, 2 : 3 ratio is optimal) (see Chapter 3, Figure 3.14, tooth #23).
  - 1 : 1 (minimum) (see Chapter 3, Figure 3.14, tooth # 25).
  - >1 : 1 (unfavorable) (see Chapter 3, Figure 3.14, tooth #24) [1].
- Patient's age: is the permanent tooth fully erupted? If not, place an Ion crown until fully erupted. If a primary tooth, place an Ion crown.
- Placement of finish line location (Table 11.1).
- Strong gag reflex? Large strong tongue?
- High esthetic demands? Does the patient have realistic expectations? If so, consider custom shade match at the dental lab.
- Cost.

Table 11.1 Finish line placement: advantages and disadvantages.

Finish line placement	Advantages	Disadvantages
Supragingival	Easier to obtain the margins when making a final impression Easier to remove excess cement Preferred for gingival health; will not violate the biologic width Most cleansable (hygienic) for the patient Easily accessible for the dentist at recall appointments to check for recurrent decay	Esthetics if in the esthetic zone If recession and vital, may have root sensitivity
Equigingival	Esthetic until the gingiva recedes More cleansable for the patient than a subgingival finish line	Harder to obtain margins when making a final impression, requires cord retraction More challenging to remove excess cement Less accessible for the dentist at recall appointments to check for recurrent decay with the explorer
Subgingival	Esthetic to hide the margin and for emergence profile, until the gingiva recedes Can help improve retention when the tooth has a short clinical crown Cover sensitive roots *Note*: sometimes unavoidable due to caries, previous restorations, trauma, and esthetics	Most challenging to obtain the margins when making a final impression. Requires cord retraction, may require gingivectomy or crown lengthening Most challenging to remove excess cement Greater risk of violating the biologic width Least easily accessible for the dentist at recall appointments to check for recurrent decay with the explorer

In addition to the section Indications and Considerations for Crowns.

Indications

For indications and other options, see Chapter 4, Table 4.3.

Considerations

- Plaque control and caries risk: if high caries risk (HCR) and extensive plaque, weigh the pros and cons of placing a bridge. You may simply be moving the location for caries to develop to the gumline. If the patient does not have meticulous hygiene, the bridge will fail from caries and/or periodontal disease and the patient will end up losing more teeth than they had missing when they requested a bridge. Consider a removable appliance until the plaque control and caries risk improves. A bridge can be a disservice to a patient with HCR (Figure 11.8).
- Number of teeth being replaced
  - Ante's Law: evaluate the BWs and PAs to determine if "the root surface area of the abutment teeth had to equal or surpass that of teeth being replaced with pontics" [6].
  - More than two teeth considered high risk, the longer the less rigid and more bending [1].
  - Posterior: replace two or more teeth [1].
  - Anterior: replace up to four incisors [1].
- Abutment teeth
  - Adjacent teeth that have restorations are better candidates for a bridge than virgin adjacent teeth as you would be compromising even more tooth structure on virgin teeth.
  - If root canal treated, the tooth has a greater risk of fracture. Consider double abutment especially if a bruxer.
  - Root configuration:
    - Molars: multirooted divergent roots are better than multirooted fused roots [1].
    - Single rooted: irregular configuration or curved are better than tapered [1].
  - Secondary abutment: must have at least as much root surface area and favorable crown/root ratio as the primary abutment [1].
  - Arch curvature: when pontics lie outside of the inter-abutment axis lines, the pontics produce a torquing movement. More problematic when replacing four maxillary anteriors, thus first premolars may have to be used as secondary abutments [1].
  - Tilted molar abutments: typically seen with mandibular third and second molars. Orthodontic uprighting of the molar may be necessary for a parallel path of insertion for a bridge, which could take about three months [1]. A molar distal to the tipped molar could prevent the seating of the retainer. Other options include telescoping crowns, a proximal half crown on the tilted molar, or a nonrigid connector. Telescoping crowns and nonrigid connector require more tooth reduction [1].
  - Lateral incisors as an abutment tooth: the weakest anterior tooth [1].
  - First premolar as an abutment tooth: the weakest posterior tooth [1].
  - Canine as a pontic: considered complex. Should not replace more than one additional tooth due to the amount of stress on the bridge. If loss of a canine and two or more adjacent teeth, an RPD is recommended [1].
  - Cantilevers: meaning one end of the bridge does not have a retainer. This can be destructive to the abutment teeth. Generally, should only replace one tooth with two abutments. Scenarios where it may work are as follows:
    - Maxillary canine as an abutment replacing a maxillary lateral incisor with no occlusal contacts in centric or excursions.

Mandibular molar and second premolar as abutments replacing a mandibular first premolar [1].

Mandibular first and second premolars as abutments replacing a mandibular first molar; however, the molar pontic must be the size of a premolar to minimize stress on the abutments [1].

Esthetic zone: consider the pontic to ridge location. Will this lead to an unesthetic result?

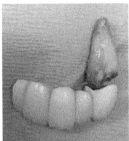
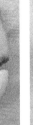

Recurrent Decay

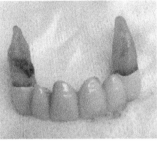

Periodontal Disease

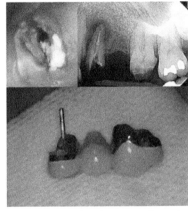

Loss of retention due to a split tooth

Figure 11.8 Examples of failed bridges.

Author's Crown Material Decision Tree

1. Patient involvement

Ask if the patient has a preference on tooth color or non-tooth color:

Tooth colored options (PFM, zirconia, all ceramic).

Non-tooth colored options (gold, cast metal).

Ask the patient if some visible metal is acceptable:

Yes (PFM with metal occlusal or lingual or metal collar, gold, cast metal).

No (PFM with no metal visible, zirconia, all ceramic).

Determine if the patient has bruxing or any other habits (e.g. nail biting, chewing pens) or if the patient's diet consists of hard foods (e.g. chewing ice).

Yes (gold, PFM with metal occlusal for posterior or lingual for upper anterior, polished zirconia).

No (PFM, zirconia layered, all ceramic).

Metal allergies? Avoid base metal (nickel often found in PFM base metal crowns).

2. Clinical exam

Supraerupted or large pulp horns?

Yes (use most conservative preps: gold, solid zirconia, or PFM with metal occlusal for posterior). Warn of possible need for RCT.

No (any crown type).

Dark abutment, buildup, or metal core that needs to be blocked out?

Yes (gold, cast metal, PFM, zirconia).

No (any crown type).

Are the adjacent teeth crowned? If so, what material type? (For best shade try to match the material.)

Opposing teeth:

Natural: consider wear of material on opposing tooth; porcelain and glazed zirconia are abrasive on opposing enamel, so consider use of an occlusal guard. Request from the lab polished (not glazed) zirconia to reduce abrasiveness as the glaze on glazed zirconia will wear off making the crown abrasive. See Section Lab Prescriptions.

Removable: less concerned with wear on opposing teeth; more flexibility with reduction; can easily adjust denture teeth.

Crown: try to match crown materials so similar wear coefficients. If gold, oppose with gold or metal occlusal.

Abutment teeth for RPD?

No (any type).

Yes (PFM, metal, gold, solid zirconia). If considering PFM, determine the design (see Figure 11.1).

Margin design

Metal collar/margin: most cleansable, least tooth reduction, useful if subgingival or hard to reach part of tooth with minimal reduction, and easier to adjust versus porcelain which fractures. Determine which surfaces of the tooth or 360° (better for gingival health) (Figure 11.9).

Metal–porcelain junction (disappearing margin): more esthetic.

Porcelain margin (butt-joint): most esthetic, least conservative, higher likelihood of chipping.

Metal design

Metal occlusal: for minimal tooth reduction, for short clinical crowns, and/or opposing gold/metal.

Metal lingual: for minimal tooth reduction or for maxillary anteriors (centric stop should be ≥1.5 mm from the metal–porcelain juncture). Better gingival health.

Metal rest seats as indicated: for cast metal RPD (to avoid porcelain fracture).

Figure 11.9 A lingual metal collar was used on the PFM at the hard to reach places along the distal and lingual surfaces.

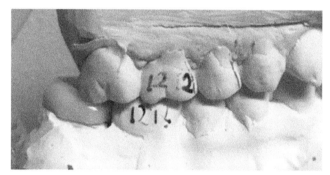

Buccal

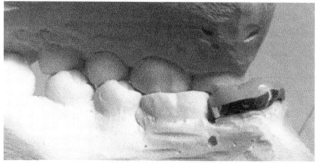

Lingual

3. Consider crown material properties (Table 11.2)

Crown material properties.

Crown material	Advantages	Disadvantages	Indications	Contraindications	Miscellaneous
Gold	Minimal tooth reduction Gentle on opposing teeth Longevity Strength Well-sealed margins Almost no material failures	Not tooth colored (while some patients may prefer gold colored)	Bruxer Cast metal RPD design Short clinical crown Dark abutment	Metal allergy	
Cast metal	Well-sealed margins Almost no material failure Minimal tooth reduction	Esthetics (silver color)	Dark abutment	Metal allergy	
Stainless steel	Inexpensive Does not require sending to a lab to be fabricated	Temporary Easily perforated Not custom made Margins not well sealed	Pediatric teeth Immature permanent teeth until tooth fully erupted	Metal allergy	
Zirconia (monolithic/solid)	Minimal tooth reduction (more tooth preservation) Strength Less likely to fracture compared to layered zirconia or PFM	More opaque looking than layered zirconia and lithium disilicate More difficult to section if removing or replacing crown Unable to use nonrigid connectors for bridges Abrasive if not well polished or if glazed once the glaze wears off	Bruxer Short clinical crown Limited interocclusal space Dark abutment		High biocompatibility despite being a metal Translucent zirconia is not as strong and can fracture when adjusting limit only to anteriors 3Y to 4Y to 5Y increases in translucency and decreases in strength

Material	Pros	Cons	Indications	Contraindications	Considerations
Zirconia (layered)	• More esthetic than solid zirconia	• Requires more tooth reduction • Porcelain (layer) can fracture off exposing metal coping • More difficult to section if removing/replacing crown	• Dark abutment • More esthetic than solid zirconia		
PFM	• Tooth colored • Well-documented longevity	• Requires more tooth reduction • Porcelain can fracture off exposing metal coping • More opaque looking	• Bridges • Bruxer, only if metal occlusal on posteriors or metal lingual on anteriors • Cast metal RPD abutment tooth • Dark abutment	• Metal allergy	• Porcelain is feldspathic • Select metal type: base (non-precious), noble (semi-precious), high noble (precious) • Going from non-precious to precious increases in quality, cost, better marginal seal, greater gold content, biocompatability • Determine margin design • Determine metal design
Lithium disilicate (all ceramic, e.g. e.Max)	• High esthetic demands • Most translucent, similar to enamel, with option of requesting more opaque to block out darker stump	• Susceptible to fracture • Requires the most tooth reduction	• Anterior teeth	• Bruxer • Deep overbite • Edge-to-edge bite • Dark abutment	

Notes:
This is not an all-encompassing list of crown materials and others exist.
When it comes to selecting the right crown materials, typically either strength or esthetics will be compromised.

4. Review the crown reduction guidelines (Table 11.3).

Table 11.3 Crown reduction guidelines.

Crown material	Reductions	Margin design
Gold/cast metal	• Functional cusp: 1.5 mm • Nonfunctional cusp: 1 mm	• Chamfer circumferentially: 0.5 mm • Feather edge is OK
Stainless steel crown	• Occlusal: 1–1.5 mm • Buccal/lingual: reduce occlusal one-third and mesial buccal bulge • Round all corners	• Subgingival feather-edge finish line with no ledge
Zirconia (monolithic)	*Anterior/posterior* • 1.0 mm ideal reduction, 0.6 mm minimum [7] • Recommend at least 1 mm reduction; if 0.5 mm and adjustment is required, can easily perforate	• Rounded shoulder 1 mm or chamfer circumferentially preferred. Feather edge is OK • Rounded internal line angles
Zirconia (layered)	*Anterior* • Incisal: 1.5–2 mm • Axial: 1–1.5 mm *Posterior* • Occlusal: 1.5–2 mm • Axial: 1–2 mm [8]	• 1 mm Chamfer • Rounded internal line angles
PFM	*Anterior* • Incisal: 1.5–2 mm • Facial: 1.2–1.5 mm • Axial: 1.2–1.5 mm (P), 1 mm (M) • Lingual: 1 mm *Posterior* • PFM occlusal: – Functional cusp: 2 mm – Nonfunctional cusp: 1.5 mm – Buccal: ≤1.2 mm – Lingual: <0.6 mm • Metal occlusal: – Functional cusp: 1.5 mm – Nonfunctional cusp: 1 mm	• Porcelain butt-joint: 1.2–1.5 mm shoulder • Metal–porcelain junction: 0.5 mm chamfer (the reason this junction is the same reduction amount as M is because the lab technician can thin the amount of materials used) • Metal collar: 0.5 mm chamfer

Lithium disilicate (all ceramic, e.g. e.Max)

Anterior

- Chamfer
  - Facial: 1.5–2 mm
  - Lingual clearance: 1–1.5 mm
  - Incisal: 1.5–2 mm
  - Gingival margin: 1–1.5 mm

Or

- Shoulder: 1 mm
- Lingual reduction: 1 mm
- Incisal: 2 mm
- Labial: 1.5 mm [9]

- Chamfer or
- Rounded shoulder 1 mm circumferentially [9]

Some approaches for crown reduction include the following (Figure 11.10).

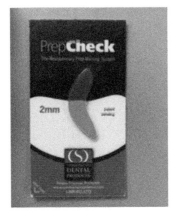

Reduction Tabs

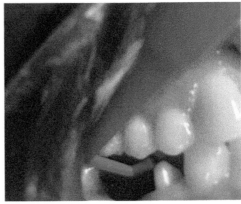

Hand Instruments

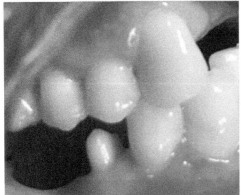

"Eyeballing it"

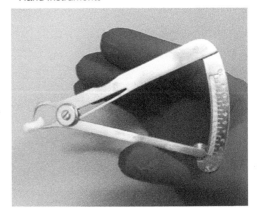

Measuring a temporary crown with calipers

Figure 11.10 Some examples for evaluating crown reduction.

Reduction bite tabs: have the patient bite and pull to see if adequate clearance and place interproximally (e.g. Flex Tabs). Some bite tabs also mark the tooth (e.g. PrepCheck) (see Figure 11.10).

Hand instruments, e.g. PrepSure (see Figure 11.10).

"Eyeball it": this is the least accurate approach and may result in over- or under-reduction (see Figure 11.10).

"Eyeball it" and fabricate a temporary crown: before the final impression, measure it with calipers for adequate reductions and inspect it for any perforations (lack of adequate reduction).

Fabricate a temporary crown and measure with calipers: if inadequate reduction, for example on the facial of an anterior, the lab may overbulk the crown which would be unesthetic, or the crown will be too thin, or opaque porcelain will be used (see Figure 11.10).

Bur thickness: knowing the exact thickness of the burs and using these to place depth cuts in the tooth, and then connecting these depth cuts.

Putty matrix: create two putty matrixes of the tooth. Inspect to ensure all the anatomy is recorded.

On one, use a blade to slice it mesiodistally along the center of the occlusal/incisal to create a facial and lingual half.

One the other putty matrix, use a blade to slice it buccolingually.

Use these putty matrix cross-sections to evaluation amount of reduction.

Can visualize amount of reduction and/or measure with a periodontal probe.

Occlusal reduction burs

Bite registration: place bite registration over the occlusal and have the patient bite into maximum intercuspation (MICP). Once set, measure the bite registration with calipers for adequate reductions and inspect it for any perforations (lack of adequate reduction).

Green wax: 0.5 mm thick, can fold in half so it becomes 1 mm thick.

5. Review triple tray verses full arch impressions (Table 11.4).

Table 11.4   Triple tray versus full arch impressions.

Tray type	Advantages	Disadvantages	Indications	Contraindications
Triple tray[a]	• Less chair time • Less impression material (saves money) • Less likely to cause gagging • Note that the stiffer the tray, the more accurate as it will not flex	• Less accurate • The filament between the upper and lower teeth will distort the occlusal anatomy of the unprepared teeth and can cause the patient to shift their teeth preventing biting in MICP [10] • Provides the lab technician with less information, e.g. does not provide the anatomy of the contralateral tooth if trying to match the anatomy for esthetic purposes • Inaccurate bite from the patient biting on the plastic or not biting properly can lead to inaccurate occlusion • Does not provide enough information for the lab technician to accurately check occlusion, including lateral excursions. This will lead to more adjustments at the delivery appointment • Flimsy: this leads to distortions when the laboratory pours the models leading to crown redos. Also, during handling and multiple pours not as strong [11] • Can only obtain MICP, cannot obtain excursions or centric relation (CR)	• One to two crowns	• Lack of a posterior stop (need teeth for the lab technician to articulate the models) • Esthetic cases • When crowning the most distal tooth in the arch. The second molar provides anatomy and cusp inclination to guide the anatomy of teeth anterior to it [10] • Best if lab has contralateral second molar as a guide

(Continued)

Table 11.4 Triple tray versus full arch impressions.

Tray type	Advantages	Disadvantages	Indications	Contraindications
Full arch tray[b]	More accurate Allows lab technician to accurately check occlusion including MICP and excursions if full arch trays are obtained with a facebow Strength: leads to less distortions when the lab technician pours the models	More impression material (higher cost)	Three or less crowns Bridges	

[a] Recommend adhesive material on the tray. This will help the impression material adhere to the tray during multiple pours, reducing distortion for the lab technicians [12].
[b] Recommend sending a bite registration over the prepared tooth (e.g. Blue Moose or something comparable).

Bite Registration

- In addition to the final impression (and opposing impression if not using a triple tray), send the laboratory a bite registration so that it can verify the patient's bite.
- Rehearse having the patient bite into MICP [13]. If the patient cannot reliably bite into MICP, you will have to extrude the bite registration onto the prepared tooth and opposing tooth [13].
- Only obtain a bite registration of the prepared teeth/opposing teeth [13]:
  - Full-arch bite registration is less accurate and a waste of material [13].
  - The goal is for all other teeth to be in MICP (i.e. no bite registration material between the other teeth) [13].
- Once the bite is set, trim the bite registration and try it back in the mouth to verify the patient is in MICP [13]. Trim with a scalpel to:
  - Remove any material contacting soft tissue.
  - Remove any material contacting teeth other than the prepared tooth/teeth and opposing tooth.
  - Remove enough material so that only the occlusal or incisal half of the prepared tooth/teeth and opposing tooth is covered [13].

Referrals

Refer if the treatment needs are beyond your training and skill level (e.g. changing VDO, full mouth rehabilitation).

Consents

- Contact your liability insurance for written consent forms for crown and bridge.
- Consent may be verbal and/or written.
- Discuss and document in the patient's chart.
- Informed consent should include:
  - Recommended treatment.
  - Treatment alternatives including no treatment.
  - Advantages, disadvantages, risks, and costs of all options.
- For discussion on treatment options, see Chapter 4, Table 4.3.
- Patient has the right to making an informed decision.
- Initial crown: anytime a crown is to be prepped, warn the patient of the risks:
  - Need for RCT, crown lengthening, post and core, core buildup, in addition to crown.
  - Tooth can still become decayed at the crown margin. Oral hygiene is critical.
- Crown replacement: anytime a crown is to be removed (e.g. recurrent decay, an open margin, fractured), warn the patient of the risks:
  - On the radiograph it is not possible to see through the crown to determine the amount of tooth structure remaining.
  - Tooth may be deemed nonrestorable (e.g. could be fractured at the gumline, could be deeply decayed beneath) and require extraction (see Figure 11.26).
  - RCT may be needed or an existing root canal may need to be redone.
  - Tooth may require crown lengthening, post and core/core buildup, and crown.
- Bridge: when planning for a bridge, warn the patient of the need for meticulous hygiene including special cleaning aids (e.g. Superfloss, floss threaders, Proxabrushes, Waterpik) as he or she will not be able to floss as easily. If the bridge is not well maintained, the patient can end up losing abutment teeth and having more missing teeth than when the bridge was planned. Crowns and bridges should not be placed until caries and hygiene are under control.

Shade Selection

Figure 11.11   At the delivery appointment for a #21 zirconia crown, the crown was tried in and the patient was handed the mirror. The patient (and the dentist) were not happy with the shade. A photo was taken for the lab with the desired shade A3 clearly visible.

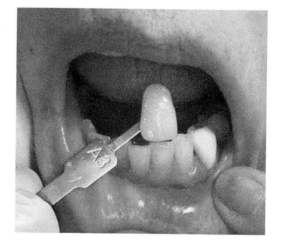

Background

- Obtain a shade match of the hydrated teeth, but not after preparation as the neighboring teeth are also desiccated, which changes the shade.
- Value: degree of lightness or darkness (decreases along the shade guide from A to D).
- Hue: name of the color (e.g. yellow).
- Chroma: saturation (increases within the letter, e.g. A1, A2).
- With age, value decreases and chroma increases.
- If unsure, choose a lighter shade as you can send it back to the lab to stain.
- Very common to have multiple shades in different parts of the mouth. Always take the shade in the area of the crown being made.
- Different shade guides exist, so on the lab prescription write which one was used (e.g. Vita Classical).

Steps

- Determine shade before prepping the tooth (for accuracy, teeth shade should be determined on hydrated teeth, not after prepping as all the adjacent teeth are desiccated).
- Patient should remove any lipstick, sunglasses, and anything else brightly colored which can interfere with shade selection.
- Prophy polish the tooth and rinse.
- Sit between the patient and a natural light source (e.g. window). Natural light is the best light spectrum to use for shade selection.
- Quickly scan the shade guide across the patient's teeth.
   - Do not spend more than five seconds analyzing as the eye will fatigue and not be able to discriminate between shades. Look away at an object that is blue.
   - Value is the most important. Squint your eyes when selecting.
- When deciding between two shades, hold one on each side of the tooth [1].
- Place the shade tab body-to-body and then edge-to-edge on the tooth.
- Consider sending a photo to the lab with the shade tab label visible. Note: not as exact as a custom shade match.
- Whitening: if patient wants teeth whiter, inform them that tooth whitening should be completed two weeks prior to shade selection. If whitening is carried out later, the crown/bridge will not whiten.
- Approval: At two points in time, consider having the patient sign approvals for shade:
   - before having crown/bridge fabricated
   - before permanently cementing crown/bridge (See Figure 11.11).
   - The Dental Insurance Company recommends dentists get written esthetic approval on all restorations, including bridges, dentures, partials, crowns, and veneers.

Procedural Steps

Crowns

Appointment 1: Prep/Temp/Final Impression
- Complete a clinical and radiographic exam.
- Complete treatment planning considerations.

- Local anesthesia.
- Obtain preliminary impression/matrix for temporary crown fabrication.
  - If any recession or abfractions, trim or drill this out of the matrix to prevent a thin brittle temporary material along the margin (want it adequate thickness/strength).
  - Trim or drill out areas where cusps or filling material may be missing to allow temporary crowns to have as normal contour as possible.
- Obtain tooth shade and approval from patient.
- Check occlusion with articulating paper (to match the dots on the temporary crown).
- Prep to ideal (see Table 11.3).
- Obtain stump shade if zirconia or lithium disilicate.
- Remove any decay and place a core buildup if necessary (see Section Core Buildups) and finalize preparation.
- Pack cord if there is a subgingival or equigingival finish line.
  - Cord size depends on pocket depth and tissue thickness.
  - Cord should have been previously soaked in appropriate hemostatic agent.
  - One cord or two cord technique:
    - If one cord, use the largest cord that fits.
    - Thinner cord is packed first and should be the exact circumference of the tooth. If needed, thicker cord is placed over thinner cord and may be overlapped.
    - Prior to taking the impression, if using two cords be sure to reposition the more apical cord after the top cord is removed. The deeper cord often comes out when the top cord is removed and can cover the margin, interfering with the impression capturing the margin accurately.
  - Place cord for eight minutes.
- Refine prep (smooth sharp edges, smooth uneven margin, remove any "J" lip margins that could fracture later creating an open margin). For a smooth cavosurface carefully adjust with a flat-end diamond bur (e.g. end cutting bur) and no water with feather light pressure on the tooth to prevent overheating.
- Verify that the entire margin is on natural tooth structure and not on the core buildup.
- Fabricate the provisional crown (before the final impression, as it helps spot problem areas that can be adjusted before the final impression). Rehearse the seating of the matrix. Verify the matrix seats and take note of the position.
  - If the abutment has composite or buildup, place separating agent (e.g. Vaseline) on the composite or buildup material to prevent the temporary crown from chemically bonding to the material.
  - If the adjacent teeth are temporary crowns, place separating agent (e.g. Vaseline) on those temporary crowns to prevent the temporary crown from bonding.
- Dispense provisional crown material into matrix and seat.
- Remove prior to complete setting/polymerization for bench setting.
- Trim off excess (with large acrylic burs) or cut with scissors when soft. If multiple adjacent crown units, option to splint with adequate gingival embrasure for oral hygiene or separate units.
- If separate units, trim gingival and occlusal/incisal embrasure and bend to snap, then smooth interproximal but do not touch the flat/shiny portion to maintain contacts
- Check retention: retentive or nonretentive (risk of swallowing/aspiration)?
- Check proximal contacts: if open, leads to food impaction and tooth migration; if too tight, leads to discomfort. Floss should have adequate resistance and be accessible.
- Check marginal integrity: if open, leads to sensitivity, food trapping, and recurrent decay; if under-contoured, leads to gingival overgrowth and food trapping; if over-contoured, leads to inadequate access for hygiene, and gingivitis.

Check contour: marginal ridges should be same height, gingival and occlusal/incisal embrasures. Is there clearance for the interdental papilla? If not will cause gingivitis (Figure 11.12).

Check occlusion: if hypo-occlusion, can drift; if hyperocclusion, tooth becomes sore and can fracture. Check other side of arch. If need for adjustment, measure the thickness with the calipers to prevent perforating or weakening the crown (minimal thickness 1 mm). If thin, reduce more on preparation as long as no exposure of the pulp; if risk of exposure, consider enameloplasty on the opposing tooth. Only alter preparation prior to taking the final impression.

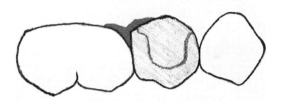

Figure 11.12   Illustration of a poorly contoured temporary crown #4 causing gingivitis.

Evaluate the provisional crown to determine if crown prep refinement is necessary (Figure 11.13). If thin walls or occlusal, consider more reduction for adequate reduction to prevent brittle temporary and definitive crown.

Final impression

Pumice the adjacent teeth to remove plaque and any calculus (if calculus is captured on the impression, the lab may process a crown with inaccurate contours and proximal contacts).

Caution: check for bony undercuts and existing FPDs. PVS can cause tray to become locked in the mouth. To prevent this, dry and place rope wax.

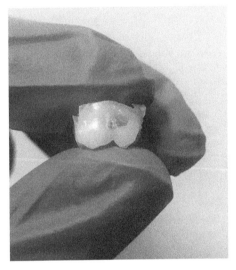

Figure 11.13   Temporary crown reveals a thin buccal wall due to under-reduction.

Sit the patient up prior to making the final impression to prevent excess impression material from being swallowed or inhaled.

Inform the patient that "we need to capture a very accurate impression for the lab, hopefully it comes out on the first try but we may have to retake it until it comes out well."

Check fit of impression tray (see Table 11.4).

Check working and setting time of impression materials.

Rehearse path of light body tip around tooth into the sulcus, keeping syringe in contact with the tooth margin in one continuous motion.

Wet the cord (to prevent tearing the tissue and causing bleeding) and remove the cord and dry the tooth. If bleeding occurs, place hemostatic agent for 10 seconds and then rinse off.

The assistant loads tray with PVS heavy body as you dispense PVS light body around margin, gently blow air aimed into sulcus, then continue adding PVS light body around tooth. Can try PVS medium body as it is less likely to blow off tooth instead of PVS light body. (Light body is water, medium body is more viscous, and heavy body is the most viscous.)

Seat the tray and set the timer. If using a triple tray, tell the patient to "bite tightly" in their "normal bite" and "You can still swallow, I will support your chin until the material sets."

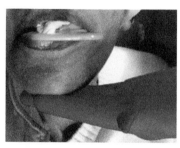

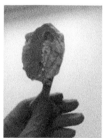

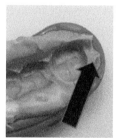

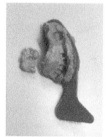

Support the chin until the impression material sets completely

Hold the triple tray up to the light to verify the patient bit into occlusion.

Make sure the patient did not occlude on the plastic.

Send the triple tray with a bite registration for the lab technician to confirm the bite.

Figure 11.14   Advice for using a triple tray.

Support the chin the entire time to ensure the individual's jaw does not relax thus distorting the impression (Figure 11.14).

Remove tray and inspect

Hand the patient a paper towel to wipe the mouth.

Check for:

Voids.

A clearly defined finish line (removes the guesswork for the lab technician).

Presence of flash if the margin is equigingival or subgingival (Figure 11.15).

Anatomy of the abutment tooth, adjacent and opposing teeth.

No evidence of biting on the plastic tray.

Biting into occlusion (adjacent teeth should have contacted creating thin spots or perforations while adequate occlusal clearance between the abutment tooth and the opposing tooth).

Bite registration: obtain to verify the bite in MICP (as patients can bite differently with the triple tray), dispense over abutment so the material contacts opposing tooth, and have patient bite and support his or her chin until bite registration sets (see Figure 11.14). CR bite is for more complex prosthesis.

Cement the provisional crown.

Dry tooth but don't desiccate, dry intaglio of provisional.

Place lubricant (e.g. Vaseline) on the cameo of provisional to prevent cement from sticking (for easier cleanup).

If concerned about breakage of the buildup at removal during Appointment 2, mix separating agent (e.g. Vaseline) with temporary cement.

Line walls of intaglio with temporary cement.

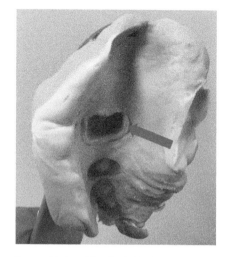

Figure 11.15   Clearly defined crown margins and flash.

Seat the temporary (an even amount of excess cement should extrude from the temporary crown margins) and verify that:

the bite feels the same to the patient

margins are sealed.

If posterior: patient bites firmly (to counteract hydrostatic pressure).

If anterior: hold in place and maintain pressure (to counteract hydrostatic pressure).

After one minute (when the cement is in the rubber phase) remove excess temporary cement with floss (pulling floss out the side) and an explorer in the sulcus. Have the dental assistant press on the occlusal or incisal surface while clearing away the excess cement to prevent the temporary crown from lifting.

Make sure there are no cords remaining in the sulcus (can lead to a periodontal abscess, discomfort, recession).

See Section Postoperative Instructions.

See Section Lab Prescriptions.

Evaluate the Case Prior to Appointment 2

Check the fit of the crown on the master cast and working die (Figure 11.16).

If problems with the case, you may have to return the crown to the lab and reschedule Appointment 2.

If problems with the case, may require a new final impression at Appointment 2.

Inspect the intaglio for any blebs or undercuts. If blebs are present, remove with smallest round bur without contacting the margin.

If porcelain, check finish and integrity of the porcelain.

Examine and become familiar with the path of insertion.

Crown

Check for any blebs on the margins (preventing seating) and on the intaglio (prevents seating and causes rocking).

Master Cast

Check proximal contacts

Check occlusion

Working Die

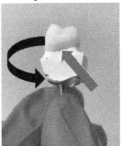

Spin the die and evaluate the margins and contours. In this case, there was an open margin.

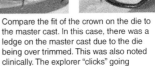

Compare the fit of the crown on the die to the master cast. In this case, there was a ledge on the master cast due to the die being over trimmed. This was also noted clinically. The explorer "clicks" going from the crown to the tooth structure.

Figure 11.16 What to look for when the case comes back from the lab.

Appointment 2: Delivery

Carefully remove the provisional crown with a curved hemostat along the long axis of the tooth (to avoid fracturing the tooth or buildup) and temporary cement with spoon excavator and pumice on prophy angle. Important to confirm with the explorer that all the subgingival cement is removed. Pumice adjacent teeth to remove plaque.

Determine if local anesthesia necessary; best not to use in order for the patient to check if the bite feels normal. Can test sensitivity by blowing air.

Try-in

Caution the patient not to swallow or aspirate. Use a throat pack (gauze) or a C-sponge.

Inform the patient: "Don't swallow, that is a natural reflex and the crown is not yet cemented. If this goes down the airway, sit up and cough." If the crown is not retrieved, a radiograph needs to be taken to determine if the crown was aspirated or ingested. Aspiration is much more serious and requires medical intervention.

Familiarize yourself with the path of insertion. Can the crown rotate? If so, learn how to seat without rotating and opening the margins.

For multiple crowns (Figure 11.17), try in individually. Seat crowns in an order which ensures complete seating and cement in the same order.

If crown has poor retention, add denture adhesive (e.g. Poligrip) or fit checker to intaglio to seat. All ceramic crowns have had hydrofluoric acid etch. For these use rope wax on the cameo to the adjacent teeth to hold in place.

Check retention: retentive or nonretentive (risk of swallowing/aspiration)?

Check proximal contacts:

Shredding or snagging the floss? Could be a tight contact or an overhang on the crown (a plus margin).

Open? If not open on the cast from the lab, make a new final impression and send to the lab. If open on the cast and clinically, send the case back to the lab to add contact.

Too heavy? This can prevent the crown from seating. Spray the contact with Occlude, seat, remove and check for burn-through. Adjust burn-through with a diamond bur. Or check by rubbing articulating paper on the floss and trying to floss; this will mark the proximal contact (SpotIt Contact Finder already colored). Adjust where it is marked. Adjustments needed until the crown seats. Beware not to open the contact by overadjusting (Figure 11.18).

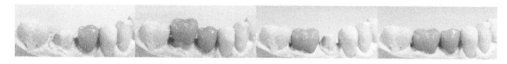

Figure 11.17   Determining the order in which multiple adjacent crowns will seat. In this case, crown #30 must be cemented prior to Crown #29.

Figure 11.18   After using SpotIt Contact Finder to locate the heavy contact for adjustment.

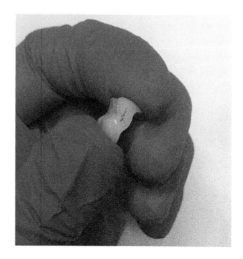

Tip: adjust the crown on the die for support and to prevent nicking the margin (See Figure 11.25).

If you lose contact: return crown, master cast, and working die to lab to add a contact as long as the open contact is reproducible on the master cast. If not, make a pickup impression for the lab to add contact, unless it is solid zirconia (new final impression).

Internal adaptation: if you suspect the crown is not seating completely, use Fit Checker, line the intaglio surface, and seat the crown. Wait for the material to set, remove the crown and inspect. Any areas of burn-through (i.e. perforation) can be marked with a red pencil or memorize the location and adjust with a bur and repeat. Adjust with a carbide bur (Figure 11.19).

Margins:
  Open? Explorer "clicks" from tooth to crown and from crown to tooth and the tip of the explorer is able to get underneath the crown margin.
  Flush (ideal)?
  Bulky (plus)? Explorer "clicks" from tooth to crown.
  Under-countoured (sub)? Explorer "clicks" from crown to tooth.

Contour: anatomy, marginal ridges at the same height as adjacent teeth, embrasure space, emergence profile are consistent with adjacent teeth.

Occlusion: crown must be in occlusion. Do not adjust occlusion until certain the crown is fully seated. Check contacts on the other side of arch. The new crown should not alter the bite. Adjust before polishing. If need for adjustment, measure the thickness with the calipers to prevent perforating or weakening the crown. If thin, consider enameloplasty of the opposing tooth.

Take a BW to check for closed margins after all adjustments and polishing has been completed.

Obtain patient shade approval prior to cementation.

Select cement type (Table 11.5).

Cementing:
  Have the dental assistant line the intaglio with cement. Do not fill the crown with cement like filling a bathtub with water and immediately wipe off the cement from the cement mixing spatula.

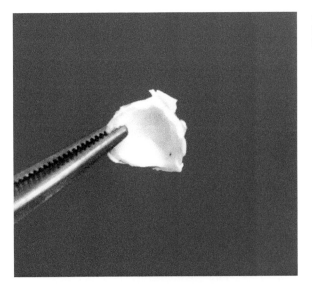

Figure 11.19 Perforation noted when using the Fit Checker that required adjustment for the crown to seat.

Seat the crown and verify:

Seat and with fingers rotate and inspect with explorer that the margins are sealed (crowns can rotate in the wrong direction and end up with open contacts that are filled with cement and at the recall appointment the cement has washed away and the open margin is visible).

Excess cement should extrude around the entire margin.

Verify the bite feels the same to the patient.

If posterior: patient bites firmly on cotton roll (to counteract hydrostatic pressure).

If anterior: hold in place and maintain pressure (to counteract hydrostatic pressure) along the long axis of the tooth.

After one minute (at the rubber phase) remove excess temporary cement with floss and an explorer in the sulcus. Remove the cotton roll after seating and have the patient confirm bite and clench firmly. Cotton rolls can shift crowns.

See Table 11.6.

See Section Postoperative Instructions.

Bridges

Very similar to the procedural steps for crowns, with the following differences.

Diagnostic Appointment

See Section Indications and Considerations for Bridges.

Assessment

Has tooth been extracted?

Yes:

Is there tooth migration of the adjacent and opposing teeth?

Is there a horizontal and/or vertical bony defect?

No:

Is the plan to extract and place a temporary bridge to aid with healing?

(a) Can prep the adjacent teeth and temporize.

(b) Extract the tooth and replace the temporary crowns with a temporary bridge.

(c) Have the extraction site heal about two to three months. A periodontal consultation may be needed to improve the gingival architecture.

(d) Make the final impression.

(e) Deliver the bridge. Can temporarily cement the bridge for a month to verify the papilla looks good as it continues healing (no black triangles, no space beneath the pontic). If everything looks good, permanently cement. If it does not, send to the lab to add porcelain.

Evaluate the smile line to determine if the pontic tooth/teeth will be visible.

Obtain diagnostic impressions and a bite registration, and pour up the models.

Evaluate the occlusion:

Need for enameloplasty of any opposing supraerupted teeth?

Crossbite? Maintaining or changing the crossbite?

Determine the bridge design:

See Ante's Law.

Consider placing retention grooves on the buccal and lingual (Figure 11.20).

Bridge dislodging forces tend to be mesiodistal [1].

Consider placing retention grooves on the mesial and distal for single crowns (if lacking retention). Crown dislodging forces tend to be in the faciolingual direction [1].

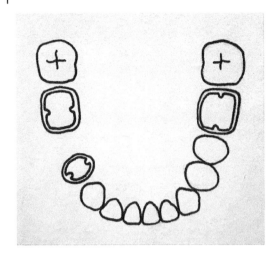

Figure 11.20 Illustration of retention grooves for a bridge and a crown.

- Determine the pontic design (see Section Lab Prescriptions).
- Create the pontic tooth/teeth using a denture tooth, or waxing up a tooth or using a temporary Ion crown.
- Duplicate the model with the pontic tooth/teeth.
- Fabricate a matrix for the bridge, such as a putty matrix.
- Can also fabricate a custom tray for an accurate impression.

Appointment 1: Prep/Temp/Final Impression

- Determine which tooth to prep first. Prep the smaller tooth first because to match the parallelism of the other tooth, better to have more room for error on the larger tooth with less risk of a pulpal exposure.
  - Can prep both together for parallelism, such as 30 D then 28 D, then 30 M then 28 M, then 30 B, then 28 B, and so forth so that the bur is held at the same angle.
  - Alternatively, you can roughly prepare the walls straight, then work on the parallelism of the reciprocal walls.
- When prepping abutment teeth be sure to create parallelism with the preps. Hover with a mirror to check for parallelism and no undercuts with one eye closed to detect. To verify parallelism and no undercuts, consider making an impression and pouring up with quick setting stone (e.g. Snapstone).
- Recommend full arch impressions.
- Obtain a bite registration in MICP over the preps.
- Fabricate the provisional bridge. For pontic shape, see Section Lab Prescriptions.
- Verify adequate gingival embrasure space for the patient to floss and space for floss below the pontic.
- When temporarily cementing the bridge, wrap floss around the connector for easier cleanup once the bridge is seated and the cement has set (Figure 11.21).
- Request a metal framework from the lab for a PFM bridge (see Section Lab Prescriptions).

Figure 11.21 Technique for easier cement removal when cementing a bridge.

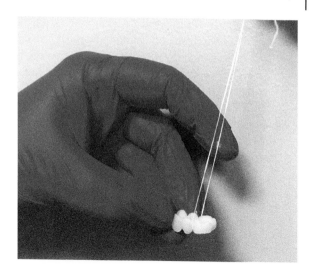

Visit Between Appointments 1 and 2: PFM Bridge Framework Try-in

- Evaluate the metal framework on the models (Figure 11.22).
- Remove the provisional bridge, and clean off the excess cement.
- Try in the bridge framework and check the following:
  - Seating: verify the pontic is not interfering with complete bridge seating.
    - May have to use Fit Checker to hold the framework in place.
    - Should be passive and not pushing teeth apart/together.
  - Internal adaptation: if you suspect the bridge is not seating completely, can use Fit Checker, line the intaglio surface, and seat the bridge. Wait for the material to set, remove the bridge and inspect. Any areas of burn-through (i.e. perforation) can be marked with a red pencil or memorize the location and adjust with a bur and repeat. Adjust with a carbide bur (see Figure 11.19).
  - Pontic to ridge relationship: is there adequate clearance for porcelain (1 mm minimum, 1.5 mm for good esthetics). Verify the pontic is not preventing the bridge from seating (use Fit Checker or Occlude). Check for blanching gingiva from heavy contact.
  - Proximal contacts: these will be open to allow space for porcelain.
  - Margins: verify closed margins on the abutments. If you plan on a porcelain butt-joint, make sure the lab has the metal coping reach the margins for the framework try-in to verify seating. Later the lab can remove the metal.
  - Contour:
    - Emergency profile.
    - Verify adequate clearance for the gingival papilla.
    - Verify adequate clearance for floss and Proxabrushes in the gingival embrasures.
  - Occlusion: the bridge should not be in occlusion, unless you requested metal occlusal surfaces.
  - Verify adequate occlusal clearance for the 1.5 mm of porcelain.
    - If the bridge is in occlusion when the plan is to have porcelain covering the surface, consider the following:
      - Adjust the metal with a carbide bur, but first measure the thickness with a caliper to avoid perforating or creating a thin metal coping.
      - Enameloplasty of the opposing teeth.

▫ Refining the preps to create more occlusal clearance and making a new final impression and redoing the bridge framework try-in appointment.

▫ Check protrusion, lateral excursions, and retrusion to verify that the lab will have enough clearance to add porcelain, unless some areas are planned for metal occlusal or metal lingual.

◦ Take a BW to evaluate the margins.

◦ Obtain a bite registration in MICP over the framework and verify proper mounting.

◦ If the framework does not fit, make a new final impression and send to the lab.

◦ Optional: bisque bake try-in appointment.

▫ Rationale: verify the PFM bridge fits, and allow for adjustments with a bur before the bridge is glazed. If adjusting at delivery and sending back to the lab to re-glaze, the properties will become less translucent and more brittle.

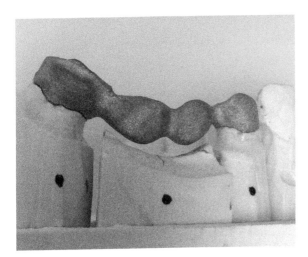

Figure 11.22 PFM metal framework.

Appointment 2: Delivery

◦ Try-in (Figure 11.23)

▫ Check pontic to ridge relationship: verify the pontic is not interfering with complete bridge seating (use Fit Checker or Occlude or a thin piece of articulating paper). Check for blanching gingiva from heavy contact. Inspect and feel the pontic and tissue-contacting areas (connector) outside the mouth to verify smooth porcelain against the gingival tissue.

▫ Check proximal contacts: floss should have adequate resistance and be accessible.

▫ Check margins:

‣ Open? Explorer "clicks" from tooth to crown and from crown to tooth or the tip of the explorer can get under the margin.

‣ Flush (ideal)?

‣ Bulky (plus)? Explorer "clicks" from tooth to crown.

‣ Under-countoured (sub)? Explorer "clicks" from crown to tooth.

▫ Check contour:

‣ Emergency profile.

‣ Verify adequate clearance for the gingival papilla.

‣ Verify adequate clearance for floss and Proxabrushes in the gingival embrasures.

▫ Accessible for the patient to clean (Figure 11.24).

Verify adequate gingival embrasure space for the gingival papilla and for the patient. to floss. If not, the bridge will be cemented and the patient will not be able to maintain proper oral hygiene.

Marginal ridges should be same height, gingival and occlusal/incisal embrasures present. Not over- or under-contoured.

Check occlusion:

Check the occlusion without the bridge and then with the bridge in to verify the same.

If in hypo-occlusion the teeth can drift; if in hyperocclusion, the teeth can become sore and the bridge can fracture.

Esthetics: does the patient approve? Make sure before cementing.

- Take a BW to evaluate the margins.
- Select cement type (see Table 11.5).
- When cementing the bridge, wrap floss around the connector for easier cleanup once the bridge is seated and the cement has set (see Figure 11.21).
- See Table 11.6.

Figure 11.23 PFM bridge.

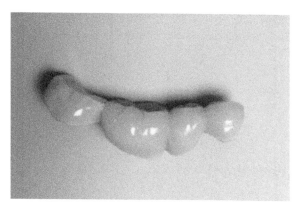

Figure 11.24 Bridge with inadequate clearance for the interdental papilla. Unfortunately, the patient was unable to fit any floss or Proxabrushes in the gingival embrasures to maintain proper hygiene.

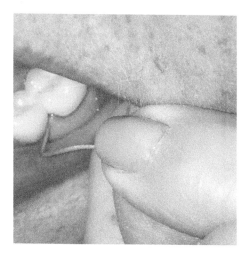

Table 11.5 Crown/bridge material and cement types.

Crown/bridge material	Cement and special instructions
PFM/metal/gold	RMGI cement, GI cement
Zirconia (monolithic, layered)	After trying in, decontaminate the intaglio by sandblasting or with Ivoclean. Spray water and dry. Cement with RMGI cement or resin cement system (for nonretentive tooth prep or veneers) [14] or GI cement
Lithium disilicate	After trying in, rinse the intaglio with 5% hydrofluoric acid for 20 seconds, water spray and dry, use a silane primer on the intaglio and air thin, and cement with RMGI cement or resin cement (for nonretentive tooth prep or veneers) [14]. 5% Hydrofluoric acid reinforces the lab's etch and cleans
Leucite-reinforced ceramic	Resin cement
Stainless steel crown	RMGI or GI cement

Notes:
Bonding the crown with resin cement will make future removal more challenging compared with luting (with RMGI) [14].
Check the manufacturer's instructions for indications and instructions.

Table 11.6 Adjusting crown/bridge materials.

Crown/bridge material	Adjustments
PFM	Occlusal and proximal adjustments with a fine diamond (e.g. football diamond) followed by the porcelain polishing burs. Carbide for the metal if the occlusal is metal. Warn the patient that adjusting may expose the metal coping beneath the porcelain. If patient does not want any metal visible and you're concerned about the amount of reduction leading to visible metal, consider adjusting the opposing tooth with the patient's consent
Metal/gold	Carbide bur at high speed, then brownie and then greenie at slow speed
Zirconia (monolithic, layered)	Adjust with a fine-grit diamond with light pressure. Football-shaped bur for occlusal, tapered bur for cusps or proximal contacts, and a round bur to adjust a cusp and fossa. Even though zirconia is a metal, use the ceramic polishing burs or zirconia polishing burs using light pressure with no water. Polishing zirconia is critical. If it is not well polished it is very abrasive to the opposing teeth. Glaze is not the same as it wears off
Lithium disilicate	Cement or bond into place before adjusting. Use a fine diamond with water and air to avoid overheating the crown. Polish with a pink (and gray) rubber wheels (or points) and diamond polishing paste [9]. Keep adjustments minimal to prevent microfractures
Stainless steel crown (SSC)	Do not adjust SSC, as this will cause perforation. Instead adjust the abutment and/or have patient bite down to deform the SSC

Figure 11.25   To adjust the crown, place the crown on the die for support and to prevent nicking the margins.

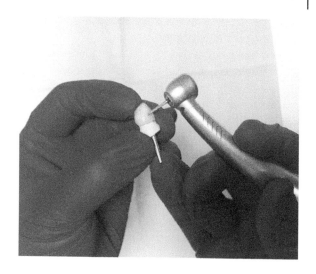

Alternative Steps

Removing ("Sectioning") a Crown

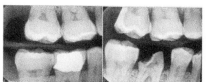

Removal of #30 PFM crown. The build up came out with the sectioned crown. The abutment had extensive decay and was deemed non-restorable.

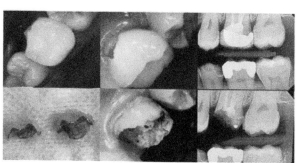

Removal of #14 PFM crown. Same outcome as #30 PFM crown.

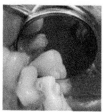

Removal of #13 PFM crown. The abutment had only a small amount of decay on the buccal surface and was deemed restorable.

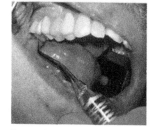

Removal of #3 PFM crown. The condition of the abutment is to be determined.

Figure 11.26   Examples of crown removal cases.

Discuss the risks involved (see Section Consents).

Evaluate the radiographs.

Clinical pearl: if there is a post, or a large buildup, assume that there is a greater chance that the tooth is nonrestorable since the last dentist had to place a post and/or buildup as the tooth was already compromised.

Anesthetize.

Make a preliminary impression for the future temporary crown.

Use a fresh bur:

Gold/metal/stainless steel crown: carbide (thick, coarse carbide crown-removing burs work best). For gold crowns, give the pieces back to the patient in a bag if they are interested in selling their gold for cash.

PFM: coarse diamond for the porcelain, carbide small round bur for the metal.

Zirconia: coarse diamond.

Lithium disilicate: coarse diamond.

Take care not to injure the soft tissue and avoid the patient aspirating or swallowing the bur (oftentimes the bur breaks).

Isolate the tooth: especially with PFM or ceramic crowns, large pieces can fly off the tooth and become swallowed or aspirated.

Section the crown with the high-speed bur from buccal to lingual.

Check often to make sure you are not drilling into tooth structure. Note that amalgam under a crown can mimic the metal coping of the crown. If the material is easier to cut through, it is amalgam so don't cut deeper.

Keep the cut as narrow as the bur (if too wide there is nothing to wedge apart).

Be sure to cut all the way to the crown margin.

Caution when using nitrous oxide and oxygen sedation, as there is a risk of creating a fire (see Chapter 18).

Place the crown spreader instrument into the narrow cut on the occlusal surface and twist.

Remove with a curved hemostat.

Assess restorability: may have to take a new radiograph to check for recurrent decay.

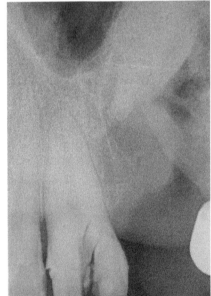

Figure 11.27 Iatrogenic damage to tooth #8.

A cautionary tale (Figure 11.27)

A colleague sectioned a gold basket crown because it had an open margin. Once the tooth was sectioned, the colleague placed the crown splitter on the tooth and twisted it. At this point the tooth was deemed non-restorable and was extracted and the patient received an implant at no charge for the error. The dentist's mistake was thinking that the facial of the gold basket crown was porcelain when it was in fact enamel. This should have been prevented.

Removing ("Sectioning") a Bridge

- Discuss the risks involved (see Section Consents).
- Will the patient accept leaving the office with one or more missing teeth? Or should you fabricate a stayplate ahead of time? (Figure 11.28)
- Determine if you have to remove the entire bridge or maintain a portion.
- If removing an entire bridge, follow the instructions in the preceding section (Removing a Crown) for each retainer.
- If maintaining a portion, section the bridge at the connector and err on the side toward the pontic so you don't nick or perforate the remaining crown. Once sectioned, contour, smooth and polish the proximal surfaces of the remaining abutment crowns. If you do not err on the side toward the pontic, you may remove too much crown material on the proximal side of the crown (Figure 11.29). If a PFM bridge, warn the patient beforehand that the proximal surface of the tooth where the connector was sectioned will be metal and not tooth colored (Figure 11.30).

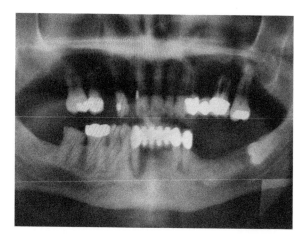

Figure 11.28 In preparation for sectioning a bridge, consider which teeth will be missing at the end of the appointment and if you need to prepare ahead of time with an immediate partial.

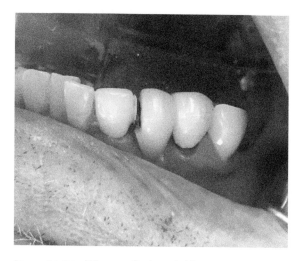

Figure 11.29 When sectioning a bridge, err on the side closer to the pontic to avoid damaging the crown being retained.

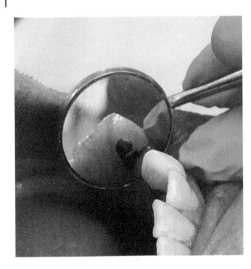

Figure 11.30   When sectioning a PFM bridge, warn the patient that the connector which is metal (i.e. silver in color) will show. This may be unesthetic (depending on the location in the mouth) and the patient may want the crown redone.

Seven Scenarios Involving Removable Partial Dentures/Complete Dentures

Scenario 1: Replacing an Abutment Crown of an Existing RPD in a Patient Willing to be Without their RPD for Several Days

- Determine if the RPD should be replaced.
- Warn the patient:
    - The RPD was made prior to the crown and will try our best to make the RPD fit the new crown; however, a new RPD may have to be fabricated.
    - When replacing a crown there is no guarantee the tooth can be saved as we do not know if the tooth is decayed or fractured beneath.
    - You will be without the RPD for several days.
- Make a diagnostic impression and fabricate a custom tray. Drill a hole in the tray over the major connector. This way you can hold an instrument in place to verify the RPD is fully seated during the final impression (Figure 11.31).
- Prep the tooth and pack a cord.

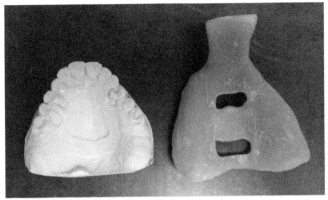
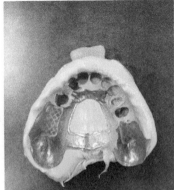

Figure 11.31   A custom tray for a pickup impression of #5 PFM crown.

- Bite registration.
- When ready, remove the cord and dispense light body PVS over the abutment. Seat the RPD with the clasps engaged. Dispense light body over the clasp covering the abutment tooth. Load the tray with heavy body and seat. Push an instrument handle through the window in the custom tray with pressure to seat the RPD until fully set.
- Verify the partial can seat completely with the temporary crown and that there is some clearance between the clasps and the temporary crown to prevent dislodgement of the temporary crown when the patient removes the partial.
- Send the lab the opposing full arch impression, full arch final impression with RPD, and bite registration.

Scenario 2: Replacing an Abutment Crown of an Existing RPD in a Patient Not Willing to be Without their RPD for Several Days

- The most accurate way is to have a pickup impression for the lab (patient will be without the RPD). The RPD can be picked up the next day from the lab, but then the lab needs the RPD again for a final check. Alternative is the following.
- Only possible if there are vertical stops. If with the RPD out of the mouth the VDO collapses, it will require construction of wax occlusal rims and sending these along with diagnostic casts.
- In this case you must create an adaptation pattern.
- Prep the tooth. Pack cord. When ready, remove the cord. Place Duralay (not bite registration as it is too flexible) over the prep, seat the RPD with the clasps engaged and wipe the bite registration so the metal clasp is visible. Once set, remove the RPD and the Duralay. Trim the adaptation pattern so that the intaglio is intact (showing the shape of the abutment) and the cameo shows the clasp/rest design.
- Obtain a full arch final impression.
- Send to the lab the full arch final impression, adaptation pattern, and opposing full arch impression.
- Verify the partial can seat completely with the temporary crown and that there is some clearance between the clasps and the temporary crown to prevent dislodgement of the temporary crown when the patient removes the partial.

Scenario 3: Crowning a Non-abutment Tooth with an Existing RPD

- Determine if the RPD should be replaced.
- Determine if the RPD has an intimate relationship with the non-abutment tooth. If not, the patient should not have to go without the RPD. If the framework contacts the non-abutment tooth, best to follow Scenario 1.

Scenario 4: Survey Crowns of an Abutment Tooth Planned for an RPD

- First design the RPD (see Chapter 13).
- Determine the design of the crown for the lab prescription:
    Rest seats and their locations.
    Undercut amount necessary:
        0.01 inch (0.25 mm) for chrome cobalt cast retainer
        0.02 inch (0.5 mm) cast gold retainer
        0.03 inch (0.75 mm) for wrought wire
    Prep the crown with additional reduction for mesial/distal rest seats. For cingulum rests on the lower canines, a shelf can be created to the crown. For cingulum rests on upper canines, prep deeper as it can interfere with the opposing teeth.

Scenario 5: Crown on a Tooth with an Existing Stayplate

- Apply lubricant (e.g. Vasoline) on the cameo.
- Prep pack cord, remove cord, light body, seat the stayplate, and seat the tray loaded with heavy body. Carefully remove the stayplate from the final impression.
- Send the lab the opposing full arch impression, full arch final impression, and a bite registration.

Scenario 6: Crown Opposing an Existing Complete Denture

- Check the occlusion between the teeth and complete denture.
- Determine if the complete denture requires replacement (see Chapter 12).
- Obtain an impression of the denture extraorally.
- Prep the crown.
- Obtain a full arch final impression.
- Obtain a full arch bite registration.
- Send the lab the full arch final impression, bite registration, and opposing model.

Scenario 7: Crown Opposing an Arch Planned for a Complete Denture

- Appointment 1:
  - Diagnostic impressions of both arches.
  - Evaluate the study models to determine if enameloplasty or buildups of teeth are required for an ideal occlusal scheme, and if necessary complete this first.
  - Fabricate a wax occlusal rim for the edentulous arch. May require a wax occlusal rim for a partially edentulous arch.

- Appointment 2: determine the proper VDO with the wax occlusal rim(s).
- Appointment 3:
  - Prep the crown.
  - Make a full arch final impression.
  - Obtain a bite registration of the entire arch with the patient in VDO with the wax occlusal rim(s).
  - Send the lab the full arch final impression, bite registration, opposing model, and wax occlusal rim(s).
- Appointment 4: deliver the crown.
- Appointment 5: obtain a final impression for the RPD.
- Appointment 6: RPD framework try-in and wax occlusal rims/bite/tooth shade/gum shade/form of ID.
- Appointment 7: tooth try-in.
- Appointment 8: delivery.

Core Buildup

- Assess restorability (see Figure 11.6).
- Core buildup needed when there is not enough tooth structure for the crown.
- Core material options (from strongest to weakest):
  - Amalgam: strongest, but do not prep crown same day as placing amalgam because it needs to set completely.
  - Composite: bonds to enamel, some release fluoride (e.g. ParaCore, CompCore), and requires good isolation.
  - RMGI: bonds to dentin, releases fluoride (e.g. Fuji II LC).
  - GI: bonds to dentin, releases fluoride, weakest (e.g. Fuji IX).
- Shade: if the permanent crown material is not translucent, it is advantageous to *not* match the shade of the dentin. Some buildup material colors come in white or blue. This helps you distinguish between the natural tooth and the core buildup when prepping the crown to ensure placement of the margin on natural tooth structure. Crown materials that are translucent include lithium disilicate and solid zirconia crowns (3Y to 4Y to 5Y increase in translucency and decrease in strength).

Post and Core

- A post may be needed to retain the core (buildup) if there is inadequate tooth structure for mechanical and/or chemical retention.
- See Figure 11.6 for post length.
- Tooth first requires adequate ferrule (see Figure 11.6).
- Indications for post
  - Root canal-treated tooth.
  - If in addition to the ferrule there are none or one wall remaining, or two adjacent walls remaining.
- Post recommendations
  - Place the post in the largest and straightest canal:
    - Maxillary molars: the palatal root.
    - Mandibular molars: the distal root.
  - Select passive fitting parallel (not tapered) nonmetal posts (metal if small diameter). Nonmetal posts prevent the fracture problem associated with metal posts, are bonded in the canal, and have some degree of flexibility similar to dentin [5].
  - Use a preformed post, unless the canal is very wide.
  - Steps:
    - Heat and melt the gutta percha in the coronal two-thirds of the root leaving 4–5 mm of gutta percha for the apical seal.
    - Measure the depth in the canal with a periodontal probe.
    - Try in the post.
    - Take a PA prior to cementing to verify depth of post.
    - Cement the post.
    - Complete the buildup ("core").

Lab Prescriptions

- Dentists use lab prescriptions to communicate to the lab technicians their requests for fixed or removable prostheses.
- Figure 11.1 is a collage of various lab prescriptions addressing crown and bridge.

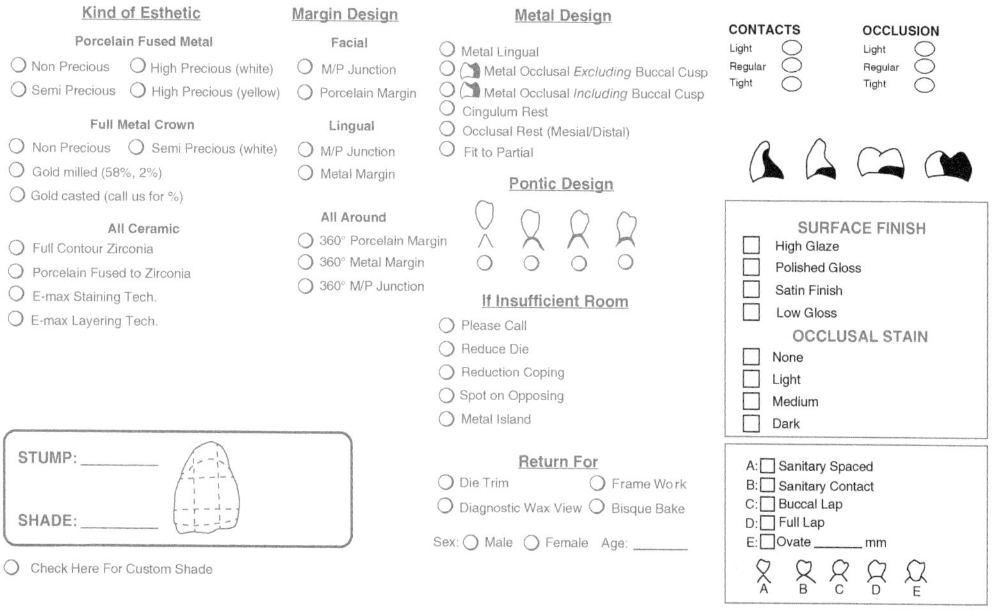

Kind of Esthetic
Porcelain Fused Metal
Non Precious
High Precious (white)
Semi Precious
High Precious (yellow)
Full Metal Crown
Non Precious
Semi Precious (white)
Gold milled (58%, 2%)
Gold casted (call us for %)
All Ceramic
Full Contour Zirconia
Porcelain Fused to Zirconia
E-max Staining Tech.
E-max Layering Tech.

Margin Design
Facial
M/P Junction
Porcelain Margin
Lingual
M/P Junction
Metal Margin
All Around
360° Porcelain Margin
360° Metal Margin
360° M/P Junction

Metal Design
Metal Lingual
Metal Occlusal *Excluding* Buccal Cusp
Metal Occlusal *Including* Buccal Cusp
Cingulum Rest
Occlusal Rest (Mesial/Distal)
Fit to Partial

Pontic Design

If Insufficient Room
Please Call
Reduce Die
Reduction Coping
Spot on Opposing
Metal Island

CONTACTS
Light
Regular
Tight

OCCLUSION
Light
Regular
Tight

SURFACE FINISH
High Glaze
Polished Gloss
Satin Finish
Low Gloss

OCCLUSAL STAIN
None
Light
Medium
Dark

STUMP: ________
SHADE: ________
Check Here For Custom Shade

Return For
Die Trim
Frame Work
Diagnostic Wax View
Bisque Bake
Sex: Male Female Age: ______

A: Sanitary Spaced
B: Sanitary Contact
C: Buccal Lap
D: Full Lap
E: Ovate ______ mm
A B C D E

Figure 11.1 Collage of lab prescriptions.

Below is a sample of a detailed template for writing a crown and a bridge lab prescription. If a dentist does not provide adequate crown reduction the lab will communicate this to the dentist (Figure 11.32).

CROWN

Please fabricate _____ [Select crown material]

Shade: _____ using [insert shade guide. Draw diagram if using multiple shades]

Stump shade: _____ using [insert guide; necessary for all porcelain crowns and solid zirconia]

Margin design: _____ [if PFM]

Metal design: _____ [if PFM]

Contacts: _____ [Select type]

Occlusion: _____ [Select type]

Surface finish: _____ [Select type]

Occlusal stain: _____ [Select type]

Additional notes: _____

[For zirconia crowns request "polished" not "glazed." Glazed zirconia increases wear of opposing enamel once the glaze wears off and the unpolished zirconia beneath is exposed. It is acceptable to have glaze on nonoccluding surfaces for esthetics. For metal crowns indicate if you want it matte or finished (shiny)]

BRIDGE

In addition to the Crown Lab Prescription add:

Pontic design: _____ [Select type] [See Figure 11.1]

   Sanitary spaced (i.e. hygienic): _____ [Easiest for oral hygiene. Unesthetic]

   Sanitary contact (i.e. conical): _____ [Easier for oral hygiene. Poor esthetics]

   Buccal lap (i.e. modified ridge-lap): _____ [difficult for oral hygiene. Esthetic]

   Full Lap (saddle-ridge-lap): _____ [Not recommended, not easy to clean]

   Ovate ___ mm: [Most esthetic. Difficult for oral hygiene. The space for the millimeter value refers to how deep the socket will be for the pontic to rest on. The lab technician will trim the model to the depth provided. However this is not always necessary. The socket depth can be formed with an immediate provisional bridge (right after the extraction)]

Return for: _____ [Select which one]

   Framework Try-in _____ [For PFM bridges only, when checking the fit of the bridge including the margins and occlusal reduction]

   Bisque bake _____ [For PFM bridges only, for making adjustments before the bridge is glazed]

   Delivery

Reduction Coping

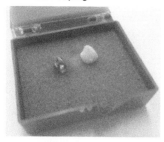
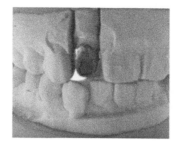
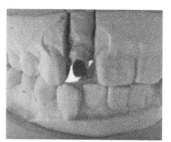

Spot on Opposing

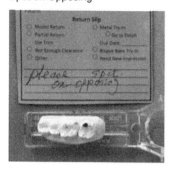

Figure 11.32 Example of how the lab may communicate to the dentist when there is inadequate clearance on a crown.

Postoperative Instructions

Consider providing both verbal and written instructions.

Temporary crown/bridge

- This is temporary, may last 30 seconds to 30 days, just as the name implies.
- Avoid hard food as it can break the temporary crown, which is weaker than a permanent crown. Avoid anything you might imagine could break a hard acrylic.
- Avoid sticky food as it can pull off the temporary crown, which is not permanently cemented.
- Continue with proper oral hygiene, brushing after breakfast and flossing and brushing before bed. Take care when flossing to not pull off the temporary crown; instead pull the floss out the side.
  - For bridges use a floss threader and floss (or Superfloss) to clean beneath the bridge, taking care not to pull up on the temporary bridge.
- Contact us as soon as possible for a replacement if the temporary falls off or breaks. This is important because:
  - The temporary protects the tooth beneath and if that tooth breaks/chips the permanent crown may not fit.
  - The opposing tooth and neighboring teeth can migrate before the next appointment and then the permanent crown will not fit.
  - The gum can start to grow over the prepared tooth and the permanent crown will not fit and the excess gum will have to be removed surgically.
  - You will experience tooth sensitivity to hot and cold, unless the tooth has been root canal treated.
- Do not use superglue. It is hard to remove and will require drilling the temporary off, which can damage the tooth underneath.

Recommend OTC pain medication if needed as gums may be sore (e.g. cord packing, gingivectomy) and tooth may be sensitive from the trauma (i.e. drilling). See Chapter 16.

Contact us if any pain/discomfort persists or increases.

Permanent crown/bridge

Do not eat anything for the first hour as the cement is still setting. Be careful during the first 24 hours, as you were with the temporary crown. After 24 hours you can treat the newly crowned tooth like you would with any other tooth when it comes to chewing and flossing.

Continue with proper oral hygiene, brushing after breakfast and flossing and brushing before bed. Oral hygiene is especially important with crowns because the tooth can still become decayed at or below where the crown meets the tooth. For this reason, it is important to direct the toothbrush bristles toward the gumline to clean this vulnerable juncture where plaque accumulates.

Even though the edge of the crown feels very smooth to you and I, microscopically, the level we are talking about with bacteria, there is a huge ledge at the crown margin that needs extra attention to be kept clean.

Contact us if any pain/discomfort persists or increases. A tooth can always feel a bit sensitive after cementing a crown.

Stainless steel crown

See Chapter 17.

Clinical Pearls

Troubleshooting

Crown preps

Detecting undercuts: these must be avoided in crown/bridge preps.

Close one eye when evaluating a preparation to detect undercuts.

Can also hold a periodontal probe against the axial wall and slowly move it from the most occlusal spot on the abutment to the margin. If the tip of the probe disappears there is an undercut.

Another sign of an undercut is when fabricating a provisional crown: when it is removed from the abutment it will break.

To remove the undercut, one must either add buildup material (e.g. composite, glass ionomer) or taper the prep until the undercut is relieved.

Poor retention (see image of bowl in Figure 11.6): consider subgingival margins (i.e. lengthening the walls of the preparation), retention grooves, ensuring the walls are parallel and not tapered, and roughening the prep.

If the adjacent tooth has been nicked: first try to prevent this (see Section Tips). If deep, restore with composite. If shallow, smooth and polish and make sure when you wrap floss around the nicked tooth that the floss does not shred or snag. Needs to be done before the final impression is made.

Fixing a leaning crown prep (picture the Leaning Tower of Pisa): this will interfere with the path of draw/insertion. Recommend building up the side that is over-tapered and refine the other side to remove the undercut.

Fixing undercuts from adjacent teeth

If adjacent teeth are tipped creating an undercut which the temporary locks beneath, this may require enameloplasty of the tipped tooth before making the final impression. If severely tipped, may require orthodontic uprighting, or a telescopic crown.

Temporary crowns

Breaks when removing from the tooth? The abutment likely has an undercut, or the adjacent teeth have an undercut. If the prep has an undercut it requires buildup material or refining the prep to remove the undercut. If the adjacent tooth has an undercut, dry the tooth, wrap rope wax around it, and with a plastic instrument make the contour parallel to the long axis.

Breaks and sticks to the tooth? Was a separating agent (e.g. Vaseline) not placed over the core buildup or composite? The temporary crown likely chemically bonded to the restorative material.

Repairs: do not waste time repairing with bonding agent (placing, drying, light curing) and flowable or packable composite (light curing). Often it is faster to redo the temporary and a solid temporary is stronger than one with patches of composite. However, make sure the problem is not with the abutment (e.g. undercuts, inadequate amount of reduction, bonding to the restorative material) or adjacent teeth (tipped, locking in the material).

Early loss of temporary crown and the gum grew over the abutment margin and the teeth migrated: at the crown delivery appointment the crown may not seat. You may be able to move the gingiva out of the way by placing a cord temporarily during the crown delivery appointment and pulling it out immediately after verifying that the bite feels normal before the permanent cement sets. If excess growth, removal of the gingiva may be necessary with a laser, scalpel, or high-speed bur. If the tooth migrated, the definitive crown will require adjusting; if still unable to seat after adjusting, you will have to make a new final impression, a new temporary crown, and reschedule for a delivery appointment.

Crown (temporary or permanent) lost so long ago the abutment now occludes with the opposing tooth: the opposing tooth may require enameloplasty, or the supraerupted abutment tooth may require endodontic treatment if prepping the crown will expose the pulp. Orthodontic intrusion may be another option. If the supraeruption is severe, the tooth may require extraction.

Making a temporary from a tooth missing the crown. First check the occlusion: if the tooth has supraerupted or the opposing has supraerupted, there will not be enough occlusal clearance for a temporary crown. Place an Ion crown (SSC harder and more difficult to work with) over the tooth and make a preliminary impression. Then fabricate the temporary crown.

Making a temporary from a broken tooth missing anatomy: make a preliminary impression/ matrix. Once made, use a high-speed bur to drill out the anatomy to create the shape of the tooth. Alternatively, place composite (without etching and bonding) for the missing anatomy and light cure. Then fabricate the matrix.

Temporary crown with a posterior open bite: fabricate the temporary crown and roughen the occlusal. Add temporary crown material to the occlusal and have the patient bite. Once set, remove the temporary crown. Mark with a pencil the areas the cusps contacted to keep as the fossas and trim the temporary creating the anatomy of the cusps.

Temporary crown missing material at the margin: this can happen if there was recession or abfraction. In these cases be sure to create space for more bulk in the matrix with the high-speed drill.

Unsure where to adjust the proximal contacts: do not adjust the shiny contact point or will lose contact, but it is acceptable to smooth around it. If multiple splinted temporary crowns, use a separating disc at the gingival and occlusal embrasure and bend the temporary until it snaps, then smooth around the shiny contact point to keep contacts.

Temporary crown with poor retention: evaluate the prep to discover if it is overly tapered or too short. Do not recommend cementing with permanent cement as the cement can match the color of the abutment and will have to be drilled off later, with the risk of damaging the abutment at the crown delivery.

Fear of removing a temporary crown and breaking the buildup: section temporary but not to the margin to avoid damaging and altering the prep and split with a hand instrument.

Difficulty removing a temporary crown with the hemostat: try gently twisting back and forth (clockwise and counterclockwise) in small quick movements to loosen the temporary crown from the abutment and then you should be able to remove the temp.

Crown at delivery will not seat

Check and adjust if the proximal contact is too heavy.

Check for gingival ingress. May require anesthetizing and packing a cord, or removal of tissue with a laser, bur, scalpel, or Electrosurge.

Crown delivery and multiple crowns will not seat

Try the crowns on the master cast for sequencing. Seat one at a time to verify the margins are sealed. Try seating multiple crowns in different orders to get them all to seat (see Figure 11.17). Be sure to cement in the same order. Recommend to cement one crown at a time and remove all the excess cement before cementing the next crown. (Remember that when trying to cement too many crowns at once, the cement material may partially set and will not allow complete seating.)

If the crowns are still not seating completely together, adjust the proximal contacts.

Crown delivery and there is an open proximal contact

Do not cement as this is substandard treatment.

See how many Mylar strips fit into the open proximal contact and inform the dental lab (e.g. three Mylar strips thick). You can also dispense bite registration material into the open proximal contact and send the lab to show the size of the open proximal contact.

Check the fit of the crown on the master cast from the lab, which was poured from the final impression (not the die, which has been trimmed/altered).

If the crown on the master cast has an open proximal contact, send it back to the lab and request they add proximal contact by adding more porcelain. Porcelain can be added to solid zirconia, layered zirconia, lithium disilicate, and PFM. If it is a gold crown, the crown will have to be remade.

If the crown on the master cast does not have an open proximal contact, retake the final impression as the teeth may have shifted and/or the impression may be distorted.

Bridge delivery with an open margin

Use Occlude or Fit Checker under the pontic to verify it is not contacting the edentulous ridge prematurely (adjust the pontic if it is). If not interfering, may have to adjust the proximal contacts.

Shade off at delivery

Show the patient using the mirror. If the patient does not approve of the shade, do not permanently cement the crown. Take photos with shades and the shade tab next to the tooth (body-to-body and edge-to-edge) and send the case back to the lab with the photos. Consider a custom shade match. The patient can be sent to the lab.

Prep to ideal and then remove the decay, or remove the decay and then prep to ideal?

If determining restorability, remove the decay first.

If the tooth is deemed restorable, prep to ideal and then remove the decay as the decay will be easier to access and less will have to be removed once prepped to ideal. Then build up the voids (i.e. core buildup) and refine the prep.

Trouble obtaining a good final impression of multiple crowns

Try the two-step technique, which in a way customizes the tray. Pack cords around abutments. Load a tray with heavy body PVS or PVS putty and cover with a layer of plastic wrap (from the grocery store). Set the tray; once set, remove the tray and peel off the plastic wrap. Then remove the cords and dispense light body around the abutments from distal to mesial tooth.

Load the tray with light body only where the preps are. Seat the tray and apply firm pressure both anteriorly and posteriorly (if not done, you will obtain two distinct levels of material affecting the occlusion).

Rocking bridge at the framework try-in

First verify that the pontic is not prematurely contacting the edentulous ridge. If rocking allows only one side to seat at a time, this could be due to blebs or shrinkage in processing the metal. This may require sectioning the bridge and placing a resin (e.g. Duralay) at the site connecting the framework and holding it in place until it sets to send back to the lab. Recommend another try-in appointment. Use Fit Checker to hold the bridge in place before adding resin.

Treating fractured porcelain on a PFM

Can attempt to repair with a porcelain bonding kit and packable composite or replace the crown. Consider replacing with a solid zirconia crown to prevent a repeat.

Strong tongue in the way while prepping

Retraction using the mirror may not cover enough surface area, which can lead to cutting the tongue with the bur. Instead use a tongue depressor to retract, or isolate (e.g. rubber dam, Dryshield).

Broken core buildup at the crown delivery

If it is small to medium, fill the crown with more cement.

If it is big, check retention. Is the crown loose? Recommend a new buildup, refine the prep, and final impression.

Tips

Creating a smooth flat crown prep margin without a "lip" or "J" margin: to refine the prep at the end, use a diamond end cutting (a non-side-cutting) bur without water to lightly touch the tooth for short periods at a time (to avoid heating the tooth) to smooth the uneven margin. Alternatively, you can use hand instruments (e.g. hatchet, hoe).

Any time you enameloplasty (e.g. spot reduce the opposing tooth) apply topical fluoride varnish (to remineralize the tooth and to decrease sensitivity).

Esthetic cases: you or the lab could wax up the models and from there you can fabricate the matrix for the provisionals. The patient can provide feedback on the esthetics of the provisional. You can adjust as necessary and make a new impression to send to the lab to duplicate the adjusted provisionals for fabrication of the definitive restorations.

Prepping with core buildups: any buildup restorative material (or existing restorative materials such as composite or amalgam) is much softer than tooth structure. Take care, as it is easy to over-reduce in areas of the core buildup when prepping a crown.

Perforation warning: consider recession and/or abfraction as part of the existing reduction on a crown prep. If not considered, can easily cause a mechanical pulpal exposure when reducing in these areas for the crown prep.

Checking prep margin: apply pressure with a periodontal probe to check the margin; if it slips then the margin is not very defined (i.e. will occur with a feather-edge margin). Also run the periodontal probe around the margin circumferentially to check it is smooth and to check it "connects." If this is not checked, you may make a final impression and upon evaluation see that the margin in one area does not "connect" to the rest of the margin (Figure 11.33).

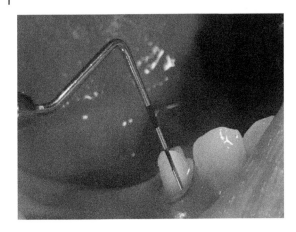

Figure 11.33 Check the prep margin circumferentially with a periodontal probe before the final impression.

How to avoid nicking the adjacent tooth: protect the adjacent tooth from being nicked.

Use a proximal protector (e.g. FenderWedge, Wedgeguard) (see Chapter 7, Figure 7.12). Caution: it is still possible to drill through this.

Alternatively, you can pre-wedge with a wooden wedge. Then cut the proximal contact with a narrow diamond bur and leave a thin shell of enamel and remove with hand instruments (e.g. hatchet, hoe).

Packing cord: lasso the tooth with the cord and pull it into the sulcus. With the cord packer hold for three seconds and move to the next segment of the cord and hold for three seconds, and so on (Figure 11.34).

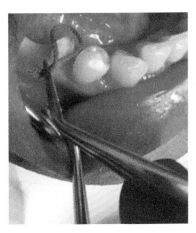
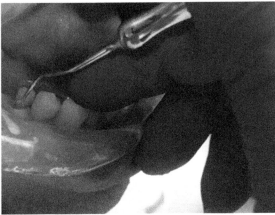

Figure 11.34 Packing cord.

Multiple crown delivery: to reduce confusion, write on the tray table the crown numbers so that when trying the crowns in and before cementing you can tell the crowns apart (Figure 11.35).

Figure 11.35 Tip for reducing confusion when delivering multiple crowns.

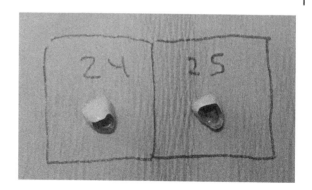

If abutment is exposed don't use 20% topical benzocaine: patients will complain of discomfort, so instead skip the topical and use local anesthetic.

Don't use clear temporary cement, use the white kind: dentist or assistant may not realize there is excess subgingivally or interproximally and patient will complain of discomfort later.

Don't have patient wear temporary crown for more than two weeks: the occlusal will wear and the abutment and opposing will supraerupt and the definitive crown will be too high and will require adjustment of the entire occlusal.

Use fresh diamond burs: single-use burs cut better and produce less heat than dull burs.

Enamel pearl: place margin above as the pearl could have a pulp horn inside.

Vertical nontapered axial walls: hold the bur as perpendicular as you can to the occlusal surface, check from various angles with the mirror, and begin to prep.

Remove blebs on "opposing" casts: if not done, will interfere with occlusion of the restoration.

CDT billing code tips

Only bill BW if it is diagnostic. Do not bill BW if a working radiograph (e.g. the pre-cementation BW at the crown delivery appointment).

Use the D2740 Porcelain/Ceramic substrate code for zirconia crowns even though zirconia is a metal. (Similarly, use the ceramic polishing kit for zirconia crowns and not the metal polishing kit, even though zirconia is a metal.)

If doing "herodontics" to save the tooth, warn the patient there is no second chance, as this is a last ditch effort to save the tooth. This will set their expectations so that the next time the crown fails the patient hopefully recalls the discussion (which should always be documented).

For proper infection control, do not send the lab the final impression with cotton rolls attached as these cannot be disinfected. Carefully cut the cotton rolls off (don't pull off as this can distort and tear the impression) (Figure 11.36).

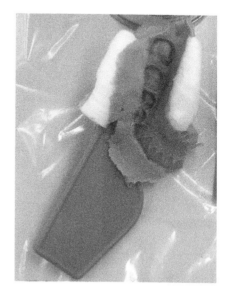

Figure 11.36 Cotton rolls cannot be properly disinfected. Remove before sending the final impression to the lab.

Real-Life Clinical Scenarios Answered

Dental Students' Questions

"How do we know if the tooth needs a filling, or a buildup, or a crown?"
  See Section Indications and Considerations for Crowns.
"I'm not good at shade selection. Any advice?"
  See Section Shade Selection.
"Doctor, did I invade the biologic width?"
  See Section Biologic Width.
"Do I send the patient for crown lengthening before I prep the crown?"
  See Section Treatment Planning.
"What is flash?" (See Figure 11.15)
  In a crown/bridge final impression, flash is the portion of the PVS material that enters the sulcus around the tooth. This is only necessary if the prep has an equigingival or subgingival margin in order for the lab technician to know exactly where to place the margin of the crown.
"Do I take a bitewing before and after cementing the crown?"
  A pre-cementation bitewing (or PA for anteriors) is recommended to check the crown for sealed margins interproximally before permanently cementing the crown.
"How do I check for interferences?"
  See Chapter 7, section Real-Life Clinical Questions Answered: "Where should the dots go on the composite when checking occlusion? Should there not be any dots on the filling?"

Dental Students' Comments

"I'm doing a crown because it was treatment planned by the last student."
  Not a good answer. What is the diagnosis and the indication for the crown?
"For crowns, I always treatment plan PFMs."
  Why? What is the indication for this material versus another material? See Table 11.2.
"I've never cut off a crown before, I hope the tooth is OK underneath."
  Be sure to discuss the risks involved with the patient (see Section Removing a Crown). You will not know unless you remove the crown if it is indicated.
"Today I am prepping a survey crown."
  Have you designed the RPD? Do you know the metal design for the crown (e.g. rest seat locations)? Do you know how much more to prep at the rest seats? Do you know how much of an undercut to ask the lab to make? See section Seven Scenarios Involving Removable Partial Dentures/Complete Dentures.

Dental Assistant's Questions

"Doc, every time I make the temporary it breaks and sticks on the tooth."
  See Section Troubleshooting.
"At the crown delivery appointment I just took the temporary crown off and the buildup broke. What should I do?"
  Let me check if the tooth is still restorable. If it is, we will have to build it up again, refine the prep, and make a new final impression to send to the lab, as it will be impossible to retrofit the existing crown to the new buildup.

To avoid this happening again:

- Place a separating agent (e.g. Vaseline) on the core buildup when we fabricate the new temporary crown.
- Hallow out the crown a little bit.
- Mix Vaseline with the temporary cement when cementing the temporary crown.
- When you remove the temporary crown at the next appointment (i.e. the crown delivery appointment) be very gentle and use the curved hemostat to remove the temporary along the long axis of the tooth (no rocking motion).

Patients' Questions

- You section off an existing crown and determine the tooth is not restorable. The patient yells "You're telling me now I have to get the tooth pulled when I thought I was just getting my crown replaced?"

  Everything we do involves informed consent so that the patient can make an informed decision with an understanding of the risks and benefits (see Section Consents).

- "Doc I cannot afford a crown right now but I just had a root canal done and the specialist said I need a crown. How long can I wait?"

  While I cannot provide you with a specific length of time you can wait, I can tell you that the longer you go without the crown, the greater the risk that this tooth will fracture and we will have to extract the tooth. There are many factors including how much tooth structure is remaining, the opposing teeth, and how much wear and tear the teeth get (e.g. diet, grinding or clenching). Studies show that for premolars and molars full coverage crowns are recommended and as time passes the risk of failure increases [15].

- "Which type of crown will last the longest?"

  I can provide you with a ballpark estimate, but there are many variables that affect how long a crown will last. Variables include caries risk, periodontal risk, oral hygiene, oral habits (e.g. bruxism, clenching, wear and tear), diet (e.g. eating yogurt vs. chewing on ice cubes), dental materials, and skill level of the dentist. There are no guarantees in dentistry and nothing artificial is as durable as natural dentition. Also, with esthetics and strength, typically one is compromised.

  Gold crowns are typically considered to last the longest (40 years). PFM crowns have good survival rates (in one study, high gold-based metal-ceramic crowns placed by prosthodontists had about an 85% survival rate at 25 years) [16]. Long-term studies are needed for zirconia crowns, lithium disilicate crowns, and other newer crown materials. Stainless steel crowns have the shortest lifespan.

  Additionally, in any tooth where the root canal (the "living" portion of the tooth) has been removed, the remaining tooth structure is more brittle. It can break and we cannot predict how it will break. It can break in such a way that you could lose the tooth.

  See Table 11.2 to weigh the pros and cons of different crown materials.

- "The temporary broke again, should I sleep with my partials in until I get the permanent crowns?"

  Normally I would not recommend sleeping with partials in. However, in a case like this in which we are fabricating a crown because the filling and tooth continue to break due to nighttime grinding, it would be a good idea to sleep with the partials in until we deliver the permanent which will be much stronger. I'd recommend removing the partials when you can during the day to allow for more blood circulation to the gingiva.

When fabricating a new temporary crown, be sure to check for clearance between the temporary crown and partial to prevent dislodgement of the temporary crown when the patient. removes the partial. If a stayplate, it may require adjusting the acrylic.

"How do you know if I have a cavity under the crown? Can you pull the crown off to see and then put it back on?"

Sometimes the cavity will appear on the radiograph at the crown margin or root surface. Sometimes it is detectable clinically. Sometimes an open margin is detected clinically and one can assume if the tip of the explorer can fit inside, then microscopic cavity-causing bacteria have already entered and caused decay. Sometimes the crown falls off the tooth because of the extent of decay, or the decay causes the abutment to fracture. Sometimes a patient complains about food getting trapped beneath the crown or complains that the tooth becomes symptomatic. However, there is no way of knowing the extent of the decay unless the crown is removed.

It is not possible to remove the crown to inspect what is beneath and then cement it back on because the process of removing the crown destroys it (see Section Removing a Crown).

"Do you recommend a bridge or an implant?"

It depends on the case. There are many variables including advantages disadvantages, risks, and costs (see Chapter 4, Table 4.3).

Crown not seating at the delivery appointment and patient said "The temporary crown fell off the next day but I figured I'd see you in a week for the permanent crown and it wasn't bothering me so I didn't call."

The crown may not be seating because the gingiva grew over the margin and/or because the adjacent teeth migrated toward the abutment. The crown may have to be adjusted or remade with a new updated final impression. This also means you did not sufficiently emphasize to the patient the importance of the postoperative instructions (see Section Postoperative Instructions).

At the crown delivery appointment, patient said "Doc, this tooth is so sensitive to cold."

It is not uncommon for teeth to be sensitive with temporary crowns. Temporary crowns do not fit the tooth as closely as permanent crowns. It's not the sensitivity but the progression that's important. If the sensitivity is getting worse, an evaluation (endodontic diagnostic testing) is needed. If the sensitivity is the same, recommend leaving the temporary on for one to two weeks longer and pain generally decreases. If still not improving after being in a temporary crown for an additional one to two weeks, recommend evaluating the tooth again (endodontic diagnostic testing) or temporarily cementing the permanent crown. We need to be sure the tooth is asymptomatic prior to permanently cementing the permanent crown to avoid the tooth needing RCT through the brand-new crown. Better to have the root canal done without damaging the new crown.

"My crown fell off and I just need you to glue it back on."

See Chapter 10, section Real-Life Questions, Concerns, and Demands Answered.

"When are we supposed to worry about incisal or anterior guidance?"

When prepping anterior crown cases, it is good practice to obtain and send preoperative impressions to the lab in addition to the final impression. This way the lab can duplicate the patient's anterior guidance for the new crowns. The lab technicians can also determine the size of the teeth with a golden proportion gauge, and by evaluating the wear facets. Its also a good idea to send preoperative photos of the patient's entire face and smile to aid in determining the shape of the teeth. In addition, a Koise Dento-Facial Analyzer can be used and sent to the lab as a facebow transfer to communicate the facial midline and the occlusal plane parallel to the pupils.

Scenarios

- A dental student tries on a crown and no open margins are detected. Once the student cements the crown, the crown now has an open margin on the buccal.
  - This can be from allowing cement to harden while biting on a cotton roll.
  - This can be from overfilling the intaglio with cement versus lining the walls.
  - This can be from the cement setting too quickly while seating the crown.
  - This can be from the crown rotating during placement.
    - It is important to familiarize yourself with the path of insertion before cementing a crown. Can the crown rotate? If so, this could create an open margin if rotated in the wrong direction.
- A dental student permanently cemented a crown on the patient without showing the patient how it looks in the mirror for shade selection approval.
  - See Section Consents.
- The dental assistant loads the crown with Fuji IX instead of Fuji CEM.
  - Know the materials you use, know the manufacturers' instructions, and always confirm what is being handed to you by the dental assistant. In this case the crown was loaded with a restorative material, not a cement material. It was immediately wiped with multiple microbrushes before the material set.
- A dental student makes a full arch final impression and it becomes locked in beneath a bridge.
  - It is important to always check for undercuts such as buccal exostosis or presence of bridges in the mouth before making an impression with PVS as it can become locked in the mouth and then the tray has to be drilled in half and removed. If undercuts are detected, dry the area and block out with rope wax.

References

1 Shillingburg, H.T., Sather, D.A., Wilson, E.L. et al. (2012). *Fundamentals of Fixed Prosthodontics*, 4e. Chicago: Quintessence Publishing.

2 Wassell, R.W., Steele, J.G., and Welsh, G. (1998). Considerations when planning occlusal rehabilitation: a review of the literature. *Int. Dent. J.* 48 (6): 571–581.

3 Ingber, J.S., Rose, L.F., and Coslet, J.G. (1977). The "biologic width": a concept in periodontics and restorative dentistry. *Alpha Omegan* 70: 62–65.

4 DHCS (2021). *Medi-Cal Dental*. Medi-Cal Dental Provider Handbook. https://www. dental.dhcs.ca.gov/MCD_documents/ providers/provider_handbook/handbook.pdf (accessed 18 May 2021).

5 American Association of Endodontists (2020). *Treatment Standards*. Chicago: AAE. Available at https://www.aae.org/specialty/wp-content/ uploads/sites/2/2018/04/TreatmentStandards_ Whitepaper.pdf (accessed 1 May 2021).

6 Ante, I.H. (1926). The fundamental principles of abutments. *Mich. State Dent. Soc. Bull.* 8: 14–23.

7 Glidewell (2020). BruxZir Full-Strength Zirconia. https://glidewelldental.com/solutions/crown-and-bridge/zirconia/bruxzir-full-strength-solid-zirconia (accessed 1 May 2021).

8 Glidewell (2020). Lava Crowns and Bridges. https://glidewelldental.com/solutions/crown-and-bridge/zirconia/lava-crowns-and-bridges (accessed 1 May 2021).

9 Glidewell (2020). IPS e.max. https://glidewelldental.com/solutions/crown-and-bridge/glass-ceramics/ips-e-max (accessed 1 May 2021).

10 Winter, R. (2012). When to use triple tray impressions. https://www.speareducation.com/spear-review/2012/10/when-to-use-triple-tray-impressions (accessed 1 May 2021).

11 California Dental Arts (2020). The advantage of a full arch impression tray. http://www.caldentalarts.com/the-advantage-of-a-full-arch-impression-tray (accessed 2 May 2021).

12 California Dental Arts (2020). How to improve the outcome of your triple-tray impressions. http://www.caldentalarts.com/triple-tray-impressions (accessed 1 May 2021).

13 DiTolla, M. and Cash, M (2006). Bite registration 101. https://glidewelldental.com/education/chairside-dental-magazine/volume-1-issue-2/bite-registration-101 (accessed 2 May 2021).

14 Gordon J (2014). Christensen Clinicians Report. How to prepare zirconia and IPS e.max restorations for cementation. http://www.cliniciansreport.org/uploads/files/146/CR-Special-Report.pdf (accessed 2 May 2021).

15 Nagasiri, R. and Chitmongkolsuk, S. (2005). Long-term survival of endodontically treated molars without crown coverage: a retrospective cohort study. *J. Prosthet. Dent.* 93 (2): 164–170.

16 Walton, T.R. (2013). The up to 25-year survival and clinical performance of 2,340 high gold-based metal-ceramic single crowns. *Int. J. Prosthodont.* 26 (2): 151–160.

12

Complete Dentures

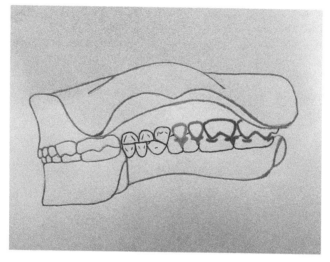

Figure 12.1 Position of the maxillary lingual cusps relative to the mandibular teeth.

Chapter Outline

- Real-Life Clinical Questions
- Relevance
- Setting Realistic Expectations
- Clinical and Radiographic Exam
    - Evaluation of Existing Dentures for Replacement
    - Evaluation of Edentulous Patient Prior to Denture Fabrication
    - Evaluation of Dentate Patient Prior to Denture Fabrication
- Treatment Planning
- Consent Forms
- Complete Denture Procedural Steps
    - Appointment 1: Preliminary Impressions
    - Appointment 2: Final Impression
    - Appointment 3: Wax Occlusal Rims

Clinical Dentistry Daily Reference Guide, First Edition. William A. Jacobson.
© 2022 John Wiley & Sons, Inc. Published 2022 by John Wiley & Sons, Inc.

Real-Life Clinical Questions

Patients' Requests

- "I need a new lower denture, mine is too loose."
- "I need a new denture because when I chew food on one side my denture gets loose."
- "My front tooth came out sucking on a lollipop. Can you replace it?"
- "My denture was made in another state. Can you adjust it?"

Patients' Concerns

- "Is it OK for me to swallow this [alginate]?"
- "How do I prevent bone loss under my dentures?"

Patients' Questions and Comments

- "Why are you recommending pulling a healthy tooth for a denture to fit?"
- "I'm going to eat a nice steak tonight with my new dentures."
- "This denture is making me gag, can you trim the back?"
- "How much glue should I put on the denture?"
- "I need to keep my dentures moist? Why is that?"
- "How long do I soak it with one of those tablets?"
- "My previous dentist never told me I am supposed to take my teeth out at night!"

"It falls out when I talk."

"I get food stuck under my dentures."

"How long will it take for my sore spot to heal?"(Figure 12.2)

"I had a sore spot so I stopped wearing it for a week. Can you adjust it?"

"Before a tube of denture glue would last me eight weeks, now it lasts three weeks."

Figure 12.2   Traumatic ulceration from a denture.

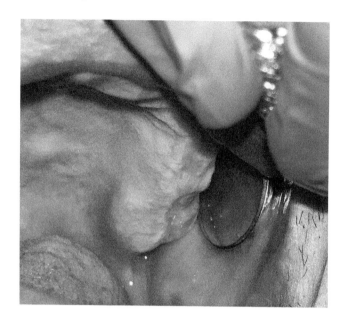

Relevance

You may not be a denture wearer, but your patients will rely on *you* for your expertise.

Setting Realistic Expectations

Explain the following facts about dentures to the patient.

Dentures are removable appliances and not fixed to the gums. The dentures will move and food will get underneath them.

A denture is a prosthesis, or artificial body part, similar to a prosthetic leg. Some people with prosthetic legs can run marathons, some can only walk, and some cannot accept the prosthesis as their own. Dentures are no different.

No matter how well the dentures are made, some people will adapt well to chewing, speaking, smiling, and wearing their dentures. Some will only wear their dentures in public for appearance, and some will choose not to wear their dentures. In my experience, patients who have optimistic outlooks and are "patient" are the most adaptive.

Dentures will not feel like your original teeth and the biting force is significantly reduced, at best only 20–40% of the force compared to your natural teeth [1].

Dentures may never feel like the "old set" of dentures. Dentures may feel different and require a period of adjustment.

It will still be important to maintain good hygiene by cleaning your gums, tongue, and dentures to prevent fungal infections and removing the dentures at night to help preserve the ridge [2].

It is common to get sore spots that will require adjustments by the dentist. First there will be big sore spot adjustments, then little sore spot adjustments, and then dialing down the bite. Some people experience gagging (usually disappears within a few days) [2].

It will take time to adapt to chewing and speaking with the dentures.

Clinical and Radiographic Exam

1) Evaluation of existing dentures for replacement.
2) Evaluation of an edentulous patient prior to denture fabrication.
3) Evaluation of a dentate patient prior to denture fabrication.

1. Evaluation of Existing Dentures for Replacement

The American College of Prosthodontics recommends that dentures and partial dentures be evaluated for replacement when at least one of the following conditions occurs:

1) Signs of chronic irritation.
2) Denture adhesives required to eat, retain dentures, or applied more than once daily.
3) Patient cannot wear dentures.
4) Denture has degraded leading to "instability, loss of retention, loss of esthetics, loss of support, inability to eat, or if the prosthesis or prosthetic teeth are discolored, cracked, broken, or missing" [3].
5) Teeth are lost.
6) Prosthesis in function for more than five years, recommend consult with dental provider for their prosthesis to be examined regularly [3].

Ask the Patient

- What problems are you experiencing with your current dentures?
- When were the dentures made?
- How many sets of dentures have you had?
- Do you recall ever having these dentures relined or repaired?
- How much adhesive are you placing on the dentures? More than previously?
- How do you feel about the tooth and gum shade?
- Pleased with tooth shape/size/characteristics? Make study models of existing dentures as a reference for the lab technician (Figure 12.3).
- Any things you would like differently in the new set of dentures?

Evaluate the Patient

- Denture hygiene (Figure 12.4).
- Amount of adhesive on denture (Figure 12.4).
- Amount of occlusal wear of acrylic teeth (Figure 12.5).
- Broken or missing teeth.
- Denture base fractured or perforated.
- Form of identification present?

Figure 12.3   Study model of denture.

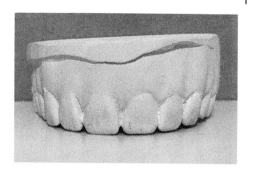

Figure 12.4   Note the patient's poor denture hygiene. Also note the color difference of the denture base on the facial gingiva compared to the right flange, evidence of a previous reline. Note the excessive amount of denture adhesive (bright pink).

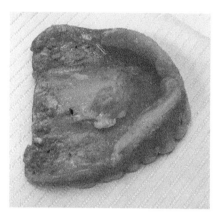

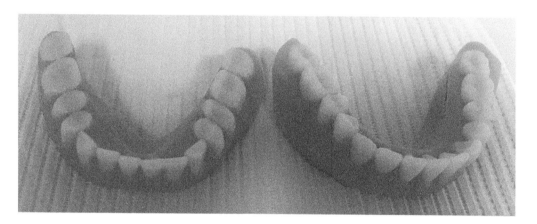

Figure 12.5   Patient's five-year old denture (left) and new denture (right). Note the occlusal wear on the previous denture. Wear amount varies based on diet, habits, and amount of use.

- Difference in base colors for evidence of previous reline (Figure 12.4).
- Try dentures in and evaluate retention, stability, and support (Figure 12.6).
  - Retention: resistance to the removal of the denture from the tissue
    - Loose? Underextended flanges? Overextended flanges?
  - Stability: resistance to horizontal and lateral movement (e.g. rotates).
  - Support: resistance to movement toward the denture-bearing tissue.

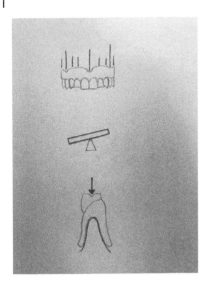

Figure 12.6   Retention, stability, and support.

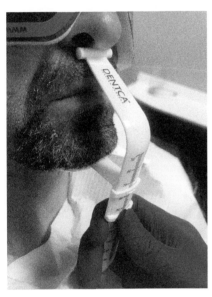

Figure 12.7   Dentca Jaw gauge.

- Vertical dimension of occlusion.
  - Ideal? Does it appear collapsed (nose too close to chin, skin fold at commissures) or excessive (nose too far from chin, clicking with speech)?
  - Measure VDO and make necessary changes to new denture (Figure 12.7).
- Adaptation to tissue: check with pressure-indicating paste (PIP) (see Section Appointment 5: Denture Delivery).
- Incisal display at rest: tooth/gum display when smiling. Ideal, inadequate, excessive? (See Section WOR Checklist)
- See also following section.

It is important to remind the patient not to use denture adhesive prior to future dental visits, in order for the dentist to have a clean ridge for each appointment.

2. Evaluation of Edentulous Patient Prior to Denture Fabrication

- Extraoral exam, intraoral exam, and oral cancer screening (see Chapter 2).
- Panoramic radiograph (see Chapter 3). Check for:
  - Retained root tips to extract (Figure 12.8).
  - Unerupted teeth. May choose to monitor. As bone resorbs, tooth may become exposed. Unlikely if covered in bone, no pathology, and/or over 40 years old.
  - Pneumatized sinuses. If maxillary tuberosity reduction or alveoplasty needed, could cause perforation.
  - Pathology: refer to specialist.

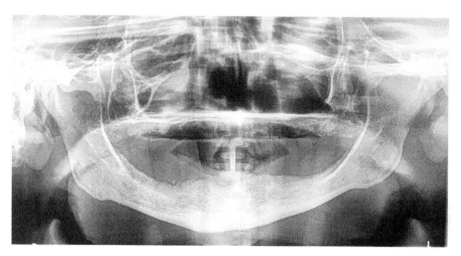

Figure 12.8   Retained root tip noted on panoramic radiograph.

- Examine the oral cavity:
  - Moisture: dry mouth will have reduced retention and is more susceptible to sore spots. Thick-ropy saliva is more mucin "sticky" but is not well distributed, whereas thin-watery saliva spreads better but is not as sticky, so a normal combination is best for retention. Discuss dry mouth treatment. See Chapter 5.
  - Edentulous ridge
    - Relationship: Class I, Class II, Class III, and crossbite affect esthetics, function, stability, support and retention.
    - Ridge height: adequate (high), moderate, or poor (flat, atrophied) (Figure 12.9). The higher the ridge, the better for retention, stability, and support (see Figure 12.6).
    - Texture:
      - Firm smooth (Figure 12.10).
      - Firm uneven (Figure 12.11).
      - Buccal exostosis: interferes with denture adaptation and causes tender areas overlying exostosis.
      - Flabby (hyperplastic replacement): possible surgical removal unless extreme atrophy of entire ridge. Modified impression technique if kept. See Section Troubleshooting.

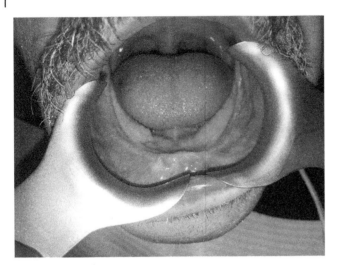

Figure 12.9   Atrophied ridge.

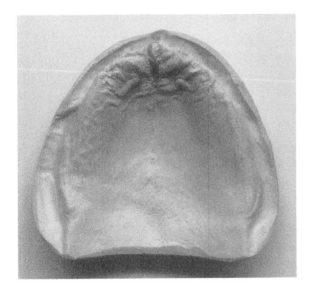

Figure 12.10   Smooth ridge.

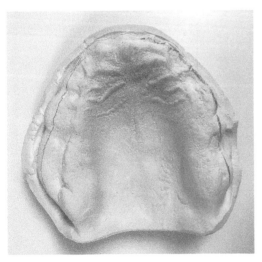

Figure 12.11   Uneven ridge.

Color
  Healthy soft tissue.
  Erythematous or white spots: possible fungal infection requires treatment (Figure 12.12).
  Pathology: refer to specialist (see Chapter 2).
Signs of chronic irritation: includes epulis fissuratum (Figure 12.13), oral ulcerations, or treatment-resistant *Candida*-related denture stomatitis [3].
Frenum: high frenum attachment (labial, buccal, lingual) to ridge. If high, can lead to poor retention and traumatic ulcerations unless the denture is adjusted or frenectomy is performed.
Palate depth: deep (better retention) versus shallow (poor retention).
Tori
  Palatal tori: impingement on the posterior palatal seal (PPS) affects retention. Location may interfere with PPS.

Figure 12.12 Fungal infection.

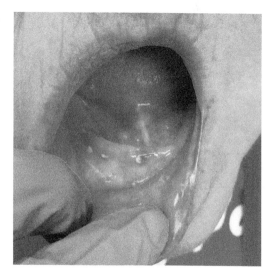

Figure 12.13 Epulis fissuratum. The patient's denture was able to rest in three different positions.

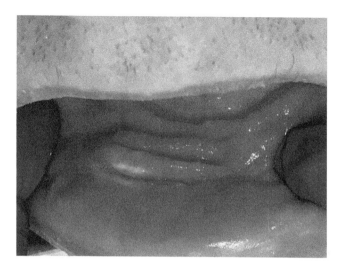

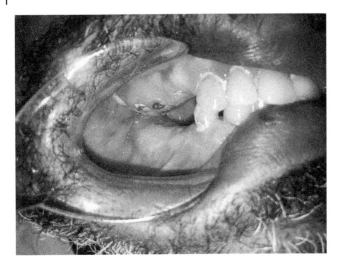

Figure 12.14   Inadequate space for opposing teeth.

- Mandibular tori are usually removed.
- Removal is carried out for improved stability/retention/adaptation of dentures and the prevention of fulcrum. Undercuts from the tori prevent the flanges from extending to a desired length. Tender areas overlying the tori can develop.
- Maxillary specific:
  - Prominent anterior ridge with undercut requires alveoplasty. Prominent ridge can cause poor esthetics with excessive lip support. Deep undercut prevents denture adaptation, whereas slight undercut can aid in retention.
  - Maxillary tuberosity (Figure 12.14) may impinge on the space for denture teeth in posterior. Need a minimum of 10 mm between ridges for denture teeth/bases.
  - Maxillary tuberosity undercut may cause interference when seating denture.
  - Palatal vault: shallow leads to poor stability. too deep to poor support.
- Pre-prosthetic surgery checklist:
  - Extractions
  - Sinus lift
  - Evaluation/treatment of radiographic of pathology
  - Evaluation/treatment of fungal infections or other pathology
  - Surgical removal of hyperplastic tissue or epulis fissuratum
  - Frenectomy (specify location)
  - Alveoplasty of each quadrant of irregular/uneven/undercut boney areas (specify location)
  - Maxillary tuberosity reduction.
  - Maxillary tuberosity undercut removal
  - Palatal and/or mandibular tori removal (specify location)
  - Buccal exostosis removal (specify location)
  - Sedation
  - Other.

- Extraoral exam, intraoral exam, and oral cancer screening (see Chapter 2).
- Full-mouth radiographic series and/or panoramic radiograph (see Chapter 3). Check for:
  - Indication for extraction of all teeth (confirm clinically). Document diagnosis of each tooth justifying need for extraction. For example, #2 retained root, #3 deep MODB caries to pulp, #7 periodontally compromised with grade 3 mobility, #9 removal for prosthodontic purposes.
  - Unerupted teeth: may choose to monitor.
  - Pneumatized sinuses: if maxillary tuberosity reduction or alveoplasty could perforate.
  - Pathology: refer to specialist.
- Examine oral cavity
  - Teeth findings: confirm radiographic findings, add additional clinical findings.
  - Comprehensive periodontal charting (see Chapter 6).
  - VDO:
    - Ideal? Does it appear collapsed (nose too close to chin, skin fold at commissures) or excessive (nose too far from chin, clicking with speech)?
    - Measure VDO and make necessary changes to new denture (see Figure 12.7).
  - Measure amount of incisal display of upper and lower incisors.
  - Occlusion: Class I, Class II, Class III, and crossbite affect esthetics, function, stability, support and retention.
  - Esthetics:
    - Tooth shade.
    - Amount of incisal display at rest and smiling.
  - Saliva production.
  - Frenums, tori, exostosis, hyperplastic tissue, uneven ridge, ridge with undercuts.
- Make study models: as reference for tooth shape/size/characteristics (see Figure 12.15).
- Pre-prosthetic surgery checklist:
  - Extractions
  - Sinus lift

Figure 12.15 Preoperative study model.

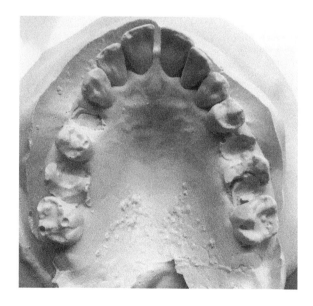

Evaluation/treatment of radiographic of pathology
Evaluation/treatment of fungal infections or other pathology
Surgical removal of hyperplastic tissue or epulis fissuratum
Frenectomy (specify location)
Alveoplasty of each quadrant of irregular/uneven/undercut boney areas (specify location)
Maxillary tuberosity reduction.
Maxillary tuberosity undercut removal
Palatal and/or mandibular tori removal (specify location)
Buccal exostosis removal (specify location) (Table 12.1).

Treatment Planning

Table 12.1   Treatment planning.

Comprehensive oral evaluation
Oral cancer screening (see Chapter 2)
Periodontal evaluation (see Chapter 6)
Radiographs (see Chapter 3)
Decide on the treatment option[a]

Treatment options	Sequence
Complete dentures	• Reline[b] every three to five years [4]: depends on the patient, when the denture becomes loose
	• Replace[b] every 5–10 years [4]: replace for tooth wear, or esthetics
Pre-prosthetic surgery	• Immediate complete dentures with soft reline for three to six months
Immediate interim dentures	• Change soft reline as necessary, depending on severity of irritation [5] and longevity of materials used
Complete dentures (best option)	• Hard reline at six months
	• Replace with new set of dentures at 6–12 months
Pre-prosthetic surgery	• Heal two to three months (8–12 weeks) prior to impressions for dentures
Healing period	
Complete dentures (second best option)	• Complete denture
	• Hard reline at 6–12 months if indicated
Pre-prosthetic surgery	• Immediate complete dentures with soft reline for three to six months
Immediate dentures (third best option)	• Change soft reline as necessary, depending on severity of irritation and longevity of materials used [5]
	• Hard reline at the earliest six months if indicated

Denture adjustments

Periodic oral evaluation (recall exam)

Radiographs (if indicated) (see Chapter 3)

Relines, repairs, replacements

[a] Even if a patient cannot afford implants, recommend and document.
[b] According to the American College of Prosthodontists there is "currently no evidence to determine the frequency of denture relines, rebases, or remakes of removable complete or partial dental prosthesis" [3].

Consent Forms

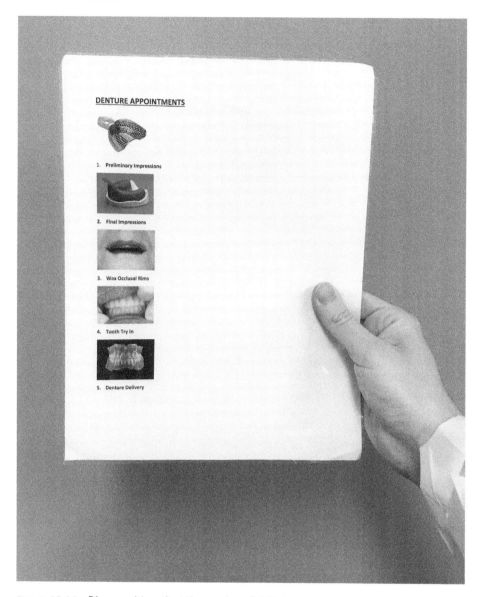

Figure 12.16 Discuss with patient the number of visits to expect.

- Informed consent is governed by state law.
- Contact your professional liability carrier and/or attorney for specific guidance and forms.
- Examples of the Denture Consent Form and Prosthesis Processing Consent Form are shown below. Note that the purpose of the Prosthesis Processing Consent Form is to encourage the patient to carefully evaluate the tooth set-up and prevent him or her from demanding a new prosthesis at delivery. Complaints to be avoided at delivery could include "These teeth are too yellow," "This looks like I have fake teeth," and "I need this remade."

Time Frame
- Typical six to eight appointments include: preliminary impressions, final impressions, wax rim, tooth try-in, delivery, adjustments [Figure 12.16]
- Two weeks between each appointment to allow turnaround time for lab.
- Possible delays:
  - Need for additional surgery (alveoplasty, tuberosity reduction, frenectomy, etc.) which will require more healing time.
  - Need for lab to make adjustments to cases.

Immediate Dentures
- Involve extraction of the teeth and insertion of the denture on the same day.
- These are transitional dentures and may have to be relined or remade six months following insertion.
- Fees for relines or remakes are not included/covered.
- Minor adjustments and temporary (soft) relines may be required and are included the first six months.
- Advantage: elimination of 8–12 week period without teeth.
- Disadvantage: no opportunity to have a tooth try-in appointment to check the esthetics, phonetics, fit and occlusion (bite).

Conventional Dentures
- After removal of teeth, 8–12 weeks for healing prior to the first step in fabricating the dentures (the more time spent healing, the better the denture fit).
- Advantages:
  - Opportunity to have a tooth try-in appointment to check the esthetics, phonetics, fit and occlusion (bite).
  - Typically, fewer adjustments.
  - Reline or remake of dentures may not be required as soon.
- Disadvantage: 8–12 week period without teeth.

I Understand:
- Teeth will be removed and a prosthesis made.
- Typically five steps included but may be more: preliminary impressions, final impressions, wax rim, tooth try-in, delivery, adjustments.
- All denture patients will have an adjustment period to learn how to speak.
- "Teeth" no longer held in by roots. Instead muscles, ridge, suction hold them in.
- Lower denture has no suction, so harder to keep in place.
- Front teeth are just for "show" and I need to learn to bite and chew on back teeth where ridge can support the biting force.
- I must remove the prosthesis eight hours every day or I will cause harm to gum, bone and mouth; if not:
  - Increased chance of fungal infection.
  - Shorter life of the denture.
  - Bony ridge supporting denture will resorb and erode under the constant compressive forces.
  - Bone resorption will continue throughout my lifetime making subsequent denture construction more difficult, less satisfying and less comfortable for me than my previous denture experience.
- I must keep my dentures clean.
- I must come in for recall exams for checkups and oral cancer screenings.

- Dentures have their own challenges and are not a complete solution to my dental needs.
- Issues with dentures include: difficulty speaking and/or eating, food under dentures, functional problems, loose dentures, feeling of fullness, sore spots (especially with dry mouth) or excessive salivary production (temporary), need for future relines and remakes.
- There is NO guarantee I will be able to successfully and comfortably wear a well-constructed denture.
- Dentures are not considered a replacement for teeth but a replacement for no teeth.
- Dentures at best will end up with significantly less chewing force as compared to my natural teeth.
- Patient Name: _____
- Medical Record Number: _____
- Patient (or Patient's Representative) Signature: _____
- Date: _____
- Dentist name: _____
- Dentist Signature: _____ [4]

Prosthesis Processing Consent Form

Type of Prosthesis [check boxes]
- Maxillary Complete Denture
- Mandibular Complete Denture
- Maxillary Resin Partial Denture
- Mandibular Resin Partial Denture
- Maxillary Cast Metal Partial Denture
- Mandibular Cast Metal Partial Denture
- Other: _____

Today I've had the opportunity to try in my prosthesis at the wax try-in stage. At this stage the teeth are set in wax to evaluate the appearance and bite of the prosthesis.
I am satisfied with the following:

- Shape, size, color, position, angulation, and overlap of teeth
- Amount of teeth and gum shown at rest and when I smile
- Lip support (not strained, too full, or too flat)
- Bite (feels good, even, and teeth contact on both sides)
- Pronunciation of words (teeth are not clicking together or too far apart when speaking)

I consent to having my prosthesis sent to the lab for final processing.
I understand that once my prosthesis is processed, my prosthesis may require several adjustments; however any major alterations to the appearance and bite of the prosthesis will be made at my own expense.

- Patient Name: _____
- Medical Record Number: _____
- Patient (or Patient's Representative) Signature: _____
- Date: _____
- Dentist name: _____
- Dentist Signature: _____

Complete Denture Procedural Steps

Appointment 1: Preliminary Impressions

- Goal is to capture anatomy necessary to create custom trays.
- Inform patient that it may take several attempts for an accurate impression and the better the impression sent to the lab, the better the final product will be.
  - Select edentulous stock trays 5 mm wider to accommodate alginate [5] (Figure 12.17).
    - High palatal vault? Build palate with rope wax so alginate reaches palate.
    - High ridge? Build up tray periphery with rope wax.
  - Tell patient to "keep cheeks/lips as loose and relaxed as possible, I will pull and wiggle your cheeks and lips so that the impression captures all the anatomy."
  - Mandibular (start with lower first as less gagging, better tolerated and familiarizes patient with procedure):
    - Insert front to back, telling patient to "lift tongue up, stick your tongue out of your mouth, now try reaching your left ear, then your right ear, repeat a few times." Then pull the cheek up/out/around, and pull lip out/up/around, telling patient to "pucker, smile."
  - Maxillary:
    - Insert front to back, making sure some material is expressed posterior of tray. Pull cheek out/down/around, pull lip out/down/around, telling patient to "pucker, smile, move jaw side to side. You can sit up and look down at your shoelaces if it makes you more comfortable." Mouth mirror can be used to wipe away excess material going down soft palate.
- Inspect accuracy of impressions, and retake if necessary.
- If patient wears dentures:
  - Make impressions of dentures outside the mouth as a reference for tooth shape/size/characteristics.
  - Inform patient not to wear for 12–24 hours prior to the next visit (final impression).
- Once impressions poured, evaluate preliminary models for any additional pre-prosthetic surgery needed such as alveoplasty.
- See Section Lab Prescriptions.

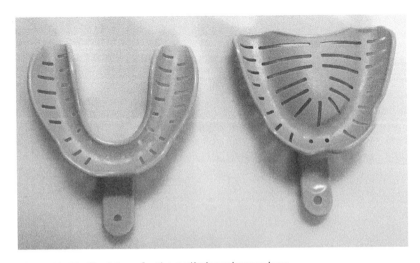

Figure 12.17   Stock trays for the preliminary impressions.

- Goal is to make accurate impressions using custom trays (Figure 12.18) to determine the contours, height, and width of the borders for the dentures.
- Inform patient it may take several attempts for an accurate impression and that the better the impression sent to the lab, the better the final product.
- Place petroleum jelly on any facial hair present to prevent PVS light body from sticking to hair.
- Border molding: aim is to determine the contours, height, and width of the borders for the complete dentures by shaping the impression material via manipulation of the tissues and musculature (Figures 12.19 and 12.20) adjacent to the borders of the impression trays.
  - Try in maxillary and mandibular custom trays.
  - Verify tray flanges are 2–3 mm short of vestibule/frenula and 2 mm beyond the vibrating line ("aaah"); if overextended, adjust with acrylic bur.
  - Apply adhesive to custom trays.
  - Caution: block out undesirable undercut with rope wax applied to dried tissue to prevent impression from locking into mouth.
  - Border mold with heavy body PVS or green compound stick (either at once or in sections at a time). Compound stick requires the wax spacer to be maintained on the intaglio of the custom trays while border molding. Compound stick must be heated in order to apply to periphery of custom tray, but should be dipped in hot water bath (140°F, 60°C) for three to five seconds to temper the wax to avoid burning the patient. This extends the malleability of the compound while inserting and border molding. After border molding the wax spacer must be removed (wax spacer preserves the space for the PVS light body wash).
  - Mandibular:
    - Border mold: pull the cheek up/out/around, pull lip out/up/around, telling patient to "pucker, smile" (Figure 12.21).
    - Have patient rinse with Listerine to dry the mouth and then swish with cold water (reduces saliva).
    - PVS light body wash: tell patient to "lift tongue up, stick tongue out of your mouth, now try reaching your left ear, then your right ear, repeat a few times." Then pull the cheek up/out/around, pull lip out/up/around, telling patient to "pucker, smile" (Figure 12.22).
  - Maxillary: close slightly so no knife edge,
    - Border mold: pull cheek out/down/around, pull lip out/down/around, telling patient to "pucker, smile, move jaw side to side" (Figure 12.23).
    - Have patient rinse with Listerine to dry the mouth and then swish with cold water (reduces saliva).
    - PVS light body wash: pull cheek out/down/around, pull lip out/down/around, telling patient to "pucker, smile, move jaw side to side" (Figure 12.24).
- Inspect accuracy of impressions: make sure maxillary final impression has captured the hamular notch.
- Defining the PPS
  - PPS: "positive shape on the most posterior extent of the intaglio surface of the maxillary complete denture, shaped like cupid's bow" [4].
  - Function is to "create positive tissue contact, keep food away from the intaglio surface of the denture, increase retention" [4].
  - Works "as a valve seal, creates soft tissue displacement at the junction of the movable and non-movable tissue, depresses glandular tissue, expresses air [and creates] suction" [4].
  - Identifying PPS landmarks
    - Maxillary soft palate at rest (Figure 12.25).

Posterior extent of the denture (the "aaah" line or vibrating line): the posterior vibrating line is the area that dictates the distal palatal extension. Have the patient say "aaah" and mark the line from hamular notch to hamular notch (Figure 12.26).

Anterior extent (blow line, Valsalva line) of the palatal seal: the anterior vibrating line is at the junction of the hard and soft palate. Have the patient perform a Valsalva maneuver (pinch their nose while patient blows gently out of nose; Figure 12.27), and the Valsalva line will appear as "Cupid's bow" (Figure 12.28).

Mark the posterior and anterior extent with the Thompson stick (Figure 12.29).

Seat maxillary final impression to transfer the PPS location to impression.

Send to lab. If not sending to lab to pour master cast and fabricate wax occlusal rims (WORs):

Bead, box and pour impressions

Mix pumice and mounting plaster with water, place on tile and raise up to 2 mm below vestibule of impression with tray seated in the pumice/plaster mix. Once set, trim short of 4 mm from the vestibule for the land area. Place Alcote or Vaseline on the land area to prevent stone from bonding to pumice/plaster mix. Wrap in boxing wax. Pour stone into impression. Once set remove model from impression. Trim master cast for a land area of 3–4 mm, depth of 1–2 mm, ridges parallel to tabletop, and minimum 15 mm thick base.

Carve the PPS onto the maxillary master cast (see Figures 12.30 and 12.31 for dimensions).

See Section Lab Prescriptions.

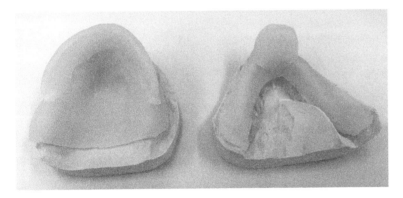

Figure 12.18 Custom trays.

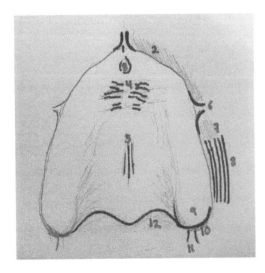

Figure 12.19 Maxillary anatomy: 1, labial frenum; 2, labial vestibule; 3, incisive papilla; 4, rugae; 5, median palatine raphe; 6, buccal frenum; 7, buccal vestibule; 8, buccinator; 9, maxillary tuberosity; 10, hamular notch; 11, pterygomandibular raphe; 12, posterior palatal seal area.

Figure 12.20   Mandibular anatomy: 1, retromolar pad (denture should cover anterior half); 2, masseter; 3, buccal vestibule; 4, buccinator; 5, depressor anguli oris; 6, buccal frenum; 7, labial vestibule; 8, mentalis (denture should cover only superior third); 9, labial frenum; 10, lingual frenum; 11, genioglossus; 12, mylohyoid; 13, residual alveolar ridge; 14, mylohyoid ridge; 15, buccal shelf.

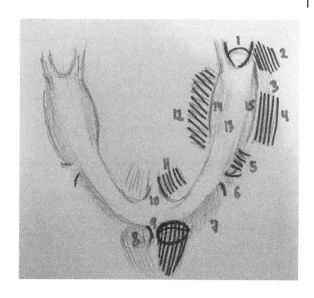

Figure 12.21   Mandibular border molding.

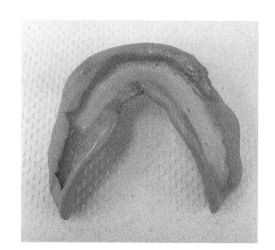

Figure 12.22   Mandibular wash.

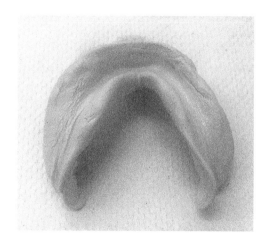

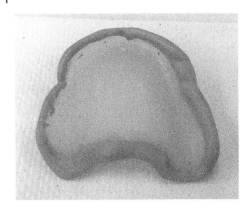

Figure 12.23   Maxillary border molding.

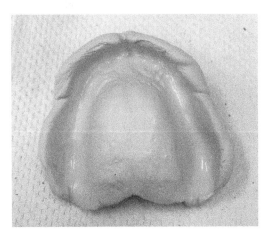

Figure 12.24   Maxillary wash.

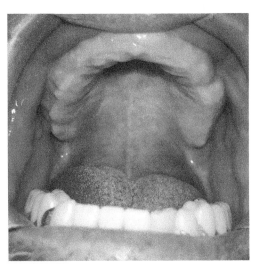

Figure 12.25   Maxillary soft palate at rest.

Figure 12.26 The vibrating line.

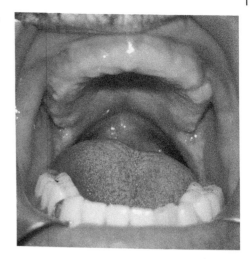

Figure 12.27 The Valsalva technique.

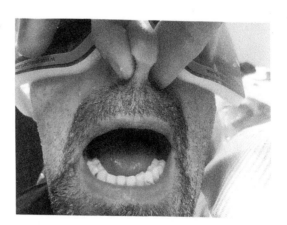

Figure 12.28 Valsalva line.

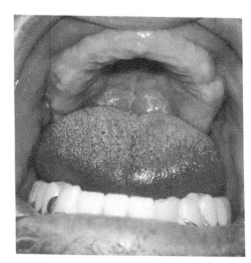

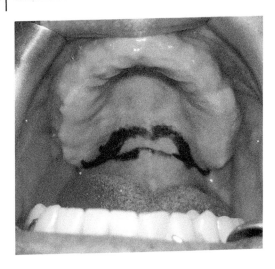

Figure 12.29 PPS marked with the Thompson stick (also known as indelible marker).

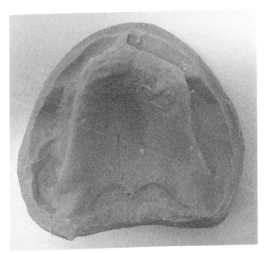

Figure 12.30 PPS carved into the master cast.

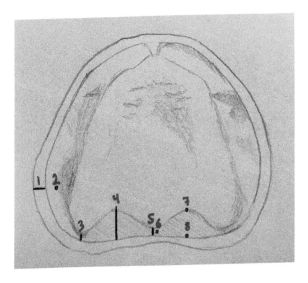

Figure 12.31 Dimensions of the cast. (1) Land area 3–4 mm long; (2) Depth 1–2 mm; (3) Length 1 mm; (4) Length varies 4–8 mm; (5) Length 2 mm; (6) Depth 0.5 mm; (7) Depth 0.5 mm and gradually deepens to (8) Depth 1.5 mm.

- Goal: to record the maxillomandibular relationship to properly set teeth.
- Patient may be concerned by:
  - The bulkiness of the WORs. Inform the patient that this is to provide stability for record making; teeth will take up less space.
  - The looseness of the dentures. The lab blocks out the undercuts with wax on the master cast which results in a loose fit at both the WOR and teeth try-in appointment. The processed denture base will have a more intimate adaptation to the gums.

WOR Checklist

1) On model, check if WORs are centered over ridge in posterior and can see vestibule (for denture stability) (Figures 12.32 and 12.33).
2) Insert maxillary WOR only
   a) Labial/buccal/palatal overextended? Trim as needed.
   b) Posterior contacting palate? If not, take a PVS light body wash impression (Figure 12.34). (Note that lab technician may prefer PVS light body wash be taken at the tooth try-in visit when patient is able to bite hard into occlusion. If not biting hard, wash could increase VDO and lead to excessive incisal display which is unesthetic and affects phonetics.)
   c) Frenum clearance? If not, deepen notch.
   d) Use tongue depressor to check if WOR is parallel to pupils.
   e) Use tongue depressor to check if WOR is parallel to ala tragus line.
   f) Maxillary incisal display:
      i) Determine amount of incisal display (Figures 12.35–12.37).
      ii) With age the lip gets longer and covers more teeth and teeth wear in the front.
      iii) Consider age: >60 years, above lip line; age 40–60 years, at lip line; <40 years, 2 mm display.
      iv) Add or remove wax.
3) Remove maxillary WOR and insert mandibular WOR.
   a) Labial/buccal/lingual overextended? Trim as needed.
   b) Frenula clearance? If not, deepen notch.
4) Determine vertical dimension at rest (VDR).
   a) Remove mandibular WOR and insert maxillary WOR.
   b) Mark the tip of the nose and the chin with Thompson stick, or use a sticker.
   c) Tell patient to "inhale, wet your lips and say mmmmmm" and measure distance from nose to chin with tongue depressor. This measures VDR. Repeat three times to confirm equal measurements (Figure 12.38).
   d) Insert mandibular WOR.
   e) Tell patient to "inhale, wet your lips and say mmmmmm." Is measurement the same? If longer must reduce WOR and repeat until same VDR measurement is obtained.
5) Determine the VDO
   a) Compare to previously measured VDO obtained with previous dentures or teeth (see Figure 12.7).
   b) Tell patient to bite down. Measurement should be 2–4 mm less than VDR.
   c) Adjust wax as needed until accurate.

d) Tell patient "Can you close comfortably when you bite or do the muscles feel strained?" Reduce VDO with the wax rim former if excessive/strained mentalis (Figure 12.39). If ideal incisal display of maxillary, then reduce WOR on mandibular.

6) Mandibular WOR level with lower lip at canine/premolar area.

7) Verify maxillary/mandibular WORs contact evenly (smooth).

8) Evaluate phonetics (repeat at tooth try-in) (see Figure 12.55).

    a) Tell patient to say "Mississippi" or to count from 60 to 70. Is there freeway space (closest speaking space 1–3 mm, upper lower incisal edges should almost touch)? If not, reduce VDO (remove wax).

        i) If "S" sounds like a whistle, reduce VDO (remove wax) or diastema between upper central incisors.

        ii) If "S" sounds like "Sh" increase VDO (add wax).

        iii) If "S" sounds like "th" (lisp), due to excess space between lateral borders of tongue and upper premolars (broad arch), narrow the space by adding ledge of wax/acrylic adjacent to upper premolars. Could be due to excessively narrow arch or to excessive overjet, or the presence of diastemas.

    b) Tell patient to say Fs (Example: "Fearless fire fighter in San Francisco") and to count from 40 to 50. Is maxillary incisal edge contacting lower lip wet/dry line? If so, may have to add projection or height.

    c) Tell patient to say "peanut butter." Lips should contact. If not, reduce VDO (remove wax).

9) Determine esthetics

    a) Profile/lip support: ideal 90° nasolabial angle. Convex? Concave? Adjust wax as needed.

    b) Tell patient "Smile as BIG as you can or denture will have a gummy smile."

        i) Inscribe the midline.

        ii) Inscribe the upper and lower lip smile line. (Set necks of teeth at or above the upper smile line.)

        iii) Inscribe the distal canine (in alignment with alas) (Figure 12.40).

10) Determine centric relation (CR is "a maxillomandibular relationship, independent of tooth contact in which the condyles articulate in the anterior–superior position against the posterior slopes of the articular eminences; in this position, the mandible is restricted to a purely rotary movement; from this unstrained, physiologic, maxillomandibular relationship, the patient can make vertical, lateral or protrusive movements; it is a clinically useful, repeatable reference position" [6]).

    a) Remove WORs. Create nonparallel notches in WORs (Figure 12.41).

    b) Lay patient supine in chair.

    c) Insert WORs.

    d) Dispense bite registration over mandibular WOR.

    e) Tell patient to place tongue to back of throat and gently bite down until back teeth are almost touching (1 mm apart) [5]. Take two bite registrations and compare. Tell patient not to bite hard or it will distort the wax decreasing VDO. Support patient's chin as bite registration sets to prevent movement (Figures 12.42 and 12.43).

11) Determine tooth/gum selection

    a) Characteristics of teeth (e.g. photo of previous teeth, study models of teeth before extraction, diastema size, ideal teeth, special characteristics, study model of existing denture, radiographs of teeth).

    b) Tooth shade (squint to check value; avoid shade whiter than sclera of eye, as eyes should be noticed before teeth). Specify the tooth shade guide used (Figure 12.44).

   c) Gingiva shade (communicate shade guide used) (Figure 12.45).

   d) Evaluate WORs with bite registration on models:

      i) Select 0° monoplane teeth if underbite (Class III), posterior x-bite (Figure 12.46). Unable to reproduce bite, atrophied ridge (vs. 15° lingualized teeth). Monoplane (no cusp to fossa relationship, just flat teeth for stability).

12) Facebow transfer and protrusive record. (Optional but recommended for occlusal accuracy. Purpose of the facebow transfer is to record the relationship of the TMJ to the maxillary arch to mount the master casts accurately on the articulator. Protrusive bite record made to set condylar guidance.)

13) Identification (full name) or patient declines ID. If declining, patient signs in chart.

14) Bring friend/relative to next visit for the tooth try-in?

15) See also Section Lab Prescriptions.

Figure 12.32   Maxillary WOR.

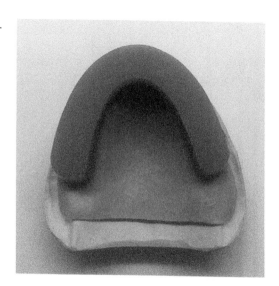

Figure 12.33   Mandibular WOR.

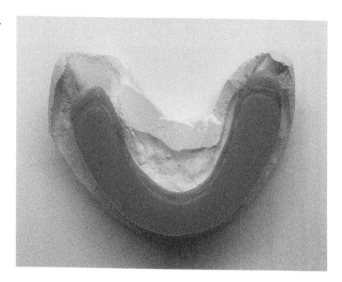

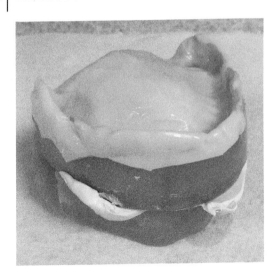

Figure 12.34 Wash at the WOR appointment, but preferred at the tooth try-in visit as the patient can bite hard into occlusion.

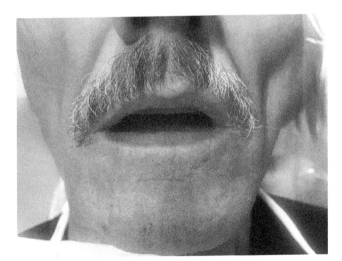

Figure 12.35 This amount of incisal display was ideal for this patient.

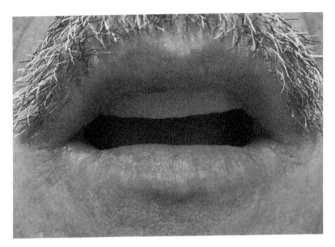

Figure 12.36 This would lead to too much incisal display and a gummy smile. Melt the wax with the wax rim former.

Figure 12.37 This may lead to too little incisal display, but may be indicated in certain cases.

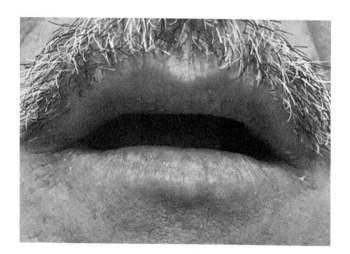

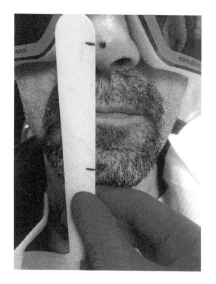

Figure 12.38 Obtaining VDR.

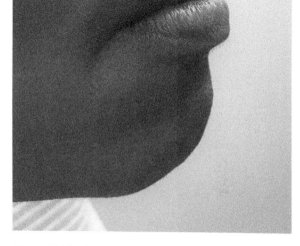

Figure 12.39 Strained mentalis muscle.

Figure 12.40 Inscribe the midline, smile line, and the alas (side of the nose which is for the distal aspect of the canines).

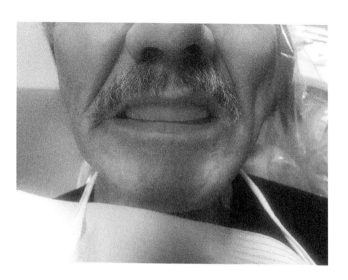

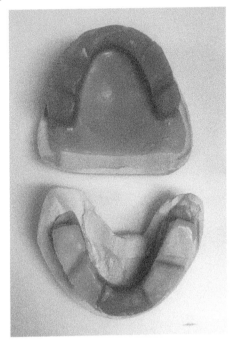

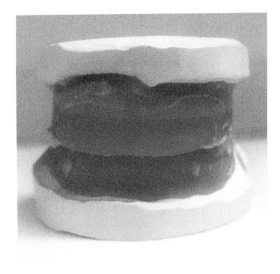

Figure 12.42   WORs ready for mounting.

Figure 12.41   Nonparallel notches on the WORs.

Figure 12.43   WORs ready for mounting.

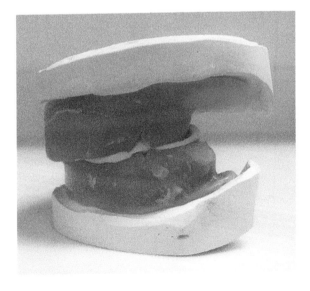

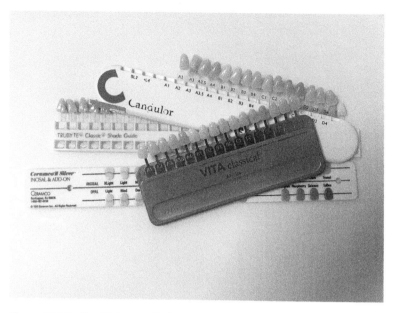

Figure 12.44   Specify the tooth shade and which tooth shade guide is being used.

Figure 12.45   Specify the gum shade and which gum shade guide is being used.

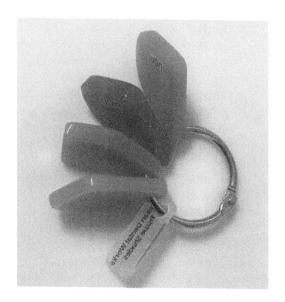

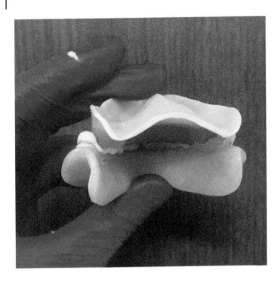

Figure 12.46   Note the posterior crossbite of the WORs.

Teeth Setting Guidelines

Teeth setting may be completed by you or by lab technician. If lab technician, prescribe and evaluate teeth setting.

- Set teeth in the following order: upper anterior, lower anterior, lower posterior, upper posterior.
- Landmarks on master cast
  - Upper:
    - Line through incisal papilla to facial land area marks midline.
    - Line perpendicular to this one from posterior portion of incisive papilla, marks maxillary cusp tips [5].
  - Lower:
    - Mark halfway up the retromolar pad, distal of occlusal plane of last molar.
    - Straight line along center of residual alveolar ridge (maxillary lingual cusps set over this) extending to the land area. This line marks the central fossas for the mandibular posterior teeth extending to the distal of mandibular canine incisal edge.
- Anterior teeth:
  - Facial surface of maxillary central incisors 8 mm from incisive papilla (teeth not set directly over edentulous ridge).
  - Set necks of upper teeth at/above upper smile line.
  - Maxillary lateral incisors 0.5 mm shorter than maxillary centrals and canines.
  - Maxillary anterior overjet 1.5–2 mm, overbite 0.5 mm (if monoplane: 2 mm overjet, 0 mm overbite to prevent tilting) (Figure 12.47).
  - Slight distal tilt of all anteriors at the necks of the teeth except lower central incisor (Figure 12.48).
  - From the incisal view the most prominent third varies from middle (M), incisal (I), or gingival (G) (Figure 12.48).
- Posterior teeth: set teeth in lingualized occlusion/balanced occlusion (Figure 12.49).
  - This provides improved stability by maintaining contacts bilaterally on excursions (Figure 12.50).
  - Set teeth over the ridge for stability (i.e. when the patient is chewing).
  - Maxillary lingual cusps centered over mandibular residual alveolar ridge.
  - Curve of Spee with maxillary M 1D cusps and maxillary M2 cusps (no curve if monoplane teeth).
  - Maxillary lingual cusp locations (see Figure 12.1).
    - Maxillary PM 1L cusp → mandibular PM1 DMR and mandibular PM2 MMR.

Maxillary PM 2L cusp → mandibular PM 2 DMR and mandibular M1 MMR.

Maxillary M ML cusp → mandibular M1 central fossa.

Maxillary M DL cusp → mandibular M1 DMR and mandibular M2 MMR.

Maxillary M2 ML cusp → mandibular M2 central fossa.

Maxillary M2 DL cusp → mandibular M2 DMR.

Check occlusion on the articulator with articulating paper (Figure 12.51).

Make sure no teeth contact in anterior in CR (location teeth set).

Reposition teeth if teeth not contacting or major adjustment required.

Adjust teeth with bur if minor changes are required, there are contacts on incline planes or contacts in right location but not even weight (bullseye is heaviest, adjust to lighten) [5].

Check centric contacts in one color (e.g. blue).

Check if maxillary lingual cusps contact mandibular marginal ridges and/or central fossa; if not, deepen mandibular fossa first. If maxillary lingual cusps on mandibular incline plane, adjust maxillary lingual cusp second [5].

Check excursion in different color (e.g. red). Do not remove centric contacts (e.g. blue) which you have already addressed [5].

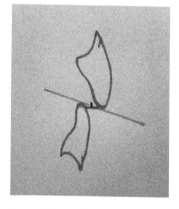

Figure 12.47 Overjet and overbite. Red, overjet; black, overbite; green, incisal guidance.

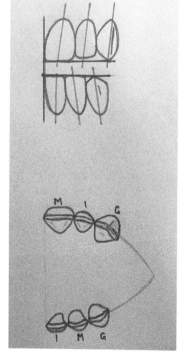

Figure 12.48 Tilts of teeth and prominent thirds.

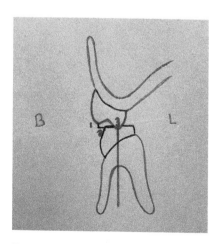

Figure 12.49 Lingualized/balanced occlusion. Note the amount of overbite (1) and overjet (2), and that the biting forces (3) are directly over the center of the ridge for stability.

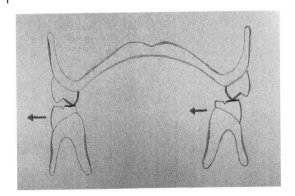

Figure 12.50 Lateral excursions with lingualized/balanced occlusion.

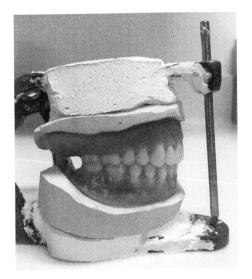

Figure 12.51 Check occlusion with articulating paper.

Appointment 4: Tooth Try-in

1) Evaluate occlusion on the articulator from all angles, including from inside (tongue perspective) (Figure 12.51).
2) Anterior tooth set-up.
3) Insert individually to check overextensions; if overextended anywhere, adjust and seat on the cast and draw a line outlining the denture on the cast so that the lab technician knows how much to trim the denture flanges.
4) Maxillary denture may require denture adhesive to prevent it falling out as it is (i) in denture base material with poorer fit to ridge than denture acrylic will be and (ii) it does not have PPS.
5) Is posterior contacting palate? If not, take a PVS light body wash impression and have patient bite hard into occlusion to prevent increase in VDO. Consider second tooth try-in appointment to verify VDO has not changed and incisal display has not changed.
6) Check occlusion intraorally

a) Check occlusion with articulating paper. Have patient bite on posterior left side and tug, then repeat on right side. Patient's teeth should prevent paper from being pulled. Articulating paper should come out in the anterior; if it doesn't, adjust. Anterior occlusion can cause tipping of the posterior.

b) If teeth are not occluding properly (Figure 12.52):

 i) Reposition teeth as necessary by heating wax and try in.

 ii) If major changes are required, obtain bite registration of only the areas teeth are not occluding. Communicate to lab to remount case and reposition teeth into occlusion and return for a second tooth try-in appointment.

7) Evaluate esthetics

 a) Profile/lip support: Convex? Concave? Flat? Adjust wax as needed.

 b) Face patient at eye level to evaluate.

 c) Confirm midline matches face.

 d) Check incisal display at rest (Figure 12.53).

 e) Check smiling esthetics, and have patient approve (Figure 12.54).

 i) Upper lip line even with upper gumline.

 ii) Necks of upper teeth at or above lip line (not gummy smile).

 iii) Upper incisors match lower lip line.

 f) Without providing any feedback, first ask and listen to patient's input on the appearance [5].

 g) Friend or relative input to the try-in.

 h) Have patient approve tooth shade (if unhappy with shade, select new shade with patient, send case back to lab for a second tooth try-in until patient approves shade).

8) Evaluate phonetics (Figure 12.55).

 a) Tell patient to say "Mississippi." Is there freeway space (closest speaking space 1–1.5 mm, edge-to-edge almost touching). Upper/lower posterior should not contact.

 i) If "S" sounds like a whistle, reduce VDO or add wax to rugae.

 ii) If "S" sounds like "Sh" increase VDO.

 b) Tell patient to say Fs (Example: "Fearless fire fighter in San Francisco") and to count from 40 to 50. Is maxillary incisal edge contacting lower lip wet/dry line?

 i) If "F" and "V" sound alike, upper anteriors are improperly positioned either vertically or horizontally. If "V" sounds like "F" the anteriors are too short. If the "F" sounds like "V" the anteriors are too long.

 c) Tell patient to say "peanut butter." Lips should contact. If not, reduce VDO.

 d) Tell patient to say "this, that, there."

 i) Tongue should stick out 3 mm between upper/lower anteriors. If >6 mm, the teeth are too lingual; if <3 mm, the teeth are too labial.

 ii) If "T" sounds like "D" upper anteriors too lingual. Reposition.

 iii) Tell patient to say "Dad walked the dog on a dreary day."

 iv) If "D" sounds like "T" upper anteriors are too labial. Reposition.

9) Contours: concave on B/L to allow room for tongue/cheek.

10) Prosthesis processing consent form (see Section Consent Forms). If you and/or the patient are unsatisfied with tooth set-up, send case back to lab and schedule second tooth try-in appointment. May require a third tooth try-in appointment. Repeat until you/patient are satisfied.

11) See also Section Lab Prescriptions.

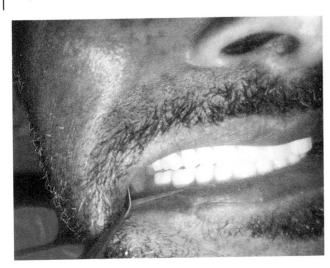

Figure 12.52 Posterior teeth not occluding properly.

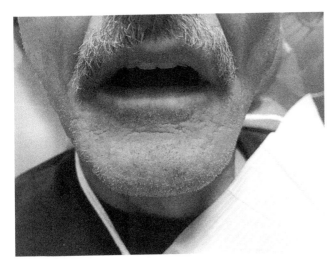

Figure 12.53 Evaluate the amount of incisal display at rest (can tell the patient to mouth breathe and to pretend they are watching television).

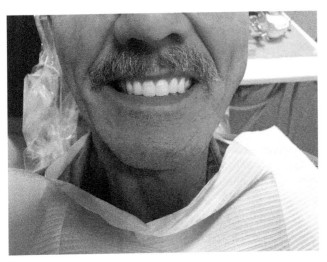

Figure 12.54 Evaluate the amount of tooth and gum display when smiling.

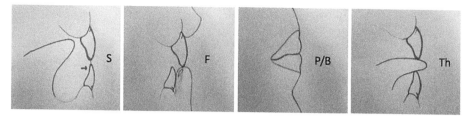

Figure 12.55   Tongue, teeth, and lip position for proper phonetics.

Appointment 5: Denture Delivery

Prior to inserting in patient's mouth check the following.

- Presence of PPS on upper denture (Figure 12.56). If not present, see Section Troubleshooting.
- Undercuts: will pinch tissue, cause sore spots, and prevent seating (Figure 12.57). Slight maxillary anterior undercut can aid in retention if not pinching.
- Blebs: feel for surface irregularities (Figure 12.58) with finger on cameo and intaglio. Some spots may only be detected with gauze (Figure 12.59).
- Sharp edges on flanges: smooth these with acrylic bur.
- Hand articulate dentures and make sure posterior pink acrylic of upper and lower are not contacting. If contacting, adjust.
- Check if the maxillary denture extends to the hamular notch (for retention).
- Check maxillary posterior border for taper ending 2–3 mm thick, not too thick or sharp edge [5].
- Assess mandibular denture: adjust distolingual flange if posterior to retromolar pad; if not adjusted will cause pain on swallowing [5].
- Try dentures in.
  - Insert maxillary denture.
  - Any discomfort? Any resistance to seating (i.e. pops up)?
  - Check if there is adequate clearance for the frenum.
    - Regardless, add PIP. Place thin layer with visible brush strokes (Figure 12.60), seat and apply pressure on occlusal surfaces of molars, then remove and check for burn-through (Figure 12.61). Adjust burn-through with acrylic bur, reapply PIP, and repeat until no burn-through occurs. May have to adjust flanges until denture seats completely.
    - Remove PIP with gauze or alcohol wipe.
  - Repeat process with mandibular denture: ask the patient to stick out their tongue, and toward their left and right ear. Check for dislodgement. May have to adjust overextended flanges.
- Check occlusion:
  - Have the patient bite on cotton rolls for one minute (one cotton roll on each side in the posterior). This will compress the denture-bearing tissues, simulating the position of the denture when it is worn for a longer period of time.
  - Have patient bite with back teeth and pull the articulating paper through the anteriors. Should be able to pull from canine to canine (anterior teeth not in contact). If unable to pull, contact is heavy, so adjust until out of occlusion for improved denture stability.
  - Have patient tap teeth a few times with articulating paper (CR, not excursions).
    - Remove spots on Upper Buccal cusp tips and Lower Lingual cusp tips (remember as "No BULL").
    - Remove from incline plane so marks are on upper lingual cusp tips and lower central fossas/marginal ridges in CR (if not, teeth will "slide into place" causing tipping and making denture unstable).

- Check phonetics (see Section Appointment 4: Tooth Try-in).
- Check esthetics (see Section Appointment 4: Tooth Try-in).
- Verify that patient can insert and remove dentures.
- Postoperative instructions: provide verbal and written instructions to patient (see Section Postoperative Instructions).
- Provide denture brush, denture container, adhesive samples, cleaning samples, soft toothbrush and tongue scraper (Figure 12.62).
- Label denture container with patient's name.
- Show patient how to apply denture adhesives. Various types exist, such as cream (i.e. Poligrip, Fixodent), powder (i.e. Poligrip, Fixodent), strips (i.e. Poligrip Adhesive Seals, Sea-Bond Denture Adhesive Seals).
  - Follow manufacturer's instructions.
  - For adhesive cream, dry the denture and apply three to four drops (Figure 12.63). Tell patient that "less is more."
  - For adhesive powder, wet the denture and apply powder. Tap to remove excess (Figure 12.64).
- Discuss nutritional counseling for denture wearers (see Chapter 5).

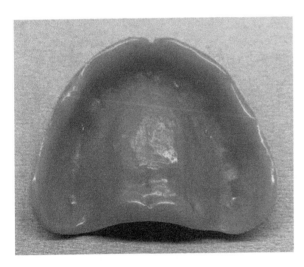

Figure 12.56 Clearly defined PPS (i.e. post dam).

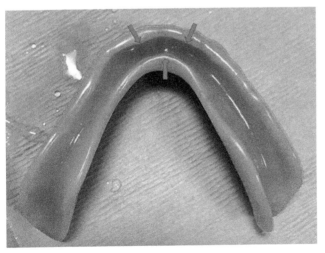

Figure 12.57 Undercuts.

Figure 12.58 Bleb on intaglio of the denture. This can lead to a sore spot.

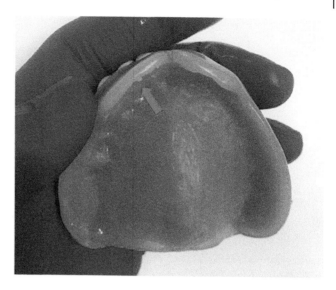

Figure 12.59 Check for rough spots on the intaglio with gauze. These can lead to sore spots.

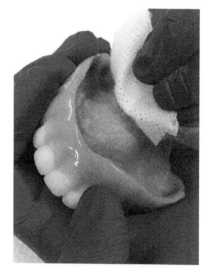

Figure 12.60 Apply PIP with the brush creating brush strokes.

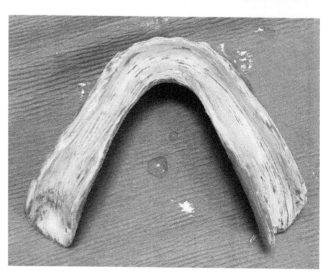

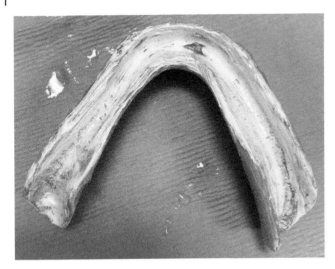

Figure 12.61 Check for burn-through (i.e. missing PIP) and adjust as necessary.

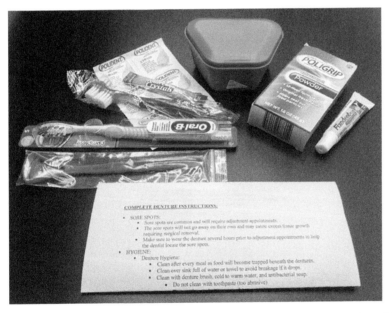

Figure 12.62 Oral hygiene supplies and postoperative instructions to review with the patient and to place in their goody bag.

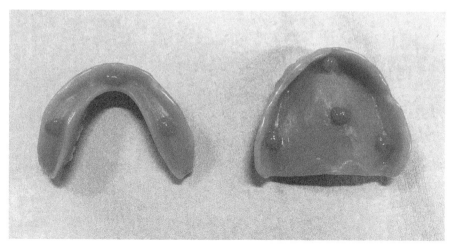

Figure 12.63 Application of the proper amount of denture adhesive cream for patient education.

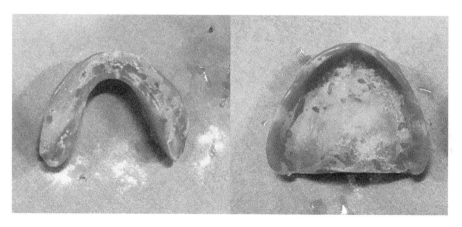

Figure 12.64 Application of powder denture adhesive for patient education.

Appointment 6: 24-Hour Follow-up

- Address chief complaint.
- Encourage/reassure the patient that it will take several weeks [6–8] to adapt [5].
- Check all intraoral surfaces for traumatic ulcerations.
  - If traumatic ulceration, mark with Thompson stick, seat denture to transfer mark, remove denture, adjust with acrylic bur, seat denture and ask patient for percentage improvement.
  - Inform patient it may take 10–14 days for healing. Swishing with warm salt water reduces the swelling. Can also apply a topical anesthetic for palliative treatment (e.g. 20% benzocaine).

Appointment 7: One-Week Follow-up

Repeat of 24-hour appointment.

Appointment 8+: Denture Adjustment

Repeat of 24-hour appointment

Periodic Oral Evaluation (Recall Exam)

- Address chief complaint.
- Extraoral/intraoral exam.
- Oral cancer screening (high risk in partially edentulous and edentulous patients) [2].
- Oral hygiene instructions.
- Radiographs (only if evidence of disease) (see Chapter 3).
- Evaluation of dentures:
  - Denture base fractured or perforated.
  - Amount of tooth wear.
  - Amount of adhesive on denture.
  - Denture hygiene.
  - Evaluation of fit of dentures:
    - Retention: resistance to the removal of the denture away from the tissue.
    - Stability: resistance to horizontal and lateral movement.
    - Support: resistance to movement toward the denture-bearing tissue.
  - VDO: does it appear collapsed, adequate, or excessive?
  - Disclosing wax: check for overextensions (as ridge resorbs, denture flanges become overextended).
  - Check fit with PIP. Wipe off PIP and disclosing wax with alcohol wipe and rinse with water.
  - Check occlusion.
- Clean denture in ultrasonic denture bath (Figure 12.65).
  - Clean at recall visits (or as needed) to minimize biofilm accumulation over time [8].
  - Scrub off any calculus, food, adhesive, or other debris (Figures 12.66 and 12.67).

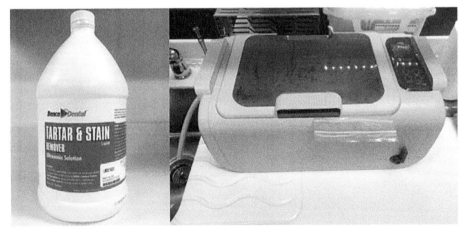

Figure 12.65   Place the dentures in a bag with tartar and stain removal cleaner. Close the bag and place it against the wall of the ultrasonic bath. The high-frequency vibrations will loosen the tartar for easy removal with a denture brush.

Complete Dentures

Figure 12.66 Maxillary denture with calculus adjacent to the patient's Stensen's duct (i.e. parotid duct).

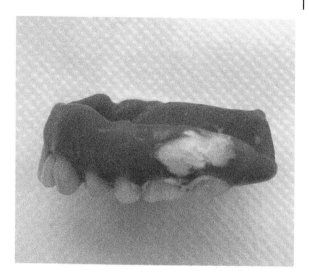

Figure 12.67 Mandibular denture with calculus adjacent to the patient's submandibular duct.

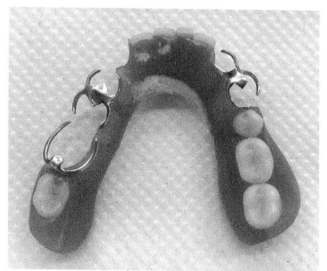

Related Procedural Steps

Interim (Temporary) Dentures

Temporary dentures are delivered immediately after oral surgery and are meant to be replaced. They are worn during the healing time (6–12 months) and will require one or more relines, and then new dentures (permanent/long term) are made after the healing process.

Immediate Dentures

Dentures delivered immediately after oral surgery meant for long-term usage and which will require one or more relines.

- For either interim immediate denture or immediate dentures warn patient that esthetics, phonetics and bite will not be ideal (Figure 12.68).

- Impressions appointment:
    - Obtain two sets of impressions (one set to alter, one to keep as reference).
    - Mobile teeth: warn patient "this may hurt or extract your teeth." Use alginate.
    - Nonmobile teeth: border mold with heavy body PVS and light body PVS wash (capture details).
    - Bite registration.
    - Obtain gshade and tooth shade.
    - Determine any esthetic changes patient wants in the teeth.
    - Determine whether there is loss of VDO; if there is, VDO must be increased.
    - Accept or decline full name for identification.
    - Send case to lab to mount and fabricate immediate dentures.
    - Optional: create vacuum form surgical stent for oral surgeon as a guide for alveoplasty.
        - Use 0.80 mm thick Biocryl.
        - Trim teeth on models, and perform alveoplasty on models for smooth rounded edentulous ridges without undercut.
        - Place cast of vacuum former, heat Biocryl until it sags 1 inch (2.5 cm), turn vacuum on, drop Biocryl over model, wait 25 seconds, remove Biocryl, and cut "V" notches around frenums.
        - Send to oral surgeon to place on ridge after extractions and alveoplasty.
        - Any gingival blanching indicates that further alveoplasty is required.
- Oral surgery day: deliver dentures (see Section Appointment 5: Denture Delivery). Inform patient to wear denture for 24 hours and not to remove as the swelling will prevent it from seating and to return after 24 hours for adjustment. Caution: DO NOT RELINE if sutures are placed, as this can rip the sutures out.
- Adjustment at 24 hours.
- Adjustment at one week.
- Alternative approach
    - Rationale: confirms VDO and is easier for the patient to chew on healed posterior ridges.
    - Sequence:
        - Extract posterior teeth except first premolars (or any two sets of opposing posterior teeth to maintain the VDO).
        - Heal for several weeks.
        - Make impressions.
        - WOR appointment to confirm the VDO.
        - Tooth try-in of posterior teeth to confirm VDO and tooth shade.
        - Process and finish denture.
        - Extract anterior teeth and remaining vertical stops and deliver the immediate denture.
        - Soft reline.
        - Hard reline at six months.
    - Extract teeth except second premolar and first molar as vertical stops. Take impressions.

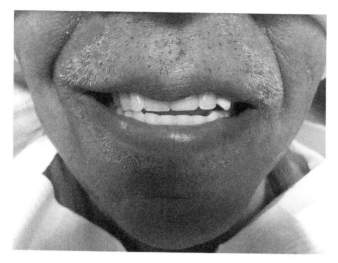

Figure 12.68 **Figure 12.68** Esthetics and occlusion can be unsatisfactory with immediate dentures as there is no opportunity for a tooth try-in appointment.

Complete Denture Opposing Cast Metal RPD

Same sequence as complete dentures except for the following.

- If the patient is happy with the apperance of the existing denture, make an impression for the lab to match the tooth shape/size.
- Preliminary impressions: evaluate the models to determine if any teeth modifications are needed (i.e. rest preps, enameloplasty) (see Chapter 13).
- Final impressions: teeth modifications as necessary prior to impressions (see Chapter 13).
- WOR appointment: try in RPD cast metal framework and verify that it seats all the way, with no interferences (see Chapter 13).
- Tooth try-in appointment: same steps as for complete dentures.
- Delivery: deliver dentures (see Section Appointment 5: Denture Delivery) and provide RPD post-operative instructions (see Chapter 13).

Complete Denture Opposing Dentition

Same sequence as complete dentures except for the following.
- Preliminary impressions: evaluate the models for any teeth modifications needed (i.e. enameloplasty of supraerupted teeth or mandibular molars with steep curve of Spee [5]).

Complete Denture Opposing Existing Complete Denture

This can occur when a patient loses their opposing denture.

- Appointment 1: obtain impression of existing denture (on the tabletop) and opposing ridge.
- Appointment 2: WOR (Figure 12.69).
- Appointment 3: tooth try-in.
- Appointment 4: delivery.

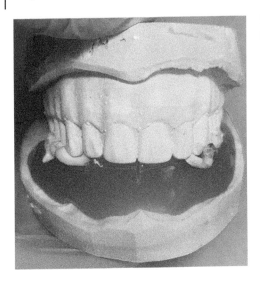

Figure 12.69 Existing denture opposing the opposing WOR.

Duplicate Existing Dentures

An option to expedite the denture process by duplicating existing in only three appointments (by skipping the final impression appointment and WOR appointment).

- First appointment: impressions using the existing dentures as custom trays.
  - Same steps as a lab reline except do *not* remove undercuts as denture will be returned to patient and some undercuts aid in retention. Place Coe-Comfort on intaglio of upper and lower dentures and have patient bite hard while the material sets. Inform the lab to pour models, mount case in existing VDO (unless worn dentition and inadequate VDO, in which case you may want the lab to increase VDO by a specified amount such as 2 mm), and return dentures to patient same day. Fabricate upper and lower denture tooth set-up for tooth try-in appointment.
- Second appointment: tooth try-in.
- Third appointment: delivery.

Repairs, Relines, Repositions, Additions, and What the Lab Needs from You

- Relines: refers to resurfacing the inside of the denture. These can be hard or soft and can be completed chairside and laboratory fabricated.
- Relines are beneficial when the ridge resorbs, causing loosening of the dentures.
- Residual ridge reduction:
  - Average: year 1 after extractions, 2–3 mm loss in maxilla, 4–5 mm loss in the mandible; 0.1–0.2 mm annually in mandible and four times less in maxilla [2].
- For laboratory repairs, relines, repositions and additions, see Chapter 13, Table 13.3.
- Chairside procedural steps
  - Chairside clean break repair
    - With sticky wax connect the dentures halves, place separating medium on the intaglio, pour model in plaster (make sure no undercuts or denture will lock in, if undercuts adjust with bur), gently remove dentures from model, use acrylic bur to remove acrylic from denture forming a 2-mm space, place separating medium on model to prevent denture from sticking to model, follow manufacturer instructions for denture repair acrylic, and polish.
  - Chairside hard reline

Follow manufacturer's instructions.

Remove undercuts and create vent holes in the denture base with a #8 round bur. Place chairside hard reline material. Caution: the material can heat up and become locked in the undercuts, so recommend frequent removal from the mouth (and open the windows as there can be noxious odors).

Chairside soft reline

Same as the chairside hard reline, except use of soft reline material (e.g. Coe-Soft, Coe-Comfort). There is minimal risk of the denture locking in, and no noxious odors.

Adding a denture tooth (Figure 12.70)

Check smile line with denture in. If gingiva is visible inform patient the repair material color may not match and this would be visible when smiling. Remove any tooth fragment (Figure 12.71) from denture (or superglue) and create room for repair material (chemical bond, thus good idea to increase the surface area for bonding) With high speed create retentive slots in denture tooth (Figure 12.72), adjust denture tooth to fit alignment/angulation with adjacent teeth and in occlusion with opposing teeth (Figure 12.73). Fill with acrylic repair material (or chairside hard reline material), allow to set, and polish (Figure 12.74). Try in, and adjust occlusion as necessary.

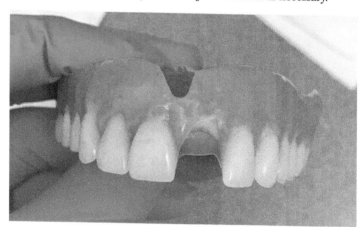

Figure 12.70 Patient arrives to the office with a missing denture tooth.

Figure 12.71 Evaluation of the denture and fragment.

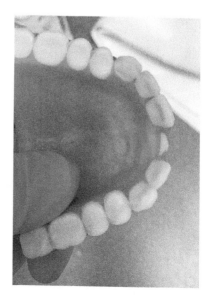

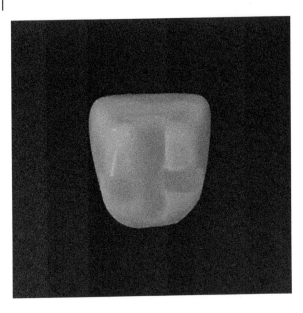

Figure 12.72 Retentive grooves made with a high-speed bur in a denture tooth. Good to have a supply of anterior denture teeth in various shades in your office for these esthetic emergencies.

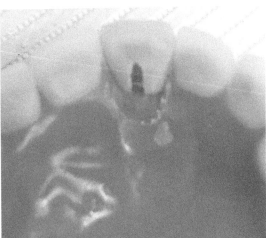

Figure 12.73 Checking the fit of the new denture tooth next to the adjacent teeth and checking occlusion.

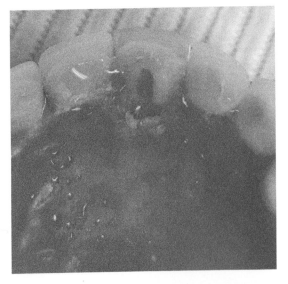

Figure 12.74 The new denture tooth has been added to the denture and polished.

Lab Prescriptions

Write requests in sequential order.

Lab Prescription (Impressions to Custom Trays)

Included maxillary and mandibular alginate preliminary impressions

1) *Please pour models*
2) *Fabricate custom trays for maxillary and mandibular denture final impressions*

Thank you

Lab Prescription (Final Impression to Wax Occlusal Rims)

Included maxillary and mandibular denture final impressions

1) *Please pour master casts*
2) *Add heavy posterior palatal seal (PPS)**
3) *Fabricate maxillary and mandibular denture wax occlusal rims*

Thank you

---

* Remember to ask the lab to add a heavy post-dam PPS; if you don't there is a risk the lab will either not supply one or make it too light. You can always trim it.

Lab Prescription (Wax Occlusal Rim to Tooth Try-in)

Included maxillary and mandibular wax occlusal rims, bite registration, and master casts

1) *Please mount case*
2) *Marked on wax occlusal rims patient's midline, smile line, distal of canines*
3) *Included _____* as a reference for selecting tooth size/shape/characteristic†*
4) *Tooth shade _____ [specify shade guide used]*
5) *Please set posterior teeth in lingualized occlusion (anatomic maxillary teeth opposing flat or shallow cusped mandibular teeth)‡*
6) *Return for tooth try-in*

Thank you

---

* Could refer to a study model of the patient before extraction, study model of patient's existing denture, photo of patient's smile, or radiograph of patient's teeth. Specify if the patient wants teeth longer/wider/rounder/shorter/ with a diastema of __ mm, etc.
† Tooth shape/size often referred to as "mold."
‡ If monoplane teeth indicated, use the following: "Please select/set monoplane teeth. In the anterior, set teeth with Max anterior overjet 2 mm and 0 mm overbite. Return for tooth try-in."

Lab Prescription (Tooth Try-in to Delivery)

Included maxillary and mandibular tooth set-up and mounted master casts on articulator. Patient approved tooth set-up

1) *Process and finish dentures*

2) Gingiva shade _____ [specify shade guide used]
3) Add patient's full name _____ to dentures for identification
4) [If applicable] Trim flanges to the line drawn on the cast
5) Return for delivery

Thank you

Postoperative Instructions

Provide patient with *both* verbal and written instructions for taking care of their oral health (see Figures 12.62 and Figure 12.75).

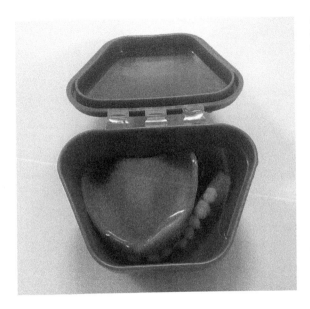

Figure 12.75 Instruct the patient to place dentures in a container at night when sleeping for eight hours a day.

Complete Denture Instructions

- Sore spots
    - Sore spots are common and will require adjustment appointments.
    - The sore spots will not go away on their own and may cause excess tissue growth requiring surgical removal.
    - Make sure to wear the denture several hours prior to adjustment appointments to help the dentist locate the sore spots.
- Hygiene
    - Denture hygiene:
        - Clean after every meal as food will become trapped beneath the dentures.
        - Clean over sink full of water or towel to avoid breakage if it drops.
        - Clean with denture brush, using cold to warm water, and antibacterial soap.
            - Do not clean with toothpaste (too abrasive).
            - Do not place in boiling water [8] (can warp).
        - If using a denture cleansing solution (such as Polident), thoroughly rinse and brush denture prior to wearing [8].

If using denture adhesives, the adhesive must be thoroughly removed from the denture and oral cavity daily [8].
- Oral hygiene:
  - Clean your gums with soft toothbrush and warm water twice a day for two minutes [5].
  - Clean your tongue with tongue scraper.
- Storage
  - Dentures are always to be removed at night, the only exception being for immediate dentures. After all the teeth are extracted, wear the immediate dentures for the first 24–48 hours. Do not remove the immediate dentures for more than 30 minutes or they may not fit due to swelling. Only remove after eating to clean and then place the dentures back in the mouth.
  - Do not wear partials when you sleep.
    - Wearing all day and all night will cause harm to the gums, bone, and mouth.
    - The gums need adequate blood circulation for eight hours a day.
    - Failure to let your gums rest will cause the ridge support to become flatter sooner and the denture and future dentures will be harder to fit properly [2].
    - You can develop fungal infections from over-wearing, especially with poor hygiene.
  - Always keep the partials moist whether:
    - in mouth
    - in a container with water (away from pets)
    - in a sealed bag with water.
  - If it becomes dehydrated it will warp and no longer fit [8].
- Chewing
  - Be patient, it usually takes six to eight weeks to adapt to a new prosthesis [5].
  - Begin with soft foods and cut the food into small pieces.
  - Chew food on both sides simultaneously to reduce denture tipping.
  - Careful with hot foods and drinks. May burn tissue.
  - Chew only with your back teeth as the front teeth can break. The front teeth are only for esthetics and to help you pronounce words.
- Speech
  - Be patient, can take two to four weeks to adapt.
  - Pronunciations such as "s" and "f" may be difficult in the beginning, so practice reading aloud in mirror.
  - May help to swallow first to "set" denture in place. You will be more aware of speech problems than other people.
- Precautions
  - Do not drop the dentures, they can break.
  - Cover your mouth when you sneeze, or the dentures can fly out of your mouth and break if they land on a hard surface.
  - Do not store the dentures in a napkin/tissue/paper towel, as these get accidently thrown away.
- Future appointments
  - Return for recall exams for:
    - Oral cancer screenings.
    - Evaluation of the gums.
    - Cleaning of the dentures.
    - Evaluation of the dentures. Dentures may require relines, repairs, and remakes. Replacement may be needed every 5–10 years.

DENTURE ANALYZER | CHAIRSIDE GUIDE

Complaints About Denture Function

Problem	Causes	Solutions
Denture seems to "move around"-Instability		

When not occluding	1 Overextension of borders and posterior limits
	2 Under-extended borders
	3 Loss of post-dam seal
	  a. Post-dam on hard palate
	  b. Post-dam not over-hamular notches
	  c. Insufficient post-dam
	4 Dehydration of tissues due to alcoholism or medication
	5 Flabby tissues displaced when taking impressions due to improper tray
		1, 2, 3, 4, 5.
		In all cases a new impression is necessary. Best to grind out the tissue side and take a wash, using compound where necessary to extend impression to include post-dam area. Rebase or refine entire denture

When chewing food	1 Loss of post-dam seal 2 Anterior teeth too far labially 3 Flabby anterior tissues 4 Improper incising habits 5 Lower posteriors set off ridge	1 Same as above 2 Remount and reset, bringing anteriors back lingually 3 Surgery to remove poor denture foundation and rebase 4 Patient education is the only answer 5 Reset and correct posterior alignment

When occluding in centric	1 Malocclusion:
	  a. Premature individual teeth hitting
	  b. High occlusion on one side of arch
	  c. Bicuspid area premature contact
	2 Upper denture 'riding' on hard palate surface
	3 Flabby tissues over ridge
	4 Teeth set too far buccally
	5 Centric occlusion not in harmony with centric relationship
		1 Malocclusion:
		  a. Remount selective grind and mill-in
		  b. Remount and reset
		  c. Try chairside mill-in or remount and reset
		2 Relieve pressure area
		3 Remove flabby tissue with surgery and rebase
		4 Remount and reset to lingual
		5 Remake on denture

General overall soreness on ridge	1 Vertical open too much 2 Totally inaccurate denture base	1 Remake one of the dentures to correct vertical, providing plane of occlusion is acceptable 2 Try a wash impression and rebase, or remake the denture after tissue treatment
Sore under lower lingual flange	1 Centric off-mastication drives lower forward 2 Lingual flange over extended 3 Posterior teeth too far distal	1 Recheck vertical and centric. Rearticulate and remove the interfering cusps or change to non-interfering teeth. 2 Shorten and repolish flange 3 Remove 2nd molars
Sore under lower labial flange	1 Too much overbite 2 Overextended labial flange 3 When masticating patient throws lower forward	1 Rearticulate and change tooth position 2 Shorten flange and repolish 3 Recheck vertical and centric. Change to centromatic posteriors. Check lingual flanges
Burning Sensations*		
Burning feeling on hard palate area	High pressure area in the acrylic base*	Locate the high area, remove and polish
Burning feeling on upper anterior ridge	Pressure on papilla and rugae area*	Relieve
Burning feeling on bicuspid area to tuberosities	High pressure area in the acrylic base*	Same as above-grind 1st bicuspid out of occlusion
Burning feeling on lower anterior ridge	High pressure area in the acrylic base*	Same as above
Complaints About Phonetics		
Whistle on "S" sounds	1 Not enough room for tongue between upper bicuspids 2 Space between centrals	1 Remount and move bicuspids to the buccal or, if room permits, grind out more room for tongue 2 Close space
Lisping on "S" sounds	1 Too much space for tongue between upper bicuspids	1 Narrow palate space between upper bicuspids by adding ledge of acrylic
"Th" and "T" sounds indistinct	1 Not enough room in dentures for tongue 2 If "Th" and "T" sound alike, the anteriors are too far lingual	1 Thin out dentures from lingual side-don't grind tissue side 2 Remount and move anteriors out to the buccal
"F" and "V" sounds indistinct	1 Improper position of upper anterior teeth-either vertically or horizontally	1 Difficult adjustment-must decide and try to correct

*Burning sensations are usually caused by pressure on a nerve as it leaves nasopalatine or by under-cured bases. (Diabetics get the burning sensations occasionally.)

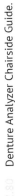

Figure 12.80 Denture Analyzer Chairside Guide.

DENTURE ANALYZER | CHAIRSIDE GUIDE

Uncomfortable Dentures

Problem	Causes	Solutions
Sore Spots		
Sore spot in vestibule area Upper or lower denture	1. Overextended borders 2. Rough spot in base	1. Shorten borders and polish 2. Smooth and refinish
Sore spot in upper post-dam area (Posterior limit of upper)	1. Post-dam too deep 2. Sharp edges on the posterior seal 3. Overextension	1. Reduce base carefully and gradually to avoid loss of border seal. Round off sharp edges. 2. Same as above 3. Same as above. Make sure the post-dam is on soft tissue.
Single sore spot on the crest of the ridge	1. Premature occlusion 2. Inaccurate denture base 3. Voids or porosity in acrylic 4. Nodules under base	1. New centric registration or accurate bite. Remount dentures on articulator and adjust bite. 2. Take a "wash" impression and rebase after tissue treatment 3. Take a "wash" impression and rebase after tissue treatment 4. Remove nodules
Seems to Feel "Interference"		

When swallowing	1. Upper: a. Overextension in the posterior buccal flange
	    b. Too thick in posterior
	2. Lower: a. Overextension in the lingual
	    b. Too thick in lingual posterior flanges
	3. Overclosed vertical
	4. Too much vertical
	5. Posteriors too far to lingual-crowding tongue
		1.Upper: a. Carefully reduce distal buccal flange
		    b. Adjust by thinning dentures from the outside, not the tissue side
		2.Lower: a. Carefully reduce the flange
		    b. Reduce from the outside–do not grind tissue side
		3. Remount and reset, correcting vertical
		4. Same as above
		5. Remount and reset opening arch to allow more tongue room

Gagging		
Immediate on insertion	1. Upper: Overextension. Too thick posterior border 2. Lower: Distal-lingual flange too thick	1. Upper: Denture must be double-post dammed and cut back to anterior post-dam. 2. Lower: Carefully reduce from the outside. Do not grind tissue side.
Delayed gagging 2 weeks to 2 months after delivery	1. Faulty post-dam allowing saliva under denture 2. Malocclusion allowing denture to loosen causes saliva, seepage	1. Grind out post-dam area and take "wash" impression for a laboratory reline. 2. Remount and mill-in. Sometimes necessary to reset the teeth.
Biting cheek and tongue		
Keeps biting cheek and/or tongue	1. Posterior teeth set end-to-end 2. Overclosed 3. Posterior teeth set too far to the lingual or buccal	1. Rearticulate and reset posteriors (Wax try-in is highly recommended) 2. Rearticulate and reset all teeth, opening bite 3. Rearticulate and reset posterior teeth
Redness of tissue		
Tissue getting red in denture-bearing area	1. Ill-fitting denture base 2. Improper cure of denture base 3. Avitaminosis	1. Take a wash impression and re-base denture. Check for prematurities in the occlusion 2. Re-base (heat-cure acrylic). 3. Prescribe vitamins
All tissues becoming fiery red including cheeks and tongue	1. Denture base allergy (extremely rare)	1. Change base material by having laboratory "jump" to a vinyl base material. All acrylic teeth must be removed and replaced. A patch test should be taken.
Pain in mandibular joint		
	1. Vertical overclosed 2. Centric relation off 3. Arthritis 4. Trauma	1. Rearticulate and reset all teeth to open bite 2. Take intra-oral tracing and reset. Retrial advised 3. Consult patient's M.D. 4. Difficult to correct. Consider TMJ treatment. Consider OF posterior teeth.

Complaints About Appearance

Too bulky under nose	1. Labial flange of upper too long or too thick 2. Upper anterior teeth set too far back	1. Reduce bulk and/or length repolish 2. Reset anteriors lingually. Try-in suggested.
Sinking in under nose	1. Upper labial flange needs more bulk 2. Upper labial flange needs more length	1. Add wax to build up proper contour and have laboratory build out base 2. Grind out tissue side of labial flange, add compound border and take "wash" impression. Reset anteriors for lip support
Upper lip sinks in too far	1. Upper anterior teeth set too far to lingual	1. Add wax on teeth to proper contour and have laboratory set teeth more to labial for lip support
Shows too much teeth	1. Vertical too great 2. Occlusal plane too low 3. Cuspids and laterals set too prominent 4. Upper anterior teeth set out too far	1. Have laboratory reset all teeth, closing vertical. Maintain esthetics by determining to raise or lower upper or lower teeth. 2. Have laboratory reset all teeth, raising occlusal plane 3. Replace cuspids and laterals with smaller teeth and rotate them in 4. Reset teeth back to ridge
Just look too false	1. Set too regular, technic type set-up 2. All teeth look the same shade 3. No gingival contouring or staggering of gingival depth	1. Try sculpturing anterior incisors to give abraded appearance. Rotate and stagger teeth in set-up 2. Change to characterized anterior teeth 3. Have laboratory process new base with anatomical finish and characterized base

Figure 12.80   (Continued)

For repairs, relines, repositions, and additions, see Chapter 13, Table 13.3.

Fungal infections (see Chapter 16).

Flabby ridge (hyperplastic replacement): surgical removal unless extreme atrophy of entire ridge. Use modified impression technique if flabby ridge kept intact. Create "window" in custom tray material. Border mold and wash with light body PVS. Add light body PVS through window to capture anatomy of flabby ridge without pressure of tray material influencing the shape of the flabby ridge.

Occlusion: molars occluding on left side only, adjust until even bite on left/right.

Soreness

Don't ask if soreness is better, ask patient to quantify in percentage terms [5].

Get good history on soreness to determine if denture requires occlusal or base adjustment:

Typical soreness related to denture base: patient feels pain when first inserting denture, discomfort even when not eating, may or may not progress through the day [5].

Typical soreness related to occlusion: pain when chewing, progresses through the day [5] (Figure 12.76).

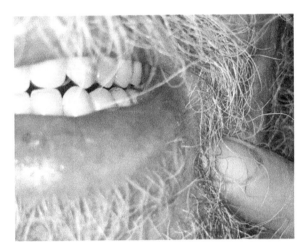

Figure 12.76   Instruct the patient to chew on a wet cotton pellet (which you provide) and if any discomfort to hold in that position and to point to the area causing discomfort. The occlusion may have to be adjusted.

Don't adjust blindly; use indicating medium to locate (articulating paper, PIP, disclosing wax) for accurate and time-efficient adjusting.

Unsure of location: patient states they have a sore spot but don't know exactly where. Inspect denture-bearing tissues for ulcerations. If no ulcerations visible, use nonmarking end of Thompson stick (Figure 12.77) to gently glide over the denture-bearing tissues. If the patient feels the sore spot, flip the stick over and mark the area. Seat the denture to transfer the mark to the denture and adjust 0.5 mm of the denture.

Do not remove too much denture material as sore spot is swollen and will result in poor adaptation if too much is removed. Usually 0.5 mm is sufficient amount to remove [5].

Sore spots in combination with xerostomia mean less lubrication and increased risk of sore spots. Provide xerostomia handout (see Chapter 5).

Soreness in sulcus: apply disclosing wax, border mold, adjust burn-through on flange (Figure 12.78).

Soreness on edentulous ridge: pressure spot from denture or occlusion related. Check with PIP for pressure spots and check occlusion with articulating paper and adjust.

Soreness when swallowing: overextension of distolingual border of mandibular denture, adjust.

Frenal soreness: widen frenal notch with acrylic bur to allow for functional movement and smooth sharp edges.

Soreness when opening wide: reduce thickness of distobuccal flange of maxillary denture, inadequate space for coronoid process.

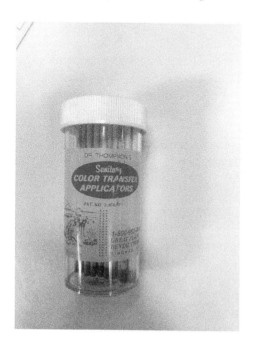

Figure 12.77   Dr. Thompson's Sanitary Color Transfer Applicators. Referred to in this chapter as the "Thompson stick" or "indelible marker."

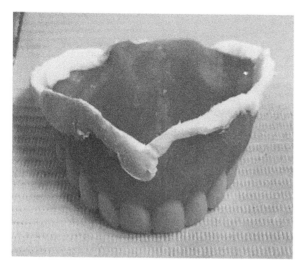

Figure 12.78   Disclosing wax on a denture prior to inserting in the mouth to check for overextended flanges.

- **VDO**: if making VDO changes, determine if upper incisal display/esthetics are ideal to determine which (or both) arches of teeth to intrude.
  - Tired facial muscles/strained mentalis/teeth "chattering": excessive VDO, so send back to lab for eventual rebase and new tooth try-in appointment with reduced VDO.
  - Visible gingiva of lower denture at tooth try-in: VDO is excessive. If esthetics of upper is good, remove all lower teeth and obtain a new CR at the correct VDO (see Section Appointment 3: Wax Occlusal Rims). Have lab mount and reset all lower teeth and return for another tooth try-in appointment.
- **CR**
  - Getting patient in CR at WOR appointment:
    - Patient should be in supine position. Tell patient: "Touch the tip of your tongue to the back of your throat and slowly close."
    - Alternatively, make a ball of wax on the posterior cameo surface of the WOR tell patient "Touch ball with the tip of your tongue as you slowly bite with your back teeth."
  - At the tooth try-in appointment patient states "I have to move my jaw way back to get it to where you want it to be." Remove all lower posterior teeth and make notches in the WOR. Obtain a new CR bite (see Section Appointment 3: Wax Occlusal Rims) and send to lab to reset the lower teeth.
- **Poor retention**
  - May be multifactorial, including anatomy, psychological factors, saliva, ill-fitting dentures, gravity, technique.
  - For the most accurate impressions polyester is recommended. The second best is PVS, and the third best option is alginate. If using alginate the cast must be poured as soon as possible to prevent distortion.
  - Denture falls out when opening wide: flanges overextended, may be impinging on frenums, too thick at maxillary distobuccal flange, or impinging pterygomandibular raphes. Check with disclosing wax and PIP. Insert denture slowly to see which part of flange touches vestibule first (premature contact) and adjust.
  - Hamular notches captured? (Figures 12.79 and 12.80).
  - Denture falls out when smiling: flange too thick in maxillary posterior buccal; adjust.
  - Loose after several hours: related to occlusion, or overextended flanges with good PPS. Check with indicating material and adjust.
  - Maxillary posterior dropping: overextended PPS, underextended PPS, inadequate (flat) PPS, or premature occlusion (check anterior contact). Mark the PPS in the mouth, seat the denture to transfer the mark, and adjust if overextended.
  - Tips when eating: try cutting up food and chewing on left and right side simultaneously.
  - Find out if any change in body weight; anecdotally, may need a reline if weight is lost.
  - Lower denture pops out when moving tongue: check for overextensions with disclosing wax and adjust.
  - Don't overadjust flanges, since both underextended and overextended flanges cause poor retention.
  - Saliva quality and quantity contributes to denture retention; if dry mouth is present, provide xerostomia handout (see Chapter 5).

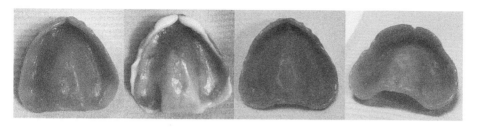

Figure 12.79 The right hamular notch was not captured during the impression appointment. The denture had poor retention. The denture was relined (with Coe-Comfort) and the right hamular notch was captured. The denture was sent to the lab for a hard reline and returned. Note the defined right hamular notch and PPS.

- **Short/underextended flange** (possibly from over-reduction/adjusting): border mold with compound or heavy body to extend and wash impression, and send to lab for hard reline. Want flange as high up as patient can tolerate while not overextended causing dislodgment with border molding. Both underextended and overextended flanges cause poor retention.
- **Esthetics**
  - If the smile looks unesthetic at the tooth try-in, send the lab photos from three angles:
    - At eye level of the patient smiling (showing nose, smile, chin).
    - A profile of the patient smiling (showing nose, smile, chin).
    - An image taken from the dentist's 12 o'clock perspective looking down at the patient smiling (showing nose, smile, chin).
  - If setting teeth for tooth try-in appointment, recommend using the rag wheel to polish the pink wax and placing Hi-Gloss Liquid Model Wax Gloss coat over the pink wax for a shiny esthetic try-in.
  - Upper teeth not flared out enough. Lab must reset all teeth to avoid diastemas.
  - Showing too little teeth:
    - Teeth must be reset. Patient may complain of appearing to have no teeth if no incisal display at rests.
    - Determine location for new placement of maxillary anterior incisal edges. If at tooth try-in appointment, reposition maxillary anterior teeth to correct incisal edge. If VDO is acceptable reposition all other remaining teeth maintaining VDO with proper anterior overjet/overbite. If VDO is deficient, determine amount of VDO to increase. If at delivery, return to lab to reset all teeth and inform lab number of millimeters of incisal display to include. Determine if size of teeth must be changed.
  - Large nose: if alas are far apart, at the WOR appointment the distal of the canines will be placed too laterally and the teeth selected will be too wide/large. Select teeth that are smaller (if possible, obtain previous photo of patient's teeth for size selection).
  - Large tongue: patient complains the tongue is too big for a denture. Inform patient that the intrinsic tongue musculature will reorganize and adapt to the new shape in the mouth with the dentures over time [2].
  - Crooked nose: to match the midline of the denture with the face, inspect the master cast for the incisive papilla and mark the midline on the WOR. See if this landmark coincides. Can also split the difference in the midline by referencing the eyes and lips. Also helps to send three photos to the lab (frontal, profile, looking down from 12 o'clock).
  - Teeth look artificial: trim incisal edges for abraded appearance, rotate and stagger teeth, include various shades.
  - Shade:

If you show patient all the shades available, they will choose the whitest shade. An option is to select two to three shades, place under patient's lip and obtain their input as guidance [5].

Patient unhappy with shade. Lab could reset all teeth in new shade and process for delivery. However, best to do a second tooth try-in appointment to prevent the financial liability and time of resetting all the teeth after delivery for another try-in and then another delivery. Do not attempt to persuade patient into being happy with the denture in order to sign the prosthesis consent; it is better to correct this at the try-in stage.

Masculine versus feminine tooth characteristics

Masculine:

Teeth: prominent incisal angles/square corners. Flat labial surface. Darker shade. Larger size teeth.

Smile line: flat.

Feminine:

Teeth: rounded incisal edges and corners, open incisal embrasures. Curved labial surface. Lighter shade. Smaller size teeth.

Smile line: curved.

Cheek biting: inadequate overjet of posterior cusps. Adjust mandibular buccal cusps on buccal so that 1–2 mm overjet and 1 mm space between buccal cusp of upper and lower (see Figure 12.49). Can also be caused by the teeth not occluding (a posterior open bite).

Reline: inform patient there is no guarantee that reline will improve retention. Patient may be upset, stating "Now I have no suction and bite is off." To avoid this, prior to reline, evaluate both the retention and occlusion. Make patient aware of any problems with retention and occlusion (e.g. show patient in mirror open bite on posterior right side). Inform patient may require denture adhesive.

Second and third relines: relieve the intaglio with acrylic bur and then reline. If you don't relieve the intaglio, the VDO will increase and will lead to unesthetic amount of gingival and incisal display. Also be sure to create vent holes with a #8 bur in the denture base.

Teeth setting: if inadequate space for posterior tooth, reduce length on distal half so it does not show in the esthetic zone. Do not reduce length on the mesial or both mesial and distal.

Temporomandibular disorders: in general, TMD prevalence diminishes with age. Promote tissue rest and "application of moist heat (10–20 minutes, four times a day) or cold application (five minutes each time), soft diet, avoidance of muscle strain (e.g. avoid gum chewing or clenching), and identification and avoidance of events that can trigger pain or discomfort." Analgesics such as NSAIDs may be needed for acute pain, along with stress management [2].

Miscellaneous Advice

Oral cancer risk: high risk in partially edentulous and edentulous patients due to association with heavy alcohol and tobacco consumption, less education, lower socioeconomic status, and poor dental health [2]. If lesion does not heal in 10–14 days refer for biopsy.

Communication

Try to avoid the word "take" in "take impression" or "take a bite" which gives patients the idea that all you do is "take" from them; instead replace "take" with "make."

Use layman's terms, such as "suction" and "better grip" with higher ridge.

Warn patients they may prefer the old denture to new denture.

Unhappy unsatisfied patient: inform patient you did your best to make a good fitting prosthesis; however, you can refer to another dentist/prosthodontist. If poor prognosis was identified early on, emphasize limitations throughout the treatment phase to set realistic expectations for the patient.

Denture hygiene

- Dentures accumulate plaque, calculus, and stains similar to teeth. Failure to clean the biofilm is associated with increased risk of denture stomatitis [8].
- Plaque disclosing solution can be used to educate patients [5].
- Patients are usually not aggressive enough when cleaning along denture gumline.
- Recommend both soaking overnight and brushing dentures.
- Stress the importance of gentle nonabrasive denture cleaners (not toothpaste).
- Dental biofilm accumulates more on rough denture surfaces than smooth dentures surfaces [8].

Removing denture adhesive cream from oral cavity. Options include rinse with warm salt water multiple times and spitting and removing excess with a soft toothbrush and a little tooth-paste. Alterntively, instead of warm salt water, rinse with a mouthrinse (e.g. Listerine).

Soft relines: try to avoid using (unless in healing phase) as the patient will become accustomed to the soft material and not adapt well to the permanent long-term denture acrylic material. Soft reline material is temporary and will degrade and peel off.

Patient refusal

- Patient refuses removal of root tips and only wants dentures. First, seek to understand why patient refusing treatment. Inform patient the root tips are a source of infection (may already be infected) that can cause systemic problems and will affect the fit of the dentures. Use the analogy "It is like keeping a pebble in the shoe and not removing it." Inform patient of your proposed treatment plan/recommendations as a dental professional and that patient has the freedom to go to another dentist for a second opinion.
- Patient not interested in scheduling a follow-up visit. Inform patient you can almost guarantee there will be a sore spot that may require adjusting. Also emphasize need for recall exams and oral cancer screenings.

Evaluate how master casts are trimmed. If the base is not parallel to the edentulous ridge (check on tabletop), the WORs may be canted in the mouth.

Baking soda: patient wants to clean teeth with baking soda. Inform patient that it is too abrasive and will cause loss of shine. Tell patient that eyes and teeth should appear shiny.

Denture (and container) identification: various states in the United States require some form of dental prosthetic identification (check with your state dental board). Purpose is to identify an individual or to identify a denture if lost, misplaced or damaged. If tooth is lost, identification can help lab (if same lab) replace with the same tooth brand, mold and shade [9]. Document form of identification in record and if patient refuses, document patient refusal. Place name on container as someone in household/community living center may grab the wrong denture container.

Removing upper denture with good retention

- Inform patient to "close lips tightly and blow to break denture seal."
- Inform patient if about to sneeze to cover mouth as the dentures may fly out.

Suction dentures: use medical-grade suction cups on intaglio (per lab technician) as a last ditch effort to aid in retention with severe ridge resorption. Recommend patient save money for implant over denture or implant-retained denture in the future.

Adjusting occlusion: save time by using high-speed bur.

Remove articulating paper marks on teeth: use alcohol wipe.

Patient eye protection: patient should always wear eye protection, even if simply adjusting denture as acrylic debris can get into patient's eyes.

Unable to satisfy a patient: one option is to explain that "I've done the best I can and for some reason I am not able to satisfy your needs, so let me give you a refund and refer you to a prosthodontist."

- "I need a new lower denture, mine is too loose."

  With a lower denture we are not able to get the same type of suction as we can with the upper, therefore the lower can be problematic. Let me first take a look and evaluate your gums and the fit of your denture.

- "I need a new denture because when I chew food on one side my denture gets loose."

  Even with a new set of dentures, chewing food on one side will cause the upper denture to drop on the opposite side. Let's evaluate the fit of your current dentures. Let me have you bite on a cotton roll on both the left and right side (Figure 12.81). Now let me have you bite a cotton roll on just the left side (denture will drop on the opposite side) (Figure 12.82). Even with new dentures I recommend cutting food into smaller pieces and learning to chew on both sides simultaneously for denture stability to prevent one side from dropping/popping out. Let me take a look and evaluate your gums and the fit of your denture.

- "My front tooth came out sucking on a lollipop. Can you replace it?"

  Where is the tooth? Determine if:

  - Swallowed or aspirated (refer for chest/abdomen X-ray).
  - Saved and available for use.
  - "We could try to repair it today for you." (See Figure 12.70)

- "My denture was made in another state. Can you adjust it?"

  See Chapter 13, section Real-Life Clinical Scenarios Answered.

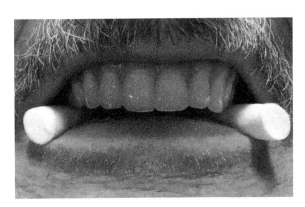

Figure 12.81   The patient is biting on cotton rolls bilaterally, stabilizing the denture.

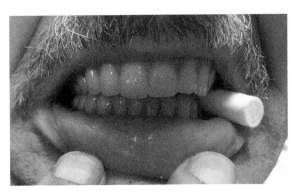

Figure 12.82   The patient is biting on a cotton roll unilaterally, causing the contralateral side of the upper denture to drop down. For this reason it is recommended to chew food on both sides simultaneously for denture stability.

Patients' Concerns

- "Is it OK for me to swallow this [alginate]?"

  Alginate is considered safe and "probably not harmful if ingested" according to the safety data sheet (of one brand of alginate) [10]. "Alginate is made up mostly of calcium and potassium alginate from seaweed (kelp, the brown seaweed in the ocean)" [11].

- "How do I prevent bone loss under my dentures?"

  Bone loss is progressive and irreversible. Poor-fitting dentures can speed up this process along with wearing dentures all day and night [2]. Return regularly once a year to check the fit of the dentures, as they may have to be adjusted, relined, or remade.

Patients' Questions and Comments

- "Why are you recommending pulling a healthy tooth for a denture to fit?"

  At times we recommend removing a tooth if the tooth is diseased, if the bone is diseased, and sometimes for functional or prosthodontic purposes.

- "I'm going to eat a nice steak tonight with my new dentures."

  While I'm happy to see your excitement with the new dentures, don't get discouraged if it is a challenge. I recommend starting slow, with soft foods and working your way up to tougher chewier foods. Cut the food into small pieces and chew on both sides simultaneously for denture stability. This adjustment takes time, like a child learning to crawl before walking and running.

- "This denture is making me gag, can you trim the back?"

  The denture must extend to a point between the hard and soft palate. Trimming the denture back will result in loss of "suction" and the denture will not be as retentive. Let me take a look to see how far back it is extended.

  Mark the PPS. Make sure it does not go beyond the posterior vibrating line; tissue should not be moving beneath the posterior border of the denture when patient says "aaah." Gagging usually disappears within a few days as you adjust to the denture [2].

- "How much glue should I put on the denture?"

  Dry the denture and apply four drops of cream to the upper and three drops to the lower (see Figure 12.63).

- "I need to keep my dentures moist? Why is that?"

  If the denture is left out and becomes dehydrated, the acrylic will warp and the denture will no longer fit the ridge properly.

- "How long do I soak it with one of those tablets?"

  Usage instructions vary with different products; some are meant for a three-minute soak and some overnight. Soaking overnight will not harm the denture. Make sure to rinse and brush after removing the denture from the container before placing it in your mouth. (You know product information if supplying patient with samples.)

  "Brushing is more effective (60–80% vs. 20–30%) for plaque removal compared to soaking alone. Combine brushing with soaking for more efficiency" [5].

- "My previous dentist never told me I am supposed to take my teeth out at night!"

  I was not there at that time so I cannot say anything; however, it is important to allow the tissues to rest overnight to allow for blood circulation. If you do not you increase the rate of bone loss [2]. As you lose bone, the ridges shrink/flatten making the denture loose and future dentures more difficult to fabricate.

- "It falls out when I talk."

Does it fall out when you open your mouth wide? The denture may be overextended (see Section Troubleshooting). Can use disclosing wax.

Does it fall out if you move your tongue? Try sticking your tongue out, toward the left and right ear. Let me see if it needs adjusting (deepen frenal notches).

"I get food stuck under my dentures."

This will happen so it is very important to remove and clean the dentures thoroughly after eating. You may find it beneficial to use denture adhesive to help prevent some food from getting under the dentures.

"How long will it take for my sore spot to heal?" (See Figure 12.2)

We need to remove the source by adjusting your denture for the sore spot to heal. In the mouth, sores usually heal within 10–14 days. It is important that we follow up with you, because it if does not heal we will need to evaluate the area further (for biopsy). (Analogy: like removing a rock from the inside of your shoe.)

"I had a sore spot so I stopped wearing it for a week. Can you adjust it?"

Do you recall where the sore spot was? Best to come in as soon as possible if you have a sore spot as the gum is typically red or ulcerated so we know exactly where to adjust rather than just guessing.

"Before a tube of denture glue would last me eight weeks, now it lasts three weeks."

Denture may be due for a reline. Check fit.

References

1 Kaul, A.S. and Goyal, D. (2011). Bite force comparison of implant-retained mandibular overdentures with conventional complete dentures: an in vivo study. *Int. J. Oral Implantol. Clin. Res.* 2 (3): 140–144.

2 Zarb, G. and Bolender, C. (2004). *Prosthodontic Treatment for Edentulous Patients: Complete Dentures and Implant-Supported Prostheses*, 12e. St Louis, MO: Elsevier Mosby.

3 American College of Prosthodontists (2018). The frequency of denture replacement. https://www.prosthodontics.org/about-acp/position-statement-the-frequency-of-denture-replacement (accessed 1 December 2019).

4 Love, C.J. (2011). PowerPoint presentations at Case Western Reserve University School of Dental Medicine.

5 Loney, R.W. (2019). *Complete Denture Manual*. Halifax, NS, Canada: Dalhousie University. http://removpros.dentistry.dal.ca/Manuals.html (accessed 27 November 2021).

6 Academy of Prosthodontics (2017). The Glossary of prosthodontic terms, 9e. *J. Prosthet. Dent.* 117 (5S): e1–e105. https://doi.org/10.1016/j.prosdent.2016.12.001.

7 Advanced Dentistry of New Providence (2020). Consent for immediate and complete dentures. https://www.adonp.com (accessed 1 December 2019).

8 Felton, D., Cooper, L., Duqum, I. et al. (2011). Evidence-based guidelines for the care and maintenance of complete dentures: a publication of the American College of Prosthodontists. *J. Prosthodont* 20 (Suppl 1): S1–S12.

9 Dental Prosthesis Identification (2020). States mandating denture identification. http://www.denture-id.com/Regulations/State-Id-Mandates (accessed 1 December 2019).

10 Dental Corporation of America (2015). Alginate. http://www.dentalcorp.com/impression/alginate.html?_ga=2.248549319.1901719269.1574226229-1846034215.1548916999 (accessed 1 December 2019).

11 Dentsply/International Dentsply/Caulk Safety Data Sheet (2013). https://www.dentsplysirona.com/content/dam/dentsply/pim/manufacturer/Restorative/Direct_Restoration/Adhesives/Etch__Rinse_Adhesives/ProBOND_All_Purpose_Total_Etch_Bonding_Agent/CAU_634255X/ProBond-Adhesive-Primer-SDS-534895-96-59bzqyv-en-1411.pdf (accessed 19 November 2019).

13

Removable Partial Dentures

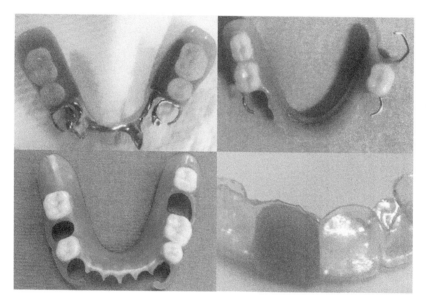

Figure 13.1 (*Upper left*) Cast metal RPD; (*upper right*) stayplate; (*lower left*) flexible partial; (*lower right*) Essix appliance.

Chapter Outline

- Real-Life Clinical Scenarios
- Relevance
- Setting Patients' Expectations
- Clinical and Radiographic Exam

Clinical Dentistry Daily Reference Guide, First Edition. William A. Jacobson.
© 2022 John Wiley & Sons, Inc. Published 2022 by John Wiley & Sons, Inc.

- Treatment Planning
  - Sequencing
  - Treatment Needs Prior to Fabricating a Partial (if Indicated)
  - Selecting Appliance Type
- Kennedy Classification and Relevant Terms
- Procedural Steps
  - Consent Form
  - Cast Metal RPDs
  - Repairs, Relines, Repositions, Additions, and What the Lab Needs from You
  - Stayplates (Also Known as Acrylic Resin Partial, Interim Partial, Treatment Partial, Transitional Partial, Flipper)
  - Flexible Partials
  - Essix Appliances
  - Immediate Partials
  - Complete Dentures Opposing Cast Metal RPDs
- Lab Prescriptions
  - Cast Metal RPDs
  - Stayplates
  - Flexible Partials
  - Essix Appliances
  - Immediate Partials
- Postoperative Instructions
- Clinical Pearls
  - Troubleshooting
  - Tips
- Real-Life Clinical Scenarios Answered
- References

Real-Life Clinical Scenarios

Dental Students' Questions

- "How do I design the RPD?"
- "When do I have to do a wax occlusal rim appointment for an RPD?"
- "What is the altered cast technique?"
- "What is the appointment sequence if I'm making a complete denture over an RPD?"

Dental Assistant's Question

- "The schedule says enameloplasty. What's that?"

Patients' Questions

- "I just broke my front tooth off at the gumline. I'm going out tonight for New Year's Eve and I can't be seen like this. Can you help me?" (Figure 13.2)
- "I want partials. Which type do you recommend?"
- "Will my loose teeth tighten up once I have partials?"

- "You need to drill my teeth? My teeth are already weak!"
- "Why are you recommending pulling a healthy tooth for a partial to fit?"
- "Why aren't my partials ready today?" [At appointment 2]
- "Doc, you're replacing one tooth, why is this partial the size of my hand?"
- "Why so many clasps?"
- "The wire broke. Can you fix it?"
- "Can you repair this?" (Figure 13.3)

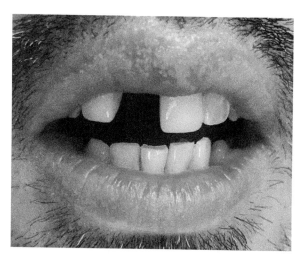

Figure 13.2 Fractured tooth #8.

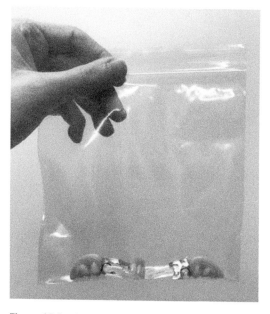

Figure 13.3 A patient brought his broken cast metal RPD in a bag.

Patients' Comments

- "I just bite it into place."
- "My last dentist made me a partial and when I got home, I had a panic attack because I couldn't take it out of my mouth!"

Patients' Demands

- "I want teeth back here." (Figure 13.4)
- "Doc, I need you to bend this wire." [Points to cast metal clasp]
- "I want you to replace my missing teeth and then you can work on my fillings."
- "My partial feels loose, it was tighter before. Now I can pop it out with my tongue."
- "I want you to adjust my partial. It was made in another state."

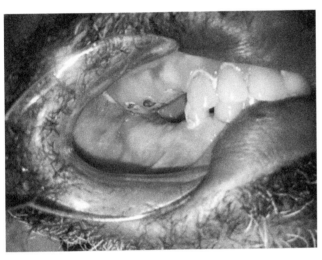

Figure 13.4 A partially edentulous patient with retained root tips on the upper right.

Relevance

As a dentist you will have patients interested in RPDs. A partial is a removable prosthesis that replaces one or more missing teeth, but not all of the teeth.

The need for a partial:
- may be urgent (e.g. patient just broke tooth #8 and plans to go out tonight for New Year's Eve);
- may be planned far in advance (e.g. patient with several asymptomatic teeth planned for extractions).

The patient may want a partial as a:
- short-term solution until receiving a fixed restoration (e.g. implant or bridge);
- interim solution until eventually transitioning to a complete denture;
- long-term solution to missing teeth.

For these reasons it is important to know the basics. This chapter addresses cast metal RPDs, stayplates, flexible partial dentures, and Essix appliances.

Setting Patients' Expectations

- Interview your patients to find out what their treatment expectations are. Are partial dentures the best option? See Chapter 4, Table 4.3.
- You must set realistic expectations for your patients when discussing partial dentures as a treatment option. If not your patients can become discouraged, disappointed, frustrated, and angry, demand a redo, file a complaint, etc.
- Movement:
  - An RPD is removable, so it will have movement.
  - Depending on how many teeth are remaining, it may feel like wearing flip-flops. If there are teeth on both sides (tooth-borne), there is less movement. If there are teeth only on one side (tissue-borne), it may be harder to adapt to wearing.
- Sore spots.
- Require removal and cleaning:
  - Since partials are not attached to the gums, food will get underneath which can irritate the gums.
  - It will still be necessary to brush and floss the teeth, with the partial out of the mouth, and it is important to clean the partial several times per day.
  - The partial will have to be removed at night when sleeping.
- Advantages: there are advantages to a partial denture versus a complete denture.
  - A complete denture can feel very loose, like marbles in someone's mouth, and can be very difficult to adapt to wearing, speaking, and eating.
  - A partial denture has clasps that wrap around natural teeth for support, reducing the amount of movement.
  - With a partial the remaining teeth still preserve some proprioception, so that the sensation of chewing is retained, making it easier to adapt to compared with a denture.
- Adapting to partials:
  - Everyone adapts differently. Some people with prosthetic legs can run marathons, some can only walk, and some have trouble accepting the prosthesis as their own. Partial dentures are no different.
  - No matter how well the partials are made, some people will adapt well to chewing, speaking, smiling, and wearing their dentures. Some will only wear their partials in public for appearance, and others will choose not to wear their partials.
  - It will take time to adapt to chewing and speaking with the dentures.
- Number of appointments:
  - The entire process may take two to six appointments.
  - Teeth may require modifications and at times pre-prosthetic surgery is required.
  - It is common to get sore spots from the new partials. This will require adjustments appointments. Some people experience gagging (usually disappears within a few days).
- See also Section Consent Forms.

Clinical and Radiographic Exam

Perform a comprehensive oral evaluation, radiographic interpretation (see Chapter 3), and periodontal evaluation (see Chapter 6).

Removable Partial Dentures

Treatment Planning

Sequencing

- Tooth replacement is typically the *last* stage of the treatment plan (see Chapter 4, Table 4.1). Some exceptions include:
  - An esthetic emergency.
  - Opening the bite (VDO) with a stayplate in order to restore the teeth (e.g. with buildups, temporary or permanent crowns). If the bite is not stable the restorations will likely fail due to the chewing forces (Figure 13.5). Once restorations are complete, then a long-term prosthesis can be fabricated.
- Usually it is "fixed before removable"; however, start with the end in mind. If crowns are planned, the partial denture design must be completed first as this dictates the crown design (see Chapter 11).
- After completion of the partial denture, the patient will return for recall visits and other treatment as indicated. The American College of Prosthodontists has stated that there is "currently no evidence to determine the frequency of denture relines, rebases, or remakes of removable complete or partial denture prosthesis" [1].

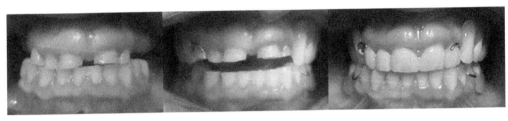

Figure 13.5 In some cases, tooth replacement is required earlier in the treatment plan to open the bite.

Treatment Needs Prior to Fabricating a Partial (if Indicated)

- Prophylaxis, fluoride varnish, and oral hygiene instructions.
- Periodontal treatment: clasping periodontally compromised teeth will increase mobility.
- Teeth bleaching.
- Direct or indirect restorations due to caries/unsatisfactory restorations/fractured teeth/uneven occlusal scheme.
- Desensitizer for hypersensitive teeth: clasping may increase sensitivity.
- Root canal treatment.
- Orthodontic treatment.
- Changes to VDO:
  - Maintain (ideal).
  - Increase (collapsed bite/no posterior stops).
  - Decrease (via extractions, enameloplasty, orthodontic intrusion).

- Preparation of teeth:
  - Rest seats.
  - Enameloplasty (for supraerupted teeth, tipped teeth, creation of guideplanes, dimpling).

- Impacted tooth:
  - Bony impacted or soft tissue covering: inform the patient that these could become exposed and then require extraction later.
  - Unerupted teeth: may choose to monitor. As bone resorbs, tooth may become exposed. Unlikely if covered in bone, no pathology, or over 40 years old.
- Oral surgery: pre-prosthetic surgery checklist
  - Extractions
  - Sinus lift
  - Evaluation/treatment of radiographic pathology
  - Evaluation/treatment of fungal infections or other pathology
  - Surgical removal of hyperplastic tissue or epulis fissuratum
  - Frenectomy
  - Alveoplasty of each quadrant with irregular/uneven/undercut bony areas
  - Maxillary tuberosity reduction
  - Maxillary tuberosity undercut removal
  - Palatal and/or mandibular tori removal
  - Buccal exostosis removal
  - Sedation
  - Other.
- Patient preferences:
  - Accepts period of time without teeth for healing? If not, provide immediate partial.
  - Accepts tooth modifications? If not, cannot offer cast metal RPD.
  - Accepts visible metal clasps? If not, flexible partial or hybrid partial (Figure 13.6).
- Metal allergies present? If so, determine which type of metal.
- Esthetic zone: take photos and determine which teeth are visible and lip line (e.g. clasp visible on premolars).
- For mandibular partial: have patient lift tongue and measure the distance of floor of mouth to lingual gingival margin.

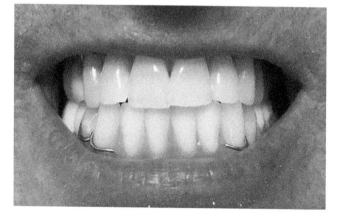

Figure 13.6 Be sure to inform the patient ahead of time that metal will be visible, as this may not be acceptable to some patients and alternatives will have to be discussed.

Removable Partial Dentures

Selecting Appliance Type

See Figure 13.1.

Table 13.1 Removable appliance types: advantages and disadvantages.

Removable appliance type (material)	Advantages	Disadvantages
Cast metal RPD (typically, cobalt chromium)	• Long-term/permanent appliance • Good retention/stability/support • Can be relined/repaired • Stronger for those with history of breaking partials • Indications include low caries/periodontitis risk and well-healed edentulous ridge	• Requires surveying and teeth modifications • Requires more appointments • Visible metal
Stayplate (also known as acrylic resin partial, interim partial, treatment partial, transitional partial, flipper and immediate partials [acrylic resin/polymethyl methacrylate and wrought wire clasps])	• Interim appliance until transitioning to a complete denture • Can be relined/repaired • Indications include high caries/periodontitis risk • Tighter fit than flexible because of metal clasps • *For immediate partials*: no period of time without teeth • May be possible to have no clasps if lingual undercuts	• Less retention/stability/support than a cast metal RPD • Short-term/temporary appliance • Breaks more easily than cast metal • Visible metal • *For immediate partials*: no opportunity for tooth try-in appointment to check occlusion, phonetics, esthetics, and loose fitting/food trap with ridge resorption
Flexible partial Different materials: Valplast and TCS (thermoplastic nylon resin), DuraFlex (ethylene propylene) [2]	• Esthetic (no visible metal) • Metal-free (metal allergies)	• Not as tight a fit as stayplate and cast metal RPD • Not as long term as cast metal RPD • Teeth mechanically retained (not chemically bonded) and can "pop" off when base flexes • Contraindicated if replacing upper anterior with deep bite (≤4 mm) (teeth can be dislodged) • Contraindicated to replace long span of teeth • Contraindicated in cases with flared teeth [3] • Can reline, repair, and add teeth; however it does not fuse well so instead recommend redoing the partial instead
Essix appliance (composite resin or a denture tooth and clear vacuform material/stent/splint typically copolyester)	• Urgent solution, can be made same day in office or in only two appointments • Temporary solution to a missing tooth in the esthetic zone	• Short-term/temporary appliance • Not for chewing food • Not for replacement of posterior teeth • Teeth will not occlude • Typically, cannot repair and requires replacement • Not indicated if bruxism, as quickly deteriorates

Table 13.1 (Continued)

Removable appliance type (material)	Advantages	Disadvantages
Hybrid partial-stayplate or cast metal RPD	• Flexible clasps in esthetic zone • Advantage of wrought wire clasps for stayplate, or cast metal clasps for RPD in posterior	• Weak acrylic–flexible junction (stayplate) or weak metal–flexible junction (RPD) as flexible material relies on mechanical bond • Flexible clasp cannot be relined, can stain, and will be thicker

Kennedy Classification and Relevant Terms

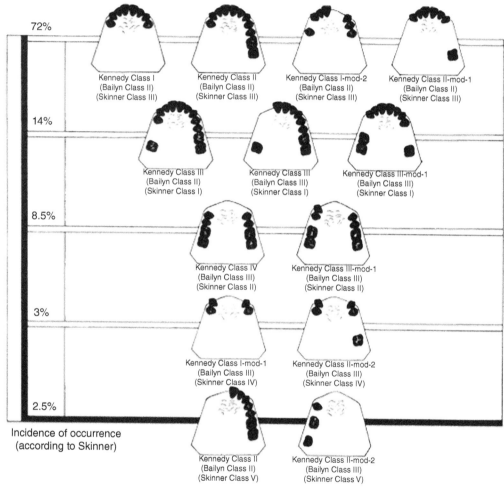

Figure 13.7 Representative examples of partially edentulous arches classified by the Kennedy method. *Source:* Carr and Brown [4]. Reproduced with permission of Elsevier.

Kennedy Classification

- See Figure 13.7.
- Classified by "class" and "mod"
  - Class: determined by the most posterior edentulous areas.
  - Mods: modifications, number of additional edentulous spans between teeth.
- Class I: posterior bilateral edentulous spaces (distal extensions).
- Class II: unilateral posterior edentulous space (distal extension).
- Class III: unilateral posterior edentulous space bound by natural teeth (tooth-borne).
- Class IV: anterior edentulous space (crossing midline) (tooth-borne) [4].
- Class I and II: considered distal extensions.
- Class III and IV: considered tooth-borne.

Relevant Terms

- **Major connector**: connect two sides of the arch together for cross-arch stability and never rests on movable tissue.
- **Minor connector**: connects the major connector to the direct and indirect retainers.
- **Direct retainer**: resists movement of RPD away from teeth (i.e. clasps).
- **Indirect retainer**: prevents rocking/teeter-totter movement. For Kennedy Class I/II it is located perpendicular to the fulcrum line (canine cingulum rests). The fulcrum line is the line from the most posterior rests. Kennedy Class III/IV do not require indirect retainers, as this is provided by other types of support such as at the rugae and lingual plate [5].

Procedural Steps

Consent Form

- See Chapter 12, section Consent Forms.

Cast Metal RPDs

Appointment 1: diagnostic casts
  - Upper/lower alginate impressions, bite registration.
  - Pour models and hand articulate (if possible).

- Evaluation: it is critical to evaluate the study models to prevent avoidable complications such as:
  - Abutment tooth with no retention, even with a clasp, because the tooth lacked an undercut (Figure 13.8).
  - Food trap due to a tipped tooth which was not recontoured (Figure 13.9).
  - Unesthetically narrow anterior denture tooth because adjacent teeth migrated and were not recontoured (Figure 13.10).
  - Unesthetic anterior open bite because the opposing teeth were not built up (Figures 13.11 and 13.12).
  - Patient complaining that her posterior teeth don't occlude when she bites (Figure 13.13).
  - Patient complaining that he hits metal when he bites down (Figure 13.14).

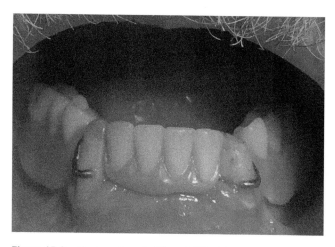

Figure 13.8 Abutment teeth (22 and 27) with no retention, even with a clasp, because the teeth lacked an undercut.

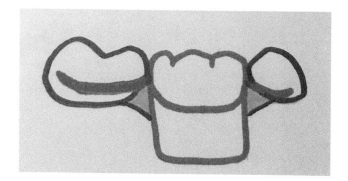

Figure 13.9 Illustration of food trap due to tipped tooth which was not recountered.

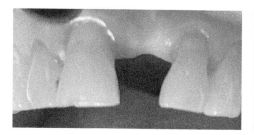 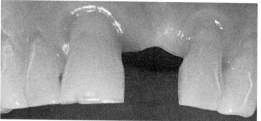

Figure 13.10 In this case, #8 mesial and #10 mesial were recontoured to improve esthetics for a proportional #9. Otherwise #9 would appear too narrow and have "black triangles.

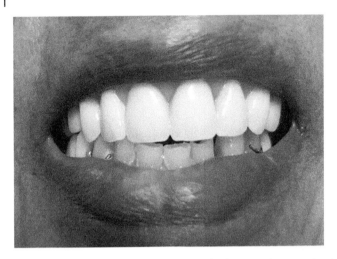

Figure 13.11   Unesthetic anterior open bite because the opposing teeth were not built up.

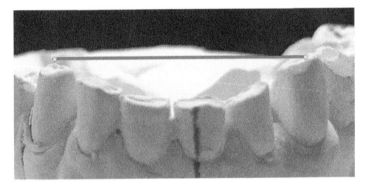

Figure 13.12   Unesthetic anterior open bite because the opposing teeth were not built up.

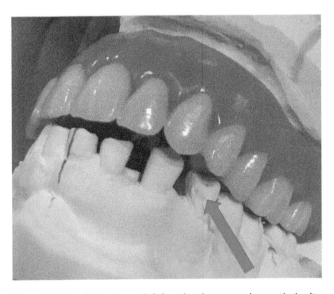

Figure 13.13   Patient complaining that her posterior teeth don't occlude when she bites.

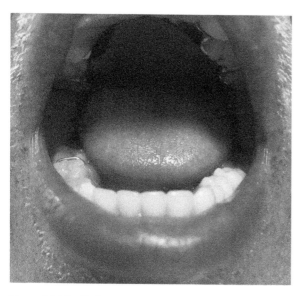

Figure 13.14   Patient complaining that he hits metal when he bites down.

Surveying

The Ney Surveyor aids in designing an RPD by determining the height of contour line (HOCL/ survey line/guide line), desirable and undesirable undercuts, and path of insertion (Figure 13.15). This step is necessary prior to crown and bridge (see Chapter 11 for crown and RPD scenarios).

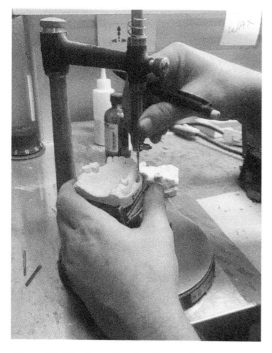

Figure 13.15   Surveying the diagnostic study model.

Steps

- Place trimmed cast on tilt-top with occlusal surface parallel to floor (0 tilt).
- Start with the canines and anteriors
  - Choose a tilt with best esthetic results: may have to compromise between esthetics and function.
- Evaluate the distal extension(s).
- Evaluate the tooth-supported area.
- Use the analyzing rod to check the following.
  - HOCL:
    - HOCL should be on the buccal middle third of the tooth and on the lingual gingival third (Figure 13.16).
    - Tilting the tilt-top can create more desirable undercuts, or teeth may have to be modified.
    - Use the carbon marker to mark the HOCL on abutment teeth:
      - HOCL too occlusal: adjust the tilt-top or enameloplasty to move the HOCL more gingivally.
      - HOCL too gingival, the clasp will infringe on the gingiva.
    - Measure undercuts with gauge:
      - 0.01 inch (0.25 mm) chrome cobalt cast retainer.
      - 0.02 inch (0.5 mm) cast gold retainer.
      - 0.03 inch (0.75 mm) wrought wire (WW) (wrought gold or wrought chrome cobalt, the most flexible).
      - If tooth does not have enough enamel, may have to crown.
      - If tooth does not have the appropriate undercut, may have to perform enameloplasty or create a dimple in the shape of the retentive tip.
  - Soft tissue:
    - Check for undesirable undercuts.
    - Check distance to floor of mouth and frenula.
    - Need for alveoplasty or tori removal?
  - Tipped teeth:
    - May require guideplanes to reduce food trap.
    - Check for lingually tipped teeth, which can interfere with major connector seating flush against soft tissue, e.g. lower molars tilted lingually.
  - Teeth adjacent to edentulous ridges:
    - Check for mesial drifting of anterior teeth, which may require enameloplasty to create space for replacement teeth.
    - Check for parallelism between the teeth adjacent to edentulous areas.
    - Check for undercuts adjacent to ridge (need for guideplanes).
- Check occlusion:
  - Supraerupted teeth?
    - Interocclusal space requirements: 7 mm for RPD, 5 mm for flexible.
    - Need for extractions, alveoplasty, enameloplasty, orthodontic intrusion?

- – Uneven occlusal scheme? See Figure 13.17.
  - – Embrasure space for ball end clasp?
  - – Adequate overjet/overbite?
- Mark the path of insertion/draw on the sides of cast. Note that an RPD designed at a tilt is less easily dislodged than one which inserts perpendicular to the plane of occlusion.
- Tripod: mark lines on the side of the cast for repositioning or create a transfer stint/jig. Mark three spots on the cast and create a plastic (e.g. triad) transfer stint form with three openings to be transferred to a master cast.

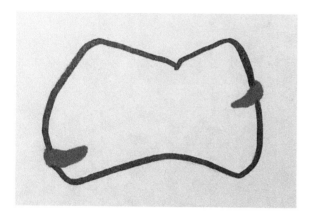

Figure 13.16 Placement of the retentive arm below the HOCL and the reciprocal arm above the HOCL.

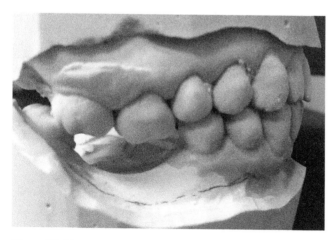

Figure 13.17 Uneven occlusal scheme due to supraeruption. If teeth #2 and #3 do not undergo enameloplasty, the opposing teeth will also be set in an uneven occlusal scheme.

RPD Design

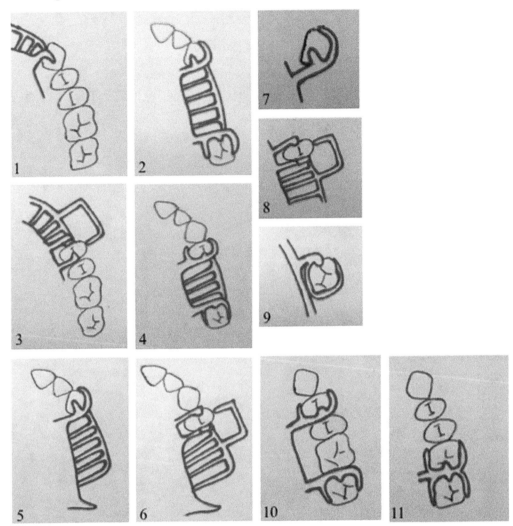

Figure 13.18 Direct retainers.

Table 13.2 Author's approach to RPD design.

Steps	Options
Assign Kennedy classification and mods	• I, II, III, or IV and modifications 1, 2, 3. . .
Determine type of maxillary major connector	• Anterior–posterior palatal strap (preferred, Kennedy I, II, II mod 1, IV, around tori) • Mid/posterior–palatal strap (Kennedy III/IV, ≥8 mm wide) • Metal palate with metal grid in post-dam for acrylic (Kennedy I, no tori) (can be relined but bulkier) • Full palatal (Kennedy I, no tori, <6 teeth, periodontal disease) • U-shaped "horseshoe"/anterior palatal strap (least preferred, Kennedy III/IV with inoperable tori)

Table 13.2 (Continued)

Steps	Options
Determine type of mandibular major connector	• Lingual bar (preferred, contacts tissue, 3–4 mm wide, 4 mm below gingival margin) • Lingual plate (contacts teeth, use if high lingual frenum/shallow floor)
Determine type(s) of direct retainers (clasps)	• Tooth-borne edentulous span mesial to canine: cingulum rest on canine (Kennedy IV). See Figure 13.18 (1) • Tooth-borne edentulous span distal to canine: C-clasps facing away from each other with guide planes. See Figure 13.18 (2) • Tooth-borne edentulous span mesial to premolar: RPI on premolar (with D rest, reverse of the normal RPI) (Kennedy IV). See Figure 13.18 (3) • Tooth-borne edentulous span distal to premolar: C-clasps facing away from each other with guide planes. See Figure 13.18 (4) • Edentulous tissue-borne (distal extension) distal to canine: cingulum rest on canine. See Figure 13.18 (5) • Edentulous tissue-borne (distal extension) distal to premolar: RPI on premolar (with M rest). See Figure 13.18 (6) • Edentulous mesial and distal to canine/isolated canine: C-clasp on canine engaging MF undercut. See Figure 13.18 (7) • Edentulous mesial and distal to premolar/isolated premolar: RPI on premolar (with M rest). See Figure 13.18 (8) • Edentulous mesial and distal to an isolated first molar with first and second molars in the opposing arch: ring clasp is preferable; see Figure 13.18 (9); however, a split clasp would also be stable both • Long posterior dentate spans: embrasure clasps on molar or C-clasps facing away from each other on premolar and molar symmetrical to contralateral edentulous space. See Figure 13.18 (10 and 11)

Additional considerations with direct retainers (clasps)	• Total number of direct retainers for retention: 4 > 3 ≥ 2 (absolute minimum) [4]
	• Abutment teeth preferences for direct retainers: molars > premolars > canines > laterals and centrals
	• Alternative to RPI (if frenum, shallow vestibule, deep soft tissue undercut):
	  - RPA: M rest, D proximal plate with C-clasp engaging the MF
	  - Back-action clasp: M rest and clasp engaging MF, for canines or premolars
	• Clasping periodontally compromised tooth: instead extend clasp to a tooth with better support
	• Avoid altering existing amalgam restorations (often fail) for rests/guide planes by using a different tooth or crown tooth [4]
	• Consider clasp visibility in the esthetic zone

Determine type(s) of indirect retainers (prevents teeter-totter/rocking)	• Cingulum rests on canine perpendicular to fulcrum line (needed for Kennedy Class I/II). Don't use central (speech) or lateral (root length) [4]
Survey the study models to determine	• If HOCL is desirable/undesirable/modifiable • Where to place rests, proximal planes, dimples
Determine tooth retentive options	• One tooth on well-healed ridge: tube teeth (cannot reline) • Two or more teeth: retentive network
Edentulous ridge retentive network	• If distal extension, include tissue stop • If maxillary distal extension, framework extent to two-thirds hamular notch and denture base around maxillary tuberosity • If mandibular distal extension, extend to two-thirds retromolar pad
Other considerations	• Aim for symmetry • Design to minimize movement for sticky and hard foods

Disclaimer: with RPD design there are different philosophies, designs, clasps, and situations (see Section Tips).
RPI: R, rest; P, proximal plate; I, I-bar.

Custom Trays

Consider fabricating custom trays for the RPD final impressions.

- Laboratory fabricated.
- In-house fabricated:
  - Two layers of base plate wax over teeth, one layer of base plate wax over soft tissue.
  - Two layer of acrylic (e.g. Triad) with a handle and cure. For the handle, make crosshatch pattern with knife before curing for better grip.
  - Remove the base plate wax except in the hard palate and mandibular edentulous ridge to act as a spacer.
  - Drill retention holes with #8 round bur.

Appointment 2: Tooth Modifications and Final Impression

- **Tooth modifications** (typically does not require anesthetic, limited to enamel)
  - Cingulum rest seat/ledge rest seat (Figure 13.19).
    - o Teeth: canines > centrals and laterals.
    - o Location: lingual surface. On mounted models, mark where lower canine contacts upper canine. Make sure cingulum rest is 1.5–2 mm cervical. Do not violate the marginal ridges, stay between.
    - o Shape: follow cingulum contour or straight if not pronounced, <90° cavosurface.
    - o Dimensions: 1 mm deep with no undercuts (1.5 mm deep if crown). If cingulum is not prominent, build up with composite or crown.
  - Occlusal rest seat (Figures 13.20 and 13.21).
    - o Teeth: molars and premolars.
    - o Location: occlusal surface, one-third of buccal–lingual.
    - o Shape: rounded triangle.
    - o Dimensions: one-third of buccal–lingual width, 2.5 mm sides of triangle, 1.5 reduction of marginal ridge, center deepest point.
      - ▪ Center deepest (<90° cavosurface) to transmit forces along the long axis and prevent partial from moving away from the abutment tooth causing orthodontic movement.
  - Embrasure rest (Figure 13.22).
    - o Teeth: molars and premolars.
    - o Location: occlusal surface, one-third of buccal–lingual.
    - o Shape: adjacent facing occlusal rests; rounded triangles with buccal and lingual reduction for minor connector and direct retainers.
    - o Dimensions: each tooth rest requires 2.5 mm sides of triangle, 1.5 reduction of marginal ridge, center deepest point, and 1.5 mm buccal and lingual.
      - ▪ Center deepest (<90° cavosurface) to transmit forces along the long axis and prevent partial from moving away from the abutment tooth causing orthodontic movement.

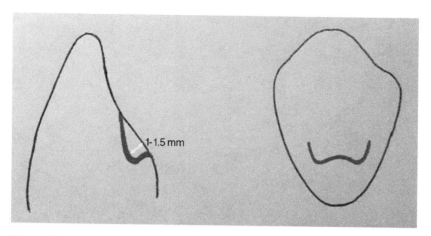

Figure 13.19   Cingulum rest seat.

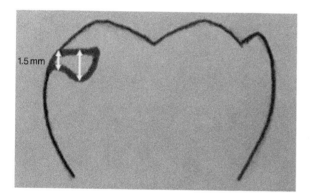

Figure 13.20   Occlusal rest seat.

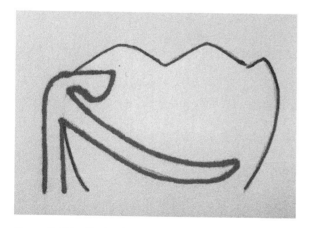

Figure 13.21   Occlusal rest and clasp.

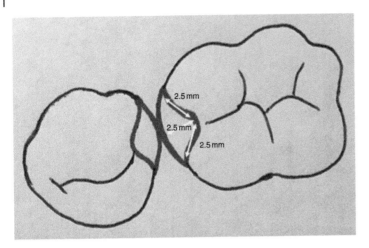

Figure 13.22 Embrasure rest seat.

- RPI (R, rest; P, proximal plate; I, I-bar) (Figure 13.23).
  - o Teeth: premolars.
  - o Location: R, mesial occlusal rest; P, distal proximal plate; I-bar, on the buccal cervical one-third of the tooth below the HOCL.
  - o Shape: M occlusal rest, D proximal guide plane.
  - o Dimensions: M occlusal rest one-third of buccal–lingual width, 2.5 mm sides of triangle, 1.5 reduction of marginal ridge, center deepest point. For I-bar on buccal if undercut not present, enameloplasty the plane or create a dimple for a 0.01 inch (0.25 mm) undercut the shape of the retentive tip.
  - o Miscellaneous: less torque on tooth versus C-clasp.
  - o Prep distal guideplane before rest seat for proper mesial–distal dimension.
  - o Contraindicated if deep soft tissue undercut, frenum, shallow vestibule use RPA or back-action clasp:
    - ▪ RPA: M rest, D proximal plate with C-clasp engaging the MF.
    - ▪ Back-action clasp: M rest and clasp engaging MF, for canines or premolars.
- Guideplanes
  - o Enameloplasty to create parallelism between adjacent teeth to an edentulous space.
  - o If placing a rest seat, first create the guideplane. If done in reverse, the rest seat will be too short mesiodistally.
- Lowering the HOCL (Figure 13.24): enameloplasty with diamond bur.
- Raising the HOCL (creating an undercut on a tooth with no undercut) (Figure 13.25).
  - o Dimpling: create a dimple in the shape of and for the retentive tip of a C-clasp at least 1 mm away from the gingival margin.
  - o Adding bulk with composite.
  - o Crowning the tooth, instructing the lab to add undercut.

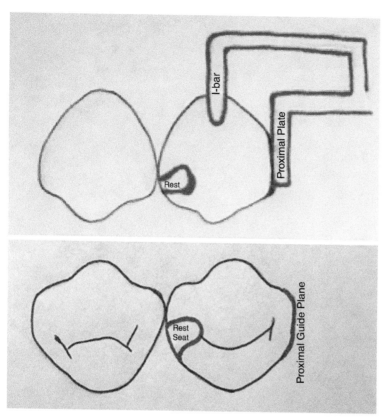

Figure 13.23 RPI.

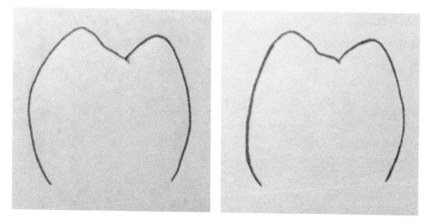

Figure 13.24 Lowering the HOCL.

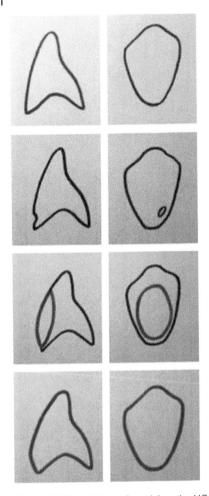

Figure 13.25 Options for raising the HOCL.

- **Final impression**
  - Remove any calculus on teeth.
  - Mark the vibrating line ("aaah") and hamular notches to transfer mark to model.
  - Check for any undercuts of the ridge and block out by drying and placing rope wax to prevent impression from locking in.
  - Border molding: only border mold edentulous areas (for both tooth supported and distal extension)
    o Final impression techniques
      ▪ With a custom tray with no wax spacer:
        a) Heavy body on periphery and edentulous areas (not teeth). Border mold moving cheeks/tongue/lips.
        b) Once set, remove tray. Place medium body over teeth, blow air to capture anatomy/ rest seats, and load tray with medium body, and seat.

- With a custom tray with wax spacer
    a) Border mold using heavy body PVS with wax spacers on intaglio of custom tray.
    b) Remove wax spacers and make impression with light body PVS.
- Evaluate the final impression
  - For mandibular Kennedy I/II: has distal extension been properly captured? If not, plan altered cast technique at framework try-in appointment.
- Fluoride varnish to decrease sensitivity of teeth with enameloplasty.
- Planning altered cast technique (mandibular Kennedy I/II)? Request from lab to place saddle on framework for distal extensions.
- Draw partial design on lab prescription form or on a duplicated model.
- Use a sharpened red/blue pencil, with red for retentive undercuts, and blue for other elements. Draw accurately so less guesswork for lab technician [4].

Appointment 3: Framework Try-In, Altered Cast Technique, WOR/Bite/Shades

Framework Try-In

- Inspect framework:
  - Remove any small blebs or artifacts with high-speed bur.
  - Check fit on model.
- Carefully seat framework.
- Tight/not seating initially.
  - Occlude spray.
  - Chloroform and rouge (only for evaluating fit of metal, not acrylic; can melt acrylic):
    o Shave with scalpel, mix with chloroform in Dappen dish.
    o Apply to framework with brush.
    o Make sure chloroform has evaporated before inserting (halothane is a safer alternative).
    o Trim burn-through with carbide bur.
    o Remove rouge with chloroform and cotton tip applicator.
- Check if there is any space between major connector and soft tissue (Figure 13.26).
- Check if the rest seats are fully engaged (Figure 13.27).
- Check if the clasps are contacting abutment teeth.
- Check if the clasps are impinging the gingiva. If so, require adjustment by dentist or repositioning by lab technician.
- Check occlusion
  - Teeth occluding?
  - Teeth occluding on metal rests/clasps? See Figure 13.14. Adjust the metal, taking care not to make it thin/brittle (not less than 1.5 mm). May have to deepen the rest seat and make a new final impression. Alternative is to adjust the opposing tooth.
- Tight/*still* not seating. Are extensive adjustments and time required for framework to seat intraorally?
  - Redo final impression. Poor fit may be from inaccurate impression, inaccurate pour, warped impression material, poured impression stood too long.

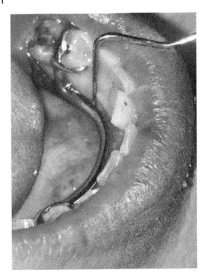

Figure 13.26 At the framework try-in appointment, a gap was noted between the lingual bar and the ridge.

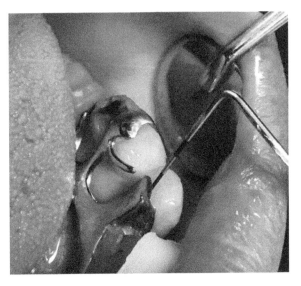

Figure 13.27 At the framework try-in appointment, the metal framework is not contacting the distal of #21 and the cingulum rest on #22 is not contacting the cingulum rest seat. Note that on some occasions there may be a space and once the patient bites down the framework might seat completely, eliminating the space.

Altered Cast Technique

- Altered cast technique is used typically for mandibular Kennedy class I/II, in which the lingual–alveolar anatomy is not properly captured (Figure 13.28).
- After ensuring good fit with framework, on the model place separating medium (e.g. Al-cote) and baseplate wax over the desired areas (distal extensions) 2–3 mm shy of vestibule. Sink the framework retentive network into the wax until the tissue stop contacts tissue. Add a layer of acrylic (e.g. Triad) over the retentive network covering the wax area to create an impression tray. Cure. Remove wax spacer, unless no tissue stop. Border mold, followed by light body PVS impression with no material between teeth and framework. Do not apply pressure on the edentulous area, only over rests. Send to lab to combine the master cast with the new model.

- Final impression:
  - Border mold
    - ○ Maxillary:
      - Open and close mouth.
      - Move jaw side to side.
      - Pull left cheek out and down.
      - Pull right cheek out and down.
      - Pull upper lip down.
      - Repeat steps.
    - ○ Mandibular:
      - Stick tongue out all the way, touch chin, reach to left ear, reach to right ear.
      - Relax mouth. Squeeze cheeks in.
      - Pull left cheek out and up.
      - Pull right cheek out and up.
      - Pull lower lip up.
      - Repeat steps.

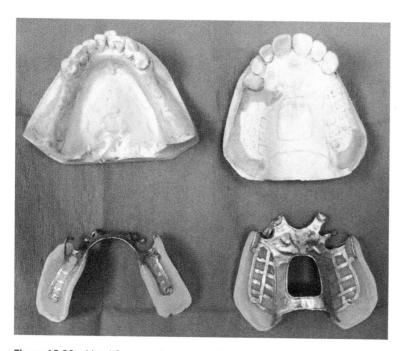

Figure 13.28 Metal frameworks were tried in to verify the fit. Acrylic was added for the edentulous areas in preparation for the altered cast impression.

WOR/Bite/Shades
- **WOR**
  - Verify the framework is fully seated.
  - In-house fabrication of WOR (Figure 13.29).
    - WOR dimensions: anterior, 6–8 mm wide; posterior, 8–10 mm wide; maxillary, 22 mm high; mandibular, 18 mm high.
  - WOR should be stable and a layer of wax should be on the intaglio of the framework retentive network. For mandibular distal extension, tissue stops should be flush with the wax (Figure 13.30).

Removable Partial Dentures

- VDO:
  - ○ If not opening VDO, adjust the wax until teeth in proper occlusion (Figure 13.31).
  - ○ If opening VDO:
    - ■ Obtain anterior overjet/overbite: 1.5–2 mm/0.5 mm. If no posterior stops present, adjust wax to obtain the following.
    - ■ Maxillary incisal display 2 mm (if young; with age, less maxillary incisal display and more mandibular incisal display).
    - ■ Mandibular occlusal plane at lower lip level.
  - ○ Patient able to close comfortably?
- Check phonetics:
  - ○ Tell the patient to say "Mississippi" and to count from 60 to 70.
    - ■ Check freeway space (closest speaking space, teeth/WOR should not occlude)
  - ○ Tell the patient to say "firefighter" and to count from 50 to 60.
    - ■ Maxillary central incisor edges should contact lower lip wet/dry line.
- Profile: convex or concave? Adjust the wax as needed.
- Ala tragus parallel to the WORs?
- Pupils parallel to the WORs?
- If anterior WOR: mark the smile line, midline, alas (distal of canines).
- Create nonparallel notches in WOR

- **Bite**
  - Obtain bite registration only of WORs and not of teeth, or will not occlude as captures too much detail in areas of opposing teeth.
- **Shades**
  - Gum shade: use the same gingiva guide the lab uses (varies by lab).
  - Tooth shade.
  - Tooth characteristics (ideal, diastema, etc.).
  - Patient approves?
  - Form of identification (ID).

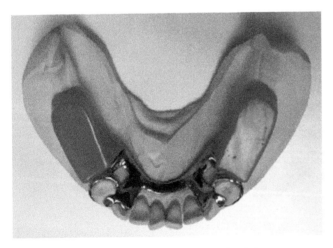

Figure 13.29 Metal framework with wax occlusal rims.

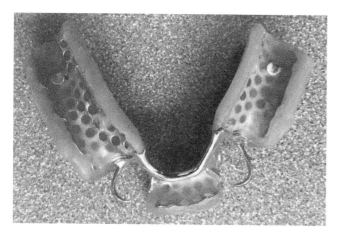

Figure 13.30   Tissue stops visible on the intaglio of the metal framework.

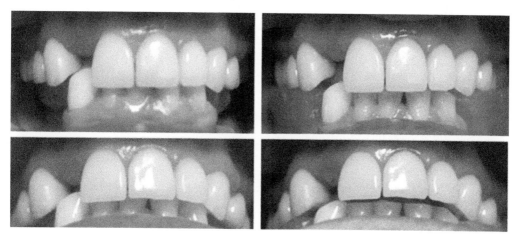

Figure 13.31   Opening the VDO with the wax occlusal rims.

Appointment 4: Tooth Try-In

- Evaluate the framework and occlusion of the tooth set up on the articulator (Figure 13.32).
- Try in the mouth and verify that the framework is fully seated.
- Check for overextended flanges. If adjustments required, adjust and seat on model and mark with pencil. Carve outline with small bur and ask lab to not remove beading on intaglio of acrylic resin. At delivery, use beading on intaglio to adjust in house.
- Check occlusion: patient bites ("tap, tap") on red/blue horseshoe articulating paper (checking MICP, or maximum intercuspation).
  - If trying to maintaining the same VDO:
    - ○ Check occlusion without partials.
    - ○ Insert one partial at a time and check if occlusion is the same as without the partial. If different, reposition denture teeth until occlusion is the same.
    - ○ Option: check occlusion without partial in one color and with partial in another color.
  - Adequate overjet of posterior teeth to prevent cheek biting?
  - Check lateral excursions: if replacing most posterior teeth, are teeth in group function?
  - With the mouth mirror make sure all posteriors are in occlusion. If not:
    - ○ Heat wax, remove the tooth, add wax, reposition the tooth and check if in proper occlusion, *or*
    - ○ Place bite registration only where teeth not occluding. Send the case back to the lab to reset those teeth and return for another tooth try-in appointment.

- Bite on articulating paper and tug on left side; repeat with right to check for even bite.
- Obtain bite registration. Compare the bite registration in the mouth to the mounted models with partials. If not the same, request the lab to remount the case.
- Check esthetics
  - Midline: off/on.
  - Profile: convex/concave/ideal.
  - Maxillary incisal display at rest: 1–2 mm (less with age).
  - Lateral incisor 0.5 mm shorter than central incisor and canine.
  - Anterior overjet/overbite: 1.5–2 mm/0.5 mm (see Chapter 12, Figure 12.47).
  - Canted? (Figure 13.33)
  - Gingival margin matches partial gumline? (Figure 13.34)
  - Size/shape of teeth match adjacent? (Figure 13.34)
  - Upper lip line at upper gingival margin (not a gummy smile).
  - Lower lip line at level of lower incisal edges.
  - Tooth shade: patient approval (not whiter than sclera of eye).
  - Patient approves esthetics?
- Check phonetics (see Chapter 12, Figure 12.55).
  - "S" sound:
    - "Mississippi," count 60–69.
    - Freeway space, closest speaking space.
  - "F" sound:
    - "Firefighter," count 50–59.
    - Teeth 8/9 at lower lip wet/dry line.
  - "Th" sound:
    - "This, that, there"
    - Tongue protruding between anteriors 2–4 mm.
  - "P/B" sound:
    - Lips close, teeth do not contact.
  - Be sure no remaining wax on teeth, or will be replaced with pink acrylic.
  - Have the patient sign the prosthesis processing consent form (see Chapter 12, section Consent Forms).

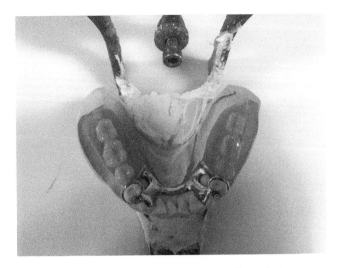

Figure 13.32 Partial denture tooth set up on the articulator.

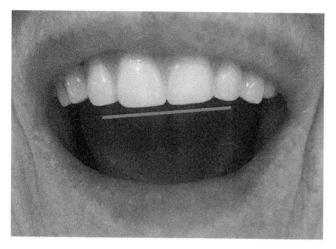

Figure 13.33 Teeth canted at the tooth try-in appointment.

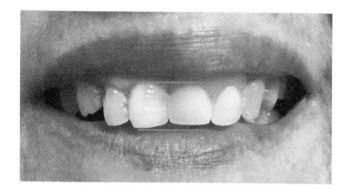

Figure 13.34 Evaluate the gingival margin and tooth shape and size at the tooth try-in appointment.

Appointment 5: Delivery

- Evaluate partial for:
  - Undercuts in the acrylic which will pinch or ulcerate the soft tissue when inserting (Figures 13.35 and 13.36).
  - Acrylic beyond the internal bevel (overlapping the major connector). This will prevent partial from seating.
  - Check for acrylic covering tissue stops on mandibular distal extensions.
- Carefully try in
  - Do not force it to seat as the partial can lock in or break.
  - Insert until encounter interference. If interference, use indicator mediums, check for burn-through, and adjust burn-through and insert.
  - Ask the patient to point to where they are feeling any pressure/pinching.
- Adjust the partial as necessary.
- Check for frenum clearance. If impinging, the patient will return with a traumatic ulceration.
- Verify patient can insert/remove. Inform patient that whichever way the partial goes in (path of insertion), it will come out the opposite.

- Schedule a one-week follow-up as it very common for patients to have sore spots which require partial adjustments.
- Provide goody bag (denture brush and container for partial; toothbrush, floss, toothpaste for dentition).
- See Section Postoperative Instructions.

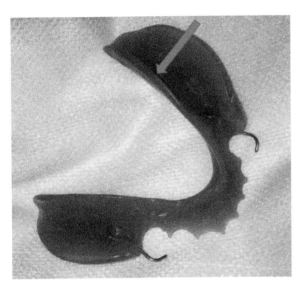

Figure 13.35 Evaluate the intaglio of the partial before seating in the mouth.

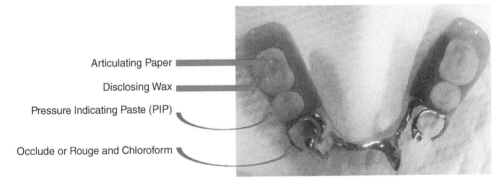

Figure 13.36 At the delivery appointment, different materials are used to evaluate different aspects of the partials: articulating paper to evaluate the occlusion; disclosing wax to evaluate the flanges; PIP for the intaglio; and Occlude or rouge and chloroform to evaluate the metal framework.

Appointment 6+: Adjustments

- Address the chief complaints.
- Ask patient if any sore spots, and adjust the partial as necessary.
- Evaluate the soft tissues.
- Locate sore spot, mark with Thompson stick, seat partial, remove to transfer mark, adjust with acrylic bur, seat, and check if relief.

Appointment: Recall Exam

- Return for recall exams and cleanings for both teeth and partials (Figure 13.37).
- Partials may require relines, repairs, and remakes (Table 13.3).

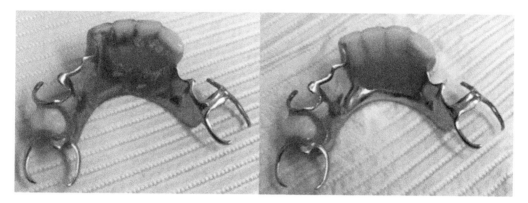

Figure 13.37 Calculus on a partial before and after removal.

Repairs, Relines, Repositions, Additions, and What the Lab Needs from You

Table 13.3 Repairs, relines, repositions, additions, and what the lab needs from you.

Repair type	What the lab needs
Repairs[a]	
Clean break of acrylic resin (Figure 13.38)	Both halves if they fit perfectly. If not, a pick-up impression
Missing piece of acrylic resin, e.g. dog bite (Figure 13.39)	Pick-up impression
Clean break of cast metal major connector (RPD) (Figure 13.3)	Pick-up impression (no opposing needed) for the lab tech to weld the metal together. This is a temporary solution (will not hold up long term) and recommend fabricating a new RPD
Clean break of cast metal minor connector Missing clasp/rest	Pick-up impression with the partial. The lab tech will attach a new minor connector
Missing half of the denture (Figure 13.40)	Lab tech could attempt to repair but may be unrepairable
Relines[b]	
Partial denture reline	Remove any undercuts on the acrylic resin and knife-edge flanges and make vent holes with a #8 round bur. Place reline material. Seat the partial and hold the metal framework. Do not apply pressure on distal extensions. Border mold (move cheeks, tongue, and lips). At reline delivery, check for frenum clearance. If impinging, patient will return with a traumatic ulceration. Check for undercuts in the acrylic, may pinch or cut the soft tissue when inserting

(Continued)

Table 13.3 (Continued)

Repair type	What the lab needs
Partial denture reline of only one area	Relieve any undercuts with acrylic bur (and knife-edge flanges) and make vent holes with a #8 round bur. Reline with material (e.g. Coe-Comfort or border mold with heavy body PVS and wash with light body PVS) only of that area and have patient bite into occlusion. Send partial to lab
Complete denture reline	Relieve any undercuts with acrylic bur (and knife-edge flanges) and make vent holes with a #8 round bur. Reline with material (e.g. Coe-Comfort or border mold with heavy body PVS and wash with light body PVS). If sending two arches place in separate plastic bags so reline material does not stick together
Functional reline (denture)	For a patient who has an old ill-fitting denture and is not ready to commit to a hard reline, can offer a functional reline. Relieve any undercuts with the acrylic bur (and knife-edge flanges) and make vent holes with a #8 round bur. And reline with material (e.g. Coe-Soft). Have the patient wear the denture in function and return. During this time do not have the patient brush the inside, but only use cold water and wet cotton to clean. The patient should use the denture brush only to clean the outside. If happy with the new fit, send to the lab for a hard reline
Repositioning[a]	
Repositioning clasp (stayplate)	Remove clasp with high-speed bur and make pick-up impression. Prescribe where to reposition clasp (e.g. impinging soft tissue, place more occlusal; or clasp not engaging tooth positioned too buccal, reposition to engage the mesial buccal of tooth)
Reposition (reset) teeth that are canted (denture) (Figure 13.41)	• At the tooth try-in visit, if the upper teeth are canted first determine which side (left or right) is at the proper height. Inscribe in the wax the ideal position for the new gumline. Helps to send photos of the case to the lab • At the delivery stage, if the upper teeth are canted, mark the new ideal position for the gumline and send back for the teeth to be set in wax again for another try-in. Helps to send photos of the case to the lab
Reposition (reset) teeth to the proper midline (denture) (Figure 13.42)	• At the tooth try-in visit, inscribe the new midline on the upper and lower wax rims and send back to reset the teeth for another try-in • At the delivery stage, if the midline is off, mark the new midline with a permanent marker[c] and send back to the lab to set the teeth in wax for another try-in
Repositioning tooth/teeth into occlusion at tooth try-in (Figures 13.43 and 13.44)	Options: • In-house melt the wax and reposition tooth before sending to the lab • Obtain bite registration only over occlusal of teeth desired to be repositioned
Repositioning tooth/teeth into occlusion after delivery	• Stayplate: section off segment of denture resin and tooth. Pick-up impression, opposing, and bite • Cast metal RPD: pick-up impression • Denture: place bite registration only in the area where the teeth do not occlude, reset teeth, and another try-in
Reposition teeth that appear intruded due to resorption after delivery of an immediate stayplate	Opposing model. Bite registration. Reline stayplate and pick-up impression of stayplate. May require new teeth for an even gingival margin
At the tooth try-in the patient feels their lower jaw is retruded or protruded (denture)	Remove all the teeth on the lower denture, add wax to obtain the proper VDO, and obtain a new bite. Send to the lab to reset the lower teeth for another try-in

Table 13.3 (Continued)

Repair type	What the lab needs
Increasing the VDO or decreasing the VDO (denture)	Determine if intruding or extruding the upper or lower teeth. If the upper gumline and incisal display is ideal, intrude, or retrude the lower teeth. • If at the tooth try-in, send to the lab to reset the teeth for another try-in • If at the delivery, send to the lab to set the teeth in wax for another try-in
Additions[a]	
Adding denture tooth due to loss of retention	Bite registration, pick-up impression, and opposing (to determine occlusion)
Adding new denture tooth/clasp after an extraction (stayplate/RPD) (Figure 13.45)	Extraction of tooth. Placement of Teflon tape over socket. Bite registration. Pick-up impression. Make opposing impression. Send to the lab to add a denture tooth and clasp
Adding a new clasp (stayplate/RPD)	Pick-up impression
Adding denture base material to an upper denture that did not reach and/or missing the PPS (denture) (Figure 13.46)	Add wax to the upper denture to support the reline material from sagging. Make vent holes with a #8 round bur. Reline the posterior with material (e.g. Coe-Comfort). Make sure the material extended to the PPS. Send to the lab for a hard reline
Miscellaneous	
Teeth are too short at the try-in (denture)	Determine if the gumline is ideal. If not, inscribe the ideal gumline level. If so determine the new tooth length by approximating how many millimeters. Keep in mind this will change the incisal display at rest and VDO. Send back to the lab to replace the teeth. Helps to send photos of the case to the lab
Teeth are too long at the try-in (denture) (Figures 13.47 and 13.48)	Determine if the gumline is ideal. If not, inscribe the ideal gumline level. Mark the teeth with a permanent marker to the desired length and send back to the lab to replace the teeth. Keep in mind this will change the incisal display at rest and VDO. Helps to send photos of the case to the lab
Gummy smile (Figures 13.49 and 13.50)	• At try-in, inscribe the desired gumline and send to lab to reset the teeth for another try-in. Note this will decrease the VDO and can change the incisal display. Helps to send photos of the case to the lab • At delivery, mark the desired gumline with a permanent marker and send to the lab to reset the teeth in wax for another try-in. Note this will decrease the VDO and can change the incisal display. Helps to send photos of the case to the lab
Ill-fitting metal framework (RPD)	Make a new impression and send to the lab for a new framework
Chairside • Clean break repair • Hard reline • Soft reline • Adding a denture tooth	See Chapter 12

Removable Partial Dentures

Contact the lab technician you work with to ask if they have any specific preferences.
See Chapter 11 for seven scenarios involving removable partial dentures/complete dentures.
[a] With any repair, reposition, or addition, check if a reline is indicated to prevent sending the prosthesis to the lab twice.
[b] Relines: with relines use a round #8 bur to drill ventilation holes into the palate of upper dentures and lingual ridge and retromolar pad of lower dentures for the excess reline material to prevent increasing the VDO. Always check the VDO before and after the reline. Depending on the type of reline material, may require an adhesive. The lab may offer a heat-cured soft reline material for patients who have no retention even after a hard reline.
[c] Permanent marker comes off the denture acrylic with alcohol.

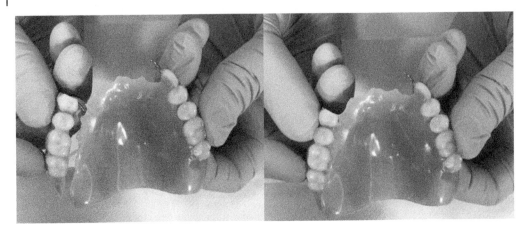

Figure 13.38   Clean break.

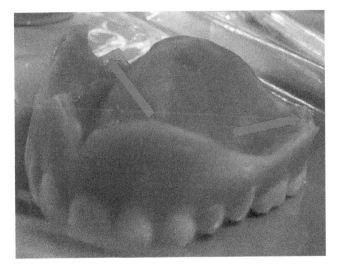

Figure 13.39   Dog bite.

Figure 13.40   Unrepairable.

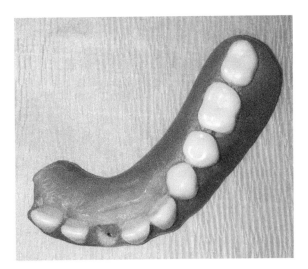

Figure 13.41 Canted teeth.

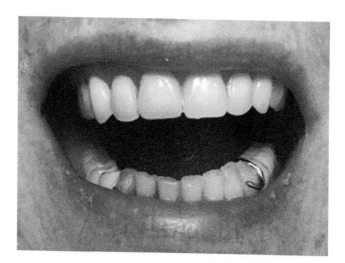

Figure 13.42 Accurate midline inscribed in the wax and marked on the model.

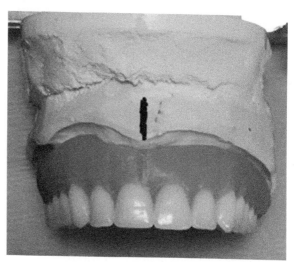

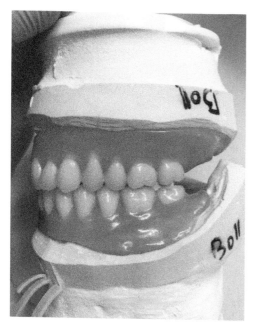

Figure 13.43 Molars not in proper occlusion.

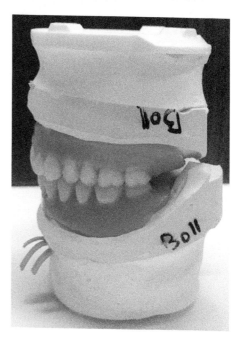

Figure 13.44 Molars now in occlusion.

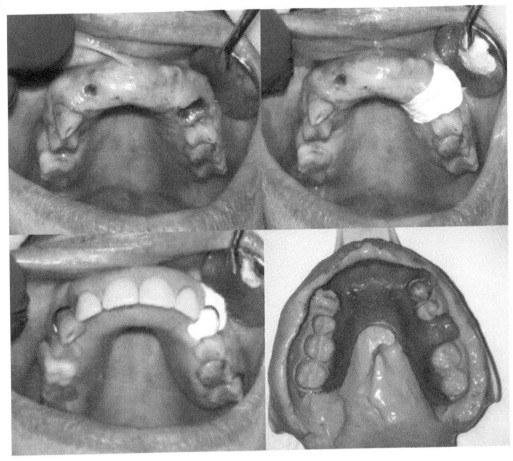

Figure 13.45 Adding a denture tooth and clasp after an extraction.

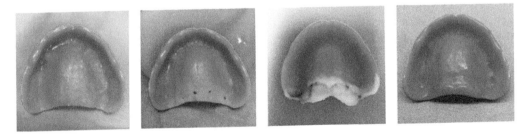

Figure 13.46 Extending the base to include the PPS.

Figure 13.47 At the tooth try-in, the teeth were too long and marked to the desired length.

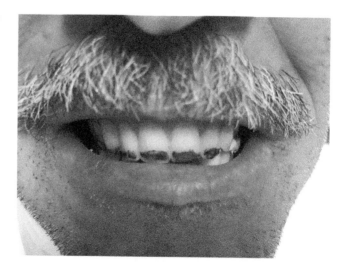

Figure 13.48 At the second tooth try-in, the teeth were at the desired length.

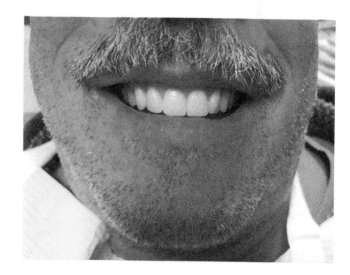

Figure 13.49 A denture and partial were delivered and at the visit the patient smiled much more than at the tooth try-in appointment. The patient now had a "gummy smile." The desired gumline was marked.

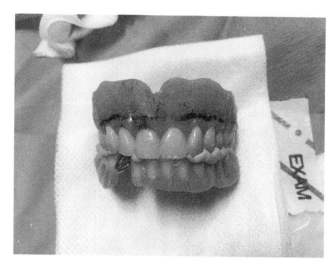

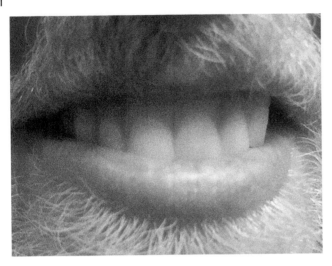

Figure 13.50   An unesthetic "gummy smile" at the delivery appointment.

Stayplates (Also Known as Acrylic Resin Partial, Interim Partial, Treatment Partial, Transitional Partial, Flipper)

- Stayplates are made of acrylic resin with wrought wire clasps. See Figure 13.51.
- Sequence options: always best to make study models (from diagnostic impression) for careful planning. Skipping this step (as a shortcut) can result in more time spent on the case.
- Stable occlusion, replacing few teeth and nonesthetic case:
  - Warn patient that there is no opportunity to try in to check occlusion, phonetics or esthetics. If unhappy with results, have to start over.
  - Appointment 1: diagnostic impressions, evaluation.
  - Appointment 2: impressions, bite, shades, ID.
  - Appointment 3: delivery. PIP and adjust burn-through (Figure 13.53), and verify patient can insert and remove (see Section Postoperative Instructions).
- Stable occlusion, esthetic case:
  - Appointment 1: diagnostic impressions, evaluation.
  - Appointment 2: impressions, bite, shades, ID.
  - Appointment 3: tooth try-in (will be loose because no clasps). Have the patient sign the prosthesis processing consent form (see Chapter 12, section Consent Forms).
  - Appointment 4: delivery. PIP and adjust burn-through (Figure 13.53), and verify patient can insert and remove (see Section Postoperative Instructions).
- Collapsed bite/replacing many teeth/supraerupted and tipped teeth/esthetic case:
  - Appointment 1: diagnostic impressions, evaluation.
    - Tooth modifications?
      - Supraerupted teeth: enameloplasty.
      - Undesirable undercuts: enameloplasty, guideplanes.
      - Adequate undercut: 0.03 inch (0.75 mm) WW.
      - Inadequate undercut: dimpling, adding composite for occlusion or crown.
      - Occlusal embrasure space for ball-end clasps?
      - Design stayplate (see Figure 13.52).
  - Appointment 2: tooth modifications/final impressions.
  - Appointment 3: WORs, bite, shades, ID.

- Appointment 4: tooth try-in (will be loose because no clasps). Have the patient sign the prosthesis processing consent form (see Chapter 12, section Consent Forms).
- Appointment 5: delivery. PIP and adjust burn-through (see Figure 13.53), and verify patient can insert and remove (see Section Postoperative Instructions).

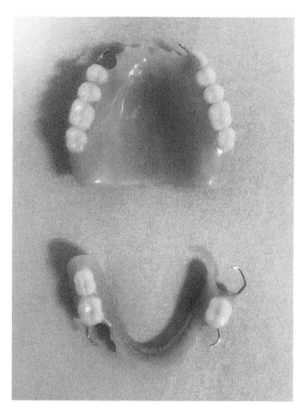

Figure 13.51 Stayplates.

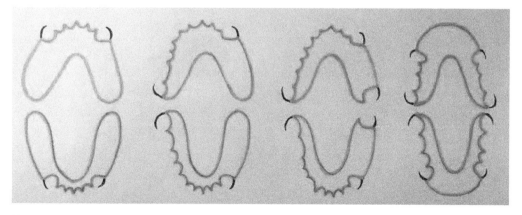

Figure 13.52 Author's stayplate designs for Kennedy Class I, II, III, and IV. For Class II/III consider also adding a ball end clasp if occlusal clearance permits.

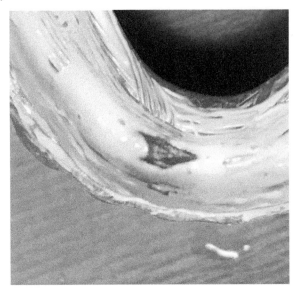

Figure 13.53 Example of burn-through requiring adjusting.

Flexible Partials

Sequence options are similar to those for stayplates (see preceding section). However, the main differences are as follows.

- Clasp types.
- Contraindications:
  - Replacing upper anteriors with a deep bite (>4 mm).
  - Flared teeth.
  - Interocclusal space <5 mm.
- Gingiva shade guide (varies based on brand).
- Diagnostic impressions and evaluation.
  - Survey abutment teeth with clasp options in mind.
    - Enameloplasty:
      - Around teeth necessary for circumferential clasps, continuous clasps, or combination clasps.
      - To create an undercut for conventional clasps. Alternative to creating an undercut with a diamond bur is to build up tooth surface (buccal or facial) with composite.
    - Consider what enameloplasty is necessary for clasp options.
- Clasps: can rest on tissue, tooth, or both.
- Clasp options (Figure 13.54):
  - Conventional clasp:
    - Similar to a WW C-clasp in shape.
    - Requires 0.5 mm (0.02 inch) or greater undercut [6].

- Circumferential clasp/ring clasp:
  - ○ 360° around the tooth.
  - ○ Must fit passively around the tooth.
  - ○ For lone standing posteriors.
  - ○ For non-lone standing posteriors: requires occlusal embrasure space or will interfere with bite. This may require enameloplasty of adjacent marginal ridges.
- Continuous circumferential clasp: surrounds multiple teeth and wraps around the most distal tooth.
- Combination clasp: circumferential clasp around an abutment tooth with a conventional clasp on the adjacent abutment tooth.
- See Section Lab Prescription.
- Delivery steps
  - Immerse in hot water for one minute, then cool for patient to tolerate. Allows smooth insertion/good adaptation.
  - Adjusting clasps (if indicated): for loose or tight clasp, immerse only the clasp in hot water and bend (Figure 13.55).
  - Adjusting the base (if indicated):
    - ○ Check fit with PIP.
    - ○ Adjustment requires thermoplastic adjusting stones, polishing kit and a scalpel to remove tags. Carbide and diamond burs will melt the partial.
  - Verify the patient can insert/remove.
  - See Section Postoperative Instructions.

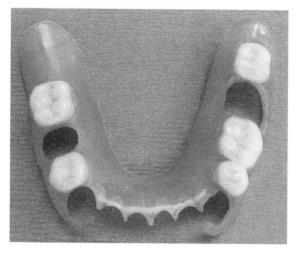

Figure 13.54 Flexible partial with both circumferential clasps and conventional clasps.

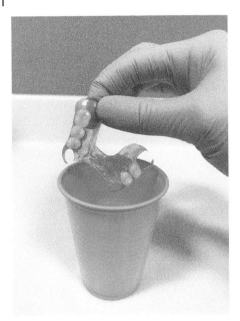

Figure 13.55 Immersing the flexible partial in hot water.

Essix Appliances

- Sequence options:
  - In-house fabrication for same-day delivery.
  - In-house fabrication for next-day delivery.
  - Lab fabricated (see Section Lab Prescriptions).
- In-house fabrication for same-day delivery (Figure 13.56).
  - Make upper and lower impressions, bite registration, tooth shade.
  - Pour and trim models.
  - Place a denture tooth to replace the missing tooth (this tooth will be retained in the Essix appliance).
    - If a denture tooth is not available:
      - Use a stainless steel crown.
      - Build up the tooth with packable composite on the model, light curing the layers.
      - Do a wax-up of the tooth, soak the model for 30 minutes and duplicate the model. If the model is not duplicated, the wax will melt from the hot vacuform stent.
  - Make sure the tooth being replaced is in proper occlusion. Hand articulate the models.
  - Use the vacuum former with a clear stent material (0.02 inch).
  - Trim the stent material 2 mm beyond the gingival margin of *all* the teeth in the arch.
  - On the model, use rope wax to block out the undercuts on the teeth adjacent to the missing tooth.
  - Fill in increments with flowable or packable composite with the matching shade and light cure.
  - Deliver and verify the patient can insert and remove the Essix appliance.
  - Optional: give the patient their model to store in case they lose or damage their Essix appliance before a long-term appliance or restoration is placed. This will save time making the replacement.
  - See Section Postoperative Instructions.

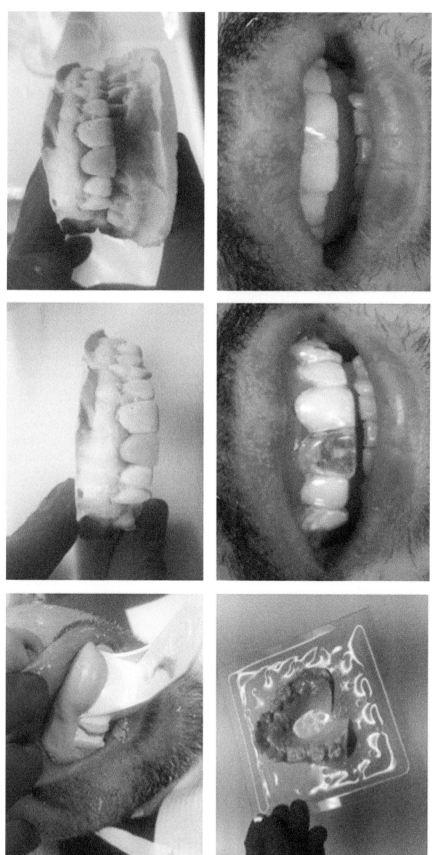

Figure 13.56 Fabricating an Essix appliance.

Immediate Partials

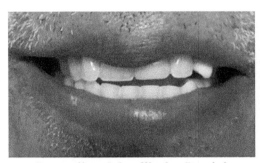 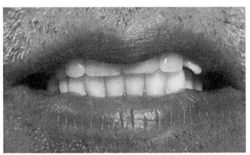

Immediate Mandibular Partial
Occlusion is off.

New Mandibular Partial
In proper occlusion.

Figure 13.57 Immediate partial and new partial.

The patient shown in Figure 13.57 was unhappy with the immediate mandibular partial because of the bite and appearance (anterior open bite). With immediate partials there is no opportunity for a tooth try-in appointment to check occlusion, phonetics, and esthetics. A new mandibular partial was fabricated which included a tooth try-in appointment and at delivery the patient was satisfied.

- Setting expectations:
  - No opportunity for a try-in appointment to check esthetics, phonetics, and occlusion.
  - The ridge will resorb (shrink) when healing and the immediate partial will become more loose over time (Figure 13.58). Recommend a reline or new partials two to three months (three is safer) after extractions. Note that most resorption will occur during the first year.
- Appointment 1: diagnostic impressions, bite, shades, ID (or final impressions)
  - Impressions (either diagnostic or final)
    - o Diagnostic impressions:
      - ▪ Evaluate to determine if teeth require enameloplasty for supraerupted teeth, tilted teeth, creation of guideplanes.
      - ▪ Prep teeth and final impression.
    - o Final impressions.
  - Obtain tooth shade, gum shade, and ID.
  - See Section Lab Prescriptions.
- Appointment 2: extractions and delivery
  - Verify the immediate partial is back from the lab and that the correct teeth have been replaced.
  - Extract teeth.
  - Try in, place PIP paste, and adjust burn-through.
  - Verify the patient can insert/remove.
  - See Section Postoperative Instructions.
- Appointment 3: adjustments.

Figure 13.58 Note the amount of space between teeth #5 and #6 and the ridge one month after extraction of #5 and #6 due to ridge resorption.

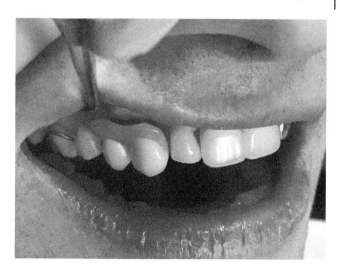

Complete Dentures Opposing Cast Metal RPDs

See Chapter 12, section Complete Denture Opposing Cast Metal RPD.

Lab Prescriptions

Cast Metal RPDs

- Impressions to custom trays
  - Pour models and fabricate custom trays for PVS final impressions
  - Return for final impressions
- Final impressions to framework/WORs
  - Pour models and fabricate the RPD metal framework
  - Follow the design as drawn:
    - o Maxillary major connectors:
      - Anterior–posterior palatal strap ___
      - Mid/posterior palatal strap ___
      - Metal palate with metal grid in post-dam for acrylic ___
      - U-shaped/horseshoe/anterior palatal strap ___
    - o Mandibular major connectors:
      - Lingual bar ___
      - Lingual plate ___
    - o Clasp type:
      - C-clasp on teeth # ___
      - RPI on teeth # ___
      - RPA on teeth # ___
      - Ring clasp on teeth # ___
      - Back action on teeth # ___
      - Other: ___ on teeth # ___
    - o [Mesial/distal] Rests on teeth # ___
    - o Cingulum rest on teeth # ___
    - o Retentive network in edentulous areas ___

- o Add tissue stop on the mandibular/maxillary distal extensions ___
- o Add metal pin/stud for tube tooth # ___
- – Fabricate WORs in edentulous areas.
- – Return for framework try-in and wax bite appointment
- Framework/altered cast impression to WORs
  - – Pour final impression of the distal extension(s)
  - – Combine altered cast model with the master cast
  - – Fabricate WORs in edentulous areas
  - – Return for wax bite appointment
- Framework/WORs to tooth set-up
  - – Mount case and set teeth # ___
  - – Tooth shade: ___
  - – Return for tooth try-in
- Tooth set-up to process
  - – Process and finish case
  - – Gum shade: ___
  - – ID: ___
  - – Return for delivery

Stayplates

- Impressions to WORs
  - – Pour models and add WORs replacing teeth # ___
- WORs/bite to tooth set-up
  - – Mount case and set teeth # ___
  - – Tooth shade:
  - – Follow design as drawn
  - – Return for tooth try-in
- Tooth set-up to process
  - – Follow the design as drawn
    - o Add WW C-clasp to teeth # ___ engaging the ___ (MF undercut, DF undercut)
    - o Add ball-end clasp between teeth # ___ and # ___ engaging the buccal gingival embrasure
  - – Gum shade: ___
  - – ID: ___
  - – Add beadline for seal
  - – Process and finish case
  - – Return for delivery

Clinical pearl: Request the lab to duplicate the master cast prior to processing the stayplate and making adjustments on the stayplate to remove any soft/hard tissue interferences to minimize adjustments and save time at the delivery. Saves time especially when replacing several nonadjacent teeth.

Flexible Partials

Similar to stayplate lab prescriptions. However, the main differences are as follows.

- Different gum shade (guide): ___
- Follow the design as drawn:
  - – Add standard clasp (C-clasp) to teeth # ___ engaging the ___ (MF undercut, DF undercut)
  - – Add circumferential clasp around tooth # ___
  - – Add continuous circumferential clasp around teeth # ___
  - – Add combination clasp around teeth # ___

Essix Appliances

- Included upper/lower impressions (or models) and bite registration
- Tooth shade: ___
- Please fabricate an Essix appliance covering all teeth in the arch replacing tooth # ___
- Return for delivery

Immediate Partials

- Please fabricate [maxillary/mandibular] immediate partial denture
- Teeth planned for extraction: #___
- Remove teeth #___ and set denture teeth #___
  - Tooth shade: ___
  - Gum shade: ___
  - ID: ___
  - Follow the design as drawn:
    - Add WW C-clasp to teeth #___ engaging the ___ (MF/MB undercut, DF/DB undercut)
    - Add ball-end clasp between teeth # ___ and # ___ engaging the buccal gingival embrasure
    - Add beadline for seal
- Return for delivery

Postoperative Instructions

Provide the patient with thorough postoperative instructions, both verbal and written, along with oral hygiene products. Products include a toothbrush, floss, and toothpaste for the dentition, and a tongue scraper for the tongue. Partial denture products include a denture container, and may include denture adhesives, and denture cleansers. See Figure 13.59.

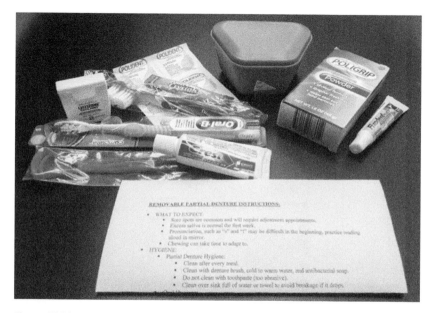

Figure 13.59 Provide the patient with both verbal and written instructions for taking care of their oral health.

Removable Partial Denture Instructions

- What to expect
  - Sore spots are common and will require adjustment appointments.
  - Excess saliva is normal during the first week.
  - Pronunciations such as "s" and "f" may be difficult in the beginning, so practice reading aloud in mirror.
  - Chewing can take time to adapt to.
- Hygiene
  - Partial denture hygiene:
    - Clean the partial after every meal
      - Clean with a denture brush, cold to warm water, and antibacterial soap.
      - Do not clean with toothpaste (too abrasive).
      - Clean over sink full of water or towel to avoid breakage if it drops.
  - Oral hygiene:
    - It is important to maintain good oral hygiene as partials increase retention of plaque and risk of getting cavities.
    - Brush after breakfast with the partials out of mouth.
    - Floss and brush at bedtime with the partials out of mouth.
- Storage
  - Do not wear the partials when you sleep. The gums need adequate blood circulation and you can develop fungal infections from overwearing, especially with poor hygiene.
- Always keep the partials moist whether:
  - In the mouth.
  - In a container with water (away from pets).
  - In a sealed bag with water.
  - If it becomes dehydrated it will warp and no longer fit.
- Precautions
  - Do not bite the partial into place: insert and remove with both hands.
  - Do not drop the partials as they can break.
  - Do not store the partials in a napkin, tissue, or paper towel as these get accidently thrown away.
  - Careful with hot foods and drinks. May burn the tissue.
  - If a partial denture is not worn regularly the teeth will migrate and the bite can change, resulting in a partial that may no longer fit. This can create a challenge for making new partials in the future and this may require additional procedures.
- Future appointments
  - Return for recall exams and cleanings for both your teeth and partials.
  - Partials may require relines, repairs, and remakes.

  If you have flexible partials
  - Cleaning:
    - Clean with cold water and antibacterial soap. Do not use hot water as the partial will warp and may no longer fit.

o Do not clean the partial with a toothbrush as it will lose its polish, become rough, and retain debris.
   - Remove at night and store the appliance in water in a container away from pets.
- **If you have an Essix appliance**
   - This appliance is to be used only for appearance and for short-term use.
   - This appliance is not to be worn when eating.
   - Cleaning:
      o Clean with cold water, antibacterial soap, and a soft toothbrush.
      o Do not use hot water as the plastic will warp and the appliance may no longer fit.
   - Remove at night and store the appliance dry in a container away from pets.

Clinical Pearls

Troubleshooting

- At the partial denture tooth try-in appointment requiring a tooth reset (or different teeth) because of esthetics and/or occlusion:
   - Obtain a new bite registration to verify the mounting, and for the lab.
   - If time permits, reposition the teeth.
   - Take photos to send to lab. If patient has high esthetic demands, ask your lab technician if the patient can schedule a "custom" tooth shape and tooth shade match.
- At the partial denture delivery appointment:
   - If heavy occlusion is on one side of the mouth at delivery, adjust on that heavy side until the teeth contact on the contralateral side and the bite feels even.
   - If some posterior denture teeth are not in occlusion:
      o Recontour the tooth anatomy by bonding composite.
      o Scrub the bonding agent on the denture tooth, dry, light cure, add packable composite to shape the tooth to ideal, light cure, check occlusion, and adjust.
   - If there is a diastema you want to close, bond composite to recontour the tooth to close (or narrow) the proximal contact.
- Trouble obtaining the distal anatomy of the last molar with alginate impressions: apply alginate with your finger behind the distal of the most distal tooth, then seat the loaded tray (with alginate) front to back.
- If a patient complains of trauma to the upper edentulous ridge opposing lower anterior teeth:
   - Consider adjusting any sharp edges on the lower anteriors.
   - Can fabricate a soft lower occlusal guard.
- Partial denture design with only one remaining mandibular tooth: request lab to fabricate a mandibular partial and instead of metal clasp encircle tooth with dual laminate hard/soft material similar to occlusal guard (Figure 13.60).
- For more examples, see Chapter 12, section Troubleshooting.

Removable Partial Dentures

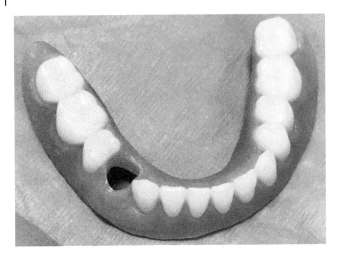

Figure 13.60 Partial denture with dual laminate material encircling the abutment tooth.

Tips

- I recommend having this book in your dental office.
  - Stratton, R.J. and Wiebelt, F.J. (1988). *An Atlas of Removable Partial Denture Design*. Chicago: Quintessence Books.
- Replace the word "take" with "make" so that the patient doesn't think of you as always taking things, like their time and money (e.g. "make an impression," "make a bite registration").
- Remove PIP from the partial with alcohol gauze wipe.
- Delivering stayplates:
  - Check with mouth mirror for any interferences preventing seating of the partial. If the contours of any teeth are prematurely contacting tooth structure, adjust.
  - Make sure the lower anterior teeth are not contacting the acrylic on the upper stayplate covering the hard palate.

Real-Life Clinical Scenarios Answered

Dental Students' Questions

- "How do I design the RPD?"
  - See Table 13.2.
- "When do I have to do a wax occlusal rim appointment for an RPD?"
  - When the patient has a collapsed bite, due to not having posterior stops, it is necessary to determine the patient's bite (VDO) with a WOR appointment. This can be done with cast metal RPDs, stayplates, and flexible partials (Figure 13.61).

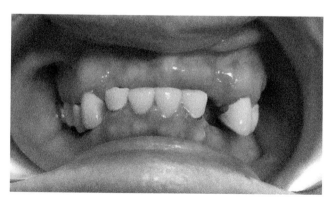

Figure 13.61 A patient with no posterior stops.

- "What is the altered cast technique?"
  - This technique is when an impression is made of the distal extension(s) using the metal framework, at the framework try-in, in order to obtain an accurate recording of the retromylo-hyoid fossa (for a better seal for retention and stability).
    - Using a custom tray or a stock tray initially for the final impression without an altered cast impression is not as accurate.
    - Indicated for mandibular Kennedy Class I/II (distal extensions).
- "What is the appointment sequence if I'm making a complete denture over an RPD?"
  - See Chapter 12, section Complete Denture Opposing Cast Metal RPD.

Dental Assistant's Question

- "The schedule says enameloplasty. What's that?"
  - Enameloplasty refers to removing small amounts of enamel to alter the shape of a tooth. This will improve the fit for the partial denture. For this procedure we will need a fine diamond bur, polishing discs with the mandrel, a high speed, slow speed, and fluoride varnish.

Patients' Questions

- "I just broke my front tooth off at the gumline. I'm going out tonight for New Year's Eve and I can't be seen like this. Can you help me?" (See Figure 13.2)
  - Evaluate the case and determine if an Essix appliance can be fabricated in-house the same day. Train your dental assistants. See Section Essix Appliances.
- "I want partials. Which type do you recommend?"
  - See Table 13.1.
- "Will my loose teeth tighten up once I have partials?"
  - Unfortunately, the damage has already been done. Your loose teeth will not tighten up. Replacing missing teeth with a partial can help distribute the chewing forces more evenly to reduce the amount of occlusal trauma. However, the clasps on partials can also loosen teeth more due to the torqueing forces.
- "You need to drill my teeth? My teeth are already weak!"

- I understand your concern. When we recontour teeth, we remove very little tooth structure ("lightly dust, recontour, smooth/polish"). Most often, patients don't even require any anesthetic as we are only adjusting the outer layer of the tooth (enamel).
- By recontouring the teeth, either by smoothing some of the surfaces that are too round or by creating dimples, it will improve the fit of the denture. Partials have unavoidable movement, but these tooth modifications will:
  o Improve retention and stability of the partial (guideplanes, changing HOCL, rest seats).
  o Help reduce food impaction (guideplanes).
  o Can improve the esthetics (create space for anterior teeth when mesially drifted anteriors).
  o Reduce orthodontic movement of teeth (rest seats).
  o Reduce trauma to the gums by acting as a stop when chewing food.
  o Create more space for the denture teeth.
- I'd like to obtain your verbal consent (and document) to recontour some of your teeth.
- "Why are you recommending pulling a healthy tooth for a partial to fit?"
  - At times we recommend taking teeth out if the tooth is diseased, if the bone is diseased, and sometimes for function.
- "Why aren't my partials ready today?" (at appointment 2)
  - Note that this is why you must set expectations ahead of time.
  - Analogy for the patient: partials are not like a pair of shoes you can buy off the rack. Partials are custom made and require various steps (appointments) for optimal results. I'm happy to explain why each step is necessary if you'd like.
- "Doc, you're replacing one tooth, why is this partial the size of my hand?"
  - Two reasons: for improved retention, and to reduce risk of aspiration and swallowing. The smaller the partial, the greater the risk. Even if you are careful, you could eat something sticky and end up swallowing the partial, which may require surgery to retrieve (Figure 13.62).

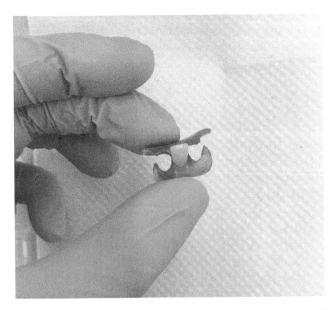

Figure 13.62 The author does not recommend partial dentures that are this small (in metal or flexible material).

- "Why so many clasps?"
  - The clasps make the partial more retentive and stable.
    - o Analogy 1: imagine moving cross-country and having to transport luggage by tying it to the roof of your car. To secure it you may need ropes, bungee cords, straps, etc. Think of the clasps as the straps.
    - o Analogy 2: imagine trying to tape a piece of paper flat on the ceiling. If you use one piece of tape, most of the paper will be hanging down. If you use another piece of tape next to the first tape, the paper will still be hanging down. If you distribute the pieces of tape, or add more, the piece of paper will stay in place.
- "The wire broke. Can you fix it?"
  - See Table 13.3.
- "Can you repair this?" (See Figure 13.3)
  - See Table 13.3.

Patients' Comments

- "I just bite it into place."
  - I do not recommend you insert your partials this way. I've had patients come in with broken partials because they thought the partial was in all the way, bit down, and broke the partials in half. Instead, insert and remove with both hands.
- "My last dentist made me a partial and when I got home, I had a panic attack because I couldn't take it out of my mouth!"
  - This is why we always verify that you are able to insert and remove the partials yourself at the delivery appointment and after any adjustments of the clasps before going home.

Patients' Demands

- "I want teeth back here." (See Figure 13.4)
  - I will have to complete a clinical exam, evaluate the radiographs, and make some study models prior to providing my recommendations. In your case, surgery will be required in order to create space for the teeth.
- "Doc, I need you to bend this wire." (points to cast metal) (Figure 13.63)
  - First examine how well engaged the clasp is to the abutment tooth.
  - Determine the type of clasp: WW or cast metal.
    - o WW C-clasps and ball-end clasps are easier to bend. However, still be careful as bending it too many times can cause it to snap (like a paperclip). Can use the bird beak pliers.
    - o Cast metal clasps can fracture despite careful bending. This includes cast metal C-clasps, embrasure clasps, and I-bars. The three prong pliers applies less pressure in one spot compared with the bird beak pliers.
    - o For bending an I-bar, you can use the edge of a desk so less stress is applied.

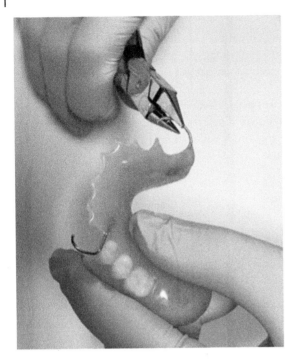

Figure 13.63 Adjusting a WW clasp on a stayplate with the bird beak pliers.

- "I want you to replace my missing teeth and then you can work on my fillings."
  – See Chapter 4, section Real-Life Clinical Questions Answered.
- "My partial feels loose, it was tighter before. Now I can pop it out with my tongue."
  – Determine if this is a stretched-out WW clasp and/or is due to resorption of the edentulous ridge.
    - If due to resorption, the partial may require a reline or remake.
    - If due to a stretched-out WW clasp, inform the patient that every time the partial is inserted and removed the clasp has to stretch over the height of contour on the tooth. Over time it will loosen and will require periodic tightening.
  – Note that a drop of denture adhesive (e.g. Fixodent, Poligrip) in each edentulous span can help.
- "I want you to adjust my partial, it was made in another state."
  – First determine if your office/clinic/school has any policy against adjusting a prosthesis made elsewhere. Once you touch it you inherit it, and any problems, as the patient may demand a replacement.
  – Check retention. Is there poor retention? Good idea to know how retentive the prosthesis is prior to avoid being accused of "Now that you adjusted my partial it feels loose."
  – Also, determine if the patient is having pain.
    - I am happy to adjust to relieve any pain. However, you may need a new partial. Often times we adjust one area and then patients become hyper aware of other problems that had already existed with the partial.
  – If you decide to proceed, show the patient the exact area being adjusted before adjusting it.

References

1 American College of Prosthodontists (2018). Position Statement. The frequency of denture replacement. https://www.prosthodontics.org/about-acp/position-statement-the-frequency-of-denture-replacement (accessed 1 December 2019)

2 Glidewell. Flexible partials. https://glidewelldental.com/solutions/removable-prosthesis/partials/flexible-partials (accessed 19 May 2021).

3 DiTolla, M. (2004). Valplast: flexible, esthetic partial dentures. *Chairside Perspective* 5 (1): http://www.drditolla.com/docs/valplast_dentures.pdf (accessed 27 November 2020).

4 Carr, A.B. and Brown, D.T. (2011). *McCracken's Removable Partial Prosthodontics*, 12the. St. Louis, MO: Elsevier Mosby.

5 Loney, R.W. (2019). *Complete Denture Manual*. Halifax, NS, Canada: Dalhousie University http://removpros.dentistry.dal.ca/Manuals.html (accessed 27 November 2020).

6 Osada, H., Shimpo, H., Hayakawa, T., and Ohkubo, C. (2013). Influence of thickness and undercut of thermoplastic resin clasps on retentive force. *Dent. Mater. J.* 32 (3): 381–389.

14

Implant Crowns

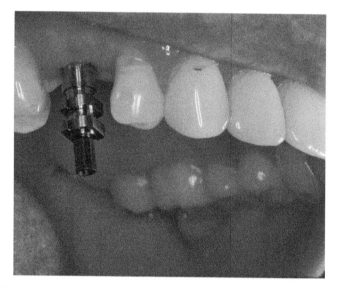

Figure 14.1 The impression coping/post fully seated for the final impression of #4 implant crown.

Chapter Outline

- Real-Life Clinical Questions
- Relevance
- Treatment Planning
  - Indications and Contraindications for Dental Implant
  - Clinical and Radiographic Exam
  - Clinical and Radiographic Dimensions for Implants
  - Cement- Versus Screw-Retained Implant Crown
  - Restorative Materials
- Referral to an Oral and Maxillofacial Surgeon or a Periodontist
- Discussion with the Oral and Maxillofacial Surgeon or a Periodontist
- Implant Parts to Order

Clinical Dentistry Daily Reference Guide, First Edition. William A. Jacobson.
© 2022 John Wiley & Sons, Inc. Published 2022 by John Wiley & Sons, Inc.

- Procedural Steps
  - Surgical Stent
  - Final Impression
  - Soft Tissue Cast
  - Provisional Implant Crown
  - Implant Crown Delivery
- Lab Prescriptions
  - Diagnostic Tooth Wax-Up and Surgical Stent
  - Soft Tissue Cast
  - Soft Tissue Cast and Screw- or Cement-Retained Provisional Crown
  - Soft Tissue Cast and Screw-Retained PFM Crown
  - Soft Tissue Cast and Cement-Retained PFM Crown
- Follow-Up
- Maintenance
- Clinical Pearls
  - Troubleshooting
  - Tips
- Real-Life Clinical Questions Answered
- References

Real-Life Clinical Questions

Dental Students' Questions

- "When should I use the open tray versus closed tray impression technique?"
- "Do you recommend cement- or screw-retained implant crowns?"
- "Should I probe around the implant when perio charting?"
- "How do I clean around the implant during a prophy?"
- "What oral hygiene recommendations should I give my patient for their implants?"

Patients' Questions

- "Do you recommend implants?"
- "Am I a good candidate for dental implants?"
- "Will I need a bone graft?"
- "If this tooth is not hurting should I wait to get it pulled with the surgeon that will place the implant so I have more bone?"
- "How long will I be without a tooth?"
- "How do my implants look on the X-rays?"
- "I don't know why a space developed between my implant crown and my tooth?"

Patient's Request

- "My other dentist placed an implant right here and I just need you to make the crown."

Relevance

As a dentist you may choose to place and/or restore dental implants. If you choose to place implants be sure to have the proper training in order to manage any surgical complications. A surgical specialist's training is much different than a weekend course or a "mini-residency" [1]. If you choose to restore implants, this chapter will provide some basics. Implants are restoratively driven, so begin with the end in mind.

Treatment Planning

Table 14.1 Treatment planning phases related to dental implants.

Treatment phase	Description (may or may not apply)
Emergency phase	Urgent treatment of pain, infection, trauma, and/or esthetic emergency
Data gathering phase	• Comprehensive oral evaluation • Medical history: medical consultation • Radiographs and interpretation • Clinical findings • Periodontal evaluation • Intraoral photographs
Stabilization phase (to control disease)	Not applicable
Definitive phase	• Tooth replacement – Implant • Occlusal guard
Maintenance phase	• Prophy or periodontal maintenance, oral hygiene instructions • Periodic oral evaluation

Indications and Contraindications for Dental Implants

- Indications
  - Missing tooth, especially with virgin adjacent teeth.
  - Patient desires a fixed tooth replacement solution (vs. removable).
- Contraindications (based on further information, the contraindications listed could fall within absolute or relative contraindications)
  - Inadequate amount of bone quality/quantity.
  - Inadequate restorative spacing (i.e. mesial–distal, interarch).

Implant Crowns

- Poorly controlled diabetes.
- Medical and psychological conditions in which elective treatment is contraindicated (see Chapter 1).
- History of radiation to the head and neck (determine amount of radiation).
- History of intravenous bisphosphonate.
- Not fully developed bones (young age).

Clinical and Radiographic Exam

- Verify the patient is free of active disease (i.e. periodontal disease and caries).
- Clinical findings:
  - Missing tooth or tooth planned for extraction?
  - High smile line?
  - Biotype (thick/thin)?
  - Adequate amount of keratinized tissue?
  - Atrophied ridge (crown will appear long)?
- Evaluate the risk factors: medical, functional, occlusal, esthetic. Determine if parafunctional habits are present; these can contribute to bone loss around the implant and would require stress reduction and night guard [2].
- Obtain radiographs:
  - Panoramic (if extraction, no sooner than three months since extraction).
  - Bitewing (not more than one year old).
  - Periapical (not more than one year old).
- Take intraoral photos.
- Obtain mounted diagnostic casts with facebow transfer:
  - Is orthodontic treatment necessary prior to implant surgery?
  - Is enameloplasty of the opposing and adjacent teeth indicated prior to implant crown final impression? (Figure 14.2)

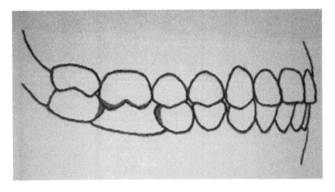

Figure 14.2 Evaluate if enameloplasty is indicated.

Clinical and Radiographic Dimensions for Implants

Table 14.2 General measurement parameters for dental implants[a].

Clinical and radiographic dimensions for implants	Minimum millimeters (mm)
Implant length (shortest)	Varies, but may be 8 or 10
Implant diameter	Varies
Implant length (longest)	Bone height to 1
Interarch space	5 (optimal 6–7)
Implant to tooth	2
Implant to implant	3
Alveolar ridge width[b]	6
Implant to buccal bone	2 (optimal 4)
Implant to lingual bone	2
Alveolar ridge height from maxillary sinus	10
Implant to maxillary sinus	2
Alveolar ridge height from inferior alveolar canal	10
Implant to inferior alveolar canal	2
Implant to mental foramen	Varies, may be 2
Depth from CEJ of adjacent teeth in esthetic zone	2–3
Gingival cuff depth	2–3 (if less, unesthetic, may display metal; if more may have difficulty with hygiene [3]

[a] Always consult with a surgeon.
[b] Note when measuring on a diagnostic cast, the thickness of the gingiva can create a false sense of adequate alveolar ridge width.

Cement- Versus Screw-Retained Implant Crown

Figure 14.3 depics a cement-retained and a screw-retained implant crown.

Table 14.3 summarizes the advantages and disadvantages of cement- vs. screw-retained implant crowns.

Screw retained is preferred.

Figure 14.3 Illustration of the components of a cement-retained implant crown (left) and a screw-retained implant crown (right).

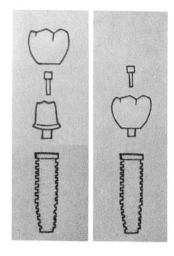

Table 14.3 Cement- versus screw-retained implant crown.

Implant crown type	Advantages	Disadvantages
Cement-retained implant crown/abutment supported implant crown	• Esthetic zone	• Potential risk of peri-implantitis/implant failure due to cement • Not retrievable
Screw-retained implant crown/implant supported crown	• Retrievable (for repair, replacement, adding material to close a newly formed open proximal contact) • Indicated when a shorter clinical crown (limited interarch space)	• Less esthetic

Restorative Materials

Is the patient opposed to having any metal visible in the mouth?

Table 14.4 Implant crown materials.

Restorative material	Advantages	Disadvantages
PFM with metal occlusal (screw retained)	• Less wear on opposing teeth • Abutment screw access hole encircled in metal to prevent fracture of unsupported porcelain [3]	• Risk of porcelain fracture (requires repair or replacement) • Esthetics (visible metal)
PFM with porcelain occlusal (screw retained)	• Esthetics	• Risk of unsupported porcelain fracture (requires repair or replacement)
Porcelain/ceramic crown (e.g. zirconia)	• Esthetics • Durability and wear on opposing varies depending on the type of porcelain/ceramic	• Durability and wear on opposing varies depending on the type of porcelain/ceramic
Base alloys (white gold)	• Less wear on opposing	• Esthetics (silver color)
Noble alloy (full cast gold)	• Less wear on opposing	• Esthetics (gold color)

Referral to an Oral and Maxillofacial Surgeon or a Periodontist

- Patient name _____
- Patient DOB _____
- Patient phone _____
- Referred by _____
- Office phone _____
- Date _____

- Referring patient for evaluation of the following:
  - Extraction(s) # _____
  - Dental implant(s) # _____
- Comments_____

Discussion with the Oral and Maxillofacial Surgeon or a Periodontist

- Communicate with the surgeon to determine:
  - When will healing be finished for me to restore the implant with a temporary or permanent crown?
  - Which implant system is being used?
  - What are the implant dimensions (to order the appropriate restorative implant parts)?

Implant Parts to Order

- The surgeon will order:
  - Implant.
  - Cover/healing screw (if two-stage).
  - Healing abutment (if one- and two-stage).
- The restorative dentist will order:
  - Impression coping/post (to transfer the position of implant to the master cast). Must specify if open or closed impression tray technique.
  - Implant replica/analog (replicates the implant for use in the cast). Lab usually provides.
  - Plastic temporary abutment and screw (for the temporary crown). Lab usually provides.
  - Abutment screw (do not use lab's screw).
  - Must also have available for use:
    - Hex driver (also known as hex tool, screwdriver).
    - Torque wrench.

Procedural Steps

Surgical Stent

Laboratory Fabricated Surgical Stent
- Make alginate impressions of both arches and obtain a bite registration to send to the lab.
- See section Lab Prescriptions.

In-Office Fabricated Surgical Stent
- See Figure 14.4 of an in-office fabricated surgical stent.
- Make alginate impressions of both arches and obtain a bite registration.
- Mount the casts.
- Wax up tooth so that it is over the ridge and in proper occlusion.
- Soak the model with the wax-up and duplicate the model (if you do not soak the model, the alginate will stick to the stone).

(a)

(b)

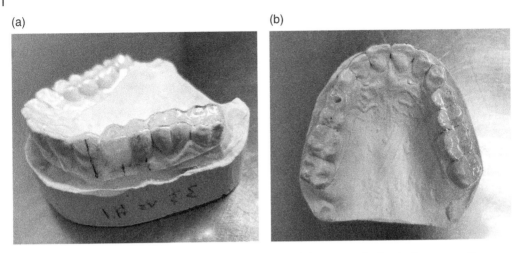

Figure 14.4 (a, b) The (untrimmed) surgical stent. This is used for communicating to the surgeon the desired implant position and as an aid during implant placement. Can be dropped off at the surgeon's office.

- Trim the duplicated model.
- Heat a thick vacuform stent over the duplicated model and form the stent.
- Trim the stent to the level of the gingiva in certain areas to provide some retention for the stent to snap on and off the teeth. Do not want it too tight or it will bind or tear or rip.
- Place lubricant on the edentulous ridge and adjacent teeth.
- Place wax up in the undercuts of the adjacent teeth (to prevent ortho resin from locking in).
- Place lubricant on a #8 round bur.
- Use the #8 round bur to drill through the stent on the occlusal of the tooth implant crown down to halfway into the ridge.
- Drill through the buccal of the stent.
- Place the #8 round bur into the occlusal and inject orthodontic resin from the buccal opening.
- Once set, remove the #8 round bur and trim the pontic so between the ridge and the pontic is a clearance of 1 mm (for the surgeon).

Final Impression

Table 14.5 Impression technique indications.

Impression technique	Indications
Open tray/direct/pick-up	• Most accurate[a] • Multiple implant case
Closed tray/indirect/transfer	• Single implant case

[a] More accurate because the heavy body stabilizes the impression coping, which remains undisturbed in the impression before master cast is poured in dental stone [3].

Open Versus Closed Tray Impression Technique

Figure 14.5 The healing abutment on #4 before removal.

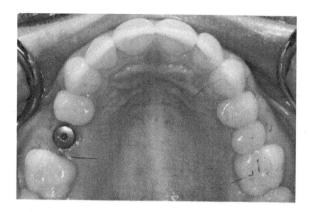

Figure 14.6 Image of the tray, using the open tray impression technique, immediately after wiping off the PVS material to expose the screw access on the impression post.

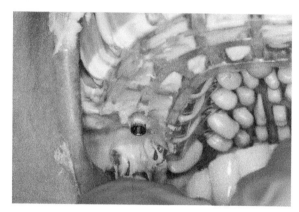

Table 14.6 Open versus closed tray impression technique steps.

Remove the healing abutment (may require anesthetic) See Figure 14.5
Or
Remove the temporary crown and temporary abutment: (the surgeon could have made a provisional at time of the delivery)

Cement-retained implant provisional crown	Screw-retained implant provisional crown
Remove the temporary crown and block out material from the temporary abutment. Unscrew the temporary abutment	Remove the access material, unscrew temporary crown/abutment

- Immediately seat and secure the impression post/coping
- If the adjacent impression copings does not seat, adjust with bur
- Take a bitewing to verify the impression post/coping is fully engaged/seated
- Determine if any enameloplasty of the opposing tooth or adjacent teeth is necessary prior to final impression. Pinpoint contacts of adjacent teeth with large gingival embrasures should be avoided; want broad contacts (see Figure 14.2)
- Obtain bite with bite registration (either with the healing abutment in or ideally with the temporary crown)
- Screw in the impression post/coping (Figure 14.1)
- Block-out access with rope wax
- Block out any bridges with rope wax (to prevent the impression from locking in)

(Continued)

Table 14.6 (Continued)

Closed tray technique	Open tray technique
• Use a stock tray • The dental assistant loads impression tray with PVS heavy body • The dentist places PVS medium body over the impression post/coping (light body allows too much movement) • Seat the tray to make the impression • Once set, remove tray from mouth	• Use a stock tray and drill a hole in the tray so the impression posts/copings protrude out of tray (passive seat) • The dental assistant loads impression tray with PVS medium body • The dentist places PVS heavy body over the impression post/coping. Heavy body minimizes any movement when the tray is removed (opposite to closed tray technique) [3] • Seat the tray and immediately wipe off the PVS material to expose the impression post/coping screw access (Figure 14.6) • Once set, remove the block-out wax from the impression post/coping screw access. • Unscrew the impression post/coping. The screw does not have to come out as long as it disengages impression post/coping • Remove the tray from the mouth

Evaluate the impression: stable impression post/coping? Adjacent and occlusal surfaces captured?

If the impression is acceptable, remove block-out wax. Unscrew the impression post/coping	N/A

Place either the healing abutment back on with hex driver, or the provisional back on

Cement-retained implant provisional crown	Screw-retained implant provisional crown	Healing abutment
Screw on the temporary plastic abutment, blocking out the access, and recement the provisional crown with temporary cement	Screw the screw-retained temporary crown back on. Block out the access hole with cotton, or Teflon, and PVS	Screw the healing abutment back on with the hex driver

Make the opposing impression

Obtain the tooth shade and gum shade (if necessary)

Send to lab for the soft tissue cast or fabricate in-house

Soft Tissue Cast

The soft tissue cast is indicated for the fabrication of the implant crown (provisional and final) to create a proper emergency profile. Without the soft tissue cast (i.e. if the model is poured up completely in stone), it will restrict access to the implant analog for the lab technician (or dentist) to create an ideal restoration.

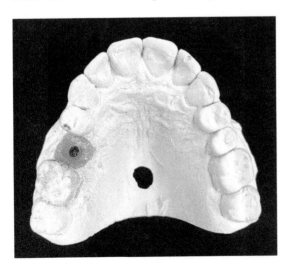

Figure 14.7 The soft tissue cast for implant crown #4.

Laboratory Fabricated Soft Tissue Cast
- Send the final impression to the lab (using either an open or closed tray impression technique) for fabrication of the soft tissue cast and provisional crown.
- See section Lab Prescriptions.

In-House Fabricated Soft Tissue Cast
- See Figure 14.7 of an in-house fabricated soft tissue cast.
- Secure the impression post/coping to the implant analog into the final impression securely as one unit.
- Use a soft tissue material, in this example GI-MASK.
- Place GI-MASK spray in the area where soft tissue material will be applied (prevents adherence to final impression).
- Dispense GI-MASK soft tissue material around the implant analog (up to the bottom of the bevel).
  - Be sure the soft tissue replica material does not enter into the impression of the adjacent teeth.
  - Create undercuts in the soft tissue material for better retention in the master cast.
- Pour the model in stone.
- Pour the opposing model.
- Mount the casts.

Provisional Implant Crown

Laboratory Fabricated Provisional Crown
- Obtain tooth shade.
- Send the final impression to the lab (using either open or closed tray impression technique) for fabrication of the soft tissue cast and provisional crown.
- See section Lab Prescriptions.

In-House Fabricated Provisional Crown
- Fabricate the implant crown matrix (clear stent) from the diagnostic wax-up (on the model used for fabricating the surgical stent).
- Remove the healing abutment with the hex driver.
- Immediately (to prevent tissue collapse) insert the plastic temporary abutment and finger tighten with ligated hex driver.
- Check occlusion and trim the plastic temporary abutment with a carbide bur for adequate occlusal clearance.
- *Screw-retained implant provisional crown* (almost always screw retained for ease of retrievability and less risk of cement)
  - Use the clear matrix (stent) with a hole for access. Place a cotton applicator (stick end) through the clear matrix into the plastic temporary abutment hole.
  - Fill the matrix from a hole in the buccal with temporary crown material. Once set remove the cotton applicator. Unscrew the plastic temporary abutment.
  - Check the proximal contacts.
  - Check and adjust the occlusion: goal is light to no occlusion. Shimstock should pull through unless biting down hard.

Implant Crowns

- Refine the shape of the provisional crowns and polish.
- Screw in provisional crown with the hex driver and torque at 15 N/cm with the torque wrench.
- Seal access with cotton roll (or Teflon tape) and PVS light body (or Fuji IX).
- Minimum four weeks between the provisional crown and making the final impression (for soft tissue adaptation).

Implant Crown Delivery

Table 14.7 Implant crown delivery steps.

Lab work evaluation (at least one day prior)

- Evaluate the mounted models, abutment, and implant crown (Figures 14.8 and 14.9)
- Make note of orientation of the abutment in order to maintain the same orientation in the mouth
- Verify you are able to seat the crown and able to insert the screw with the hex driver. (Sometimes excess porcelain prevents the screw from seating. In this case, adjust with a diamond bur as necessary)
- Check the occlusion with shimstock (must have some occlusion)
- Evaluate the crown contour including the emergence profile. Similar gingival margin to the adjacent teeth?
- Any visible porcelain fractures?
- Missing glaze on porcelain in any areas?
- Interproximal contacts adequate?
- Shade acceptable?
- Margins sealed?
- If a poor fit or defective, send the case back to lab and cancel the patient's appointment

Implant crown delivery steps

- Place a throat pack
- Ligate the hex driver with floss (cut tip of floss at an angle so narrow enough to fit)
- Remove the healing abutment or temporary crown/temporary abutment
- Irrigate debris with chlorhexidine

Cement-retained crown	Screw-retained crown
Seat the abutment	Seat the abutment/crown (connected as one unit) (Figure 14.10)

Immediately (to prevent tissue collapse) tighten with the hex driver using a brand-new screw for the final delivery. The screw will be sent from the lab or you will have ordered it. (Not the lab screw by which the abutment is attached to the master cast)

Seating difficulty:

- If blanching wait 10 minutes before retightening to fully seat. If still blanching the emergence profile is causing too much pressure
- If the proximal contacts are too heavy to seat, check with Occlude spray or floss (wrap in articulating paper so floss marks crown) and adjust to fully seat with porcelain polishing kit. If gold/metal, adjust with brownie then greenie
- If time is spent adjusting, make sure the tissue does not collapse. Place the healing abutment back in to prevent this from occurring

Table 14.7 (Continued)

Verify the patient approves the crown shade

Take a vertical bitewing of the abutment (cement retained) or abutment/crown (screw retained). The bitewing must capture abutment–implant interface (Figure 14.11)

Interpret the bitewing to verify the crown is fully seated:
- Inspect the platform–abutment interface for open margins
- If an open margin is detected, tighten more and take another bitewing to verify no open margins

Cement-retained crown	Screw-retained crown
N/A	• Check occlusion to verify the crown is fully seated
	• If high occlusion in mouth but normal on the model, there could be a bone interference, as the gap in the implant restoration interface may not be visible radiographically
	• If the crestal bone adjacent to the implant is preventing the abutment/crown from seating, replace the healing abutment and send back to surgeon to adjust the bone
	• Check occlusion with the articulating paper and shimstock; want stable occlusion with cusp to fossa relationship (not on the incline planes, no lateral forces)
	• Check the contours, proximal contacts, and margins
Once fully seated, torque abutment to 35 N/cm	Once fully seated, torque abutment/crown to 35 N/cm

Caution: Be sure to use the torque wrench properly; if used incorrectly it can strip the screw or fracture the screw within the implant

• Seat the crown	• Place cotton (or Teflon tape) into the access hole
• Bitewing to verify the crown is seated: if an open margin is noted, it may be due to tight proximal contacts; adjust as needed, or excess material on the intaglio of the crown	• Seal the occlusal 2 mm with composite
	• Alternatively, instead of placing composite use Teflon and PVS, then one to two weeks later, retorque and seal with Teflon and 2 mm of composite (as the screw can loosen)
• Place cotton (or Teflon tape) and PVS light body into abutment access and keep it flush with surface	
• Place Fit Checker on the intaglio of crown, seat, remove, and adjust any burn-through areas	
• Check the occlusion and adjust as needed	
• Check the occlusion with articulating paper and shimstock; need stable occlusion with cusp to fossa relationship (not on incline planes, no lateral forces)	
• Check the contours, proximal contacts, and margins	
• Seat the crown with permanent cement and hold while cement is setting. Use a radiopaque cement	
• Remove all excess cement	

Measure and document the pocket depths as a baseline

Review oral hygiene instructions

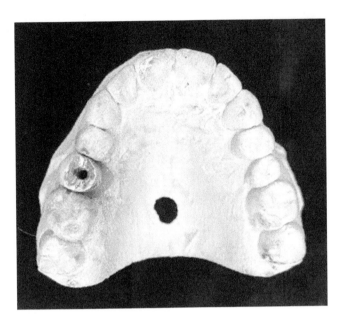

Figure 14.8 Occlusal view of the #4 screw-retained PFM implant crown on the soft tissue cast.

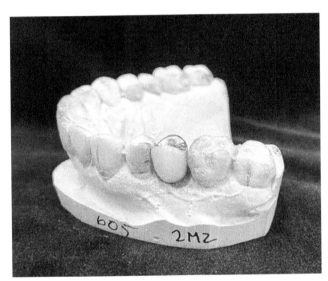

Figure 14.9 Buccal view of the #4 screw-retained PFM implant crown on the soft tissue cast.

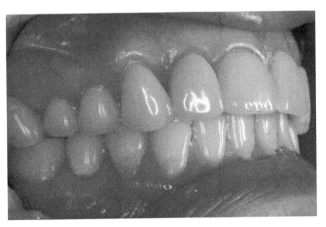

Figure 14.10 Seat the #4 screw-retained PFM implant crown and evaluate clinically.

Figure 14.11 Vertical bitewing of the #4 screw-retained PFM implant crown.

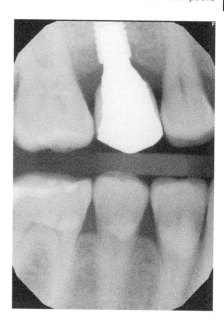

Lab Prescriptions

Diagnostic Tooth Wax-Up and Surgical Stent

- Please pour up the diagnostic casts, mount, and fabricate:
  - A diagnostic tooth wax-up in proper occlusion of tooth # ___
  - Surgical stent for the placement of an implant for tooth # ___
- Included are the following: upper/lower alginate impressions and bite registration

Soft Tissue Cast

- Please pour up final impression and fabricate a soft tissue master case of implant crown # ___
- Included are the following: final impression, opposing impression, bite registration, impression coping/post, and implant replica/analog [lab usually provides]

Soft Tissue Cast and Screw- or Cement-Retained Provisional Crown

- Please pour up final impression and fabricate a soft tissue master case of implant crown # ___
- Fabricate screw-retained or cement-retained provisional crown # ___
- Tooth shade ___
- Included are the following: final impression, opposing impression, bite registration, impression coping/post, implant replica/analog, and plastic temporary abutment and screw [lab usually provides]

Implant Crowns

Soft Tissue Cast and Screw-Retained PFM Crown

- Please pour up final impression and fabricate a soft tissue master case of implant crown # ___
  Fabricate PFM noble metal screw-retained implant crown # ___
  - No metal visible, or
  - Abutment screw access hole encircled in metal
- Tooth shade ___
- Included are the following: final impression, opposing impression, bite registration, impression coping/post, and implant replica/analog [lab usually provides]

Soft Tissue Cast and Cement-Retained PFM Crown

- Please pour up final impression and fabricate a soft tissue master case of implant crown # ___
- Fabricate PFM noble metal cement-retained implant crown # ___ with a custom abutment
- Tooth shade ___
- Included are the following: final impression, opposing impression, bite registration, impression coping/post, and implant replica/analog [lab usually provides]

Follow-Up

- Annual radiographic and clinical evaluation.
- Radiographic evaluation
  - Obtain baseline radiographs and annual radiographs. If new patient with existing implants, obtain radiographs from previous office to assess changes in bone levels [4].
  - Use BW or PA that does not include the apical portion of the implant with good paralleling technique with clear depiction of threads on both sides.
  - Evaluate for crestal bone loss. Radiograph will only show crestal bone loss on the mesial and distal (early bone loss is usually facial) [2].
- Clinical evaluation
  - Pain: pain scale 0–10.
  - Pain on percussion (horizontal and vertical)? Pain may occur, after healing, on percussion if there is inflamed tissue, a mobile implant, or implant impinges on a nerve [2].
  - If a screw-retained implant crown, check the screw access is well sealed.
  - Periodontal charting
    o Probe depths:
      ▪ Probe gently.
      ▪ Probe with plastic or titanium periodontal probe [2]. When titanium surface is present within the peri-implant sulcus, recommend probing with a plastic probe. If gold, metal, or porcelain is placed to the fixture level, use of a metal probe is acceptable [5].
    o Bleeding on probing?
    o Suppuration on probing?
    o Recession?
    o Mobility? Check for screw loosening; if retrieved, evaluate screw threads and replace as needed.
  - Occlusion adequate?

- Proximal contact present?
  - o Interproximal contact loss increases over time and is more common in the posterior and in the mandible [6].
  - o Mesial drift of natural dentition will result in open contact, as the implant is in a static position.
  - o Recommend gap closure by repairing porcelain (adding), redoing the crown, or adding composite to adjacent tooth and use of retainers.
  - o Open proximal contact can cause food impaction, leading to caries of adjacent teeth, and bone loss.
- Plaque control.

- Diagnosis
  - Diagnose the peri-implant diseases and conditions (Table 14.8).

Table 14.8 Peri-implant diseases and conditions.

Diagnosis	Definition/signs	Treatment	Etiology
Peri-implant health	Absence of erythema, BOP, swelling, and suppuration. Probing depths are usually greater than with teeth with healthy periodontal tissue. Range of probing depths are not defined for health. No increase in probing depths compared to the previous exams. No bone loss beyond the crestal bone level changes from the initial bone remodeling [4]	None	N/A
Peri-implant mucositis	Gum inflammation around the soft tissue of the dental implant with no signs of bone loss. A precursor to peri-implantitis [7]. Erythema, swelling and/or suppuration. Increase in probing depths due to swelling or decrease in probing resistance. With or without increase in probing depths compared to previous exams. No bone loss beyond the crestal bone level changes from initial bone remodeling [4]	Reversible if caught early [7]. Can be resolved in three weeks with plaque/biofilm control [4]	Strong evidence plaque is the main etiologic factor [4]
Peri-implantitis	Gum inflammation around the soft tissue of the implant with bone loss [7]. Clinical signs of inflammation: BOP and/or suppuration, increased probing depths from previous exams and/or recession of the mucosal margin and radiographic bone loss. In the absence of previous exams, BOP and/or suppuration, probing depths of ≥6 mm, bone level ≥3 mm apical to the most coronal portion of the intraosseous part of the implant [4]	Usually requires surgical treatment [7] Treatment decreases inflammation and suppresses disease progression [4]	Plaque [4] There is an increased risk if a history of severe periodontitis, poor plaque control, and/or no regular maintenance Data on smoking and diabetes are inconclusive. Some limited evidence of post-restorative submucosal cement and positioning of implants which make oral hygiene and maintenance difficult [4]

Implant Crowns

(Continued)

Table 14.8 (Continued)

Diagnosis	Definition/signs	Treatment	Etiology
Hard and soft tissue deficiencies	As a result of the healing process following tooth loss. Recession of the mucosa may be due to malpositioned implants, lack of buccal bone, thin biotype, lack of keratinized tissue, surgical trauma, and periodontal health of adjacent teeth. Keratinized tissue improves patient comfort and ease of plaque removal [4]	Requires surgery	Various causes: diminished dimensions of alveolar ridge following extraction healing site, loss of periodontal support, endodontic infections, longitudinal root fractures, thin buccal bone plates, buccal or lingual tooth position, traumatic extractions, injury, pneumatized maxillary sinus, medications, systemic diseases, congenitally missing teeth, pressure from removable prosthesis, and combinations [4]

Maintenance

- **At the dentist: prophylaxis**
  - The goal of prophylaxis is the removal of plaque biofilm without creating pits or scratches on the titanium implant.
  - Instrumentation:
    - If the implant titanium is not accessible in the sulcus and the implant restoration is porcelain, gold, or a nontitanium metal, gentle use of metal instruments is acceptable [5].
    - If the implant titanium is accessible in the sulcus, it is detrimental to use metal scalers, metal curettes, USS with metal tips, and sonic scalers with metal tips [5]. Instead use:
      - Nonmetal hand instruments: plastic, nylon, or special alloy for implant debridement that will not alter the implant surface [5]. Options include titanium, nonmetallic, graphite, nylon, carbon, and Teflon-coated instruments.
      - USS with plastic [5] or rubber sleeve is safe (see Chapter 6, Figure 6.4).
  - Prophy polish using toothpaste, fine prophy paste, flour of pumice, or tin oxide.
  - Irrigate the deposits gently with chlorhexidine. Do not insert cannula to the base of the sulcus which may gauge and cause distension of tissue.
  - Fluoride varnish: if placing topical fluoride on teeth, select a neutral sodium fluoride. Avoid acidic fluoride varnishes which may alter the titanium [2].
  - Provide oral hygiene instructions.
- **At home: oral hygiene instructions**
  - Proper oral hygiene for dental implants is critical.
  - Regular toothbrushing, flossing, and check-ups from dental professionals are required, as for natural teeth [7].
  - Optional adjunctive cleaning aids include:
    - End tufted brushes (especially if large embrasures).
    - Interdental brushes (especially if large embrasures).

    ○ Toothpicks.
    ○ Oral irrigators (set to the lowest setting and aimed interproximally to avoid pressure on the tissue cuff can alter tissue and induce bacteremia).
    ○ Chlorhexidine can be rinsed or applied to area with swab/brush [2].

Clinical Pearls

Troubleshooting

- Unsure if you should plan for immediate or delayed implant placement? Leave it up to the surgeon.
- Unsure if you should plan for immediate or delayed loading (of the crown)? Leave it up to the surgeon.
- Loose (mobile) implant crown noted at a follow-up visit? See Table 14.9.

Table 14.9 Diagnosis and treatment for loose implant crowns.

Differential diagnosis	Peri-implantitis	Detorqued screw	Fractured screw
Radiographic signs	Bone loss	• Gap between the restorative abutment and implant platform (open margin)	• Possible radiolucent fracture line in the screw
Treatment	• Refer to surgeon for evaluation and possible implant removal • Treatment plan new tooth replacement options	• Eval screw for stripping and replace with a new screw	• Retrieve the fractured screw and replace with a new screw • If unable to retrieve the fractured part, place a healing cap to support the soft tissue. Refer • If bruxing, fabricate an occlusal guard

Tips

- Time frames:
  - Extraction site healing time ranges from three to six months and is affected by tooth size, number of roots, and extent of trauma. The radiographic sign of socket regeneration is when the lamina dura is no longer present [2].
  - Osseointegration can take three to six months. Usually three months for mandible and four to six months for maxilla [3].
  - Socket preservation: three months; block graft: eight months; ortho extrusion: varies and requires enameloplasty until the tooth comes out.
- Shade selection
  - In highly esthetic cases, send the patient to the lab for a custom shade match.
  - If it is a multiple unit case with defects in the gingiva, obtain a gingiva shade.

Implant Crowns

Real-Life Clinical Questions Answered

Dental Students' Questions

- "When should I use the open tray versus closed tray impression technique?"
  - See section Open Versus Closed Tray Impression Technique.
- "Do you recommend cement- or screw-retained implant crowns?"
  - See section Cement- Versus Screw-Retained Implant Crown.
- "Should I probe around the implant when perio charting?"
  - Yes.
  - It is important to establish a baseline after the restoration is placed and monitor for any changes over time.
  - Gently probe around the implant to:
    - o monitor probe depth changes
    - o check for bleeding (or exudate) on probing
    - o measure mucosal margin migration [4].
  - This is important because you want to diagnose any changes as early as possible which may require additional treatment.
  - See section Follow-Up.
- "How do I clean around the implant during a prophy?"
  - See section Maintenance.
- "What oral hygiene recommendations should I give my patient for their implants?"
  - See section Maintenance.

Patients' Questions

- "Do you recommend implants?"
  - So many factors, not a simple yes or no.
  - See Chapter 4, Table 4.3.
- "Am I a good candidate for dental implants?"
  - I will have to review your health history and treatment goals, evaluate the radiographs, make study models, and perform a clinical exam.
- "Will I need a bone graft?"
  - I can take a look at your radiograph and look in your mouth to get an idea. However, the surgeon will have to determine if there is enough quantity (height and width) and quality of bone for an implant, and whether or not there is adequate distance from other anatomic structures. This will involve having a CBCT followed by the surgeon's assessment of the radiographic findings. CBCT provides more information than the two-dimensional radiographs we normally take as cross-sections of the jawbone can be seen, similar to sliced bread.
- "If this tooth is not hurting should I wait to get it pulled with the surgeon that will place the implant so I have more bone?"
  - Correct, any time a tooth is extracted there is bone loss.
  - If the tooth is asymptomatic I can refer you to the surgeon for evaluation to see if an immediate implant is an option. This means the tooth will be extracted and the implant will be placed at the same appointment.
  - If the tooth becomes symptomatic some options include:

- ○ Removal of decay, root canal treatment, and a temporary filling.
        - ○ Removal of decay, pulpectomy, and a temporary filling.
        - ○ Root canal treatment and coronectomy followed by fabrication of a stayplate.
- "How long will I be without a tooth?"
    - – Typically, the time it takes for the implants to heal on the lower is three months and for the upper four to six months. However, this can vary depending on several factors and will be up to the surgeon.
    - – During the healing phase we can temporarily replace the missing tooth. Options include:
        - ○ An Essix appliance, which is similar to wearing a clear aligner.
        - ○ A stayplate, which may or may not have metal wires for retention.
        - ○ A flexible partial, which has no metal.
- "How do my implants look on the X-rays?"
    - – See section Follow-Up.
- "I don't know why a space developed between my implant crown and my tooth?"
    - – The implant is fixed in place while the other teeth can potentially migrate, leading to interproximal contacts opening. This is a common problem with single implant crowns and the tooth mesial to it drifts mesial or buccal. This occurs more in some people than others with age or time.
    - – Treatment to restore the contact includes redoing the implant crown, adding contact to the implant crown, or adding restorative material to the adjacent tooth.

Patient's Request

- "My other dentist placed an implant right here and I just need you to make the crown."
    - – Find out why the patient is seeing you and not the restorative dentist that worked with the surgeon.
    - – Determine your comfort level for working on the case.
    - – Contact the patient's surgeon to understand the history of the patient and the implant.

References

1 Reznick, J.B. (2020). The importance of proper education in implant surgery. https://www.dentaltown.com/magazine/article/8048/needful-things (accessed August 2020).

2 Misch, C.E. (2008). *Contemporary Implant Dentistry*, 3e. St. Louis, MO: Mosby.

3 Shillingburg, H.T., Sather, D.A., Wilson, E.L. et al. (2012). *Fundamentals of Fixed Prosthodontics*, 4e. Chicago: Quintessence Publishing.

4 Berglunh, T., Armitage, G., Araujo, M.G. et al. (2018). Peri-implant diseases and conditions: consensus report of workgroup 4 of the 2017 World Workshop on the Classification of Periodontal and Peri-Implant Diseases and Conditions. *J. Clin. Periodontol.* 45 (Suppl 20): S286–S291.

5 Rose, L.F. and Mealy, B.L. (2004). *Periodontics: Medicine, Surgery, and Implants*. St. Louis, MO: Elsevier Mosby.

6 French, D., Naito, M., and Linke, B. (2019). Interproximal contact loss in a retrospective cross-sectional study of 4325 implants: distribution and incidence and the effect on bone loss and peri-implant soft tissue. *J. Prosthet. Dent.* 122 (2): 108–114.

7 American Academy of Periodontology (2020). Peri-implant diseases. https://www.perio.org/consumer/peri-implant-disease (accessed 11 October 2020).

Implant Crowns

15

Occlusal Guards

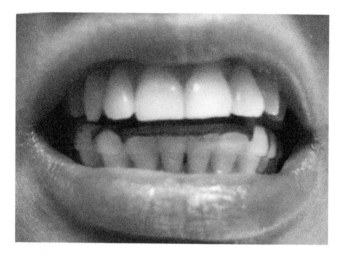

Figure 15.1   Hard occlusal guard.

Chapter Outline

- Real-Life Comments and Questions
- Relevance
- TMD Terminology
- Occlusal Guards and TMD
- The Patient Interview
- Clinical and Radiographic Exam
  - Extraoral Exam
  - Intraoral Exam
  - Dentition
  - Radiographic Exam

Clinical Dentistry Daily Reference Guide, First Edition. William A. Jacobson.
© 2022 John Wiley & Sons, Inc. Published 2022 by John Wiley & Sons, Inc.

- Treatment Planning
- Referrals
- Informed Consent
- Oral Appliances: Indications and Types
- Maxillary Versus Mandibular Arch
- Procedural Steps for Occlusal Guards, Dual Flat Plane Occlusal Appliances, Athletic Mouthguards, and QuickSplints
- Lab Prescriptions
- Postoperative Instructions
- TMD Self-Care Tips (Adjunctive Treatment)
- Clinical Pearls
  - Troubleshooting
  - Tips
  Real-Life Comments and Questions Answered
- References

Real-Life Comments and Questions

Dental Student's Question

- "What type of occlusal guard is better for patients? Hard, soft, or hard/soft?"

Patients' Comments

- "I wake up with headaches."
- "I play football at school."
- "I don't know if I grind my teeth because I'm asleep."
- "I get lockjaw."

Patients' Questions

- "Should I just get an over-the-counter nightguard or have one made at the dentist?"
- "How soon will my symptoms go away with an occlusal guard?"
- "How long will this nightguard last?"
- "I just need a nightguard during the day when driving in L.A. [Los Angeles, California] traffic."
- "How do I clean it and store it?"
- "What do I do if I wear a retainer at night but I also need a nightguard?"
- "What causes that sound in my TMJ?"
- "My child grinds his teeth. Does he need a nightguard?"

Relevance

Temporomandibular disorder (TMD) is extremely common, with 33% of the population reporting at least one symptom [1]. As a dentist you will encounter patients with TMD seeking treatment. While there is no cure for TMD, an occlusal guard and adjunctive treatment can help improve TMD symptoms.

TMD Terminology

- **Temporomandibular joint (TMJ):** "the articulation between the temporal bone and the man-dible. It is a bilateral diarthrodial, bilateral ginglymoid joint" [2].
- **TMD:** "heterogenous group of musculoskeletal and neuromuscular conditions involving the temporomandibular joint complex, and surrounding musculature and osseous components" [3].
  - "Cardinal signs and symptoms for TMD are pain in the masseter muscle, TMJ, and/or tempo-ralis muscle regions; mouth-opening limitations; and TMJ sounds" [1].
  - TMD symptoms are significantly correlated with worry, stress, irritation, frustration, and depression [3].
- **Myofascial pain:** "regional myogenous pain condition characterized by local areas of firm, hypersensitive bands of muscle tissue known as trigger points. . . . The most common effect is referred pain, often described by the patient as a tension-type headache" [4].
- **Parafunctional habits:** "unproductive movement habits; in relation to TMD, these would be oral habits, e.g. lip biting, cheek biting, grinding teeth, clenching teeth, and pursing lips" [1].
- **Occlusal appliance:** "a removable device, usually made of hard acrylic, which fits over the occlusal and incisal surfaces of the teeth in one arch, creating precise occlusal contact with the teeth in the opposing arch" [4]. The appliance decreases joint loading and protects the teeth.
  - Synonyms: occlusal guard, nightguard, mouthguard, occlusal splint, oral appliance, stabiliza-tion appliance, bite guard, bite splints, and stabilization device.

Occlusal Guards and TMD

- There is no cure for TMD.
- No single treatment has been proven to be totally effective [1].
- Recommend an occlusal guard and self-care tips/adjunctive treatment. Most patients receiving oral appliances report improvement (except 10–20%) [1].
  - "TMD patients generally report a decrease in morning symptoms, masticatory muscles become less tense and the TMJ inflammation reduces" [1].
- If there is no improvement after several weeks, reevaluate if non-TMD-related condition [1]. Consider referral.

The Patient Interview

- Questions related to TMD and mouthguards from the health history form
  - Do you have earaches or neck pains?
  - Do you have any clicking, popping, or discomfort in the jaw?
  - Do you brux or grind your teeth?
  - Do you participate in active recreational activities (i.e. sports, think need for an athletic mouthguard)?
  - Have you ever had a serious injury to your head or mouth (e.g. any jaw trauma)?
- Follow-up questions
  - Which sports do you play?
  - Any history of treatment for TMD?
  - Describe your symptoms.

Occlusal Guards

- Where is it located?
- When did the pain start?
- Rate your current pain level from 0 to 10.
- Rate the worst pain you felt in the last month from 0 to 10.
- Rate the least pain you felt in the last three months from 0 to 10.
- How long does the pain last?
- How often is the pain?
- What does the pain keep you from doing?
- What makes it feel better?
- Are you taking any medications to manage the pain?
- What makes it feel worse?
- Is your jaw ever locked closed or open?
- Questions related to daytime habits
  - Do you notice an increase in pain in the end of the day (daytime parafunctional habits)?
  - How often at rest are your teeth touching (percentage of day)? (Teeth should only touch lightly and quickly when swallowing about four to eight minutes out of 24 hours.)
  - How is your posture?
  - Do you find yourself in the forward head posture?
  - Do you find yourself clenching your teeth?
  - Any oral habits such as chewing pens, pencils, biting nails?
  - Any gum chewing and how often?
  - Do you eat hard foods?
  - Do you drink caffeinated products?
  - Do you cradle a telephone against your shoulder?
  - Do you rest your chin on your hand?
- Questions related to sleep
  - Do you wake up with headaches, tension in the jaw, or trouble opening wide?
    - Morning headaches are also a sign of obstructive sleep apnea.
  - Anyone report hearing sounds of teeth grinding at night?
  - Do you sleep on your stomach?
- Questions about mental state
  - Are you busy, frustrated, irritated, or holding tension in your muscles? Avoid using the word "stress" as TMD patients often deny being stressed [1].

Clinical and Radiographic Exam

Extraoral Exam

- Ask for the patient's permission to palpate their face and neck. The purpose of palpating the neck muscles during the extraoral exam is to determine if soreness is present. Sore neck muscles can refer pain to the masticatory structures, which can add to TMD symptoms or be the sole cause. If this is the case, it may require a referral to an orofacial pain specialist or to a physical therapist [1].
- Have a witness in the room during the exam (e.g. a dental assistant) See Figure 2.1.

- Note if fingernails appear chewed (oral habits).
- Measure the range of motions.
  - Measure range of motions before palpating muscles, as the pain from palpation can limit range of motions [1].
  - This provides a baseline for comparison at future visits.
  - Note any movements that cause the patient discomfort; if present, ask patient to point to where it hurts.
  - Measure opening:
    - Normal opening: 40–55 mm [5].
    - Measure comfort (Figure 15.2)
      - "Open comfortably without pain" [5].
    - Measure active
      - "Open as wide as you can."
      - If the patient opens to 55 mm, do not obtain a passive opening [5].
    - Measure passive
      - From active opening, push the mouth open further with your thumb on the maxillary centrals and index or middle finger on the mandibular centrals.
      - Do not have the patient open beyond 60 mm [5].
    - Measure lateral
      - Normal lateral: 8–12 mm [5].
    - Measure protrusive
      - Normal protrusive: 8–12 mm (move jaw forward like a bulldog, measure both overjet and the amount of protrusion beyond centric and record as two numbers, e.g. 2 + 8) [5].
- Limited opening? May be due to:
  - Possible trismus.
  - Possible anterior disc displacement without reduction, meaning the articular disc is anterior to the condyle and when opening the condyle is not able to slide forward and onto the disc because the disc is blocking the path.
  - Lateral pterygoid myospasm [1].

Figure 15.2 Measuring comfort.

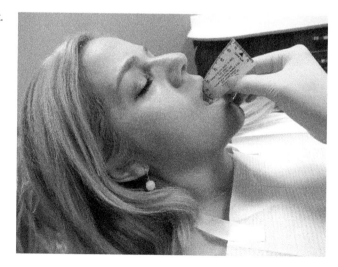

- Evaluate the path of opening.
  - Is the patient aware of this?
  - Deviation: as the mouth opens the mandible moves toward side of anterior disc displacement with reduction (if unilateral) and back to the midline (Figure 15.3).
  - Deflection: as the mouth opens the mandible moves toward side of anterior disc displacement without reduction (if unilateral) (Figure 15.4).

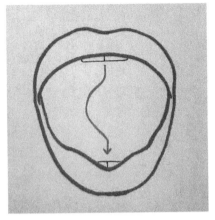

Figure 15.3 Deviation.

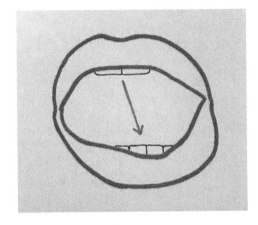

Figure 15.4 Deflection.

- Evaluate for TMJ sounds.
  - Is the patient aware of these sounds?
  - Note if unilateral or bilateral.
  - Popping/clicking (Figure 15.5). Anterior disc displacement with reduction, meaning the articular disc is anterior to the condyle, and when opening the condyle goes onto and, on closing, off the articular disc making a sound. The noise alone does not need to be treated [1].
  - Crepitus: grave sound most common in patients with osteoarthritis [6].

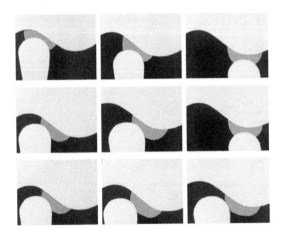

Figure 15.5 Side view of the condyle–disc–fossa relationship upon opening: posterior is to the left and anterior is to the right. Row 1: healthy articular disc and condyle relationship upon opening. Row 2: anterior disc displacement with reduction (clicking/popping). Row 3: anterior disc displacement without reduction (limited opening).

- Palpate for tenderness.
  - Palpate caudal to cranial since pain usually refers cranially.
  - Palpate in the following sequence:
    - Trapezius
    - Splenius capitis
    - Sternocleidomastoid: clavicular and sternal heads
    - Superficial masseter
    - Deep masseter
    - Temporalis
    - Medial pterygoid
    - Condyle:
      - With the patient's mouth closed, palpate the lateral pole of the condyle.
      - With the patient's mouth open, palpate the depression posterior to the condyle and pull forward to load the posterior aspect of the condyle [1]. If tender, the patient has TMJ arthralgia.

Intraoral Exam

- Check for the presence of linea alba, buccal mucosa trauma (from a cheek chewing habit), and a scalloped tongue.

Dentition

- Check for presence of attrition (severity and appropriate for age), abfractions, gingival recession, lost restorations, cracked teeth/restorations, tooth sensitivity, mobility, and secondary occlusal trauma.

Radiographic Exam

Check for the following:

- Widened PDL (on PAs) and attrition (visible clinically and on BWs).
- Panoramic radiographs:
  - Limits in image quality and superimposed images (zygoma, skull base).
  - Not to be used as sole imaging modality.
  - Gross changes of the TMJ may be seen with various conditions, including traumatic fractures, asymmetries, extensive erosion, tumors, osteophytes, changes in shape/size/opacity, and developmental abnormalities [7].
- CBCT: evaluate for osteoarthritis (decreased joint space, osteophytes, sclerosis) [6].

Occlusal Guards

Treatment Planning

Table 15.1   Treatment planning phases related to occlusal guards.

Treatment phase	Description (may or may not apply)
Emergency phase	Urgent treatment of pain, infection, trauma, and/or esthetic emergency
Data gathering phase	• Medical history • Extraoral exam, intraoral exam, and oral cancer screening • Parafunction and/or habits • Referrals to specialists
Stabilization phase (to control disease)	Not applicable
Definitive phase	• Occlusal guard
Maintenance phase	• Annual exam/periodic oral evaluation including oral cancer screenings • Evaluation of removable appliances (possible adjustments, repairs, relines, and replacements)

Referrals

If you are unable to manage the pt's TMD related pain (severe and persistent) or the diagnosis and treatment is out of your scope, refer to an Orofacial Pain Specialist (Diplomate of the American Board of Orofacial Pain. www.Abop.net) or to an Oral and Maxillofacial Surgeon.

In the referral include:

- Patient's chief complaint.
- Pain level 0–10.
- Initial signs/symptoms
- Treatment rendered.
- Adjunctive treatment.
- Medications prescribed (if any).
- Date and duration of treatment:
- Current pain level 0–10.
- Current signs/symptoms.

Informed Consent

- Informed consent is governed by state law.
- Contact your professional liability carrier and/or attorney for specific guidance and forms.

Oral Appliances: Indications and Types

Table 15.2   Oral appliances: indications and types.

Indications	Type
Clicking/popping of TMJ with no pain and no other signs of bruxism or clenching	**Hard occlusal appliance** if the clicking can be reduced when stacking one, two, or three tongue blades in the patient's mouth while they open and close (see Figure 15.1). Otherwise no occlusal appliance necessary
Clicking/popping of TMJ with pain and other signs of bruxism or clenching Osteoarthritis TMJ pain	**Hard occlusal appliance** (see Figure 15.1)
Severe grinders with holes and/or cracks in their oral appliances Patients on SSRIs Patients with excessive attrition Patients with occlusal dysesthesia Patients with full-mouth reconstruction (pressed or fired ceramics which are harder than enamel and quickly wear occlusal guards)	**Dual flat plane occlusal appliance** Since the appliances are flat and oppose each other they do not wear and can last a lifetime (Figure 15.6)
Diagnostic usage to determine if occlusal guard is indicated Interim occlusal guard when not ready to fabricate a definitive occlusal guard due to timing/treatment plan sequencing Same-day treatment for acute jaw pain Protection of breaking temporary veneers or crowns Reduce postoperative pain after periodontal or endodontic surgery	**QuickSplint** Temporary anterior bite plane (two to four weeks usage) to keep posterior teeth from contacting, reducing the amount muscles contract (www.quicksplint.com) (Figure 15.7)
Jaw muscle pain and/or limited range of motions	**Gentle Jaw** Purpose is to relieve jaw muscle pain with daily stretching (30 seconds four to six times/day). These muscles (i.e. superficial masseter, deep masseter, medial pterygoid, and temporalis) are sore from frequent contraction due to clenching/grinding (www.gentlejaw.com) (Figure 15.8)
Prevention of dental trauma (crown and root fracture, avulsion, displacement) from sports including boxing, football, hockey, lacrosse, soccer, baseball, basketball	**Athletic Mouthguard** The advantage of custom-made vs. OTC includes retention (don't have to bite to hold in place). Better retention means better protection, more comfortable custom fit, easier to breathe and speak, and less gagging [8]. The American College of Prosthodontists recommends the use of custom-made mouthguards [9]. Only one OTC sports mouthguard exists at this time accepted by the ADA[10]

SSRIs, selective serotonin reuptake inhibitors.

Occlusal Guards

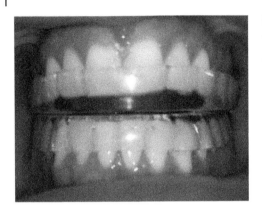

Figure 15.6 Dual flat plane occlusal appliance.
Source: Courtesy of Rich Hirschinger, DDS, MBA.
Board-certified Orofacial Pain Specialist. Inventor of
Gentle Jaw®.

Figure 15.7 QuickSplint.

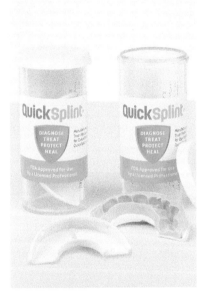

Figure 15.8 Gentle Jaw.

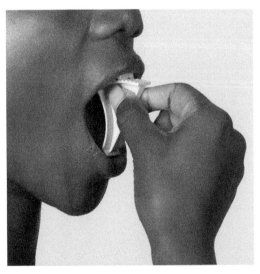

Maxillary Versus Mandibular Arch

- Occlusal guards should be full coverage (covering all the teeth in one arch) and contacting all the teeth in the opposing arch to prevent occlusal changes (e.g. supraeruption of any opposing teeth) [1]. Dual flat plane appliances are the exception, covering both arches.
- The mandibular arch is preferred as the occlusal guard is smaller, takes up less tongue space, does not obstruct the airway, is more comfortable, and is good for severe gaggers (see Figure 15.1).
- Other factors to consider include the arch with the most missing teeth, the arch with the most uneven incisal edges, the arch with the most periodontally compromised teeth, daytime usage and speech inteferences [1].
- For athletic (i.e. sports) mouthguards, the maxillary arch is preferred unless the patient is prognathic, in which case the mandibular arch is preferred.

Procedural Steps for Occlusal Guards, Dual Flat Plane Occlusal Appliances, Athletic Mouthguards, and QuickSplints

Occlusal Guards, Dual Flat Plane Occlusal Appliances, and Athletic Mouthguards

- Impressions appointment
  - Make alginate impressions of both arches.
  - Inspect for accurate impressions capturing the anatomy of *all the teeth* free of tears, bubbles, or voids. For an athletic mouthguard impression, inspect carefully to ensure you have captured the soft tissue, especially the vestibules, for retention and protection.
  - Obtain a bite registration by:
    - o Placing two cotton rolls behind the canines and instructing the patient to swallow and bite.
    - o Inject bite registration into both posterior openings and the anterior opening.
  - Send to the lab.
- Delivery appointment
  - Inspect and feel for any sharp areas that may require polishing.
  - Seat in the patient's mouth without applying too much pressure or it may be difficult to remove.
  - Ask the patient to point to any areas that feel tight/pressure or pinch and adjust as needed.
    - o May have to adjust the "fins" on the intaglio.
    - o Determine location of tight spots: place articulating paper (e.g. Accufilm) on the intaglio and seat the occlusal guard to mark the heavy spots [1] or apply Occlude spray to the intaglio to check for burn-through.
    - o Adjust as necessary: check with the lab, as some occlusal guards are thermoplastic and the manufacturer recommends placing in hot water for one minute prior to trying in the patient's mouth to improve the fit (e.g. CLEARsplint).
  - Check occlusion:
    - o Apply petroleum jelly to the red articulating paper (for the marks to show) and have the patient bite several times.
    - o Adjust until even posterior and anterior contacts (no open anterior bite).
  - Polish with an acrylic polisher and a rag wheel.
  - Verify the patient can insert and remove the appliance.
  - Provide patients with their models wrapped in bubble wrap in case they lose the occlusal guard.
  - See Sections Postoperative Instructions and TMD Self-Care Tips.

Occlusal Guards

- Follow-up appointment (one to three months from delivery)
  - Patient interview:
    - When and how often are you using the occlusal guard?
    - Which adjunctive treatment is being used and how often?
    - Symptom improvement?
    - Pain level 0–10?
    - Changes in bite? (May be due to lateral pterygoids. If there is suspicion of bite changes from osseous changes or soft tissue growths, refer for a CBCT and/or MRI.)
  - Extraoral exam.
  - Occlusal guard evaluation:
    - Check for cracks and holes.
    - Check for calculus, and remove with ultrasonic scaler if present.
    - Check occlusion with the occlusal guard and adjust if necessary.

QuickSplints

- Impression and delivery appointment: follow the instructions on www.quicksplint.com.
- Follow-up appointment (two to four weeks from delivery)
  - Evaluate the patient for decreased TMD symptoms.
  - Evaluate the QuickSplint for bite marks (signs of clenching and grinding).
  - Repeat the extraoral exam and compare to the initial extraoral exam.
  - Determine if an occlusal guard is indicated.

Lab Prescriptions

- Mandibular hard occlusal guard: ask lab to fabricate a hard acrylic mandibular stabilization appliance, no anterior guidance, no clasps.
- Dual flat plane appliance: ask lab to fabricate two hard acrylic flat plane occlusal appliances, no hardware connecting appliances, no clasps, same thickness for the upper and the lower.
- Athletic mouthguard: ask lab to fabricate maxillary mouthguard. If the patient is prognathic, request fabrication of mandibular mouthguard.

Postoperative Instructions

Oral Appliance Delivery Acknowledgment
I have just had my full coverage oral appliance delivered and acknowledge the following:

- The appliance is made to protect and stabilize my jaw muscles, joints, and teeth [1].
- The appliance is to be worn only at night except when working out with weights or when taking a nap.
- My bite on the appliance is even on both sides.
- Each morning I need to check my bite without the appliance and confirm that I can bring my teeth together so that my bite is the same as it is today.

- I will immediately schedule an appointment with Dr. _____ if I notice that my bite, with or without the appliance, is not the same as today.
- Dr. _____ is the only person who can adjust the appliance.
- I need to bring my appliance to every future appointment I have with Dr. _____.
- After taking my appliance out in the morning, I should brush the appliance with a toothbrush using only water, or mouthwash, to clean it.
- I should not use toothpaste to clean the appliance since it is abrasive and can scratch the appliance.
- About once a week, I should soak my appliance for a few hours with the biting surface face down in either a denture cleanser such as Efferdent or in white vinegar to remove any tartar deposits that could build up on the appliance. Brush the appliance well after soaking. The amount of time the appliance is soaking is not critical.
- The appliance should never be placed in hot water.
- The appliance needs to be in one or two places, either in my mouth or in the case dry.
- If I have pets, I have been informed that the appliance must be kept in a safe place away from where my pet can find the appliance since many pets, especially dogs, like to use the appliance as a chew toy.
- My appliance should be checked by Dr. _____ one month after delivery, three months, and then every six months thereafter.
- I acknowledge I have been given my plaster models, which I need to keep in a safe place and bring with me in case my appliance breaks, and it can be repaired or replaced. If I have the models, it will save me the cost of an office visit.
- Any dental treatment (such as fillings, crowns) may cause the occlusal guard to not fit properly and the guard may have to be replaced. I am responsible for the replacement fees.
  _____ (Patient Name)
  _____ (Patient Signature)
  _____ (Date)

Source: Courtesy of Rich Hirschinger, DDS, MBA. Board-certified Orofacial Pain Specialist. Inventor of Gentle Jaw®.

Athletic Mouthguard Postoperative Instructions

- When to wear
  - *Always* wear when playing sports.
- Cleaning
  - Wash daily in cold or room temperature water. Do not wash in hot water.
  - Rinse with mouthwash to improve taste.
- Storing
  - Store in a container dry when not in use. Keep it out of the heat.
  - Keep the container away from pets as dogs will use the mouthguard as a chew toy.
- Wear and tear
  - Inspect regularly for any distortions, splits, or perforations. If detected, a new mouthguard will have to be made for your protection [8].

TMD Self-Care Tips (Adjunctive Treatment)

Recommended in conjunction with the occlusal appliance.

- Exercises
  - Jaw stretching with Gentle Jaw (www.gentlejaw.com) See Figure 15.8.
  - Exercise for 20–30 minutes three to four times a day with cardiovascular low-impact exercises and/ or weight training. For weight training, limit overhead lifting if you experience neck symptoms.
- Massage
  - Your jaw and temple muscles, especially where you feel tight bands.
- Relax
  - Participate in relaxing activity each day.
- Break habits
  - Break parafunctional habits (e.g. clenching, grinding, nail biting, cheek biting, chewing objects).
  - Your teeth should only touch lightly and quickly when swallowing (only four to six minutes in each 24-hour day) and be apart the rest of the time.
  - Analogy: Patients often cross their ankles in the dental chair. If you had knee pain which was aggravated by crossing the ankles you would need to break this habit. This is similar to daytime clenching/grinding. Try "tongue up and teeth apart" [1] (same as the "N rest" position [11]).
  - When yawning, limit opening with your hand.
- Diet
  - Avoid hard and chewy foods to rest the jaw muscles and joints. Chew slowly and cut the food into smaller pieces.
  - Avoid biting with your front teeth, which compresses the jaw joints.
  - Avoid chewing gum.
  - Reduce caffeine intake (maximum one cup of coffee/day, or two cups of tea/day) [1].
- Medications
  - NSAIDs (initially on as-needed basis, not for long-term usage).
  - Voltaren gel (1% diclofenac sodium), an OTC topical NSAID gel: apply a small amount (size of two peas) to sore areas such as shoulders, neck, jaw, and/or temples three to four times a day as needed.
  - Ethyl chloride spray: prescription refrigerant spray to reduce head and neck muscle pain every three to four hours followed by jaw stretching with the Gentle Jaw.
- Hot and cold compress
  - If mild to moderate pain, apply moist heat for 15–20 minutes.
  - If new injuries, severe pain, or re-injuries, apply cold for 5–10 minutes.
- Posture
  - Improve your daytime posture (posture exercises). Avoid resting your chin in your hand.
  - If you sleep on your stomach, change your sleep posture to sleeping on your back or your side. Sleeping on your stomach puts strain on your neck and jaw.
- Therapy
  - Cognitive therapy for stress reduction and reduction of daytime clenching/bruxing.
  - Physical therapy to improve daytime/sleep posture, neck symptoms, range of motions, TMJ function [1].

Clinical Pearls

Troubleshooting

- If the patient reports removing the occlusal guard at night while sleeping, determine if the appliance is too loose, too tight, not well adjusted, or too bulky [1].

- Lab-fabricated or in-house occlusal guard not fitting? Check model for any fractured incisal edges; may have to relieve the intaglio of the occlusal guard or remake. Consider wrapping model in bubble wrap if sending to a lab.
- Trouble seeing articulating paper marks on the occlusal guard? Cover the red articulating paper with a thin layer of petroleum jelly, have the patient bite and grind. For contrast, place the occlusal guard on a white paper towel on the countertop to see the red marks.
- Occlusal guard design with only anterior teeth present: ask the lab to fabricate guard "with distal extension to premolar 2 area to help prevent aspiration."

Tips

- Occlusal adjustments: only recommend this as treatment if TMD symptoms are due to placement of a restoration [1].
- Useful analogy for communicating with patients: jaw muscles are tight like arm muscles from being overworked at the gym. Imagine big arms that are tight and not very flexible unless you intentionally make sure to stretch.

Real-Life Comments and Questions Answered

Dental Student's Question

- "What type of occlusal guard is better for patients? Hard, soft, or hard/soft?"
  - Only recommend lab-fabricated hard occlusal guards.

Patients' Comments

- "I wake up with headaches."
  - You may be clenching and/or grinding your teeth at night or have obstructive sleep apnea. Let's see if there are other signs and symptoms.
- "I play football at school."
  - Has anyone talked to you about the importance of a mouthguard? Do you wear a mouthguard when you practice? Is it comfortable? Was it made by a dentist? I highly recommend we make you a custom-fitted soft mouthguard to protect your teeth from potential damage, which can be very painful, time-consuming, expensive, and challenging to repair after an accident.
- "I don't know if I grind my teeth because I'm asleep."
  - I will perform an exam, evaluating the TMJ, the muscles of your face and neck, your range of motions, your tongue, and your teeth and let you know if I see any signs of teeth grinding. I will also ask you some specific questions to help us determine if we should be concerned.
- "I get lockjaw."
  - When you say "lockjaw" do you mean you are unable to close your mouth, or unable to open your mouth? When does this occur? How often? How do you get your mouth to close or open?
    - ○ For TMJ dislocation (inability to close)
      - ■ Since you are predisposed to this, we will take precautions during your dental visits and make sure you don't open too wide. We will also take breaks during the exam and treatment. Try to avoid opening very wide. When you need to yawn, curl your tongue to the roof of your mouth. This will limit the opening but allows you to yawn. (Can also teach

the patient's family how to unlock the patient's jaw by pushing down and back to get the condyle off the anterior wall of the eminence.)
  ○ For acute TMJ disc displacement (inability to open or "closed lock")
    ▪ Instruct the patient to unlock their jaw by moving their jaw forward to get the condyle on the disc and then opening from that protruded position. May require an anterior reposi-tioning appliance to keep the condyle on the disc for a week or two but not recommended for long-term use (see Figure 15.5).

Patients' Questions

- "Should I just get an over-the-counter nightguard or have one made at the dentist?"
  - I do not recommend OTC nightguards since they are soft. As a result of being soft, they do not fit well and can promote grinding/clenching as you try to find a stable bite. This can worsen the TMD symptoms. I recommend one made at the dentist.
- "How soon will my symptoms go away with an occlusal guard?"
  - Symptoms should improve within a few days to a few weeks.
  - Most people with TMD are between the ages of 20 and 40, as it usually resolves. It is recom-mended to keep wearing even if you find it is not needed as you may periodically have some flareups.
- "How long will this nightguard last?"
  - Occlusal guards can last from a couple of years to a lifetime. This depends largely on the amount of wear and tear you put on the appliance (Table 15.3).

Table 15.3 Type of patient and lifetime expectancy of the appliance.

Type of patient	Lifetime expectancy of the appliance
Clenchers (only applying vertical force)	Many years
Grinders with natural dentition	A few years
Grinders with restorations harder than enamel (e.g. pressed or fired ceramics)	About two years
Patients wearing dual flat plane occlusal appliances for extreme bruxing, those taking SSRIs, excessive attrition, occlusal dysesthesia, and/or full-mouth reconstruction with restorations harder than enamel	A lifetime

- "I just need a nightguard during the day when driving in L.A. [Los Angeles, California] traffic."
  - I would prefer you break the habit of clenching while driving than have to rely on an oral appliance. If you catch yourself clenching, immediately think "tongue up and teeth apart" or the "N rest" position (say the letter "N"). When the tongue is in this position it will separate the teeth, with the lips together, and relax the jaw muscles [11].
- "How do I clean it and store it?"
  - See Section Postoperative Instructions.
- "What do I do if I wear a retainer at night but I also need a nightguard?"
  - A hard nightguard acts as a passive retainer so it will prevent the teeth in that arch from moving.
- "What causes that sound in my TMJ?"

- Between the jaw condyle and fossa is a disc. Normally the disc covers the condyle as your jaw opens and closes. If the disc is anterior to the condyle and the condyle has to step onto the disc and off the disc as you open and close, it makes a clicking or popping sound. If it sounds like "Rice Krispies cereal," then it is likely due to osteoarthritis, which requires CBCT to diagnose.
- If this is your only symptom (clicking or popping), then no treatment is usually necessary.
- If other symptoms exist and we fabricate an occlusal appliance, one-third of patients report significant noise reduction or elimination, one-third have minor improvement, and one-third have no noise improvement [1].
- "My child grinds his teeth. Does he need a nightguard?"
  - Most children grind their teeth and wear down their primary canines and molars [2]. Usually no intervention is necessary and children outgrow this by 12 years of age. If not, a nightguard can be made once the child has adult teeth.
    - Only rarely is it so extensive that it endangers the pulp and the child requires stainless steel crowns to prevent exposure of the nerves and subsequent tooth sensitivity [2].
    - Most likely a child will not tolerate the nightguard and it will have to be refitted as the teeth grow.
    - Teeth near the age of exfoliation are less of a concern; grinding in adult teeth is more of a concern.

References

1 Wright, E.F. (2005). *Manual of Temporomandibular Disorders*. Ames, IA: Blackwell Munksgaard.

2 Academy of Prosthodontics The Glossary of Prosthodontic Terms, Ninth Edition. *J. Prosthet. Dent.* 117 (5S): e1–e105. https://doi.org/10.1016/j.prosdent.2016.12.001.

3 Gauer, R.L. and Semidey, M.J. (2015). Diagnosis and treatment of temporomandibular disorders. *Am. Fam. Physician.* 91 (6): 378–386.

4 Okeson, J.P. (2012). *Management of Temporomandibular Disorders and Occlusion*, 7e. St. Louis, MO: Mosby Elsevier.

5 Hirschinger, R. (2017). TMJ muscle range of motion measurements. https://www.beverlyhillstmjheadachepain.com/blog/2017/06/27/tmj-muscle-range-of-motion-measurements (accessed 10 April 2021).

6 Little, J.W., Falace, D.A., Miller, C.S. et al. (2013). *Little and Falace's Dental Management of the Medically Compromised Patient*, 8e. St. Louis, MO: Elsevier Mosby.

7 White, S.C. and Pharoah, M.J. (2009). *Oral Radiology: Principles and Interpretation*. St. Louis, MO: Mosby Elsevier.

8 Casamassimo, P., Fields, H., McTigue, D., and Nowak, A. (2013). *Pediatric Dentistry: Infancy through Adolescence*. St. Louis, MO: Elsevier.

9 American College of Prosthodontists (2018). Position Statement. Mouthguard use in sports. https://www.prosthodontics.org/about-acp/position-statement-mouthguard-use-in-sports (accessed 11 April 2021).

10 American Dental Association (2020). Sports mouthguard. https://www.ada.org/en/science-research/ada-seal-of-acceptance/ada-seal-products/product-category?category=Sports+Mouthguard (Accessed 11 April 2021).

11 Hirschinger, R (2020). N rest, and stretching exercises for jaw muscle pain. https://www.beverlyhillstmjheadachepain.com/tmj-muscle/myofascial-pain/treatment-of-myofascial-pain/n-rest-gentle-jaw-stretching-exercises (accessed 10 April 2021).

16

Dental Pharmacology

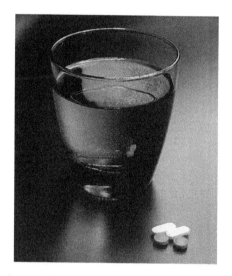

Figure 16.1   400 mg of ibuprofen and 1000 mg of acetaminophen.

Chapter Outline

- Real-Life Comments, Demands, and Questions
- Relevance
- Clinical and Radiographic Exam
- Informed Consent
- ACIID
- Prescription Writing Advice
- Adult Medications
  - Preventative

Clinical Dentistry Daily Reference Guide, First Edition. William A. Jacobson.
© 2022 John Wiley & Sons, Inc. Published 2022 by John Wiley & Sons, Inc.

- Local Anesthetics
- Antibiotics
- Analgesics
- Fungal Infections
- Viral Infections
- Anxiolytics
- Pediatric Medications
  - Preventative
  - Pediatric Local Anesthetics
  - Child Antibiotics
  - Child Analgesics
- Clinical Pearls
  - Troubleshooting
  - Tips
- Real-Life Comments, Demands, and Questions Answered
- References

Real-Life Comments, Demands, and Questions

Dental Students' Comments and Questions

- "My patient says she is allergic to penicillin."
- "When should I avoid using epinephrine in local anesthetics?"
- "My patient is not getting numb but I don't want to overdose him on lidocaine."
- "I will recommend my patient take ibuprofen."
- "I think my denture patient may have candidiasis."

Dental Assistant's Question

- "The patient wants to know if you can give her something strong after you pull out her tooth."

Patients' Demands and Questions

- "I want a refill on my chlorhexidine."
- "I need antibiotics for this."
- "Doc I rarely take antibiotics, so don't worry about antibiotic resistance. Can I have some?"
- "Do I need to take any precautions when taking this antibiotic?"
- "Can I take this medicine on an empty stomach?"
- "Can I drink beer when I'm taking this medicine?"
- "Can I take Excedrin for my toothache?"
- "I need something stronger than ibuprofen, like Norco."
- "I'm allergic to Tylenol but I can take Norco, can you prescribe me some?"
- "Can I get some tramadol after this deep cleaning?"
- "You ripped this tooth out of my skull and now you're telling me you are only going to give me ibuprofen and Tylenol?"

- "I need prednisone because that is the only thing that has worked."
- "My four-year-old has an abscess and is crying all day, can you prescribe something?"

Relevance

Whether you recommend an OTC drug, administer a drug, or prescribe a drug, it is your responsibility to understand the drug and how it will affect your patient.

Clinical and Radiographic Exam

- Review the medical history (see Chapter 1).
- Perform a thorough clinical and radiographic exam.
- Determine the diagnosis or indication prior to prescribing any medication.
- During the exam, be on the lookout for any of the four signs and symptoms of systemic involvement of an odontogenic infection in which antibiotics would be indicated.
  - Malaise, or fatigue and reduced energy [1].
  - Fascial space swelling [1].
  - Fever (>100.4°F, 38°C) [1, 2].
  - Lymph node involvement (enlarged/tender) [1] (Figure 16.2).

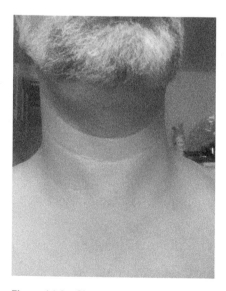

Figure 16.2 Photo taken by the patient on a weekend prior to going to the ER with a toothache. Note the submandibular lymphadenopathy on the patient's right side. Infection requiring incision and drainage would appear more diffuse and not well delineated like lymphadenopathy. Both could be tender.

Informed Consent

- Written informed consent is important when prescribing anxiolytics for dental treatment.
  - Contact your malpractice carrier for oral sedation consent forms.

– The oral sedation consent form should include the drug name, dosage, indication, instructions, side effects and precautions, patient's signature, date, the name of the driver and the patient's relationship to the driver, and the dentist signature and date.

ACIID

Before you prescribe a medication, think **ACIID** (my acronym).
- **A**: Allergies
  – Determine if a true allergy exists (e.g. hives, itching, wheezing, trouble breathing or swallowing, throat swelling) or if an adverse drug reaction exists (e.g. upset stomach).
- **C**: Contraindications
  – Determine if the medication can be safely taken considering the patient's health history.
- **I**: Interactions
  – Check for any interactions between this medication and the patient's current medications (e.g. using the Epocrates phone app interaction check).
- **I**: Indications
  – Determine if it is appropriate to prescribe this medication.
- **D**: Dosage
  – Determine the appropriate dose (neither under-medicating nor overdosing).

Prescription Writing Advice

- Provide:
  – Patient information: name, date of birth (DOB), home address.
  – Doctor's information: name, office address, signature, NPI (National Provider Identifier), state license number, DEA (Drug Enforcement Administration) Registration Number (needed for controlled substances).
  – Drug name.
  – Dosage.
  – Directions (Sig).
  – Quantity.
  – Refills (if none write 0).
- Review the prescription with the patient or the patient's caregiver.
- Precautions when writing prescriptions:
  – Avoid abbreviations.
  – Always use a leading zero for numbers below 1 (e.g. 0.5 mg) and don't use trailing zeros (e.g. 2 mg not 2.0 mg).
  – For *geriatric* patients, provide the pharmacist with the patient's age.
  – For *pediatric* patients:
    o Provide the patient's age and weight.

o Provide the intended daily weight-based dose so that the dosage can be confirmed by the pharmacist (e.g. mg/kg daily) [3].

o Write the dosage units in milliliters, not as "teaspoons" or "tablespoons." Oral medication syringes and measuring cups are recommended rather than household spoons for accurate measurements (Figure 16.3).

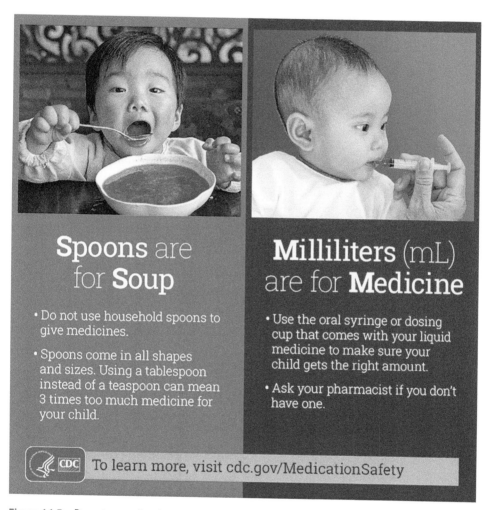

Figure 16.3 Do not prescribe dosage units as "tablespoons" or "teaspoons" as there is too much room for misinterpretation which can lead to under- or over-medicating the patient. *Source:* Centers for Disease Control and Prevention [64].

Adult Medications

Preventative

Two commonly prescribed medications for lowering caries risk are prescription strength fluoride toothpaste (Table 16.1) and Chlorhexidine (Table 16.2).

Table 16.1 Prescription-strength fluoride toothpaste.

Drug	1.1% Sodium fluoride toothpaste
Prescription	Dispense: one tube Sig: Apply a thin ribbon (or pea-sized amount) of toothpaste to toothbrush. Brush two minutes twice a day and expectorate. Do not eat, drink, or rinse for 30 minutes
Indications	Age 6+, aids in caries prevention, strengthens enamel and help reverse white spot lesions
Contraindications	0–5 years old
Pregnancy/lactation	May be used, no human data available, risk not expected [4]
Precautions	Age 6–16 years: expectorate after use and rinse Adults: expectorate after use
Miscellaneous	Contains four times the amount of F as OTC toothpaste. Contains fluoride, calcium, and phosphate (i.e. Clinpro) [5, 6]

Table 16.2 Chlorhexidine.

Drug	0.12% Chlorhexidine gluconate
Prescription	Dispense: 473 ml Sig for gingivitis: swish 15 ml for 30 seconds and expectorate (spit) twice a day Sig for caries management: swish 15 ml for one minute and expectorate (spit) twice a day for one week per month. Should be one hour apart from toothbrushing [7]
Indications	Gingivitis Age 6 through adult with high and extreme caries risk Preprocedural mouth rinse (reducing salivary bacterial load by 90% and minimizing aerosol contamination associated with dental procedures) [8]
Contraindications	Alcohol-containing formula (e.g. Peridex) contraindications include religion, alcohol recovery, xerostomia. Instead prescribe alcohol-free formula (e.g. Paroex)
Pregnancy/lactation	May be used, no human data available, risk not expected [9] Safe [10]
Precautions	Tooth staining, calculus formation, and taste alterations. Not for long-term use [8]. Taste alteration are temporary, stains teeth yellow to brown [11]. Stains can be permanent on restoration (caution with anterior composites), typically reversible on enamel
Miscellaneous	Antimicrobial rinse [8] Mouthrinse should be no sooner than two hours after toothbrushing

Local Anesthetics

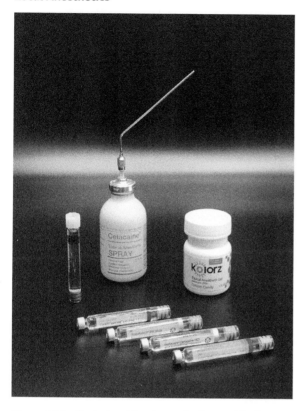

Figure 16.4   Topical and local anesthetics used in dentistry.

$$\underline{}\text{lbs} \times \frac{1 \text{ kg}}{2.2 \text{ lbs}} = \underline{}\text{kg} \times \frac{\text{MRD}}{\text{kg}}\text{mg} \times \frac{1 \text{ cartridge}}{\# \text{ mg}} = \underline{}\text{cartridges}$$

Figure 16.5   Formula for calculating the maximum dosage for local anesthetics based on the patient's weight. The patient's weight in pounds (lb), divided by 2.2 to convert to kilograms (kg), multiplied by the maximum recommended dose (MRD) which varies by drug, divided by the number (#) of milligrams per cartridge, which varies by drug, equals the total number of cartridges for the maximum dosage.

- This section reviews commonly used topical and local anesthetics (Figure 16.4), how to calculate maximum dosages (Figure 16.5), and provides max dosage tables with relevant information.
- If a patient claims to be allergic to local anesthetics, see Chapter 1, "Allergies."
- The "max dose" in Tables 16.3–16.8 are based on the manufacturers' maximum recommended dosages (Figure 16.6). This is different from the recommendations of the AAPD. The duration of action of local anesthetics is shown in Figure 16.7. See also Section Pediatric Local Anesthetics.

Anesthetic	Maximum dosage		Maximum total dosage	mg/1.7ml cartridge
	mg/kg	mg/lb		
Lidocanie 2% 1:200 000 epinephrine	7.0	3.2	500 mg	34 mg
Mepivacaine 3% plain	6.6	3.0	400 mg	51 mg
Articaine 4% 1:200 000 epinephrine	7.0	3.2	None Listed	68 mg
Prilocaine 4% plain	6.0	2.7	400 mg	68 mg
Bupivacaine 0.5% 1:200 000 epinephrine	2.0	0.9	90 mg	8.5 mg

Figure 16.6 The maximum recommended dosage of local anesthetics. *Source:* Dentalcare.com [58].

Anesthetic	Pulp	Soft tissue
Lidocaine 2% 1:200 000 epinephrine	60 minutes	180–240 minutes
Mepivacaine 3% Plain I (infiltration)	5–10 minutes	90–120 minutes
Articaine 4% 1:200 000 epinephrine 1:100 000 epinephrine	45–60 minutes 60–75 minutes	180–240 minutes 180–300 minutes
Prilocaine 4% plain Infiltration Block	10–15 minutes 60–120 minutes	40–60 minutes 120–240 minutes
Prilocaine 4% + epi 1:200 000 epinephrine	60–90 minutes	180–480 minutes

Figure 16.7 Duration of action of injectable local anesthetics. *Source:* Dentalcare.com [58].

Table 16.3 Benzocaine.

Drug	20% Benzocaine
Prescription	Dispense: one tube Sig: apply to mucosa max. four times per day [12]
Indications	Relief of soft tissue discomfort Topical anesthetic prior to local anesthetic injections or cleanings
Instructions	Dry the oral mucosa and place topical anesthetic for two minutes prior to injection [13]
Contraindications	Under two years old unless under supervision of healthcare professional [14]
Pregnancy/lactation	Avoid if pregnant/nursing [10]
Miscellaneous	Sold OTC, can prescribe, and used by dentists prior to anesthetizing

Table 16.4 Lidocaine.

Drug	Lidocaine HCl 2% and epinephrine 1:100 000					
Max dose	7.0 mg/kg or 3.2 mg/lb					
Max dose by weight[a]	Pounds	20	40	6	80	100	120–200
	Cartridges	2	4	6	8	10	11
Indications	Local anesthesia Hemostasis					
Contraindications	When sodium bisulfite or epinephrine are contraindicated					
Pregnancy/lactation	Safe for pregnancy/nursing with or without epinephrine [10]					

[a] *Source* for max dose by weight, adapted from Malamed [13].

Table 16.5 Articaine.

Drug	Articaine hydrochloride 4% and epinephrine 1:200 000 (or 1:100 000)									
Max dose	7.0 mg/kg or 3.2 mg/lb									
Max dose by weight[a]	Pounds	20	40	60	80	100	120	140	160	180	200
	Cartridges	1	2	3	4	5	6	7	8	9	10
Indications	Profound local anesthesia Superior to lidocaine when used for local infiltration in the mandible Hemostasis									
Contraindications	When sodium bisulfite or epinephrine are contraindicated									
Pregnancy/lactation	Pregnancy: risk C, use caution, consult physician Lactation: safety unknown [15]									

[a] *Source* for max dose by weight, adapted from Malamed [13].

Table 16.6 Mepivacaine.

Drug	Mepivacaine hydrochloride 3% (plain)						
Max dose	6.6 mg/kg or 3.0 mg/lb						
Max dose by weight[a]	Pounds	20	40	60	80	100	120	140–200
	Cartridges	1	2	3	4.5	5.5	6.5	7.5
Indications	When avoiding/minimizing epinephrine: sodium bisulfite allergy, blood pressure >200/115 mmHg, uncontrolled hyperthyroidism, severe cardiovascular disease (<6 months from a heart attack/stroke/CABG, unstable/daily angina, arrhythmias), taking nonspecific beta-blockers, monoamine oxidase inhibitors, or tricyclic antidepressants [13]. When shorter duration of anesthetic is desired						
Pregnancy/ lactation	Pregnancy: risk C, use caution, consult physician Lactation: safe [10, 15]						

[a] *Source* for max dose by weight, adapted from Malamed [13].

Table 16.7 Bupivacaine.

Drug	Bupivacaine hydrochloride 0.5% and epinephrine 1:200 000					
Max dose	2.0 mg/kg or 0.9 mg/lb, maximum 90 mg					
Max dose by weight[a]	Pounds	20	40	60	80	100–200
	Cartridges	2	4	5	6	10
Indications	Long-acting anesthetic for long procedures and postoperative pain management					
Contraindications	Children/elderly (risk of self-injury trauma) When sodium bisulfite or epinephrine are contraindicated					
Pregnancy/ lactation	Pregnancy: risk C, use caution, consult physician Lactation: safe [10, 15]					
Miscellaneous	Pulpal anesthesia duration about 3 hours (vs. 1 hour with lidocaine) and soft tissue for 4–12 hours (vs. 3–5 hours with lidocaine) [13]					

[a] *Source* for max dose by weight, adapted from Malamed [13].

Table 16.8 Cetacaine.

Drug	Cetacaine topical anesthetic spray Benzocaine 14.0%, Butamben 2.0%, Tetracaine Hydrochloride 2.0%
Max dose	Spray in excess of two seconds is contraindicated. Max dosage not listed
Indications	Gag reflex, topical anesthetic of mucosa
Contraindications	Under two years old
Pregnancy/ lactation	Safety has "not been established with respect to possible adverse effects upon fetal development" [16]. Lactation information not listed. Includes benzocaine 14.0%, which we avoid if patient is pregnant/nursing [10]
Miscellaneous	Rapid onset (30 seconds), duration 30–60 minutes Tissue does not need to be dried prior to use Autoclavable cannula for spray [16], also sell disposable cannulas Banana flavored

Author note: I use cetacaine for patients with strong gag reflexes (e.g. when making impressions, taking radiographs) by spraying the soft palate for one second and providing a cup for the patient to spit in. I inform the patient they can still swallow but will not feel the sensation of swallowing, which may cause some distress to an anxious patient if not forewarned. Alternatively, for controlling the gag reflex, you can have the patient lift their foot the entire time of gag-inducing procedure (e.g. alginate impression), have the patient drink a glass of cold water prior, or place salt on the patient's tongue.

Antibiotics

Indications

- If there is systemic involvement of an odontogenic bacterial infection, antibiotics are indicated with referral for treatment, or as an adjunct to pulpotomy, pulpectomy, nonsurgical RCT, or incision for drainage of abscess [1] (extractions not addressed in the guidelines).
- Systemic involvement includes:
  - Malaise (fatigue, reduced energy) [1].
  - Fascial space involvement (facial swelling) [1]. Refer to the ER for intravenous antibiotics if swelling causes difficult breathing/swallowing, cellulitis lower than inferior border of the mandible, involves the eye, or if anatomy is distorted (patient does not look human).
  - Fever (>100.4°F, 38°C) [1, 2].
  - Local lymph node involvement [1] (see Figure 16.2).
- Severe pain is not an indication for antibiotics [1].
- If no systemic involvement, warn the patient that if symptoms worsen or malaise/facial swelling/fever/tender or swollen lymph nodes become evident, they may require antibiotics.
- Consider pertinent antibiotic drug information when prescribing (see Table 16.9).

Patient Discussion about Antibiotics

Discussion with the patient should focus on the following issues.

- Prescription only applies to one course of antibiotics, so the patient should not call for refills.
- This is not an alternative to treatment (e.g. extraction or RCT).
  - The source of the infection needs to be removed.
  - If the source of the infection is not removed the infection will persist.
- There are risks involved with antibiotics:
  - Risk of anaphylaxis, opportunistic infections such as *Clostridium difficile*, and antibiotic resistance.
  - The World Health Organization is predicting that by 2050 without intervention there will be 10 million deaths annually due to superbugs [17]. This may be a leading cause of death.
- Precautions when taking antibiotics
  - Allergic reaction: if patients break out in hives they should take Benadryl (25 mg every four to six hours; caution with elderly due to falls and sedation), stop taking the antibiotic, and call the dental office. If patients have trouble breathing they should call EMS and use an EpiPen if they have one.
  - *C. difficile*: if patients develop a fever, abdominal cramping, or have three or more loose bowel movements a day, they should contact their medical provider [1].
  - Need for switching antibiotics: if no resolution of symptoms within three days, patients should call the dental office as the antibiotic may have to be changed.
  - Possible yeast infections in women: if this occurs, they should contact their medical provider.
  - Other side effects.
- Dosage frequency: effective treatment requires a constant level of the drug in the blood. Best to take medication spaced out as much as possible during waking hours.
- Follow-up
  - Reevaluate or follow up with the patient after three days to assess if there is resolution of systemic signs/symptoms.

- If the signs/symptoms begin to resolve, instruct the patient to discontinue antibiotics 24 hours after complete resolution (irrespective of reevaluation after three days) [1]. "Little to no evidence supporting the common belief that a shortened course of antibiotics contributes to antimicrobial resistance" [1].
- If no prompt response to antibiotics, consider adding oral metronidazole or discontinuing and prescribing amoxicillin/clavulanate to enhance efficacy against Gram-negative anaerobic organisms [1].

Table 16.9   Antibiotic drug information.

Antibiotic	Drug information
Amoxicillin	• Preferred over penicillin (more effective against various Gram-negative anaerobes and lower incidence of gastrointestinal side effects) [1] • Pregnancy/lactation: safe [18]
Penicillin V K	• Patient must be more compliant (four times daily vs. three times daily with amoxicillin) • Pregnancy/lactation: safe [19]
Metronidazole	• Alcohol should be avoided during, or for three days after, completion of antibiotics [3]. Interactions may be severe and fatal [20] • Different antibiotic class than penicillin and clindamycin, if allergic/contraindicated to take both • Pregnancy/lactation: may use but possible risks/caution [21] • Miscellaneous: will darken urine
Amoxicillin/ clavulanate	• Amoxicillin plus added resistance to penicillinases • "Big guns" for bad facial swelling, when other antibiotics are ineffective, when sinus exposed/infected • Pregnancy/lactation: safe [22]
Azithromycin	• Bacterial resistance rates are highest with this antibiotic [1] • Different antibiotic class than penicillin and clindamycin, if allergic/contraindicated to both • Pregnancy/lactation: may use but possible risks/caution [23]
Clindamycin	• Substantially increased risk of developing *C. difficile* even after a single dose • Patients should call PCP if they develop fever, abdominal cramping, or have three or more loose bowel movements per day [1] • Pregnancy/lactation: safe [24]
Cephalexin	• 1–5% cross-reactivity between penicillins and cephalosporins when allergic reaction is delayed. If history of anaphylaxis with penicillins, then cephalosporins are contraindicated [3] • Pregnancy/lactation: safe [25]

Antibiotic Selection Algorithm

Table 16.10 is adapted from the evidence-based clinical practice guideline on antibiotic use for the urgent management of pulpal- and periapical-related dental pain and intraoral swelling for immunocompetent patients 18 years and older [1].

Table 16.10 Antibiotic selection algorithm.

Antibiotic allergy	Antibiotic of choice
No penicillin allergy	• Amoxicillin 500 mg three times daily for 3–7 days, *or* penicillin V potassium 500 mg four times daily for 3–7 days • If first-line treatment fails, complement with metronidazole 500 mg three times daily for 7 days, *or* discontinue first-line treatment and take amoxicillin/clavulanate 500/125 mg three times daily for 7 days
Penicillin allergy and a history of anaphylaxis, angioedema, or hives with penicillin, ampicillin, or amoxicillin	• Azithromycin (loading dose 500 mg on day 1, followed by 250 mg for an additional 4 days), *or* clindamycin 300 mg four times dail for 3–7 days • If first-line treatment fails, complement with metronidazole 500 mg three times daily for 7 days
Penicillin allergy and *no* history of anaphylaxis, angioedema, or hives with penicillin, ampicillin, or amoxicillin	• Cephalexin 500 mg four times daily for 3–7 days • If first-line treatment fails, complement with metronidazole 500 mg three times daily for 7 days [1]

Antibiotic Premedications

- For indications, see Chapter 1.
  Blood levels:
  - It is important for the antibiotic to reach adequate blood levels.
  - If patients forget to take their premed, the antibiotic may be administered up to two hours after the procedure.
- If the patient is already taking antibiotics for another condition, select an antibiotic from a different class [26].
- Tables 16.11–13 provide pertinent information for the following premedications: Amoxicillin, Clindamycin, and Azithormycin.

Table 16.11 Amoxicillin premed.

Drug	Amoxicillin 500 mg
Prescription	Dispense: four tablets times number of appointments Sig: take four tablets (2 g) 30–60 minutes before dental procedure [11]
Indications	Prevention of bacterial endocarditis or orthopedic implant infection
Contraindications	Serious hypersensitivity to amoxicillin or other beta-lactams (e.g. penicillin) [3]
Pregnancy/lactation	Safe [10]. Pregnancy risk B [3]
Precautions	Dose and/or frequency modified in renal impairment Prolonged use may result in risk of fungal or bacterial superinfection, including *C. difficile* [3]
Miscellaneous	With or without food

Table 16.12 Clindamycin premed.

Drug	Clindamycin 150 mg
Prescription	Dispense: four tablets times number of appointments Sig: take four tablets (600 mg) 30–60 minutes before dental procedure [11]
Indications	Prevention of bacterial endocarditis when allergic to penicillin
Contraindications	Hypersensitivity to clindamycin, or lincomycin [3]
Pregnancy/ lactation	Safe [10]. Avoid if breastfeeding [3]
Precautions	1% of clindamycin users develop *C. difficile* [3]
Miscellaneous	*C. difficile* has never occurred with the one- dose regimen used to prevent bacterial endocarditis [3]. With food may cause less stomach upset

Table 16.13 Azithromycin premed.

Drug	Azithromycin 500 mg
Prescription	Dispense: one tablet times number of appointments Sig: take one tablet (500 mg) 30–60 minutes before dental procedure [11]
Indications	Prevention of bacterial endocarditis, or orthopedic implant infection, when allergic to penicillin
Contraindications	Hypersensitivity to azithromycin, erythromycin, other macrolide antibiotics [3]
Pregnancy/ lactation	Pregnancy risk B [3] Lactation: may use but check risks, consult obstetrics/gynecology
Precautions	Use caution if liver disease. Prolonged use may result in risk of fungal or bacterial superinfection, including *C. difficile* [3]
Miscellaneous	With food to decrease stomach upset [3]

Analgesics

- "Consider both the medication's potential to provide pain relief and its potential to cause harm" [27].
- "When comparing the efficacy of nonsteroidal anti-inflammatory medications with opioids in relation to the magnitude of pain relief, the combination of 400 mg of ibuprofen plus 1000 mg of acetaminophen was found to be superior to any opioid-containing medication or medication combination studied. In addition, the opioid-containing medications or medication combinations studied were all found to have higher risk of inducing acute adverse events" [27] (Tables 16.14 and 16.15; see also Figure 16.1).
- Anticipated pain following dental procedures:
  - Mild: SRP, subgingival restoration, RCT, simple extraction.
  - Moderate: surgical extraction, implant placement.
  - Severe: partial or full bony impaction surgery, periodontal surgery, complex implant [28], or dry socket.

Table 16.14 Ibuprofen.

Drug	Ibuprofen 400 mg
Prescription	Dispense: amount varies Sig: take one tablet every six hours as needed for pain
Max dose	3200 mg/day
Indications	Pain and swelling Mild to moderate pain [30] First-line therapy for patients in pain
Contraindications	Hypersensitivity to ibuprofen, asthma or urticaria to aspirin or other NSAIDs [3]. History of bariatric surgery. History of peptic ulcer disease/gastrointestinal bleeding [3]; determine history of ulcers, i.e. healed vs. active or recent ulcers (higher risk with ibuprofen). Avoid use in advanced renal disease [3]. Avoid if liver cirrhosis (but acceptable with hepatitis). Uncontrolled diabetes, kidney failure, taking lithium, taking methotrexate, bleeding disorders, blood thinners; if taking aspirin take ibuprofen two hours after aspirin or eight hours before so as not to interfere with antiplatelet action
Pregnancy/lactation	Avoid in pregnancy [10]. NSAID of choice while breastfeeding [31]
Precautions	Ibuprofen can interfere with the antiplatelet effect of aspirin 81 mg, diminishing its cardioprotective effect. Discuss with patient's physician [3]. Can prolong bleeding time in some patients, but less/shorter duration/reversible compared to aspirin [3]. Unlikely to lead to significant bleeding following extractions in most patients [32]. Consider a selective cyclooxygenase-2 inhibitor (e.g. celecoxib) for patients at risk for bleeding (e.g. on anticoagulant) [33]
Miscellaneous	Sold over the counter as 200 mg, have patient take two (400 mg total). Consider preoperative loading dose one hour prior to procedure. Provide postoperative ibuprofen prior to anesthesia wearing off: "better to stay out of pain then get in pain and dig yourself out." The 800 mg pills are large and may be harder to swallow for some patients; 800 mg is a large dose and may be hard on the kidneys and stomach. The patient must be well hydrated, have good renal function, and take pills with food to minimize stomach upset.

Table 16.15 Acetaminophen.

Drug	Acetaminophen 500 mg
Prescription	Dispense: amount varies Sig: take two tablets (1000 mg) every six hours as needed for pain
Max dose	1000 mg/dose and 4000 mg/day (maximum 4 g/day under the direction of a healthcare provider) [3]. Over 4 g/day is associated with acute liver failure [30]. If hepatitis/cirrhosis, maximum 2000 mg/day
Indications	When an NSAID is contraindicated
Contraindications	Hypersensitivity to acetaminophen, severe hepatic impairment or severe active liver disease [3]
Pregnancy/lactation	Drug of choice during pregnancy and lactation No known risk of fetal/infant harm with short-term use [34]
Precautions	Do not take with alcohol Do not combine with other acetaminophen-containing products (e.g. NyQuil) [11]
Miscellaneous	Take with or without food 1000 mg pill not available, patient must take two 500 mg pills

- Inform the patient that the goal is to be as comfortable as possible knowing that some discomfort is normal and may still occur [27]. Pain level of 0 is not a realistic goal [29] – dentistry is not pain-free.

Opioid Overview
- What are opioids?
  - Opioids are natural or synthetic chemicals that interact with opioid receptors on nerve cells in the body and brain, and reduce the intensity of pain signals and feelings of pain.
  - Because they produce euphoria in addition to pain relief, they can be misused [35].
- The dangers of opioids
  - "Prescription opioids can be addictive and dangerous. It only takes a little to lose a lot."
  - Every day in the United States more than 46 people die from prescription opioid overdoses [36].
- Who regulates opioids?
  - Manufacture, importation, possession, use, and distribution of controlled substances is regulated by the United States federal government [37].
  - To prescribe controlled substances, you must be registered with the DEA.
- Drug schedules
  - There are five categories of controlled substances (Schedule I–V). I has the highest potential for abuse and dependency and V has the least potential for abuse [38].
  - Schedule I has no medical use, e.g. heroin [39].
- ADA statement on the use of opioids:
  - "Dentists should consider NSAIDs as first-line therapy for acute pain management."
  - Supports multimodal pain strategies for sparing the need of opioids.
  - Opioid duration of no more than seven days for acute pain [30].
- CDC recommendations if an opioid is warranted:
  - Prescribe the lowest effective dose of immediate-release opioids.
  - Quantity of a three-day course or less will be sufficient; more than seven days is rarely needed.
    - Rationale: physical dependence on opioids is a physiologic response in patients exposed to opioids for more than a few days [40].
    - Adolescents and young adults through 24 years: limit to 8–12 tablets [41].
- Limit the quantity of opioids and manage with ibuprofen plus acetaminophen as soon as possible [29].
- Office/clinic/school pain management policy: recommend having a pain management policy.
- Prescription Drug Monitoring Program (PDMP)
  - Access your state's PDMP database (e.g. Cures 2.0 in California) to find out if patient has a history of prescribed controlled substances. Mandatory if prescription exceeds five-day supply [63].
  - Only look up records of active patients. Everything you search is tracked, and searching for people who are not patients is a violation of the Health Insurance Portability and Accountability Act 1996 (HIPAA).
  - Print or screenshot and save report with date in patient's chart.
  - I recommend searching by name and DOB, not by address, because this will narrow the search down even further as the patient may have multiple addresses listed with different reports.
- Cannabis and opioids:
  - Used medicinally and recreationally.

- "Based on current data, it can be postulated that for most patients cannabis and opioids can be used together safely. When prescribing opioids to patients who use cannabis, a lower opioid dose should be considered due to the synergistic and opioid-sparing effects of cannabinoids . . . properly educated patients when prescribing opioids about the risks of impairment and inability to perform daily activities when simultaneously using opioids with cannabis and/or alcohol" [42].

- Precautions to communicate to the patient when prescribing controlled substances
  - Risks of opioids
    - Addiction, abuse, misuse, overdose, respiratory depression, and death.
    - Risks of overdose increase if opioids combined with alcohol or other drugs, in certain medical conditions such as sleep apnea and reduced kidney or liver function, and in those aged over 65 years [43].
      - For the dentist: 50 morphine milligram equivalents (MMEs) per day or more increases risk of death from overdose. Equivalent to 50 mg of hydrocodone (10 tablets of hydrocodone/acetaminophen 5/325) per day or 33 mg oxycodone per day [32].
  - Signs of overdose
    - Pinpoint pupils, falling asleep or loss of consciousness, slow shallow breathing, pale/blue/cold skin.
    - If suspect overdose, call EMS and administer naloxone if available [43].
  - Adverse effects: constipation, dizzy/drowsy, fall risk, impaired thinking/reactions.
  - **Do not**
    - Do not use with alcohol, benzodiazepines, or other CNS depressants. May result in profound sedation, respiratory depression, coma, and death.
    - Do not drive or operate machinery for at least six hours after taking medication.
    - Avoid making any major decisions.
    - Do not share or sell medications.
  - Storage: in a secure place where others cannot get hold of them (e.g. children, family, friends, visitors).
  - Disposal: for leftover medications follow the disposal instructions on the prescription. Not all medications should be flushed down the toilet. Use community drug take-back programs to return unused medications for proper disposal. If no disposal instructions and no take-back programs nearby, mix with something in the garbage (e.g. coffee grounds or kitty litter) to make it less appealing to children, pets, and drug seekers [29, 44].

Red Flags of Drug Seekers

- Patient tries to pressure the dentist to prescribe opioids using sympathy, guilt, or threats. This may be for the patient to use or to sell.
- Patient states which controlled substance works and which noncontrolled analgesics do not work and claims allergies.
- Patient feigns dental symptoms to support obtaining medication. Make sure there is a diagnosis. Do not prescribe if nothing is wrong.
- No interest in diagnosis (or treatment).
- Patient only interested in obtaining the controlled substance at the pharmacy and not other medications (e.g. antibiotics). Follow up with the pharmacy.
- Patient states prescription was lost/stolen or medication fell into water.

- Traveling from out of town (check driver's license/insurance card for home address).
- Demands to be seen immediately
- Schedules appointment at the end of the day or week.
- Cutaneous signs of drug abuse [29].

Multimodal Pain Management Options

- Ibuprofen 400 mg preoperative loading dose one hour prior to procedure [32].
- Palliative treatment: pulpotomy, pulpectomy, occlusal adjustment, QuickSplint.
- Long-acting local anesthetic (i.e. bupivacaine):
  - Administer at the end of the procedure to help delay the onset and severity of pain.
  - If patient has acute pain and is truly interested in immediate pain relief (not drug seeking), in my experience they will accept an injection of bupivacaine to relieve the pain.
- Cold compress, up to 15 minutes at a time to help with swelling/pain: use ice inside a towel or bag of frozen vegetables; avoid ice directly on skin (painful) [32].
- Prescription anesthetic mouthrinse:
  - Lidocaine 2% viscous: dispense 300 ml. Sig: swish 15 ml to relive pain then expectorate. Every three hours, maximum eight times daily as needed for pain.
  - Pregnancy/lactation: safe [45].
- Warm salt-water rinses to decrease inflammation and remove food debris: half teaspoon of salt per glass of warm water, gently rinse for 15 seconds and expectorate.
- Sleep propped up with a few pillows to reduce pain [32].

Opioids

Tables 16.16-18 provide pertinent information for Tramadol, Tylenol #3, and Norco.

Table 16.16 Tramadol.

Drug	Tramadol 50 mg
Prescription	Dispense: 12 tablets (three-day duration if taken every six hours) Sig: take one tablet every four to six hours as needed for pain
Max dose	400 mg/day (8 tablets/day)
Indications	When both NSAIDs and acetaminophen are contraindicated Moderate to moderately severe dental pain [3]
Contraindications	Hypersensitivity to tramadol or opioids, <12 years old, respiratory depression, bronchial asthma, gastrointestinal obstruction, concomitant use with or within 14 days of monoamine oxidase inhibitor (MAOI) [3]
Pregnancy/ lactation	Avoid
Precautions	See Section Opioid Overview
Schedule	IV
Miscellaneous	Take with or without food Prescribe immediate-release Available in 50 and 100 mg tablets

Table 16.17 Tylenol #3.

Drug	Acetaminophen 300 mg, codeine 30 mg (Tylenol #3)
Prescription	Dispense: 12 tablets (three-day duration if every six hours) Sig: take one tablet every four to six hours as needed for pain
Max dosage	360 mg/day of codeine (12 tablets/day) Do not exceed 1 g every four hours and 4 g/day of acetaminophen from all sources [46]
Indications	Moderate to severe pain
Contraindications	Any acetaminophen contraindications (liver disease). Hypersensitivity to acetaminophen, codeine, or opioids; <12 years old, respiratory depression, bronchial asthma, gastrointestinal obstruction, concomitant use with or within 14 days of MAOI [3]
Pregnancy/lactation	Avoid [3]
Precautions	See Section Opioid Overview. Caution if receiving more than one source of acetaminophen-containing medications [3]
Schedule	III
Miscellaneous	Generic form acceptable with the same ingredients: acetaminophen 300 mg, codeine 30 mg [11] Take with or without food

Table 16.18 Norco.

Drug	Hydrocodone 5 mg and acetaminophen 325 mg (e.g. Norco)
Prescription	Dispense: 12 tablets (three-day duration if taken every six hours) Sig: take one tablet every four to six hours as needed for pain
Max dosage	40 mg/day of hydrocodone (8 tablets/day) Do not exceed 1 g every four hours and 4 g/day of acetaminophen from all sources [47]
Indications	Moderate to severe pain
Contraindications	Any acetaminophen contraindications (liver disease). Hypersensitivity to acetaminophen, hydrocodone, or opioids, <12 years old, respiratory depression, bronchial asthma [3]
Pregnancy/lactation	Avoid
Precautions	See Section Opioid Overview. Caution if receiving more than one source of acetaminophen-containing medications [3]
Schedule	II
Miscellaneous	Nausea is the most common adverse effect, sedation and constipation is second [3] Alternatives drugs available combining hydrocodone with ibuprofen If prescribing hydrocodone/acetaminophen, add ibuprofen [32] Take with or without food (if nausea take with food)

Real-Life Pain Management Scenarios and Tips

- Recommend informing the patient that the "goal is to be as comfortable as possible knowing that some discomfort is normal and may still occur" [27]. The pain may not reduce from a 10 to a 0, but will attempt to lower the pain so that it is tolerable
- The author's real-life scenarios described in Table 16.19 highlight the complexities of pain management.

Table 16.19   Real-life pain management scenarios and tips.

Scenario	Tips
"I'm in pain"	Ibuprofen 400 mg + acetaminophen 1000 mg is safe and effective [27] Multimodal pain management options
"I will be in pain after this procedure."	Ibuprofen 400 mg + acetaminophen 1000 mg is safe and effective. [27] Take before the anesthetic wears off. Multimodal pain management options
"The oral surgeon is booked out two months so I need Norcos until then."	You are not responsible for providing opioids for a long duration. Unless you have special training, you only treat acute pain not chronic pain, and for no more than seven days [30]. After a few days, physical dependence develops [40]. Additionally, the patient may not show up to the appointment with the specialist (intentionally or unintentionally) Ibuprofen 400 mg + acetaminophen 1000 mg is safe and effective [27] Multimodal pain management options Consider consulting the patient's physician if pain management needed for a long duration
"I saw the oral surgeon yesterday and I'm in severe pain"	Refer patient back to the specialist. They are responsible for any postoperative pain/complications
"I'm in pain and allergic to ibuprofen."	Verify there is a true allergy (or contraindication) with follow-up questions Recommend acetaminophen 1000 mg Multimodal pain management options
"I'm in pain and allergic to acetaminophen."	Verify there is a true allergy (or contraindication) with follow-up questions Recommend ibuprofen 400 mg Multimodal pain management options
"I'm in pain and allergic to both ibuprofen and acetaminophen."	Verify there is a true allergy (or contraindication) with follow-up questions and an indication for medication Consider tramadol 50 mg Multimodal pain management options

Table 16.19 (Continued)

Scenario	Tips
"I'm in pain and I need Norcos."	Be familiar with the red flags of drug seekers. See Section Red Flags of Drug Seekers
	Ibuprofen 400 mg + acetaminophen 1000 mg is safe and effective [27]
	Multimodal pain management options
"I used to do meth and I have a toothache."	(If considering opioids) No evidence that exposure to an opioid for acute pain increases the rate of relapse. Stress associated with unrelieved (undermedicated) pain may be more likely to trigger a relapse than adequate analgesia [48]
	Ibuprofen 400 mg + acetaminophen 1000 mg is safe and effective [27]
	Multimodal pain management options
"I have a toothache" – a person with substance use disorder	(If considering opioids) To prevent the patient from using all the medications at once, write multiple prescriptions each for one day for a total of two to three days [29]
	Encourage the patient to receive substance use disorder treatment and provide contact information for local treatment options [29]
	Consider consulting the patient's physician
	Ibuprofen 400 mg + acetaminophen 1000 mg is safe and effective [27]
	Multimodal pain management options
"I'm in recovery and I have a toothache."	Patient may be taking methadone, buprenorphine, suboxone, or naltrexone
	These medications do not control acute pain (instead reduce cravings and minimize physiologic withdrawal)
	May have hyperalgesia (increased sensitivity to pain commonly associated with chronic opioid therapy)
	The hyperalgesia and analgesic tolerance may be misinterpreted as drug-seeking behavior
	Ibuprofen 400 mg + acetaminophen 1000 mg is safe and effective [27]
	Multimodal pain management options
	Consider consulting the patient's pain management doctor, or physician
"I take opioids for chronic pain and I have a toothache."	Chronic opioid does not treat acute dental pain
	If considering opioids, consult with the patient's pain management doctor
	Patient will be on a pain contract. Find out the rules of the pain contract as prescribing opioids could violate/break the pain contract
	If unable to consult due to urgency, patient may require higher analgesic dosages and at more frequent intervals, such as every three to four hours instead of every four to six [29]. Be sure to follow up with the pain management doctor
	Ibuprofen 400 mg + acetaminophen 1000 mg is safe and effective [27]
	Multimodal pain management options

Fungal Infections

Prevalence of denture stomatitis is about 50% among wearers of complete denture [49]. Clotrimazole can be prescribed for oral fungal infections. See Table 16.20.

Table 16.20 Clotrimazole.

Drug	Clotrimazole troche 10 mg
Prescription	Dispense: 70 troches Sig: remove dental prosthesis from mouth (if applicable) and dissolve one troche in mouth five times per day
Indications	Oral fungal infection, candidiasis
Pregnancy/lactation	Pregnancy category C [50]. May be used while breastfeeding [51]
Precautions	Contains sucrose (flavor), increased caries risk if usage for more than three months [11]
Miscellaneous	Max dosage: 50 mg/day (five troches/day), 14-day course Troche pronounced "trow-key" Continued use 48 hours after clinical sigs have disappeared [15] Only works while in contact with soft tissue, thus high frequency is necessary Recommend prescribing the powder form of nystatin for moist extraoral lesions and prescribing nystatin ointment or cream for dry extraoral lesions [50] *For denture/partial wearers*: For dental prosthesis, either sprinkle nystatin powder on surfaces, soak in nystatin suspension [11], or apply cream or ointment onto surfaces [50] Replace denture brush Emphasize improved denture/oral hygiene and removal of dentures at night [49] (see Chapter 12)

Viral Infections

For treating recurrent herpes labialis, see Tables 16.21–22.

Table 16.21 Penciclovir.

Drug	1% Penciclovir topical
Prescription	Dispense: 5 g Sig: apply cream every two hours while awake for four days [52]
Indications	Recurrent herpes labialis. Best results if applied at prodromal stage
Pregnancy/lactation	Safe [52]
Precautions	Caution if immune deficiency [52]
Miscellaneous	More effective than OTC docosanol [53]

Table 16.22   Valacyclovir.

Drug	Valacyclovir 1000 mg
Prescription	Dispense: four tablets
	Sig: take two tablets (2000 mg) during the prodrome followed by another two tablets (2000 mg) 12 hours later [53]
Indications	Recurrent herpes labialis. Best results if applied at prodromal stage
Pregnancy/ lactation	Safe [54]
Precautions	Refer to drug reference book

Anxiolytics

Oral sedation is a form of minimal or moderate sedation in which a medication is prescribed that has a calming effect to reduce anxiety. The patient needs to be driven to and from the appointment by someone that he or she knows. See Section Informed Consent. Triazolam (Table 16.23) is an example of an oral sedative.

Table 16.23   Triazolam.

Drug	Triazolam 0.25 mg (0.125 mg if elderly or sensitive to sedatives) [3]
Prescription	Dispense: six tablets (varies based on number of visits)
	Sig: take one tablet one hour before dental appointment [3]
Indications	Dental anxiety, preoperative sedation
Pregnancy/ lactation	Pregnancy risk factor X (avoid) [3]. Breastfeeding not recommended
Precautions	In combination with opioids can cause profound sedation, respiratory depression coma, and death [55]. Do not drive the rest of the day
Controlled substance schedule	IV [3]
Miscellaneous	Onset of action 15–30 minutes, peak within two hours, duration six to seven hours [3]
	For Sig can instruct patient to take one tablet before bed and one tablet one hour before dental appointment. Some patients have such severe anxiety (racing heart and thoughts) that they have trouble sleeping the night before a procedure
	Triazolam has the shortest half-life of all oral benzodiazepines [3]
	Steps: (i) informed consent form and inform patient you will check the ID of their driver; (ii) schedule appointment for treatment under sedation; (iii) check the ID of the driver the day of appointment
	The driver must be someone the patient knows
	Take on an empty stomach. Don't take with alcohol. Limit or avoid grapefruit juice [3, 56]

Pediatric Medications

Preventative

See Section Adult Medications, Preventative.

Dietary Fluoride

Fluoride supplements "are effective in reducing prevalence of dental caries and should be considered for children at high caries risk who drink fluoride-deficient (less than 0.6 ppm F) water" (Figure 16.8).

Age	<0.3 ppm F	<0.3 to 0.6 ppm F	> 0.6 ppm F
Birth to 6 months	0	0	0
6 months to 3 years	0.25 mg	0	0
3 to 6 years	0.50 mg	0.25 mg	0
6 to at least 16 years	1.00 mg	0.50 mg	0

Figure 16.8 Dietary fluoride supplementation schedule [57]. *Source:* Copyright © 2020 American Academy of Pediatric Dentistry and reprinted with their permission.

Pediatric Local Anesthetics

- If a patient claims to be allergic to local anesthetics, see Chapter 1, "Allergies"
- For information about specific anesthetics, see Section Adult Medications, Local Anesthetics.
- The doses in Figures 16.9 and 16.10 are recommended by the AAPD. These maximum dosages differ from the manufacturers' maximum recommended dosages (see Figure 16.6).

Anesthetic	Maximum dosage		Maximum total dosage	mg/1.7ml carpule
	mg/kg	mg/lb		
Lidocanie 2% 1:200 000 epinephrine	4.4	2.0	300 mg	34 mg
Mepivacaine 3% plain	4.4	2.0	300 mg	51 mg
Articaine 4% 1:200 000 epinephrine	7.0	3.2	500 mg	68 mg
Prilocaine 4% plain	8.0	3.6	600 mg	68 mg
Bupivacaine 0.5% 1:200 000 epinephrine	1.3	0.6	90 mg	8.5 mg

Figure 16.9 Maximum dosage of local anesthetics recommended by the AAPD. *Source:* Dentalcare. com [58].

Maximum Number of 1.8ml Cartridges					
Age	Kg	Lbs	2% Lidocaine	3% Mepivicaine	4% Articanine
1 + years	7.5	16.5	0.9	0.6	0.7
2–3 years	10.0	22.0	1.2	0.8	1.0
	12.5	27.5	1.5	1.0	1.2
4–5 years	15.0	33.0	1.8	1.2	1.5
	17.5	38.5	2.1	1.4	1.7
6–8 years	20.0	44.0	2.4	1.6	2.0
	22.5	49.5	2.8	1.8	2.2
9–10 years	25.0	55.0	3.1	2.0	2.4
	30.0	66.0	3.7	2.4	2.9
11 years	32.5	71.5	4.0	2.6	3.2
	35.0	77.0	4.3	2.9	3.4
	37.5	82.5	4.6	3.1	3.7
	40.0	88.0	4.9	3.3	3.9

Figure 16.10   Dosage chart for AAPD maximum recommended dosages. *Source:* Dentalcare.com [58].

Child Antibiotics

Pediatric Antibiotic (Dental Abscess and Premed) Dosage Tables
The calculations in this section are based on a number of parameters:

1) For children, limiting the dose to twice a day versus three times a day when it is an option for better patient (and parent) compliance.
2) Using the adult dosage once weight reahes 88 lb (or 40 kg).
3) Using milliliters (ml) instead of "teaspoon" and "tablespoon" which introduces room for error/ misinterpretation. Parents can get syringes and measuring cups from the pharmacy for accurate measurements.

4) For suspension, using a higher concentration once possible to decrease volume prescribed.
5) Rounding to the milliliter, not the milligram, so less deviation from the calculated dosage.
6) The following calculations are based on the lowest weight in the weight range (e.g. based on 20 lb for the range 20–24.9 lb; or 9 kg for the range 9–11.3 kg).
7) Clindamycin and azithromycin are not available in chewable form. An alternative for clindamycin is prescribing capsules that can be opened and sprinkled on foods (e.g. pudding, yogurt, ice cream, apple sauce). Capsules are not available for azithromycin.
8) After three chewables easier to take suspension, but can offer the option to the parent and the child.
9) The four-step formula (Figure 16.11).

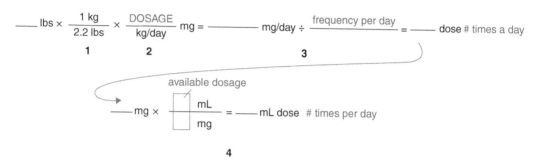

Figure 16.11 The four-step formula.

1: CONVERT POUNDS TO KILLIGRAMS

____lbs ÷ 2.2 = ____ kg *have a scale in the office, the parent may not know the child's recent weight)*

2: CALCULATE THE DOSE IN MILLIGRAMS

____kg x (Dosage)mg/kg/day

3: DIVIDE THE DOSE BY THE FREQUENCY (DOSES PER DAY)

____ mg ÷ # times per day = ____ mg per dose

4: CALCULATE IN ML OR TABLETS

FOR SUSPENSION: ____ mg ÷ (available dose per tablet) = ____ tablets X times per day *(round to nearest tablet or half a tablet)*

FOR TABLET: ____ mg ÷ (available suspension dose) x 5 mL = ____ mL X times per day *(round to the nearest 0.5 mL and for Azithromycin round to the nearest 0.25 mL)*

Amoxicillin for Dental Abscess (Table 16.24)

- 45 mg/kg daily in divided doses every 12 hours for seven days (maximum 875 mg/dose).
- Available in:
  - Suspension: 125 mg/5 ml, 200 mg/5 ml, 250 mg/5 ml, 400 mg/5 ml.
  - Chewable: 125 mg, 250 mg.

Table 16.24 Amoxicillin: pediatric dosage for dental abscess.

Weight (lb)	Weight (kg)	Dose (ml) twice daily for seven days	Dispense (ml)	Chewable(s) twice daily for seven days	Dispense (chewables)
20–24.9	9.09–11.32	4 ml (250 mg/5 ml)	56	1.5 (125 mg)	21
25–29.9	11.36–13.59	5 ml (250 mg/5 ml)	70	1 (250 mg)	14
30–34.9	13.64–15.86	6 ml (250 mg/5 ml)	84	1 (250 mg)	14
35–39.9	15.91–18.14	7 ml (250 mg/5 ml)	98	2.5 (125 mg)	35
40–44.9	18.18–20.41	5 ml (400 mg/5 ml)	70	1.5 (250 mg)	21
45–49.9	20.45–22.68	6 ml (400 mg/5 ml)	84	4 (125 mg)	56
50–54.9	22.73–24.95	6 ml (400 mg/5 ml)	84	2 (250 mg)	28
55–59.9	25–27.23	7 ml (400 mg/5 ml)	98	2 (250 mg)	28
60–64.9	27.27–29.5	7.5 ml (400 mg/5 ml)	105	2.5 (250 mg)	35
65–69.9	29.55–31.77	8 ml (400 mg/5 ml)	112	2.5 (250 mg)	35
70–74.9	31.82–34.05	9 ml (400 mg/5 ml)	126	2.5 (250 mg)	35
75–79.9	34.09–36.32	9.5 ml (400 mg/5 ml)	133	3 (250 mg)	42
80–84.9	36.36–38.59	10 ml (400 mg/5 ml)	140	3.5 (250 mg)	49
85–89.9	38.64–40.86	11 ml (400 mg/5 ml)	154	3.5 (250 mg)	49
> 90	> 40	10 ml (of 250 mg/5 ml) three times daily	210	2 (250 mg) three times daily	42

Source: Courtesy of William Jacobson DMD, MPH © 2021.

Amoxicillin for Premed (Table 16.25)

- 50 mg/kg 30–60 minutes before procedure (do not exceed adult dose of 2 g).
- Available in:
  - Suspension: 125 mg/5 ml, 200 mg/5 ml, 250 mg/5 ml, 400 mg/5 ml.
  - Chewable: 125 mg, 250 mg
    - For some of the chewable doses, I round up to prevent the risk of underdosing a serious infection.
- Total amount to dispense depends on number of visits.

Table 16.25   Amoxicillin: pediatric dosage for premed.

Weight (lb)	Weight (kg)	Dose (ml) 30–60 min before procedure	Chewable(s) 30–60 min before procedure
20–24.9	9.09–11.32	5 ml (400 mg/5 ml)	2 (250 mg)
25–29.9	11.36–13.59	7 ml (400 mg/5 ml)	2.5 (250 mg) (rounded up)
30–34.9	13.64–15.86	8 ml (400 mg/5 ml)	3 (250 mg) (rounded up)
35–39.9	15.91–18.14	10 ml (400 mg/5 ml)	3.5 (250 mg) (rounded up)
			After three chewables can provide the option to the parent and patient: do you prefer more chewables or more liquid?
40–44.9	18.18–20.41	11 ml (400 mg/5 ml)	3.5 (250 mg)
45–49.9	20.45–22.68	13 ml (400 mg/5 ml)	4 (250 mg)
50–54.9	22.73–24.95	14 ml (400 mg/5 ml)	4.5 (250 mg)
55–59.9	25–27.23	16 ml (400 mg/5 ml)	5 (250 mg)
60–64.9	27.27–29.5	17 ml (400 mg/5 ml)	5.5 (250 mg)
65–69.9	29.55–31.77	18 ml (400 mg/5 ml)	6 (250 mg)
70–74.9	31.82–34.05	20 ml (400 mg/5 ml)	6.5 (250 mg)
75–79.9	34.09–36.32	21 ml (400 mg/5 ml)	7 (250 mg)
80–84.9	36.36–38.59	23 ml (400 mg/5 ml)	7.5 (250 mg) (rounded up)
85–89.9	38.64–40.86	24 ml (400 mg/5 ml)	8 (250 mg) (rounded up)
> 90	> 40	25 ml (400 mg/5 ml)	8 (250 mg)

Source: Courtesy of William Jacobson DMD, MPH © 2021.

Clindamycin for Dental Abscess (Table 16.26)
- 20 mg/kg/day divided in three or four equally divided doses for seven days.
- Maximum daily dose of 1800 mg.
- Available in:
  - Solution: 75 mg/5 ml.
  - Chewable: not available.
  - Capsule: 75 mg, 150 mg, 300 mg (open and sprinkle on food if unable to swallow whole capsules).

Table 16.26 Clindamycin: pediatric dosage for dental abscess.

Weight (lb)	Weight (kg)	Dose (ml) three times daily for seven days	Dispense (ml)	Open ___ capsules and sprinkle on food three times daily for seven days	Dispense (capsules)
20–24.9	9.09–11.32	4 ml (75 mg/5 ml)	84	1 capsule (75 mg)	21
25–29.9	11.36–13.59	5 ml (75 mg/5 ml)	105	1 capsule (75 mg)	21
30–34.9	13.64–15.86	6 ml (75 mg/5 ml)	126	1 capsule (75 mg)	21
35–39.9	15.91–18.14	7 ml (75 mg/5 ml)	147	(Not recommend as the capsules cannot be split)	NA
40–44.9	18.18–20.41	8 ml (75 mg/5 ml)	168	(Not recommend as the capsules cannot be split)	NA
45–49.9	20.45–22.68	9 ml (75 mg/5 ml)	189	(Not recommend as the capsules cannot be split)	NA
50–54.9	22.73–24.95	10 ml (75 mg/5 ml)	210	1 capsule (150 mg)	21
55–59.9	25–27.23	11 ml (75 mg/5 ml)	231	1 capsule (150 mg)	21
60–64.9	27.27–29.5	12 ml (75 mg/5 ml)	252	1 capsule (150 mg)	21
65–69.9	29.55–31.77	13 ml (75 mg/5 ml)	273	1 capsule (150 mg)	21
70–74.9	31.82–34.05	14 ml (75 mg/5 ml)	294	(Not recommend as the capsules cannot be split)	NA
75–79.9	34.09–36.32	15 ml (75 mg/5 ml)	315	(Not recommend as the capsules cannot be split)	NA
80–84.9	36.36–38.59	16 ml (75 mg/5 ml)	336	(Not recommend as the capsules cannot be split)	NA
85–89.9	38.64–40.86	17 ml (75 mg/5 ml)	357	(Not recommend as the capsules cannot be split)	NA
> 90	> 40	20 ml (75 mg/5 ml)	560	1 capsule (300 mg) four times daily	28

NA, not applicable.
Source: Courtesy of William Jacobson DMD, MPH © 2021.

Clindamycin for Premed (Table 16.27)

- 20 mg/kg 30–60 minutes before procedure (do not exceed adult dose of 600 mg).
- Available in:
  - Solution: 75 mg/5 ml.
  - Chewable: not available.
  - Capsule: 75 mg, 150 mg, 300 mg.
- Total amount to dispense depends on number of visits.

Table 16.27 Clindamycin: pediatric dosage for premed.

Weight (lb)	Weight (kg)	Dose (ml) 30–60 minutes before procedure	Open ___ capsules and sprinkle on food 30–60 minutes before procedure
20–24.9	9.09–11.32	12 ml (75 mg/5 ml)	1 capsule (150 mg)
25–29.9	11.36–13.59	15 ml (75 mg/5 ml)	(Not recommend as the capsules cannot be split)
30–34.9	13.64–15.86	18 ml (75 mg/5 ml)	(Not recommend as the capsules cannot be split)
35–39.9	15.91–18.14	21 ml (75 mg/5 ml)	1 capsule (300 mg)
40–44.9	18.18–20.41	24 ml (75 mg/5 ml)	(Not recommend as the capsules cannot be split)
45–49.9	20.45–22.68	27 ml (75 mg/5 ml)	(Not recommend as the capsules cannot be split)
50–54.9	22.73–24.95	30 ml (75 mg/5 ml)	(Not recommend as the capsules cannot be split)
55–59.9	25–27.23	33 ml (75 mg/5 ml)	(Not recommend as the capsules cannot be split)
60–64.9	27.27–29.5	36 ml (75 mg/5 ml)	(Not recommend as the capsules cannot be split)
65–69.9	29.55–31.77	39 ml (75 mg/5 ml)	2 capsules (300 mg)
70–74.9	31.82–34.05	40 ml (75 mg/5 ml)	2 capsules (300 mg)
75–79.9	34.09–36.32	40 ml (75 mg/5 ml)	2 capsules (300 mg)
80–84.9	36.36–38.59	40 ml (75 mg/5 ml)	2 capsules (300 mg)
85–89.9	38.64–40.86	40 ml (75 mg/5 ml)	2 capsules (300 mg)
> 90	> 40	40 ml (75/5 ml)	2 capsules (300 mg)

Source: Courtesy of William Jacobson DMD, MPH © 2021.

Azithromycin for Dental Abscess (If allergic or contraindication to Penicillin and Clindamycin) (Table 16.28)

- 12 mg/kg daily on day 1, then 6 mg/kg daily on days 2–5.
- Maximum dose 500 mg/day.
- Available in:
  - Suspension: 100 mg/5 ml, 200 mg/5 ml.
  - Chewable: not available.
  - Capsules: not available.
  - Tablets: 250 mg, 500 mg.

Table 16.28 Azithromycin: pediatric dosage for dental abscess.

Weight (lb)	Weight (kg)	Dose (ml) daily on day 1	Dose (ml) on days 2–5	Dispense (ml)
20–24.9	9.09–11.32	2.5 ml (200 mg/5 ml)	1.25 ml (200 mg/5 ml)	7.5
25–29.9	11.36–13.59	3.5 ml (200 mg/5 ml)	1.75 ml (200 mg/5 ml)	10.5
30–34.9	13.64–15.86	4 ml (200 mg/5 ml)	2 ml (200 mg/5 ml)	12
35–39.9	15.91–18.14	4.5 ml (200 mg/5 ml)	2.25 ml (200 mg/5 ml)	13.5
40–44.9	18.18–20.41	5.5 ml (200 mg/5 ml)	2.75 ml (200 mg/5 ml)	16.5
45–49.9	20.45–22.68	6 ml (200 mg/5 ml))	3 ml (200 mg/5 ml)	18
50–54.9	22.73–24.95	6.5 ml (200 mg/5 ml)	3.5 (200 mg/5 ml)	20.5
55–59.9	25–27.23	7.5 ml (200 mg/5 ml)	3.75 ml (200 mg/5 ml)	22.5
60–64.9	27.27–29.5	8 ml (200 mg/5 ml)	4 ml (200 mg/5 ml)	24
65–69.9	29.55–31.77	8.5 ml (200 mg/5 ml)	4.5 ml (200 mg/5 ml)	26.5
70–74.9	31.82–34.05	9.5 ml (200 mg/5 ml)	4.75 ml (200 mg/5 ml)	28.5
75–79.9	34.09–36.32	10 ml (200 mg/5 ml)	5 ml (200 mg/5 ml)	30
80–84.9	36.36–38.59	11 ml (200 mg/5 ml)	5.5 ml (200 mg/5 ml)	33
85–89.9	38.64–40.86	11.5 (200 mg/5 ml)	5.75 ml (200 mg/5 ml)	34.5
> 90	> 40	12.5 ml (200 mg/5 ml) (adult dose 500 mg day 1)	6.25 ml (200 mg/5 ml) (adult dose 250 mg days 2–5)	37.5

Source: Courtesy of William Jacobson DMD, MPH © 2021.

Azithormycin for Premed (If allergic or contraindication to Penicillin or Clindamycin) (Table 16.29)

- 15 mg/kg 30–60 minutes before procedure (do not exceed adult dose of 500 mg).
- Available in:
  - Suspension: 100 mg/5 ml, 200 mg/5 ml.
  - Chewable: not available.
  - Capsules: not available.
  - Tablets: 250 mg, 500 mg.
- Total amount to dispense depends on number of visits.

Table 16.29 Azithromycin: pediatric dosage for premed.

Weight (lb)	Weight (kg)	Dose (ml) 30–60 minutes before procedure
20–24.9	9.09–11.32	3.25 ml (200 mg/5 ml)
25–29.9	11.36–13.59	4.25 ml (200 mg/5 ml)
30–34.9	13.64–15.86	5 ml (200 mg/5 ml)
35–39.9	15.91–18.14	6 ml (200 mg/5 ml)
40–44.9	18.18–20.41	7 ml (200 mg/5 ml)
45–49.9	20.45–22.68	8 ml (200 mg/5 ml)
50–54.9	22.73–24.95	8.5 ml (200 mg/5 ml)
55–59.9	25–27.23	9 ml (200 mg/5 ml)
60–64.9	27.27–29.5	10 ml (200 mg/5 ml)
65–69.9	29.55–31.77	11 ml (200 mg/5 ml)
70–74.9	31.82–34.05	12 ml (200 mg/5 ml)
75–79.9	34.09–36.32	12.5 ml (200 mg/5 ml)
80–84.9	36.36–38.59	12. 5 ml (200 mg/5 ml)
85–89.9	38.64–40.86	12.5 ml (200 mg/5 ml)
> 90	> 40	12.5 ml (200 mg/5 ml)

Source: Courtesy of William Jacobson DMD, MPH © 2021.

Dental Pharmacology

Child Analgesics

Analgesics recommended for children includes Ibuprofen (Table 16.12) and Acetaminophen (Table 16.13).

Ibuprofen (Medicine for pain or fever, such as Advil or Motrin)

Dosage Table

PRODUCT	CHILD'S WEIGHT (POUNDS)							
	12-17 lbs	18-23 lbs	24-35 lbs	36-47 lbs	48-59 lbs	60-71 lbs	72-95 lbs	96+ lbs
Infant's Liquid 50 mg / 1.25 mL	1.25 mL	1.875 mL	2.5 mL	3.75 mL				
Children's Liquid 100 mg / 5 mL			5 mL	7.5 mL	10 mL	12.5 mL	15 mL	20 mL
Children's Chewable 100 mg tablet			1 tab	1 ½ tabs	2 tabs	2 ½ tabs	3 tabs	4 tabs
Children's 100 mg tablet					2 tabs	2 tabs	3 tabs	4 tabs
Adult 200 mg tablet					1 tab	1 tab	1 ½ tabs	2 tabs

Chart Notes:
- **Brand names:** Advil, Motrin or store brand ibuprofen.
- **Dose:** Find your child's weight in the top row of the dose chart. Look below the correct weight for the dose based on the product you have. Adult dose is 400 mg.
- **Measure the Dose:** Use the syringe or dropper that comes with the medicine. If not, you can buy a medicine syringe at a drugstore. If you use a teaspoon, it must be a measuring spoon. Reason: Regular spoons are not reliable. Keep in mind: 1 level teaspoon equals 5 mL.
- **How Often:** Repeat every 6 to 8 hours as needed. Don't give more than 3 times a day.
- **Age Limit:** Don't use younger than 6 months unless told to by your child's doctor. Reason: For any fever in the first 12 weeks of life, your baby needs to be seen now. Also, the FDA has not approved ibuprofen for infants younger than 6 months.
- **Caution:** Do not use acetaminophen (Tylenol) and ibuprofen together. Reason: no benefit over using one medicine alone and a risk of giving too much. Exception: Your child's doctor told you to give both.

Call Your Doctor If:

- Your child looks or acts very sick
- Any serious symptoms occur like trouble breathing
- Any fever occurs if under 12 weeks old
- Fever without other symptoms lasts over 24 hours (if age less than 2 years)
- Fever lasts over 3 days (72 hours)
- Fever goes above 104° F (40° C)
- You think your child is in pain
- You think your child needs to be seen
- Your child becomes worse

Disclaimer: This health information is for educational purposes only. You the reader assume full responsibility for how you choose to use it.

Figure 16.12 Ibuprofen dosage table. *Source:* Courtesy of Barton Schmitt, MD, FAAP.

Acetaminophen (Medicine for pain or fever, such as Tylenol)

Dosage Table

PRODUCT	CHILD'S WEIGHT (POUNDS)								
	6-11 lbs	12-17 lbs	18-23 lbs	24-35 lbs	36-47 lbs	48-59 lbs	60-71 lbs	72-95 lbs	96+ lbs
Infant's Liquid 160 mg / 5 mL	1.25 mL	2.5 mL	3.75 mL	5 mL					
Children's Liquid 160 mg / 5 mL	1.25 mL	2.5 mL	3.75 mL	5 mL	7.5 mL	10 mL	12.5 mL	15 mL	20 mL
Children's Chewable 80 mg tablet			1 ½ tabs	2 tabs	3 tabs	4 tabs	5 tabs	6 tabs	8 tabs
Children's Chewable Junior 160 mg tablet				1 tab	1 ½ tabs	2 tabs	2 ½ tabs	3 tabs	4 tabs
Adult Regular Strength 325 mg tablet							1 tab	1 ½ tabs	2 tabs
Adult Extra Strength 500 mg tablet								1 tab	1 tab

Chart Notes:

- **Brand names:** Tylenol or store brand acetaminophen.
- **Dose:** Find your child's weight in the top row of the dose chart. Look below the correct weight for the dose based on the product you have. Adult dose is 500 to 650 mg.
- **Measure the Dose:** Use the syringe or dropper that comes with the medicine. If not, you can buy a medicine syringe at a drugstore. If you use a teaspoon, it must be a measuring spoon. Reason: Regular spoons are not reliable. Keep in mind: 1 level teaspoon equals 5 mL.
- **How Often:** Repeat every 4 to 6 hours as needed. Don't give more than 5 times a day.
- **Age Limit:** Don't use younger than 12 weeks unless told to by your child's doctor. Reason: For any fever in the first 12 weeks of life, your baby needs to be seen now.
- **Caution:** Do not use acetaminophen and ibuprofen (Advil or Motrin) together. Reason: no benefit over using one medicine alone and a risk of giving too much. Exception: Your child's doctor told you to give both.

Call Your Doctor If:

- Your child looks or acts very sick
- Any serious symptoms occur like trouble breathing
- Any fever occurs if under 12 weeks old
- Fever without other symptoms lasts over 24 hours (if age less than 2 years)
- Fever lasts over 3 days (72 hours)
- Fever goes above 104° F (40° C)
- You think your child is in pain
- You think your child needs to be seen
- Your child becomes worse

Disclaimer: This health information is for educational purposes only. You the reader assume full responsibility for how you choose to use it.

Pediatric Care Advice
Copyright 2000-2020 Schmitt Pediatric Guidelines LLC

Figure 16.13   Acetominophen dosage table. *Source:* Courtesy of Barton Schmitt, MD, FAAP.

Child Opioids and Anxiolytics

- The AAPD supports the FDA's safety communication which states that codeine and tramadol are contraindicated for treatment of pain in children younger than 12 years [59].
- Opioids and minors: in a study of opioid-naive adolescents and young adults receiving opioids for third molar extractions, they "were associated with a statistically significant 6.8% absolute risk increase in persistent opioid use and a 5.4% increase in the subsequent diagnosis of opioid abuse" [60].
- For anxiolytics, check with your state's dental board for permit requirements. (California requires an oral conscious sedation for minor patients permit to prescribe to dental patients under the age of 13 years).

Clinical Pearls

Troubleshooting

- Local anesthetics:
  - Difficulty anesthetizing a mandibular first molar ("hot tooth"): the mylohyoid nerve may be providing sensation to mesial root. Try to infiltrate with local anesthetic the floor of the mouth at the apex of the second molar. Also try PDL injections.
  - If heart racing with local anesthetic, epinephrine may have entered the vasculature; this will cease in a few minutes, so reassure the patient.
- Veganism and religion: if the patient is vegan or Muslim they may not take medication in a capsule (vs. tablet). Capsules are made from gelatin which are from animals. Alcohol mouthrinses may be contraindicated if the patient is Muslim, so provide alternative alcohol-free option.
- Homeless patients: you need to include an address when writing a prescription, so write "general delivery" [1]. However, controlled substances require an address, so ask for a form of identification.
- If patients report being dizzy when they have a toothache/infection, ask about their nutritional intake. They may be lacking nutrients. Recommend Boost/Ensure.
- Magic mouthwashes: many various combinations. Some pharmacies don't offer compounding, meaning they will not mix the various medications you request into one bottle. If magic mouthwash is prescribed, it must be shaken well prior to use. Recommend asking patient the percentage of improvement from using the mouthwash.
- Confused about what requires a DEA registration number and what can be electronically prescribed, phoned in, or written? See Table 16.30.

Table 16.30 DEA and prescribing clarifications.

Type of drug	Controlled substance	Non-controlled substance
Requires a DEA registration number?	Yes	No
Can be electronically prescribed (eRX)?	Yes	Yes
Can be phoned in?	Yes, if it is Schedule III, IV, V No, if it is Schedule II	Yes
Can it be on a prescription pad?	Yes, check if pad meets requirements	Yes

Tips

- CDT billing code tip: the D9110: Palliative (emergency) treatment of dental pain – minor procedure code can be used when providing local anesthesia as palliative treatment; however, do not bill this code if only writing a prescription for a medication.
- Prescription writing:
  - If the prescription pad has additional space to list more medications, crosshatch with a pen to prevent the patient from writing additional medications.
  - If you cannot edit e-RX sig, type "disregard first sig" and type your sig. Saves time so that the pharmacist doesn't have to call the dentist for clarification.
- When calling in a prescription to a pharmacy provide:
  - Patient's name, DOB, phone number, and home address.
  - Drug, dosage, Sig, quantity, number of refills.
  - Dentist's name and NPI.
  - For controlled substances provide DEA registration number.
- Drug seekers:
  - Know more than the drug seeker.
  - Avoid building a reputation as a dentist who easily prescribes scheduled drugs. Drug seekers/doctor-shoppers will come out of the woodwork and onto your schedule. Conversely, sending the message that this behavior is not tolerated will create a different type of reputation.
  - Avoid multiple extraction appointments. This only creates more postoperative pain management opportunities. Best to have all the extractions at once for one recovery.
- Patient not on record requesting anxiolytics or narcotics: if such a patient comes in with a toothache, take a step back and evaluate the entire mouth. It can become a slippery slope. Does it appear as though a lot of treatment will be required which will involve multiple prescriptions and appointments and postoperative discomfort to complete the entire treatment?
- Documentation: instead of "noncompliant" patient is "nonadherent."
- Probiotics: in a patient concerned about stomach upset due to antibiotics, suggest eating yogurt because it has probiotics. Do not eat at same time as antibiotics because they kill probiotics. Wait two hours. Can take twice daily during the antibiotic course and for one week after.

Real-Life Comments, Demands, and Questions Answered

Dental Students' Comments and Questions

- "My patient says she is allergic to penicillin."
  - What is the allergic reaction? Is it a true allergy (hives, itching, throat swelling)? Find out and document the allergic reaction in the chart for future reference as antibiotics may be indicated in the future.
- "When should I avoid using epinephrine in local anesthetics?"
  - When to avoid or minimize epinephrine usage: sodium bisulfite allergy (avoid), BP > 200/115 mmHg, uncontrolled hyperthyroidism, severe cardiovascular disease (<6 months from a heart attack/stroke/CABG, unstable/daily angina, arrhythmias), and taking nonspecific beta-blockers, MOAIs, or tricyclic antidepressants [13]. When shorter duration of anesthetic is desired.
- "My patient is not getting numb but I don't want to overdose him on lidocaine."
  - Is your patient an adult or a child? (If a child, find out the weight). Which anesthetic have you administered? How much anesthetic have you administered? Any cardiac conditions or reasons to limit dosage? What is the maximum dosage? See Section Adult Medications, Local Anesthetics.

– Do you know how to recognize the signs/symptoms of a local anesthetic overdose and how to treat this?
  ○ Epinephrine overdose:
    ▪ Signs: elevation in BP.
    ▪ Treat: administer oxygen, reassure patient, and monitor vitals. Can take 20 minutes for BP to return to normal. Call EMS if patient is deteriorating.
  ○ Local anesthetic overdose: many signs/symptoms such as anxious, confused, and rapid breathing. May lead to seizure, arrhythmia, respiratory depression, and cardiac arrest. Treatment varies. If mild administer oxygen and monitor vitals; if severe may require seizure management and basic life support [61].
- "I will recommend my patient take ibuprofen."
  – Even if you only recommend a medication, and are not writing a prescription, you want to make sure the patient does not have any contraindications to the medication. Ensure you discuss the dosage including the maximum dosage. See Sections ACIID and Adult Medications, Analgesics.
- "I think my denture patient may have candidiasis."
  – What are the signs and symptoms? See Section Adult Medications, Fungal Infections.

Dental Assistant's Question

- "The patient wants to know if you can give her something strong after you pull out her tooth."
  – It is good to make sure your dental team understands, supports, and is on board with your pain management protocols. So much of patient management is setting expectations. While the dental assistant rooms the patient, he or she can already mention that the doctor prescribes ibuprofen and acetaminophen. During informed consent for the extraction be sure to discuss the postoperative pain medications that will be prescribed. This provides the patient with the ability to make an informed decision and prevents misunderstandings after the extraction. Discuss with the patient that combining ibuprofen with acetaminophen has a synergistic effect and is both safe and effective.

Patients' Demands and Questions

- "I want a refill on my chlorhexidine."
  – Is the chlorhexidine being used for gingivitis or for caries risk management? If for gingivitis, it is not for long-term use due to side effects (see Section Adult Medications, Preventative). If for caries risk management, a refill may be indicated.
- "I need antibiotics for this."
  – Take a look and see what is going on.
    ○ Check for facial swelling, fever, tender/swollen lymph nodes, symptoms of malaise. If none of these signs or symptoms of systemic involvement are present, antibiotics are not indicated. Can cause more harm than good.
    ○ Set limits/boundaries (e.g. "I cannot," "we do not," "I am willing to").
- "Doc I rarely take antibiotics, so don't worry about antibiotic resistance. Can I have some?"
  – Antibiotic resistance is due to misuse and overuse of antibiotics. In future we may not be able to use antibiotics. And it is not the person that becomes resistant but the bacteria, which can spread to others [62].
  – Find out the community levels of resistance where you practice to avoid prescribing a medication that may have a high community resistance.

- "Do I need to take any precautions when taking this antibiotic?"
  - There are risks with antibiotics, such as allergic reactions, *C. difficile*, and antibiotic resistance. If you break out in hives, take Benadryl, stop taking the antibiotic and call the dental office. If you have trouble breathing call EMS and use an EpiPen if you have one. If you develop a fever, abdominal cramping, or three or more loose bowel movements a day, contact your medical provider [1]. If no resolution of symptoms within three days call the dental office.
- "Can I take this medicine on an empty stomach?"
  - See the tables for the specific medications in this chapter.
- "Can I drink beer when I'm taking this medicine?"
  - Do not mix alcohol with acetaminophen, opioids, or metronidazole. Consult with pharmacist for other drugs.
  - The risk is drug and patient dependent. Many factors are involved, such as the medication, the dosage, the duration, other interacting medications, any impaired clearance, etc.
- "Can I take Excedrin for my toothache?"
  - If you do not know what a drug is, look it up before providing your recommendation.
  - Excedrin contains acetaminophen, aspirin, and caffeine. Caffeine can contribute to bruxism. Aspirin can contribute to bleeding. Acetaminophen will not reduce inflammation. Recommend ibuprofen instead.
- "I need something stronger than ibuprofen, like Norco."
  - What is your current pain level on a scale of 0–10, if 0 is no pain and 10 is the worst pain imaginable? Does it come and go or is it constant?
  - What medication have you tried so far? What dosage? How many hours apart?
  - The pain is from inflammation and opioids do nothing for inflammation.
  - I recommend ibuprofen 400 mg in combination with acetaminophen 1000 mg four times a day every six hours. These two drugs work synergistically, meaning the effect is greater when combined (analogous to 1 plus 1 equals 4). See Sections Red Flags of Drug Seekers and Multimodal Pain Management Options.
- "I'm allergic to Tylenol but I can take Norco, can you prescribe me some?"
  - Acetaminophen (Tylenol) is a constituent of Norco.
  - The patient may be drug seeking. Do not become a victim. See Section Red Flags of Drug Seekers.
- "Can I get some tramadol after this deep cleaning?"
  - The pain associated with a deep cleaning is mild and for managing discomfort related to dental procedures we recommend combining ibuprofen 400 mg with acetaminophen 1000 mg. I can prescribe you that.
    - If patient is insistent, find out if the individual has tried this combination every six hours. Discuss that inflammation is causing the pain and opioids do nothing for inflammation.
    - See sections Opioids Overview, Red Flags of Drug Seekers, Multimodal Pain Management Options, and Adult Medications, Analgesics
- "You ripped this tooth out of my skull and now you're telling me you are only going to give me ibuprofen and Tylenol?"
  - This real-life quote is from a disgruntled patient demanding narcotics, using threatening body language and raising his voice in the dental office. This scenario highlights the importance of setting expectations with the patient *prior* to a procedure during informed consent.
- "I need prednisone because that is the only thing that has worked."
  - If you do not know what a drug is, look it up before providing your recommendation.

- Prednisone is a corticosteroid, which means it helps decrease inflammation but also suppresses the immune system. We do not want the immune system depressed when you have a dental infection your body is trying to fight off. We recommend combining ibuprofen and acetaminophen for pain management which will not suppress the immune system.
- "My four-year-old has an abscess and is crying all day, can you prescribe something?"
  - Diagnose the condition and determine what medication is indicated.
  - Be sure to obtain the child's weight in order to determine the proper dosage. Have a scales in the office to accurately weigh child rather than relying on the parent for an accurate weight. See Section Pediatric Medications.

References

1 Lockhard, P., Tampi, M., Abt, E. et al. (2019). Evidence-based clinical practice guideline on antibiotic use for the urgent management of pulpal- and periapical-related dental pain and intraoral swelling: a report from the American Dental Association. *J. Am. Dent. Assoc.* 150 (11): 906–921.e12.

2 Centers for Disease Control and Prevention (2020). Quarantine and isolation. http://www.cdc.gov/quarantine/maritime/definitions-signs-symptoms-conditions-ill-travelers.html (accessed 9 April 2020).

3 Wynn, R., Meiller, T., and Crossley, H. (2018). *Lexicomp Drug Information Handbook for Dentistry*, 24e. Hudson, OH: Lexicomp.

4 Epocrates (2021). Sodium fluoride (Version 21.4.1) [Mobile app].

5 3M (2020). 3M clinpro 5000 1.1% sodium fluoride anti-cavity toothpaste. https://www.3m.com/3M/en_US/company-us/all-3m-products/~/clinpro-5000-3M-Clinpro-5000-1-1-Sodium-Fluoride-Anti-Cavity-Toothpaste/?N=5002385+3294768934&rt=rud (accessed 12 April 2021).

6 Colgate (2020). PreviDent 5000 dry mouth (RX only) (1.1% sodium fluoride) toothpaste. https://www.colgateprofessional.com/products/products-list/colgate-prevident-5000-plus-rx-only (accessed 12 April 2021).

7 Featherstone, J.D.B., Alston, P., Chaffee, B.W., and Rechmann, P. (2019). Caries Management by Risk Assessment (CAMBRA): an update for use in clinical practice for patients aged 6 through adult. *J. Calif. Dent. Assoc.* 47 (1): 25–34.

8 Rose, L.F. and Mealy, B.L. (2004). Periodontics: Medicine, Surgery, and Implants. St. Louis, MO: Elsevier Mosby.

9 Epocrates (2021). Chlorhexidine (Version 21.4.1) [Mobile app].

10 Skouteris, C.A. (ed.) (2018). *Dental Management of the Pregnant Patient*. Hoboken, NJ: John Wiley & Sons.

11 Jacobsen, P.L. (2013). *The Little Dental Drug Booklet: Handbook of Commonly Used Dental Medications*, 2e. Hudson, OH: Lexicomp.

12 Epocrates (2021). Benzocaine (Version 21.4.1) [Mobile app].

13 Malamed, S.F. (2013). *Handbook of Local Anesthesia*, 6e. St. Louis, MO: Elsevier Mosby.

14 American Dental Association. Mouth Healthy. Benzocaine. https://www.mouthhealthy.org/en/az-topics/b/benzocaine (accessed 20 June 2020).

15 Little, J.W., Falace, D.A., Miller, C.S., and Rhodus, N.L. (2013). *Little and Falace's Dental Management of the Medically Compromised Patient*, 8e. St. Louis, MO: Elsevier Mosby.

16 Cetylite (2017). Cetacaine topical anesthetic spray and liquid. https://www.cetylite.com/sites/default/files/resources/Cetacaine%20Prescribing%20Information.pdf (accessed 14 June 2020).

17 Tangcharoensathien, V., Sattayawutthipong, W., Kanjanapimai, S. et al. (2017). Antimicrobial resitance: from global agenda to national strategic plan, Thailand. *Bull. WHO* 95 (8): 599–603. https://www.ncbi. nlm.nih.gov/pmc/articles/PMC5537745/.

18 Epocrates (2021). Amoxicillin (Version 21.4.1) [Mobile app].

19 Epocrates (2021). Penicillin VK (Version 21.4.1) [Mobile app].

20 Drugs.com. Metronidazole and acohol/food interactions. https://www.drugs.com/ food-interactions/metronidazole.html (accessed 20 June 2020).

21 Epocrates (2021). Metronidazole (Version 21.4.1) [Mobile app].

22 Epocrates (2021). Amoxicillin/clavulanate (Version 21.4.1) [Mobile app].

23 Epocrates (2021). Azithromycin (Version 21.4.1) [Mobile app].

24 Epocrates (2021). Clindamycin (Version 21.4.1) [Mobile app].

25 Epocrates (2021). Cephalexin (Version 21.4.1) [Mobile app].

26 American Dental Association (2020). Oral health topics. Antibiotics prophylaxis prior to dental procedures. https://www.ada.org/ en/member-center/oral-health-topics/ antibiotic-prophylaxis (accessed 12 April 2021).

27 Moore, P., Zieglar, K., Lipman, R. et al. (2018). Benefits and harms associated with analgesic medications used in the management of acute dental pain. An overview of systematic reviews. *J. Am. Dent. Assoc.* 149 (4): 256–265.e3.

28 Hersh, E.V., Kane, W.T., O'Neil, M.G. et al. (2011). Prescribing recommendations for the treatment of acute pain in dentistry. *Compend. Contin. Educ. Dent.* 32 (3): 22, 24–30. quiz 31–32.

29 O'Neil, M. (2015). *The ADA Practical Guide to Substance Use Disorders and Safe Prescribing*. Hoboken, NJ: John Wiley & Sons.

30 American Dental Association (ADA) (2020). Oral analgesics for acute dental pain. https://

www.ada.org/en/member-center/oral-health-topics/oral-analgesics-for-acute-dental-pain (accessed 20 June 2020).

31 Epocrates (2021). Ibuprofen (Version 21.4.1) [Mobile app].

32 Therapeutic Research Center (2019). Reset perceptions about treating dental pain. *Pharmacist's Letter*. https://pharmacist. therapeuticresearch.com/Content/Articles/ PRL/2019/Jan/Reset-Perceptions-About-Treating-Dental-Pain (accessed 26 June 2020).

33 Dr. Robert Bree Collaborative (2017). Dental guideline on prescribing opioids for acute pain management. https:// agencymeddirectors.wa.gov/Files/20171026F INALDentalOpioidRecommendations_Web. pdf (accessed 12 April 2021).

34 Epocrates (2021). Acetaminophen (Version 21.4.1) [Mobile app].

35 U.S. Department of Health and Human Services (2018). *Facing Addiction in America. The Surgeon General's Spotlight on Opioids*. Washington, DC: HHS https://addiction. surgeongeneral.gov/sites/default/files/ OC_SpotlightOnOpioids.pdf (accessed 16 June 2020).

36 Centers for Disease Control and Prevention (2020). CDC Rx awareness campaign overview. https://www.cdc.gov/rxawareness/ pdf/RxAwareness-Campaign-Overview-508. pdf (accessed 16 June 2020).

37 Drugs.com (2020). CSA schedules. https:// www.drugs.com/csa-schedule. html#:~:text=The%20Controlled%20 Substances%20Act%20(CSA,anabolic%20 steroids%20and%20other%20chemicals (accessed 12 April 2021).

38 DEA. Drug scheduling. https://www.dea. gov/drug-scheduling (accessed 12 April 2021).

39 U.S. Department of Justice Drug Enforcement Administration (2020). Diversion control division. Controlled substance schedules. https://www. deadiversion.usdoj.gov/schedules/#define (accessed 12 April 2021).

40 Centers for Disease Control and Prevention (2020). Providers' frequently asked questions. https://www.cdc.gov/drugoverdose/prescribing/faq.html (accessed 20 June 2020).

41 Centers for Disease Control and Prevention (2020). Dental pain. https://www.cdc.gov/acute-pain/dental-pain/index.html (accessed 20 June 2020).

42 DeFalco, A.P. and O'Neil, M. (2019). Prescribing controlled prescription medications: special considerations. *J. Calif. Dent. Assoc.* 47 (3): 171–178.

43 Centers for Disease Control and Prevention. Preventing an opioid overdose. https://www.cdc.gov/drugoverdose/pdf/patients/Preventing-an-Opioid-Overdose-Tip-Card-a.pdf (accessed 20 June 2020).

44 Mark, A.M. (2018). Just what the doctor ordered: relieving dental pain. *J. Am. Dent. Assoc.* 149 (8): 744. https://doi.org/10.1016/j.adaj.2018.05.014.

45 Epocrates (2021). Lidocaine oropharyngeal viscous solution (Version 21.4.1) [Mobile app].

46 Epocrates (2021). Tylenol 3 (Version 21.4.1) [Mobile app].

47 Epocrates (2021). Norco (Version 21.4.1) [Mobile app].

48 Alford, D., Compton, P., and Samet, J. (2006). Acute pain management for patients receiving maintenance methadone or buprenorphine therapy. *Ann. Intern. Med.* 144 (2): 127–134.

49 Zarb, G. and Bolender, C. (2004). *Prosthodontic Treatment for Edentulous Patients: Complete Dentures and Implant-Supported Prostheses*, 12e. St. Louis, MO: Mosby.

50 Newland, J., R., M., T., F. et al. *Oral Soft Tissue Diseases: A Reference Manual for Diagnosis and Management*, 6e. Hudson, OH: Lexicomp.

51 Epocrates (2021). Clotrimazole oropharyngeal (Version 21.4.1) [Mobile app].

52 Epocrates (2021). Penciclovir topical (Version 21.4.1) [Mobile app].

53 Neville, B.W., Damm, D.D., Allen, C.M., and Chi, A.C. (2016). *Oral and Maxillofacial Pathology*, 4e. St. Louis, MO: Elsevier.

54 Epocrates (2021). Valacyclovir (Version 21.4.1) [Mobile app].

55 Epocrates (2021). Triazolam (Version 21.4.1) [Mobile app].

56 Drugs.com (2021). Triazolam and alcohol/food interactions. https://www.drugs.com/food-interactions/triazolam.html (accessed 12 April 2021).

57 American Academy of Pediatric Dentistry (2020). Fluoride therapy. In: *The Reference Manual of Pediatric Dentistry*, 288–291. Chicago: American Academy of Pediatric Dentistry.

58 Schwartz, S. (2021). Local anesthesia in pediatric dentistry. https://www.dentalcare.com/en-us/professional-education/ce-courses/ce325/injectable-local-anesthetic-agents (accessed 12 April 2021).

59 American Academy of Pediatric Dentistry (2017). Policy on acute pediatric dental pain management. https://www.aapd.org/research/oral-health-policies--recommendations/acute-pediatric-dental-pain-management (accessed 12 April 2021).

60 Schroeder, A.R., Dehghan, M., Newman, T.B. et al. (2019). Association of opioid prescriptions from dental clinicians for US adolescents and young adults with subsequent opioid use and abuse. *JAMA Intern. Med.* 179 (2): 145–152.

61 Meiller, T.F., Wynn, R.L., McMullin, A.M. et al. *Dental Office Medical Emergencies: Manual of Office Response Protocols*, 5e. Hudson, OH: Lexicomp.

62 RxList (2020). Antibiotic resistance: questions and answers. https://www.rxlist.com/antibiotic_resistance/drugs-condition.htm (accessed 20 June 2020).

63 California Code (2020), Health and Safety Code 11165.4. https://oag.ca.gov/sites/all/files/agweb/pdfs/pdmp/hs-code.pdf? (accessed 20 June 2020).

64 Centers for Disease Control and Prevention (2020). Medication Safety Program. Additional resources. https://www.cdc.gov/medicationsafety/library.html (accessed 20 June 2020).

17

Pediatric Dentistry

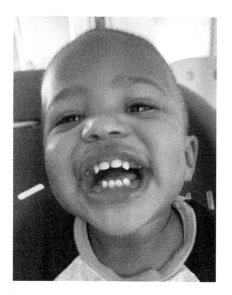

Figure 17.1   A 13-month-old child.

Chapter Outline

- Real-Life Clinical Questions and Scenarios
- Relevance
- Pediatric Medical History Form
- Clinical and Radiographic Exam
  - Clinical Exam
  - Radiographic Exam
- Teeth Eruption Charts
- Pediatric Treatment Planning
- Informed Consent
- Referrals to Specialists

- Patient Management
- Pediatric Local Anesthetic Tips
- Pediatric Medication Dosages
- Procedural Steps
  - General Remarks
  - Traumatic Dental Injuries of Primary and Permanent Teeth
  - Preventative Dentistry
  - Nitrous Oxide and Oxygen Sedation
  - Interim Therapeutic Restorations
  - Operative
  - Pulpotomies/Pulpectomies/RCT on immature permanent teeth
  - RCT on Immature Permanent Teeth
  - Primary Teeth Extractions
  - Space Maintainers
- Lab Prescriptions for Space Maintainers
- Postoperative Instructions
- Documentation
- Real-Life Clinical Questions and Scenarios Answered
- References

Real-Life Clinical Questions and Scenarios

Dental Students' Questions

- "I don't want to overdose the child, how much anesthetic can I give?"
- "I can't tell if the child is crying from fear or if the child is not numb enough?"

Dental Assistants' Questions

- "Do we perio chart on children?"
- "Hey doc, what type of X-rays do you want me to take on this five-year-old?"
- "I don't remember the tooth numbers on baby teeth."

Parents' Concerns

- "I don't know how to brush my child's teeth because she's three years old, she is my first kid and when I try she runs out of the room with the toothbrush."
- "Are my kid's teeth growing in normal? Will he need braces?"
- "How much medicine should my child take?"
- "Bump on her gums. I think she needs antibiotics." (Figure 17.2)
- "We drink well water, is there fluoride in that water?"
- "My child grinds his teeth. Does he need a night guard?"

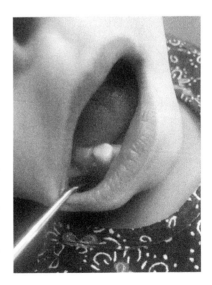

Figure 17.2 Parulis on the buccal gingiva adjacent to tooth S.

- "Is it bad she still sucks her thumb? At what age should she quit?"
- "Why does he have cavities when he doesn't eat candy?"
- "I don't want my three-year-old to have any sedation. What can you do for his cavities?"
- "Does my kid really need fillings on these teeth if they will fall out anyways?"
- "What are sealants?"
- "Loose tooth hurting him." (Figure 17.3)

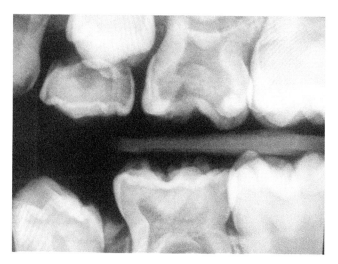

Figure 17.3   Tooth I with resorbed roots retained only by soft tissue.

Scenarios

- The parent films child in the chair receiving dental care.
- The 16-year-old brings their 10-year-old brother in for appointment.
- The parent brings the child in for an exam and cleaning and the child has braces.
- The parent wants to be in the room watching the procedure and talking to and touching the child throughout the treatment.

Relevance

Whether you treat children on a regular basis or occasionally, this chapter can serve as your go-to reference guide for your pediatric dentistry needs.

Pediatric Medical History Form

- The AAPD has a pediatric medical history form [1].
- Other child health history forms exist, including the ADA's Child Health/Dental History Form.
- Whichever form is used must be filled out by the parent or guardian, not the minor.

Clinical and Radiographic Exam

Clinical Exam

- Perform an EOE, IOE, and OCS (see Chapter 2).
  - If during the EOE you note lip licker's dermatitis, recommend breaking the lip licking habit using a lip moisturizer and prescribing topical hydrocortisone ointment. If the habit is not broken the dermatitis will recur.
- Evaluate occlusion, including midline, anterior or posterior crossbite, open bite, overjet, overbite, molar relationship, and canine relationship.
- Examine and document all existing teeth, restorations, and findings:
  - Check for normal teeth eruption patterns (see Section Teeth Eruption Charts).
  - Check for symmetry (See Figure 17.1).
  - Check for asymmetries in eruption, as these may indicated supernumerary teeth or ectopic eruption.
  - If early loss of any teeth, consider space maintainers (see Section Space Maintainers).
- Check mobilities.
- Periodontal charting
  - Periodontal probing recommended:
    o Once permanent first molars are fully erupted on a cooperative child.
    o Before this if presence or suspicion of clinical and/or radiographic signs of periodontal disease [2].
  - Recommended at initial exam (to establish a baseline) and periodic exams.
  - Early diagnosis of periodontal disease ensures greater opportunity for successful treatment.
  - Bleeding on probing is the best indicator of gingivitis.

Radiographic Exam

- Determine if radiographs are indicated and which to take.
  - See Chapter 3, section Recommendations for Prescribing Dental Radiographs.
  - The ability to take diagnostic bitewings is a good indicator for whether a child can be cooperative for treatment.
- Radiographic interpretation:
  - Count the teeth: check for supernumerary teeth or congenitally missing teeth (e.g. permanent maxillary lateral incisors), including succedaneous teeth. This may require a space maintainer (see Section Space Maintainers).
  - Check for caries.
  - Look for radiolucencies in the furcations of primary molars (unlike with permanent teeth, where the radiolucencies are usually located at the apices) (See Figure 17.4).
- Document findings.

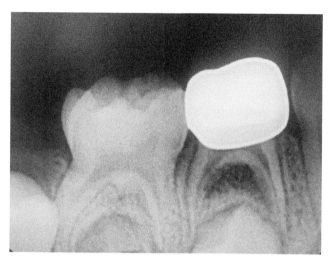

Figure 17.4   Radiolucency at the furcation of tooth S.

Teeth Eruption Charts

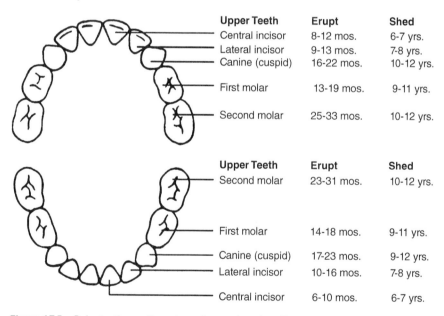

Upper Teeth	Erupt	Shed
Central incisor	8-12 mos.	6-7 yrs.
Lateral incisor	9-13 mos.	7-8 yrs.
Canine (cuspid)	16-22 mos.	10-12 yrs.
First molar	13-19 mos.	9-11 yrs.
Second molar	25-33 mos.	10-12 yrs.

Upper Teeth	Erupt	Shed
Second molar	23-31 mos.	10-12 yrs.
First molar	14-18 mos.	9-11 yrs.
Canine (cuspid)	17-23 mos.	9-12 yrs.
Lateral incisor	10-16 mos.	7-8 yrs.
Central incisor	6-10 mos.	6-7 yrs.

Figure 17.5   Baby teeth eruption chart. *Source:* American Dental Association, 2012.

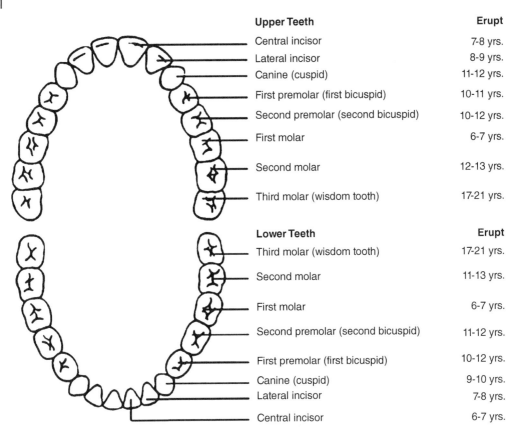

Upper Teeth	Erupt
Central incisor	7-8 yrs.
Lateral incisor	8-9 yrs.
Canine (cuspid)	11-12 yrs.
First premolar (first bicuspid)	10-11 yrs.
Second premolar (second bicuspid)	10-12 yrs.
First molar	6-7 yrs.
Second molar	12-13 yrs.
Third molar (wisdom tooth)	17-21 yrs.

Lower Teeth	Erupt
Third molar (wisdom tooth)	17-21 yrs.
Second molar	11-13 yrs.
First molar	6-7 yrs.
Second premolar (second bicuspid)	11-12 yrs.
First premolar (first bicuspid)	10-12 yrs.
Canine (cuspid)	9-10 yrs.
Lateral incisor	7-8 yrs.
Central incisor	6-7 yrs.

Figure 17.6   Permanent teeth eruption chart. *Source:* American Dental Association, 2012.

Pediatric Treatment Planning

- Sequencing restorative needs:
  1) The tooth in pain.
  2) The most serious quadrant.
  3) Permanent teeth.
  4) Primary teeth.
  5) Posterior teeth.
  6) Anterior teeth (if the anterior teeth are treated first and look good, the patient may not return for treatment on the posterior teeth).
- General considerations
  - First dental visit: "In order to prevent dental problems, your child should see a pediatric dentist when the first tooth appears, or no later than his/her first birthday" [3].
  - Exam every six months.
  - Preventive dentistry (see Chapter 5).
  - Radiographs (see Chapter 3, section Recommendations for Prescribing Dental Radiographs).
  - Primary dentition
    o Sealants on primary molars: according to the AAPD/ADA: "Sealants are effective in preventing and arresting pit-and-fissure occlusal carious lesions of primary and permanent

molars in children and adolescents compared with the nonuse of sealants or use of fluoride varnishes. They also concluded that sealants could minimize the progression of non-cavitated occlusal carious lesions (also referred to as initial lesions) that receive a sealant" [4].

  – Mixed dentition
      ○ Sealants on primary and permanent molars [4].
      ○ Check-up with an orthodontist no later than age 7 (per the American Association of Orthodontists) [5].
      ○ Involved in sports? See Chapter 15, section Athletic Mouthguards.
  – Permanent dentition
      ○ Sealants on permanent molars [4].
      ○ Involved in sports? See Chapter 15, section Athletic Mouthguards.
      ○ Evaluate third molars.
- Treatment deferral: in some cases, treatment deferral may be considered as an alternative to treating the patient under sedation or general anesthesia. Discuss the risks, benefits and alternatives, and consent must be obtained from the parent. With interim therapeutic restorations (IRT) and silver diamine fluoride, regular reevaluations and retreatments are needed (per the AAPD) [6].

Informed Consent

- Informed consent is governed by state law.
- Contact your professional liability carrier and/or attorney for specific guidance and forms (e.g. restorative treatment, extraction, nitrous sedation).
- Informed consent can be withdrawn at any time, and the dentist must comply as soon as able to safely end the procedure [7].

Referrals to Specialists

- The AAPD "believes it is unethical for a dentist to ignore a disease or condition because of the patient's age, behavior, or disabilities. Dentists have an ethical obligation to provide therapy for patients with oral disease or refer for treatment patients whose needs are beyond the skills of the practitioner."
- If beyond your skills, refer to a pediatric dentist.
- If concerned about growth patterns, malocclusion, functionality, esthetics, space maintenance issues, ectopic eruption, or crowding, consider referring to an orthodontist (Figure 17.7). The American Association of Orthodontists (AAO) recommends a check-up with an orthodontist no later than age 7 years [5].
- If an immature permanent tooth requires endodontic treatment, consider referring to an endodontist.

Pediatric Dentistry

Problems to Watch for in Growing Children

Malocclusions ("bad bites") like those illustrated below, may benefit from early diagnosis and referral to an orthodontic specialist for a full evaluation.

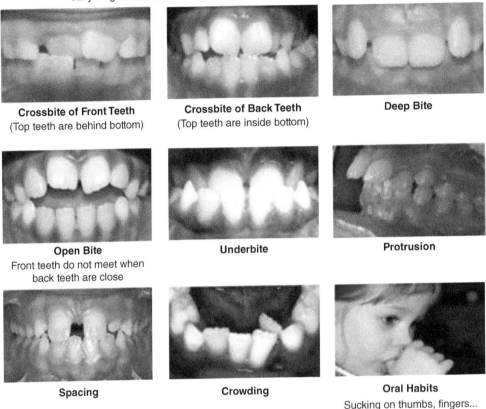

Crossbite of Front Teeth
(Top teeth are behind bottom)

Crossbite of Back Teeth
(Top teeth are inside bottom)

Deep Bite

Open Bite
Front teeth do not meet when back teeth are close

Underbite

Protrusion

Spacing

Crowding

Oral Habits
Sucking on thumbs, fingers...

Figure 17.7 Problems to watch for in growing children. *Source:* Smiles Under the Sea, https://smilesunderthesea.com/orthodontic-treatment/ [8].

Patient Management

- **Parental discussion**
  - For children age 0–2, discuss the knee-to-knee exam:
    ○ For children around age 0–2 years.
    ○ Explain to the parent how to assist you in the knee-to-knee exam. Helpful to show a photo. See Figure 5.8.
    ○ Inform the parent that it is common for children to cry out of fear, but to remember that we are not hurting the child in any way (crying will help you see the teeth).
  - Discuss cooperation level
    ○ Dentistry requires a certain level of cooperation from the patient. I will attempt to treat your child, but if uncooperative I will have to refer to a specialist as I want your child to have the most positive experience so that they are not afraid to see the dentist in the future. Every child has a different personality and some need more care.

– Discussing parent presence in the room:
  ○ Controversial and varies among clinicians.
  ○ It is recommended that the parent be in the room when you explain the findings, review oral health instructions, discuss the treatment plan recommendations, and review postoperative instructions.
  ○ It is best to encourage the parent to separate from the patient for treatment.
  ○ Rarely does having the parent in the room help.
  ○ Parents can distract the child and confuse the child, with multiple authority figures giving commands that hinder managing the child.
  ○ Parents can use the wrong language (see Child-friendly words).
  ○ The child can pick up on the parent's anxiety levels.
  ○ It is best to have a clear policy in your office about parental presence: how many in the room, including whether phones/cameras are allowed.
  ○ One approach is asking the parent their preference
    ▪ Would you like to be in the same room or the waiting room? Your child will have the same care regardless. I just ask that communication be between me, the child and the assistant. Too many voices confuses the child (multiple authority figures). We find it works best if the parent is a silent supporter/partner. We also use child-friendly words and avoid certain words that scare the child.
    ▪ We will need the child's undivided attention, and we will need undivided attention. Please be our silent partner, your presence is support [9].
    ▪ If the parent insists on being in the room, make sure the parent is siting far enough from the child that they cannot touch the child as this can be dangerous if the child moves suddenly in response.
    ▪ Another option is the parent can watch from a window or from the door.

- **Types of behavior guidance**
  – Important that dentists have a wide range of techniques to meet needs of the individual child [6].
  – Techniques have different indications/contraindications.
  – Nonpharmacological
    ○ Communication and communication guidance
    ○ Positive pre-visit imagery
    ○ Direct observation
    ○ Tell, show, do
    ○ Ask, tell, ask
    ○ Voice control
    ○ Nonverbal communication
    ○ Positive reinforcement and descriptive praise
    ○ Distraction
    ○ Memory restructuring
    ○ Desensitization to dental setting and procedures
    ○ Enhancing control
    ○ Sensory-adapted dental environments (SADE)
    ○ Animal-assisted therapy (AAT)
    ○ Picture exchange communication system (PECS) [6]
  – Pharmacological (see Chapter 18)
    ○ Nitrous oxide and oxygen sedation

- ○ Oral sedation
- ○ Intravenous sedation
- ○ General anesthesia
- **Some patient management tips**
  - Radiographs: position tube before placing film in mouth [9]. The film often causes discomfort and may cause gagging, so do not lengthen the period of time in which the patient must tolerate this.
  - Sound authoritative. For example, say "I'm going to place a bib on you" not "Can I place this bib?" as the child may refuse out of fear.
  - Open Wide mouth props are useful with pediatric and special needs patients to keep their mouth open. They are disposable and can be sent home for daily hygiene (Figure 17.8). Of note, a mouth prop in an uncooperative child is a protective stabilization that requires informed consent [7].
  - Three to four year olds: use short simple language [7].
  - Preschool age: having child assist you (e.g. hold mirror) can elicit cooperative behavior, take pride in accomplishments, and seek independence [7].
  - Be honest; don't say it won't pinch if it will, as you can lose the patient's trust.
  - Tell, show, do
    - ○ Show how the air/water blows air and tickles the patient's hand (tell, show, do).
    - ○ Let the child hold the prophy angle (to see how the tip is soft rubber) and the mouth mirror.
    - ○ Show the child, without the bur, how the high speed is noisy and squirts water to chase out the sugar bugs.

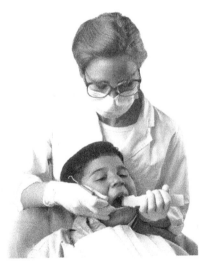

Figure 17.8   Open Wide mouth props. *Source:* courtesy of Specializedcare.com

- **Getting to know your patient**
  - How old are you?
  - What grade are you in?
  - Favorite subject in school and why?
  - What do you do for fun?

- What do you want to be when you grow up and why?
- Do you have any pets? What is your favorite part about having a pet?
- Siblings?
- Favorite show or movie?
- Fun plans for the holiday?
- **Child-friendly words**
  - Not intended to deceive the child but to create a more positive experience.
  - For older kids you can say "It's like a. . ." followed by the child-friendly word.
  - See Table 17.1.

Table 17.1 Child-friendly words.

Procedure type	Child-friendly words	Description/words to avoid
Exam	Tooth counter (and count aloud)	Explorer
	Tooth mirror (show child their reflection)	Mouth mirror
	Count teeth	Dental exam
	Tooth pictures	Radiographs
	Tooth camera	X-ray tube
	Blanket	Lead apron
	Wind and water gun	Air/water syringe (blow on child's hand)
Cleaning	Toothbrush	Prophy angle
	Tooth vitamins	Fluoride varnish
Sealant	Shields	Sealant
Anesthetic	Sleepy jelly, magic jelly	Topical anesthetic
	Sleepy juice	Anesthetic
	Weird/funny/sleepy feeling, freezing cold water, pressure, pushing, tingling, little pinch, little poke	Discomfort from needle, pain, hurt, shot
Filling	Tooth pillow	Bite block, mouth prop

Pediatric Local Anesthetic Tips

- Pediatric local anesthetic maximum dosage and dosage charts (see Chapter 16).
- Anatomic considerations
  - Inferior alveolar nerve block (IANB):
    - Use a short needle (unless second molars present).
    - Location of the mandibular foramen:
      - <8 years old: lower than occlusal plane.
      - 8.5 years old: occlusal plane.
      - Older/longer face: higher than occlusal plane [9].
    - After you give the IANB wait 10 minutes, then gently touch the labial gingiva with the side of the explorer between canine and lateral incisor to check if profound anesthesia. If not numb, administer more anesthetic.

  – Local infiltration of maxillary primary teeth: inject closer to gingival margin rather than the vestibule as done on permanent teeth.
  – Palatal injection: necessary on uppers when using rubber dam isolation, deep caries or extractions.
- Before administering local anesthetic, warn the parent that children often find the sensation of being numb more distressing than the discomfort of the injection or procedure [9].
- Administering local anesthetic
  – Place topical anesthetic ("magic jelly") for two minutes, covering the site with ligated gauze to prevent the child from tasting it.
  – Inform the patient you will give the sleepy juice which will feel weird/funny/pressure/push/little pinch.
    o Have the assistant hold the patient's hands.
    o For local infiltration, have the patient bite down during the injection [9].
    o Have the child lift their leg during the injection [9].
    o Can dispense a small amount of anesthetic and then return to the same site after about a minute to dispense more.
  – Give a water drinking break after local anesthesia to reframe the child's mindset [9].
  – When waiting for the anesthetic to set in, can tell the patient "your face feels different but you look the same" and have patient look in hand mirror.
- At the end of the procedure, place a sticker on the same side as the local anesthesia to remind the patient and the parent/guardian not to bite on that side until the numbness wears off [9].

Pediatric Medication Dosages

- See Chapter 16 for:
  – Dietary fluoride supplementation schedule
  – Pediatric local anesthetics (including maximum dosage and dosage chart)
  – Child antibiotics (dental abscess and premed)
  – Child analgesics
  – Child opioids and anxiolytics.

Procedural Steps

General Remarks

- Have everything set up and ready prior to the child arriving as you may quickly lose the child's cooperation.
- Always ligate items with floss that can be aspirated: gauze, cotton rolls, clamps.

Traumatic Dental Injuries of Primary and Permanent Teeth

- The AAPD endorses the International Association of Dental Traumatology Guidelines for the Management of Traumatic Dental Injuries [10].
- For guidelines, see Appendix A.
- For a checklist, see Chapter 10, Table 10.2.

Preventative Dentistry

See Chapter 5.

Nitrous Oxide and Oxygen Sedation

See Chapter 18.

Interim Therapeutic Restorations

- The AAPD recognizes ITR as a beneficial provisional technique in contemporary pediatric restorative dentistry.
- ITR may be used to restore and prevent the progression of dental caries in young patients, uncooperative patients, patients with special health care needs, and situations in which traditional cavity preparation and/or placement of traditional dental restorations are not feasible. ITR may be used for caries control in children with multiple carious lesions prior to definitive restoration of the teeth [11].
- Indications: uncooperative or special needs patient with asymptomatic primary teeth with caries to dentin with sound enamel margins and opportunity for follow-up and final restoration.
- Prognosis: the longevity decreases if the restoration involves multiple (tooth) surfaces compared with one surface.
- Steps:
  - Less than five minutes.
  - No local anesthetic or rubber dam.
  - Remove carious dentin with large round bur or spoon without pulpal exposure (even if partial removal of caries).
  - Cavity conditioner and dispense glass ionomer [9].

Operative

- See Chapter 7.
- Considerations with primary teeth: warn the parent the tooth may require pulpal treatment, stainless steel crown (SSC), or extraction and a space maintainer.
- Anatomy of primary teeth:
  - Thinner enamel and dentin.
  - Large pulp horns, especially the mesiobuccal pulp horns (in primary and immature permanent).
  - Mandibular primary first molar: try to maintain the transverse ridge.
  - Maxillary primary second molar: try to maintain the oblique ridge.
- Dental materials:
  - Narrow T-band matrix and wooden wedge: recommended for Class II restorations on primary teeth.
  - Amalgam
    - Retention: requires mechanical retention (undercuts).
    - Strong evidence for Class I/II in primary and permanent teeth [12].

- Composite
  - ○ Retention: bonds to enamel, thus bevel all cavosurfaces for improved retention.
  - ○ Strong evidence for the use of composite for Class I/II in primary/permanent teeth; however, for Class II in primary teeth it is based on a study of success for two years [12].
- Glass ionomer
  - ○ Retention: bonds to dentin.
  - ○ Strong evidence for RMGI cement for Class I/II in primary teeth.
  - ○ Evidence lacking to support RMGI cement as a long-term material in permanent teeth [12].

Pulpotomies/Pulpectomies/RCT on immature permanent teeth

Considerations for Pulpal Treatment on Primary and Immature Permanent Teeth

- For diagnosis evaluate the chief complaint, radiographs, clinical signs and symptoms
  - Diagnostic tests include palpation, percussion, and mobility. Percussion may confuse the child, instead press on tooth and look at child's expression [9].
  - Electric and thermal tests are unreliable on primary and immature permanent teeth [13].

- If an RCT is indicated on an immature permanent tooth, recommend referring to an endodontist.
- Determine restorability and consider alternative (extraction and space maintainer).
- Rubber dam isolation is the gold standard for pulpal treatment [13].
- Water lines: do not irrigate the pulp when exposed using dental unit water lines, since these cannot deliver sterile water because they cannot be reliably sterilized according to CDC recommendations; instead employ single-use disposable syringe for irrigants [13].
- Hemostasis control and diagnosis: the AAPD recommends that if a tooth is planned for pulpotomy and hemostasis cannot be controlled after several minutes with a damp cotton pellet, the tooth exhibits signs of irreversible pulpitis. However, inability to control hemostasis may not solely be a reliable indicator for irreversible pulpitis [14]. The inference is that you may control hemostasis but the tooth may have irreversible pulpitis and may require pulpectomy or extraction. Can dampen with chlorhexidine.
- Postoperative radiograph is recommended to check the quality of the fill and evaluate prognosis and follow-up radiographically. The success rate of pulpotomies diminishes over time and it is necessary to monitor the succedaneous tooth bud for any pathology developing [13] (e.g. furcation radiolucencies on primary which can damage the permanent tooth bud).
- Discoloration of teeth after pulpal treatment: can occur with MTA but does not influence the success rate [15]. Composite can turn gray after pulpal treatment [9].

Table 17.2 Pulpal treatment for primary and immature permanent teeth.

Diagnosis	Treatment	Details
Primary teeth		
Normal pulp	None	
Normal pulp with deep cavity preparation and caries removed	*Protective liner* (e.g. MTA, calcium hydroxide)	Monitor for postoperative pain, swelling, sensitivity, radiographic pathology (e.g. pathologic or progressive internal/external resorption, furcal or periapical radiolucency), no harm to succedaneous tooth
Normal pulp with deep caries leaving deepest caries adjacent to pulp to avoid exposure	*Indirect pulp treatment* using a liner (e.g. MTA, calcium hydroxide, RMGI) and restoration (e.g. composite, amalgam)	
Normal pulp with pinpoint exposure (≤1 mm) from cavity preparation or trauma	*Direct pulp cap* using a base (e.g. MTA, calcium hydroxide) and restoration (e.g. composite, amalgam)	
Normal pulp requiring pulpal therapy from pulp exposure with caries removal	*Vital pulp therapy/pulpotomy* only using MTA and Formacresol and not calcium hydroxide, fill with suitable base and if sufficient enamel restore with amalgam or composite; if multisurface lesion restore with SSC	
Reversible pulpitis		
Signs/symptoms: short duration of pain when provoked relieved by OTC medicine, brushing, or removal of stimulus		
Traumatic pulp exposure		
Irreversible pulpitis due to caries or trauma	*Nonvital pulp treatment/pulpectomy*	Clinical signs/symptoms should resolve within a few weeks and radiographic evidence at six months should reveal bone deposition in radiolucent area
Signs/symptoms: spontaneous unprovoked pain, sinus tract, soft tissue swelling (not gingivitis, periodontitis), furcation or apical radiolucency, internal/external resorption radiographically	Via root canal debridement with hand or rotary instruments, irrigation (sodium hypochlorite or sterile water/saline or chlorhexidine), drying canals, filling canals with resorbable material (e.g. zinc/oxide eugenol) and restoration.	
Necrosis due to caries or trauma		
Signs/symptoms: spontaneous unprovoked pain, sinus tract, soft tissue swelling (not gingivitis, periodontitis), furcation or apical radiolucency, internal/external resorption radiographically	*Or iodoform-based paste or combination paste of iodoform and calcium hydroxide [16]*	

(Continued)

Table 17.2 (Continued)

Diagnosis	Treatment	Details
Irreversible pulpitis or necrosis with root resorption on tooth to be maintained less than 12 months	Lesion sterilization/tissue repair (LSTR)	
Immature permanent teeth		
Normal pulp with deep cavity preparation and caries removed	*Protective liner* (e.g. MTA, calcium hydroxide)	No clinical signs/symptoms of sensitivity, pain, swelling, no radiographic signs of pathology, and roots should continue to develop
Normal pulp with deep caries leaving deepest caries adjacent to pulp to avoid exposure or reversible pulpitis	*Indirect pulp treatment* with two options. 1) Removal of decay as close to pulp, leaving deepest portion of caries, placing a protective liner and final restoration, or 2) Two-step process of caries excavation with interim restoration up to 12 months until removal of remaining caries and final restoration	
Normal pulp with small carious or mechanical pulpal exposure	*Direct pulp cap:* control hemostasis, cap exposure with calcium hydroxide or MTA, place final restoration	
Normal pulp or reversible pulpitis with carious exposure	*Partial pulpotomy* by removing inflamed pulp tissue beneath exposure at depth of 1–3 mm or until reach healthy pulpal tissue, hemostasis control with irrigants (e.g. sodium hypochlorite or chlorhexidine), placement of calcium hydroxide or MTA (1.5 mm thick) covered with RMGI and restoration	
Vital pulp with traumatic pulpal exposure	*Partial pulpotomy/Cvek pulpotomy:* same steps as for partial pulpotomy	
Vital pulp with carious pulpal exposure	*Complete pulpotomy* as an interim procedure to allow root development, removal of coronal vital pulp, placement of material in pulp chamber (e.g. MTA) and restoration	
Nonvital tooth with incompletely formed roots	*Apexification* to induce root end closure *Regenerative endodontics*	
Irreversible pulpitis or necrotic pulp on teeth with a closed apex	*Pulpectomy/root canal treatment*	

MTA, mineral trioxide aggregate; SSC, stainless steel crown; RMGI, resin modified glass ionomer.
Source: American Academy of Pediatric Dentistry [13].

Procedural Steps

Pulpotomy

- Indications: infected coronal pulp, but healthy radicular pulp capable of healing.
- Contraindication: signs of abscess (e.g. parulis, swelling, radiolucency at furcation, external or internal root resorption, pulp calcification, excessive bleeding from radicular stump).
- Steps
  - Obtain verbal/written consent.
  - Local anesthesia.
  - Rubber dam isolation.
  - Remove decay with bur prior to accessing the pulp (to avoid contaminating).
  - Access pulp with (different) clean large round bur and light pressure (Figure 17.9). Do not perforate the pulpal floor.
  - Remove tissue in pulp chamber with spoon.
  - Control hemostasis with moist cotton pellet for a few minutes (moist with chlorhexidine).
  - Achieve hemostasis control. If unable to control heme, see Sections Pulpectomy or Primary teeth Extractions (extractions and space maintenance is more common than pulpectomies, which are rarer).
  - Place MTA over the orifices.
  - Place restorative material.
  - Place SSC (see Section Stainless Steel Crowns).
  - Postoperative radiograph to evaluate and annually.
  - See Section Postoperative Instructions.

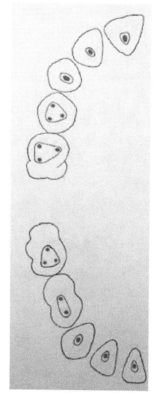

Figure 17.9 Endodontic access outline form in primary teeth.

Pulpectomy

- Indications: unable to obtain hemostasis with pulpotomy, irreversible pulpitis, necrotic.
- Steps:
  - Obtain written/verbal consent.
  - Local anesthesia.
  - Rubber dam isolation.
  - Remove decay prior to accessing pulp (to avoid contaminating).
  - Access pulp with large round bur and light pressure (see Figure 17.9). Do not perforate pulpal floor.
  - Remove tissue in pulp chamber with spoon.
  - Identify canals with endodontic explorer.
  - Use a broach to remove the pulp.
    - Estimate the working length radiographically.
    - Be sure the radiograph shows the proximity of the root to the succedaneous tooth bud.
  - Clean canals with endodontic files, stopping 2 mm short of apex.
  - Irrigate with chlorhexidine, sterile saline, sterile water, or sodium hypochlorite (must be very careful using sodium hypochlorite).
  - Dry canals with paper points.

Pediatric Dentistry

– Dry canals to achieve hemostasis.
– Fill canals with zinc oxide eugenol or iodoform-based paste, or combination of iodoform and calcium hydroxide. Examples of resorbable materials include Vitapex, Diapex, Endoflas.
– Place MTA over the orifices.
– Restorative material.
– Place SSC (see Section Stainless Steel Crowns).
– See Postoperative Instructions.

RCT on Immature Permanent Teeth

Recommend referral to an endodontist if apexification or regenerative endodontics is required.

Stainless Steel Crowns and Strip Crowns

Stainless Steel Crowns

- Indications
  - Primary posterior and anterior teeth:
    - Subgingival Class II.
    - Pulpotomy.
    - Pulpectomy.
    - One of the treatments of choice for full coronal coverage restorations in primary anterior teeth [12].
    - High-risk children with large or multisurface cavitated or noncavitated lesions on primary molars, especially when children require advanced behavioral guidance techniques including general anesthesia [12].
  - Permanent posterior teeth: SSC can be used temporarily until the tooth is fully erupted and then replaced with a definitive crown (e.g. zirconia crown, PFM) since SSCs are not custom fitting (vs. lab-fabricated crowns) and have open margins.
- Informed consent
  - The parent may disapprove of the SSC's visible metal color in the mouth.
  - Alternatives include:
    - Pre-veneered SSC or zirconia crowns: both require longer visits, better cooperation, and more reduction, and likely require vital pulpotomy especially on primary first molars [9].
    - On pulpally treated tooth: amalgam or composite if the tooth will exfoliate within two years [9].
- Steps
  - Local anesthesia.
  - Check occlusion.
  - Measure the tooth's mesial–distal dimensions and height with calipers.
  - Pre-wedge the interproximal contacts (prevents nicking adjacent tooth), especially between primary second molar and permanent first molar.
  - Reductions:
    - Occlusal: 1–1.5 mm
    - Interproximal: break contacts with feather-edge finish line subgingivally with no ledge (feel for ledge with explorer).
    - Buccal/lingual: reduce occlusal one-third and mesial buccal bulge.
    - Round all corners
  - Selecting the SSC

- ○ Chose the smallest that fits.
- ○ Size #4 then go up or down.
- ○ Seat the lingual and then buccal so it "snaps" with 1 mm into sulcus.
- ○ Check occlusion by verifying that the adjacent marginal ridges are the same height.
  - ▪ Not seating?
    - a) Inadequate occlusal reduction
    - b) Crown too long (blanching?). Scratch with explorer and cut.
    - c) Proximal contact not broken?
    - d) Proximal ledge?
- ○ Space loss due to distal decay on the primary first molar? Select SSC from opposite side and opposite arch.
- ○ Check occlusion with the opposing.
- ○ Remove the SSC with an instrument (e.g. discoid, spoon, curette).
- ○ Clean and dry the SSC.
- ○ Fill the SSC two-thirds with glass ionomer cement and seat.
- ○ Check occlusion.
- ○ Ask patient to bite hard for five seconds on the bite stick or band seater.
- ○ Clean the excess cement.
- ○ See Section Postoperative Instructions.

Strip Crowns

- Indications
  - – Primary anterior teeth:
    - ○ Esthetic tooth-colored option (vs. SSC).
    - ○ Large interproximal lesions.
    - ○ Pulpal therapy.
    - ○ Fractured.
    - ○ Discolored.
    - ○ One of the treatments of choice for full coronal coverage restorations in primary anterior teeth, in addition to pre-veneered SSCs and open-face SSCs [12].
- Steps
  - – Composite shade selection.
  - – Local anesthesia.
  - – Select the plastic crown with the same mesial–distal width (hold edge to edge) and height.
  - – Reductions:
    - ○ Incisal: 1–1.5 mm.
    - ○ Interproximal: 0.5–1 mm breaking contact. May have to go subgingivally depending on the neck of the strip crown form (e.g. wide teeth).
    - ○ Facial 1 mm with undercut at gingival one-third.
    - ○ Lingual 0.5 mm.
    - ○ Round all corners.
  - – Check the plastic crown fit: 1 mm into sulcus.
  - – Poke a vent hole on incisal corner with explorer.
  - – Etch and bond the tooth.
  - – Fill the plastic crown with composite and seat.
  - – Light cure the facial and the lingual surfaces.

Pediatric Dentistry

– Remove the plastic crown with an instrument or can cut the incisal edge with a disc and peel the plastic crown off.
– Check and adjust occlusion.

Primary Teeth Extractions

- **Preoperative evaluation checklist**
  - Are antibiotics indicated prior to the extraction appointment?
    - Any of the following: facial swelling, fever, lymphadenopathy, malaise, indurated soft tissue?
  - Will a space maintainer be needed?
  - Root anatomy evaluation:
    - Resorbed?
    - Encircles the tooth bud? If so, plan to section tooth.
    - Presence and proximity of underlying tooth bud.
    - Slender flared resorbed roots at risk of fracturing?
  - Tooth mobile?
  - Adjacent teeth mobile? At risk of unintentional extraction?
  - Parent/guardian preoperative discussion: inform parent/guardian that primary molars have thin divergent roots that are brittle, especially when weakened by resorption. Root fracture in primary molars is not uncommon [17]. If this occurs attempts will be made to remove the root, but if the risk of harming the permanent tooth bud is great, then will have to leave root and monitor.
- **Procedure**
  - Obtain written and verbal consent from the parent/guardian.
  - Local anesthesia:
    - For maximum dosages and dosage chart, see Chapter 16.
    - Walking technique around entire tooth and into sulcus [9].
  - After anesthetizing, show the patient the amount of pressure/force to be used by moving the patient's head with finger pressure.
  - For extraction steps, see Chapter 9.
  - See Table 17.3.
  - See section Postoperative Instructions in Chapter 9.
  - For postoperative pain management, see Chapter 16.

Table 17.3 Extraction forceps for primary teeth.

Teeth	Forceps	Extraction movements
A–J	150S	Palatal/buccal
C–H	1	Facial/lingual with rotation
K–T	151S	Buccal/lingual
M–R	MD3 forceps	Facial/lingual with rotation
None	Cowhorn	Do not use: contraindicated as they can damage the tooth bud

- **Troubleshooting**
  - Management of a primary molar encircling tooth bud.
    - ○ Sectioning the molar using a bur. Caution: do not cut into the furcation, which can damage the underlying tooth bud. Instead split the tooth with straight elevator.
    - ○ If the tooth bud is removed, replant and suture [9].
  - Management of a fractured primary molar root.
    - ○ Remove if it is easy to remove. If it is a very small root tip located deep in the socket in close proximity with tooth bud, or several attempts at removal have been made, leave the root tip to be resorbed. Inform the parent, document, and monitor (possible postoperative infection and delayed eruption of the permanent tooth) [17].
  - Miscellaneous: if the tooth is abscessed, expect more bleeding; gently curette to avoid damage to tooth bud. Antibiotics are not indicated and source of infection removed [9].

Space Maintainers

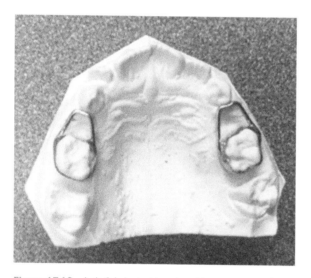

Figure 17.10 Lab-fabricated band and loop space maintainers.

- Purpose: to prevent loss of arch length, width, and perimeter [9]. If indicated but not placed, can lead to crowding, impaction, esthetic problems, and malocclusion.
- Indications:
  - Premature tooth loss
  - Space maintainer (SM) as soon as possible after tooth loss (within six months space loss occurs) [9].
  - Congenitally missing permanent tooth.
  - Ankylosis or submergence of primary tooth.
- Contraindications:
  - Permanent successor near eruption.
  - Orthodontic treatment beginning within six months of primary molar loss.

- Diagnosis:
  - Early loss of primary tooth, or congenitally missing primary (see tooth eruption charts in Figures 17.5 and 17.6).
  - On a bitewing or periapical, "about 6 months is necessary for the permanent successor to move through 1 mm of bone" [18].
  - Postpone SM until all teeth requiring extractions have been documented, since if multiple extractions are needed the design of the SM will change.
- Inform parent/guardian:
  - SM requires follow-up and good oral hygiene.
  - If loose, broken or interfering with eruption/discomfort, patient should come into the office.
  - Once tooth shows, patient should come into the office.
- SM designs:
  - Band and loop
  - Distal shoe
  - Lower lingual holding arch (mandibular)
  - Nance appliance (maxillary)
  - Transpalatal arch/palatal arch bar (maxillary).

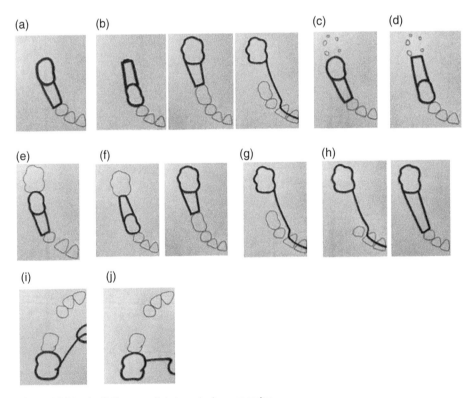

Figure 17.11   (a–j) Space maintainer design scenarios.

Table 17.4 Space maintainer scenarios.

Permanent first molar status	Arch	Missing tooth	Space maintainer
Not erupted	Maxillary or mandibular arch	Primary first molar	Band (primary second molar) and loop (distal of primary canine) (Figure 17.11a)
		Primary second molar	Distal shoe
			Once permanent first molar erupts
			Band (permanent first molar) and loop (distal of primary canine) or lower lingual holding arch with bands on permanent first molars (with permanent centrals and laterals present) or Nance (maxillary) (Figure 17.11b)
Partially erupted	Maxillary or mandibular arch	Primary first molar	Band (primary second molar) and loop (distal of primary canine) (Figure 17.11c)
		Primary second molar	Band (primary first molar) and loop (mesial of permanent first molar) (Figure 17.11d)
Erupted	Mandibular	Primary first molar	If the primary second molars are in occlusion, an SM is not needed
			If not, band (primary second molar) and loop (distal of primary canine) (Figure 17.11e)
		Primary second molar	Band (primary first molar) and loop (mesial of permanent first molar) *or*
			Band (permanent first molar) and loop (distal of primary first molar) (Figure 17.11f)
		Primary second molar and primary first molar near exfoliation	Lower lingual holding arch with bands on permanent first molars (with permanent centrals and laterals present) (Figure 17.11g)
		Unilateral primary first and second molar	Lower lingual holding arch > band (permanent first molar) and loop (distal of primary canine) (Figure 17.11h)
	Maxillary arch	Bilateral maxillary primary first molar, primary second molar, or both	Nance appliance (band maxillary permanent first molars) (Figure 17.11i)
		Unilateral maxillary primary second molar	Transpalatal arch/palatal arch bar (band maxillary permanent first molars) (Figure 17.11j)

Notes
If a primary canine is missing: extract the other canine in the same arch to prevent the midline from drifting. A SM is not needed.
If a primary incisor (centrals or laterals) is missing, an SM is not needed.

- Procedure:
  - Determine the SM type and design before extraction.
  - Different ways to fabricate the SM
    - Chairside
      - Band and loop: measure edentulous area, cut to shorten wire, insert, check fit, crimp band, glass ionomer cement.

Pediatric Dentistry

- ○ Lab fabricated (see Section Lab Prescriptions for Space Maintainers) (See Figure 17.10).
    - ▪ Option 1: fit bands and take an impression with the bands. Pour the model with the bands or send the impression with the bands to the lab for fabrication.
    - ▪ Option 2: extract the tooth and take an impression and send to lab to fabricate the SM.
  - – If distal shoe indicated: PA to see location of permanent first molar, make model before extraction, deliver at time of extraction because anesthetized, distal shoe blade goes subgingival 1–1.5 mm below the marginal ridge of the unerupted permanent first molar and a PA is taken to verify before cementing.
  - – Placement:
    - ○ Try in, check if interfering with occlusion, adjust as necessary.
    - ○ Line with RMGI cement and seat and remove excess cement.
    - ○ If tight contacts and no room for the band, place an ortho spacer (rubber) for one week and then seat the SM.
    - ○ See Section Postoperative Instructions.
- Follow-up:
  - – To verify SM is not interfering with eruption.
  - – To check if the banded tooth erupted and a new SM is needed.
  - – To check if the permanent successor has started to erupt and SM removal is needed.
  - – If a distal shoe, monitor every two months; once the permanent first molar erupts, replace with a band and loop.
- Removal:
  - – Not necessary if it falls out with the tooth.
  - – Band and loop: remove with band remover pliers and remove RMGI with a scaler.
  - – Nance/lower lingual holding arch/transpalatal arch/palatal arch bar: remove with band remover pliers.

Lab Prescriptions for Space Maintainers

- Include the impression (or poured model). Typically, the opposing is not needed as the SM should not interfere with the occlusion.

Please fabricate:
    Band and loop: band tooth _____
    Distal shoe: band tooth _____
    Lower lingual holding arch: band tooth _____
    Nance: band tooth _____
    Transpalatal arch/palatal arch bar: band tooth _____
Refer to the design
Thank you

Postoperative Instructions

- Prophy, fluoride varnish, and sealants: see Chapter 5.
- Local anesthetic:
  - – The area treated today may be numb for several hours.

- A sticker was placed on your child's shirt on the side that is numb as a reminder to avoid chewing, biting, sucking, or scratching the lips or cheek on that side.
  - Do not eat until the lip wakes up to prevent biting the lip.
  - As the area wakes up it will feel tingly.
- Composites and amalgams: see Chapter 7.
- Pulpotomies/pulpectomies/RCT on immature and mature permanent teeth:
  - Mild to moderate pain may be experienced.
  - Recommend ibuprofen and acetaminophen prior to the anesthesia wearing off.
  - If pain lasts for more than 48 hours, come in to the office.
- Stainless steel crown:
  - Gums may be red and bleeding for a few days, so recommend warm saline rinses (one teaspoon in one cup of water).
  - Recommend ibuprofen for sensitivity.
  - Avoid chewy and sticky food and gum as it can pull the crown off.
  - Brush after breakfast and at night floss and brush. If the floss gets stuck, don't pull hard or the crown can pop off; instead pull out the side
- Extractions: see Chapter 9.
- Space maintainers:
  - Diet
    - Day 1: soft food diet.
    - May be difficult to chew at first, but you will adapt over time.
    - Foods to avoid include really sticky or chewy foods, gum, and hard crunchy foods and chewing ice.
  - Gums might be sore from the band for a few days.
  - Hygiene:
    - The SM will catch food debris, so it will take extra effort to floss, rinse vigorously, and to brush around the SM.
    - If you have a Nance appliance, use a water pick or a monoject syringe to clean under.
  - Precautions
    - Do not play with the SM with your tongue. Do not try to pop it off with your tongue as this will cause it to become loose over time.
  - Return to the dentist:
    - If the SM becomes loose.
    - If the SM falls out. Be sure to store it in a safe place and bring it with you to the appointment.
    - Every six months to evaluate the fit and to check if it needs removal.
    - Once you see the white spot of an adult tooth erupting, return to the dentist for removal of the SM.

Documentation

- Always document who accompanied the child to their appointment.
- Document the child's behavior using the Frankl Behavioral Rating Scale and with objective language (Figure 17.12).

1	− −	Definitely negative. Refusal of treatment, forceful crying, fearfulness, or any other overt evidence of extreme negativism.
2	−	Negative. Reluctance to accept treatment, uncooperative, some evidence of negative attitude but not pronounced (sullen, withdrawn).
3	+	Positive. Acceptance of treatmen, cautious behavior at times, willingness to comply with the dentist, at times with reservation, but patient follows the dentist's directions cooperatively.
4	++	Definitely positive. Good rapport with the dentist, interest in the dental procedures, laughter and enjoyment.

Figure 17.12   Frankl Behavioral Rating Scale. *Source:* American Academy of Pediatric Dentistry [6].

Real-Life Clinical Questions and Scenarios Answered

Dental Students' Questions

- "I don't want to overdose the child, how much anesthetic can I give?"
  - For maximum dosages, see Chapter 16.
- "I can't tell if the child is crying from fear or if the child is not numb enough?"
  - How much time did you allow for the onset of the local anesthetic? Did you check if the patient was numb with the explorer on the gingiva before starting the procedure? If the patient feels this, then I'd recommend giving more anesthetic. If the patient is crying uncontrollably, then I'd recommend ending the treatment unless it is an emergency extraction.

Dental Assistants' Questions

- "Do we perio chart on children?"
  - See Section Clinical and Radiographic Exam.
- "Hey doc, what type of X-rays do you want me to take on this 5-year-old?"
  - See Chapter 3.
- "I don't remember the tooth numbers on baby teeth."
  - For the second primary molars, imagine two people meeting each other saying "Hey A.J." and "Hey K.T." This way you can remember teeth A, J, K and T.
  - For the canines imagine a person telling someone to be quiet by saying "shh mister" (or "chh mr") so you can remember teeth C, H, and M, R.

Parents' Concerns

- "I don't know how to brush my child's teeth because she's three years old, she is my first kid and when I try she runs out of the room with the toothbrush."
  - As the adult you know what is best for your child and you must brush their teeth twice a day. You are not asking the child's permission because it is something that has to be done. It will be challenging at first but most children will get used to it with time.
  - For small children (infant to toddlers), if there are two at home, you can do the knee-to-knee method with the child on your lap so you can brush your child's teeth. One person will hold the child's hands, as the other brushes.
  - If alone, you can sit on the floor with the child's head on your lap and brush their teeth.
  - When the child is a little older you can stand behind the child and have the child look up to the sky and brush their teeth for them, or siting on the floor with the child on your lap. This way you can have a direct view into their mouth.

- You can also make it a game, and let the child watch a show on the phone or a brush-along video.
- "Are my kids teeth growing in normal? Will he need braces?"
  - See tooth eruption charts in Figures 17.5 and 17.6.
- "How much medicine should my child take?"
  - See Chapter 16.
- "Bump on her gums. I think she needs antibiotics." (See Figure 17.2)
  - Antibiotics are indicated if a fever (>100.4°F, 38°C), facial swelling, malaise, and/or lymphad-enopathy. In this case, tooth S has a parulis on the buccal gingiva with an existing crown. Radiographic findings include a radiolucency in the furcation (see Figure 17.4). Recommend extraction, OTC pain medication, and an SM.
- "We drink well water, is there fluoride in that water?"
  - In order to determine the amount of fluoride, the private well water would have to be tested and the results obtained from a state-certified laboratory. If children in the household are under 16 years old it is recommended to test the water annually as the level of fluoride may be inadequate. If inadequate, dietary fluoride supplements are recommended or alternative water sources should be used to reduce the risk of fluorosis [19].
- "My child grinds his teeth. Does he need a night guard?"
  - See Chapter 15, section Real-Life Comments and Questions Answered.
- "Is it bad she still sucks her thumb? At what age should she quit?"
  - If using a pacifier, discontinue at age 2. If beyond age 2 or 3, may require orthodontics [9].
  - If thumb or finger sucking, discourage once the upper permanent front teeth erupt (around seven to eight years old) [9].
- "Why does he have cavities when he doesn't eat candy?"
  - Bacteria feed on the food you eat, especially sugars and starches. The bacteria produce acid as a by-product of their digesting the food and this dissolves the tooth, causing cavities. So even a diet that does not consist of sweets but consists of starches such as pasta, bread, cereal, pretzels, and crackers still leads to cavities.
  - How often does he snack? What does he like to drink? When and how often does he brush and floss?
  - See Chapter 5, section Nutritional Counseling.
- "I don't want my three-year-old to have any sedation. What can you do for his cavities?"
  - See treatment deferral in Section Pediatric Treatment Planning.
- "Does my kid really need fillings on these teeth if they will fall out anyways?"
  - If the cavity progresses it can cause pain and infection, and put the child's health at risk. In addition, if the deciduous tooth is infected, the child's permanent tooth can be discolored and brittle (Turner tooth).
    - Turner tooth: caused by periapical inflammation (infection or trauma) and will have defects ranging from brown, yellow, or white discoloration to extensive hypoplasia involving the entire crown (brittle tooth) [20]. This depends on stage of tooth development, length of infection, virulence, and host resistance. Turner tooth usually occurs in permanent premolars.
  - If the tooth is extracted, then the other teeth will migrate and prevent the adult tooth from growing in, which would require a space maintainer. The best space maintainer is a tooth.
- "What are sealants?"
  - See Chapter 5, section Sealants. Also helps to show the parents visuals (e.g. photos, models).

- "Loose tooth hurting him."
  - See Figure 17.3.
- Evaluate the radiograph to determine if the tooth is only being retained by soft tissue (i.e. no risk of fracturing the roots). If this is the case, you have the option of no treatment and your child can wiggle the tooth, or we can extract. The tooth is likely causing discomfort when the child is chewing due to the sharp edges of the enamel traumatizing the soft tissue.

Scenarios

- The parent films the child in the chair receiving dental care.
  - Decide what your policy is on cameras in the dental office. With filming, there can be HIPAA (Health Insurance Portability and Accountability Act) violations if the film (or photo) captures the dental schedule on the computer monitor or captures a conversation nearby with or regarding another patient. Also check with local state regulations, for example California has a "two-party consent" law meaning both parties must consent to be filmed as it is a crime to record any confidential communication [21].
- The 16-year-old brings their 10-year-old brother in for appointment.
  - Need to have an office policy regarding this situation.
  - Recommend calling parent/guardian asking for any change in health history. If parent/guardian signed a prior treatment plan and you now intend to deviate from the treatment plan (e.g. tooth planned for composite will now require an extraction), call the parent/guardian.
- The parent brings the child in for an exam and cleaning and the child has braces.
  - Request the orthodontist to remove the wires for the exam including radiographs and a cleaning. This will allow for diagnostic radiographs (wire not superimposed at the interproximal contacts; see Chapter 3, Figure 3.29) and allow for better access for cleaning. The ortho wire may also need to be removed for restorative treatment.
  - Review oral hygiene instructions and stress the importance of a lifelong commitment with the retainer.
- The parent wants to be in the room watching the procedure and talking to and touching the child throughout the treatment.
  - See Section Patient Management.

References

1 American Association of Pediatric Dentistry (2020). Pediatric medical history. In: *The Reference Manual of Pediatric Dentistry*. Chicago: AAPD https://www.aapd.org/globalassets/media/policies_guidelines/r_medhistoryform.pdf.

2 American Academy of Pediatric Dentistry (2020). Classification of periodontal diseases in infants, children, adolescents, and individuals with special health care needs. In: *The Reference Manual of Pediatric Dentistry*, 418–432. Chicago: AAPD.

3 American Association of Pediatric Dentistry (2020). Frequently asked questions (FAQs). https://www.aapd.org/resources/parent/faq (accessed 23 April 2021).

4 Wright, J.T., Crall, J.J., Fontana, M. et al. (2016). Evidence-based clinical practice guideline for the use of pit-and-fissure sealants: a report of the American Dental Association and the American Academy of Pediatric Dentistry. *J. Am. Dent. Assoc.* 147 (8): 672–682.e12. https://www.aapd.org/assets/1/7/G_EBD-Sealants1.PDF.

5 American Association of Orthodontists (2013). The right time for an orthodontic check-up: no later than age 7. https://www.aaoinfo.org/system/files/media/documents/Right_Time_for_Ortho-MLMS-hl.pdf (accessed 23 April 2021).

6 American Academy of Pediatric Dentistry (2020). Behavior guidance for the pediatric dental patient. In: *The Reference Manual of Pediatric Dentistry*, 292–310. Chicago: AAPD.

7 Casamassimo, P., Fields, H., McTigue, D., and Nowak, A. (2013). *Pediatric Dentistry: Infancy through Adolescence*. St. Louis, MO: Elsevier.

8 Smiles Under the Sea (2020). Orthodontic treatment. https://smilesunderthesea.com/orthodontic-treatment (accessed 23 April 2021).

9 Soxman, J.A. (ed.) (2015). *Handbook of Clinical Techniques in Pediatric Dentistry*. Ames, IA: Wiley Blackwell.

10 Bourguignon, C., Cohenca, N., Lauridsen, E. et al. (2020). International Association of Dental Traumatology guidelines for the management of traumatic dental injuries: 1. Fractures and luxations of permanent teeth. *Dent. Traumatol.* 36 (4): 314–330. https://www.aapd.org/research/oral-health-policies--recommendations/guidelines-for-the-management-of-traumatic-dental-injuries-1-fracture-and-luxations-or-permanent-teeth.

11 American Academy of Pediatric Dentistry (2020). Policy on interim therapeutic restorations (ITR). In: *The Reference Manual of Pediatric Dentistry*, 72–73. Chicago: AAPD.

12 American Academy of Pediatric Dentistry (2020). Pediatric restorative dentistry. In: *The Reference Manual of Pediatric Dentistry*, 371–383. Chicago: AAPD.

13 American Academy of Pediatric Dentistry (2020). Pulp therapy for primary and immature permanent teeth. In: *The Reference Manual of Pediatric Dentistry*, 384–392. Chicago: AAPD.

14 Coll, J.A., Dhar, V., Vargas, K. et al. (2020). Use of non-vital pulp therapies in primary teeth. *Pediatr. Dent.* 42 (5): 337–349. https://www.aapd.org/globalassets/media/policies_guidelines/g_non-vpt.pdf.

15 Dhar, V., Marghalani, A.A., Crystal, Y.O. et al. (2017). Use of vital pulp therapies in primary teeth with deep caries lesions. *Pediatr. Dent.* 39 (5): E146–E159. https://www.aapd.org/globalassets/media/policies_guidelines/g_vpt.pdf.

16 Trairatvorakul, C. and Chunlasikaiwan, S. (2008). Success of pulpectomy with zinc oxide-eugenol vs calcium hydroxide/iodoform paste in primary molars: a clinical study. *Pediatr. Dent.* 30 (4): 303–308. https://www.aapd.org/globalassets/media/publications/archives/303-8.pdf.

17 American Academy of Pediatric Dentistry (2020). Management considerations for pediatric oral surgery and oral pathology. In: *The Reference Manual of Pediatric Dentistry*, 433–442. Chicago: AAPD.

18 Simon, T., Nwabuee, I., Oueis, H. et al. (2012). Space maintenance in the primary and mixed dentitions. *J. Michigan Dent. Assoc.* 94: 38–40.

19 American Dental Association (ADA) (2018). *Fluoridation Facts*. Chicago: ADA https://www.ada.org/~/media/ADA/Files/Fluoridation_Facts.pdf?la=en.

20 Neville, B.W., Damm, D.D., Allen, C.M., and Chi, A.C. (2016). *Oral and Maxillofacial Pathology*, 4e. St. Louis, MO: Elsevier.

21 Digital Media Law Project (2021). California Recording Law. https://www.dmlp.org/legal-guide/california-recording-law (accessed 23 April 2021).

18

Nitrous Oxide and Oxygen Sedation

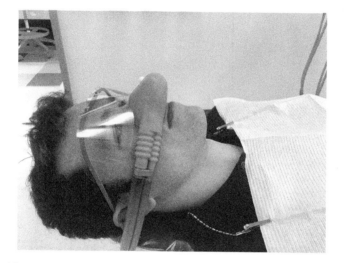

Figure 18.1   Nasal hood on the patient.

Chapter Outline

- Real-Life Questions and Comments
- Relevance
- Introduction
- Indications and Contraindications
- Signs and Symptoms of Optimal Sedation
- Signs and Symptoms of Oversedation
- Armamentarium
- Informed Consent
- Procedural Steps for Nitrous Sedation
  - Unit Set-up
  - Rooming
  - Procedure
  - Unit Shutdown

Clinical Dentistry Daily Reference Guide, First Edition. William A. Jacobson.
© 2022 John Wiley & Sons, Inc. Published 2022 by John Wiley & Sons, Inc.

- Postoperative Instructions
- Charting Template
- Clinical Pearls
  - Troubleshooting
  - Tips
  - Miscellaneous
- Real-Life Questions and Comments Answered
- References

Real-Life Questions and Comments

Student Questions

- "I haven't done nitrous in a long time, can you run me through the steps?"
- "My patient said he has a cold but he wants to get the procedure done today with nitrous. Is that OK?"
- "What do I do if my patient says his head hurts after the nitrous?"

Dental Assistant Comment

- "Hey doc, I'll get the kid started on the nitrous."

Patients' Health Concerns

- "Is nitrous safe for my child?"
- "I heard someone's mouth caught on fire using nitrous."
- "I may be pregnant. Is this safe?"

Patients' Queries

- "I am extremely anxious about this appointment today."
- "Can I get laughing gas today?"
- "What is nitrous oxide sedation?"
- "What will I feel?"
- "Can I drive home after this?"
- "I took some Valium before this."
- "How is this different from IV sedation or general anesthesia?"

Patient Comment

- "My kid is fine. He doesn't need that gas."

Relevance

- Knowing how to safely administer nitrous sedation is a valuable skill to offer your patients.

Introduction

Nitrous oxide and oxygen sedation, also known as "nitrous sedation" or "laughing gas," is a safe and effective technique to reduce anxiety and pain during dental procedures. It is a combination of two gases, nitrous oxide and oxygen, that are inhaled through the nose. The exact mechanism of action is unknown, but it depresses the cerebrum, thalamus, and midbrain functions [1]. There is no loss of consciousness and the patient receiving the treatment is still able to respond and speak. It has a rapid onset and recovery, so the patient will not need a driver, as one would with other forms of sedation.

Ambient air is 21% oxygen. We provide greater amounts of oxygen with nitrous oxide and oxygen sedation. We begin and end with 100% oxygen. Ending with 100% oxygen is done to prevent diffusion hypoxia, which is the result of a rapid release of nitrous oxide from the bloodstream diluting the concentration of oxygen. This can lead to headache, disorientation, and nausea [2]. This can be reversed with oxygen administration [3].

Indications and Contraindications

- Indications
  - Dental phobia/anxiety.
  - A strong gag reflex.
  - When profound local anesthesia cannot be obtained.
  - In a patient who refuses or is allergic to local anesthetics, nitrous will reduce the pain sensation [1] and raise the pain threshold [3]. The patient still has to be anesthetized. Nitrous will reduce pressure-induced pain but not affect pulpal sensitivity [2].
  - A cooperative child undergoing a lengthy procedure [2].
  - A short attention span or impatient for long appointments (reduced awareness of the passage of time) [1].
- Contraindications
  - Nasal obstruction: upper respiratory tract infection, allergies, deviated nasal septum, common cold [1].
  - Taking oral sedatives (unless you are trained in oral conscious sedation).
  - Those who do not like the feeling of losing control ("control freaks").
  - Chronic obstructive pulmonary disease (COPD), tuberculosis, eustachian tube blockage, other chronic respiratory disorders (excluding asthma) [1].
    - COPD: avoid with severe COPD. If you give oxygen, the patient will lose the stimulus to breathe as this depends on low oxygen levels [4].
  - A patient who declines nitrous oxide/oxygen sedation [1] (requires consent).
  - A debilitating cardiac or cerebrovascular disease. Patients who report shortness of breath or arterial blockage, and who use increased pillows for sleeping (avoid any CNS depressants) [1].
  - Uncooperative when directed to breathe through nose: children with severe behavioral issues (technique requires cooperation) [1].
  - Compulsive personalities, personality disorders (may be a negative experience, difficult to predict) [1].
  - Patients who experience claustrophobia.

Nitrous Oxide and Oxygen Sedation

– Pregnancy: first trimester (second and third trimesters are safer and when minimized to 30 minutes) [4]. Breastfeeding is safe [5] (not a contraindication).
– Neutropenia.
– Pneumothorax.
– Anecdotal: alcoholics in recovery have reported a return of "cravings" after receiving nitrous oxide [6].

Signs and Symptoms of Optimal Sedation

- Signs
  – Patient responds and follows directions, although more slowly [1].
  – Change in the patient's voice (slow and sounds "throaty" [1]).
  – Ptosis of eyelids, blank stare [3], lacrimation and/or glazed eyes.
  – Perspiration on the face [1].
  – Relaxation of the limbs, palms open, warm, and moist [3].
  – Lowered pulse [3].
  – Reduced pain response.
  – Depressed gag reflex [1].
- Symptoms
  – Pain reaction markedly reduced or eliminated [1].
  – Feeling drowsy, warm, and a floating sensation.
  – Sounds and smells are dulled [1].
  – Tingling or numbness of extremities.
  – Numbness or tingling of lips, tongue, and oral tissues: this indicates a more profound depth of sedation and permits injections of local anesthetic. After injection, reduce the nitrous oxide or turn off unless controlling anxiety [1].
  – Slight, moderate, to complete amnesia [1].

Signs and Symptoms of Oversedation

- Dreaming, hallucinating, sexual fantasy (always have a witness present, e.g. dental assistant), heaviness in chest, unable to respond.
- Anger, uncooperative, sensation of flying/falling/uncontrolled spinning [1].
- If any of these occur, stop administering nitrous oxide and administer 100% oxygen.

Armamentarium

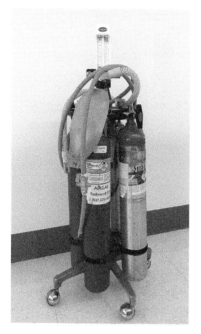

Figure 18.2 Nitrous oxide and oxygen tanks.

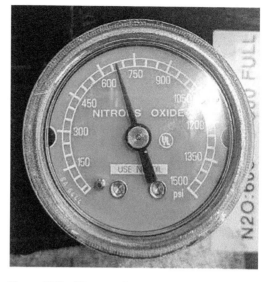

Figure 18.3 Nitrous oxide gauge.

Figure 18.4 Oxygen gauge.

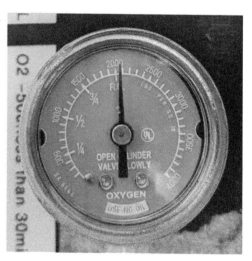

Table 18.1 Armamentarium.

	Nitrous oxide tank	Oxygen tank
Tank/cylinder color (Figure 18.2)	Blue	Green
Full tank	600–700 psi	2000–2200 psi
Gauge (Figures 18.3 and 18.4)	Inaccurate, shows full until one-quarter remaining	Accurate
State of matter	Stored as liquid, delivered as gas	Stored and delivered as gas
Miscellaneou	Sweet-smelling, colorless gas	

Informed Consent

INFORMED CONSENT FOR NITROUS OXIDE/OXYGEN SEDATION

I understand that my treatment today will include the administration of nitrous oxide and oxygen sedation.

I _____ [patient name] have been informed of the procedure and how it will benefit my treatment. This will be provided to help me feel more relaxed and less anxious.

I understand certain risks may be associated with this procedure, including but not limited to headache, dizziness, nausea, and vomiting.* Some patients, at high levels of nitrous oxide, can experience dreaming and hallucinations.

I have informed my doctor of any medications or drugs taken within the last 72 hours as these may have adverse reactions when combined with nitrous oxide and oxygen.

I have been informed of the alternatives to nitrous oxide and oxygen sedation and their associated risks.

Patient Signature: _____. Date: _____

Witness Signature: _____. Print name: _____ Date: _____

*Note that only 0.5–1.2% of patients experience nausea and vomiting. There is an increased risk with longer administration, lack of titration, increased concentration of nitrous oxide, and a heavy meal prior [2].

Procedural Steps for Nitrous Sedation

Unit Set-up

- Read the inventory tags, select the appropriate gas tanks, and update the inventory tags (Figure 18.5).
- Open the oxygen and nitrous oxide tank valves with the wrench.
- Turn the unit on (button that reads "PUSH ON").
- Press the "O_2 FLUSH" (Figure 18.6) and fill the reservoir bag two-thirds (Figure 18.7).
- Set up the nasal hood and plug it into the unit tubing.
- Plug the nasal hood tube end into the HVE (scavenger system) and start the HVE so it is barely working.
- Verify that the scavenger system is on with the scavenger indicator gauge ball (on the machine or tubing). The ball should be in the middle/green area.
- Verify that the scavenger system is working by listening to the nasal hood for suction. Step on the tube and listen for no sound for comparison of when it is not working. The scavenger system reduces occupational exposure to trace amounts of nitrous oxide.

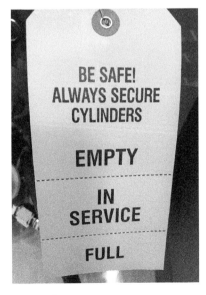

Figure 18.5 Inventory tags.

– Units with the scavenger gauge on the tubing do not require oxygen regulator levers to be up to verify the scavenger system is working.
– Units with the scavenger gauge on the unit require the oxygen regulator levers to be up to listen to and to verify the scavenger system is working.

Rooming

- Review the patient's medical history and ask for any updates.
- Check for any contraindications (see Section Indications and Contraindications).
- Review the preoperative instructions:
  – The patient should avoid having a heavy meal prior, but instead have a light meal in the two hours prior A heavy meal can cause nausea/vomiting and fasting is not required [2].
  – The patient should remove any contact lenses, as these may dry out from air leakage around nasal hood and scratch the cornea.
- Obtain the preoperative vitals (BP, pulse, respirations).
- Patient should sign the nitrous oxide/oxygen sedation informed consent form (see Section Informed Consent).
- Ask if the patient needs to use the restroom prior to beginning.

Procedure

- Explain to the patient what to expect.
- "Today we are going to be using nitrous oxide sedation to help you feel more comfortable and relaxed during your dental treatment. What you can expect is to feel relaxed, warm, your arms and legs may feel tingly, you may feel lighter, and noises may sound more distant. If you feel uncomfortable at any point please let me know. You are in complete control. Any questions?"
  – Note that if the patient is a child, don't ask if he or she is feeling any tingling sensation in his or her fingers/toes as this may lead to undesirable body movements during treatment [3].
- "I will use your name when speaking to you so that you don't have to force yourself to stay alert the entire time." [1]
- Turn up the oxygen regulator lever to 7 l/min (tidal volume) (Figure 18.8).

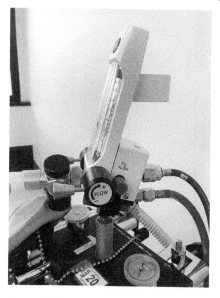

Figure 18.6 O_2 FLUSH button and FLOW levers.

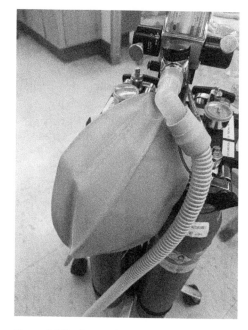

Figure 18.7 Reservoir bag.

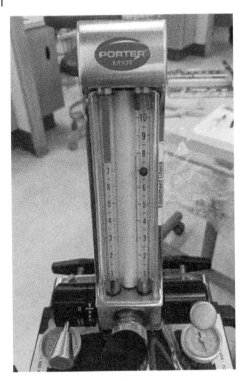

Figure 18.8 Flowmeter with the oxygen level set to 7 l/min.

- "I am going to lower your chair to the position that we will be treating you in today. Then I am going to place a mask over your nose with 100% oxygen flowing into it. I'm going to adjust the mask for a snug fit."
- Place the nasal hood on the patient (see Figure 18.1).
- "Is this comfortable? Do you feel any air leaking around the mask?"
  - If yes: adjust/tighten the mask until no air is leaking. Can place gauze between the two layers of nasal hood for a tighter seal.
- Determine the tidal volume (and maintain this for the entire procedure).
  - "You will need to breathe through your nose during the entire procedure, even when your mouth is open. Take some deep breaths in through your nose and out your nose. Inhale 1...2...3... Exhale 1...2...3..."
    - If the patient is a child you can say "Smell the happy air" [3].
- "Are you comfortable with this amount of oxygen? Does it feel like you're getting enough oxygen?"
  - Increase the tidal volume if:
    - patient reports too little oxygen
    - if the reservoir bag is deflating.
    - Decrease the tidal volume if:
      - the patient reports too much oxygen
      - the reservoir bag is fully inflated and not moving
      - May have to increase the HVE.
    - The reservoir bag should expand and contract:
      - Tidal volume for adults is around 7 l/min, for a child possibly 3–5 l/min.
- Document the tidal volume.
- "Is it OK with you to begin adding a small amount of nitrous oxide?"
  - If yes: increase the nitrous by 1 liter and decrease the oxygen by 1 liter for one minute.
- Make a note of the time to document the length of sedation.
- "[Patient's name] are you comfortable? What are you feeling? Is it OK with you to add some more nitrous oxide?" (See Sections Signs and Symptoms of Optimal Sedation and Signs and Symptoms of Oversedation.)
  - Increase the nitrous by 0.5 l and decrease the oxygen by 0.5 l for one minute.
- Continue checking in with the patient and increasing the nitrous oxide by 0.5 l and decreasing the oxygen by 0.5 l for one-minute increments until you reach the patient's baseline, or optimal level of sedation.
  - Do not increase nitrous oxide beyond the maximum of 50% nitrous oxide and 50% oxygen.
- Document the peak amount of nitrous oxide.
- "[Patient's name] do you feel comfortable? Can we start the dental procedure?"
  - If yes, begin the dental procedure.

- Complete the dental procedure.
- "[Patient's name] we have completed the dental procedure and now I am going to have you breathe 100% oxygen for the next five minutes."
- Make note of the time to document the length of sedation.
- Decrease the nitrous oxide to zero and increase the oxygen to the tidal volume for five minutes of 100% oxygen.
  - Oxygenation of five minutes for every 15 minutes of sedation, up to 20 minutes of oxygenation.
  - Make note of the time.
- [Patient's name] do you feel comfortable and back to normal? Is it OK if I remove the mask?
- Make note of the time to document the length of oxygenation.
- "How do you feel now?"
  - If the patient reports feeling dizzy, nauseous, or groggy, or has a headache, place the oxygen nasal hood on for another five minutes and then check in with the patient.
- Obtain the postoperative vitals (BP, pulse, respirations).
- Provide the postoperative instructions (see Section Preoperative Instructions).
- Dismiss the patient.

Unit Shutdown

- Close the oxygen and nitrous oxide tank valves with the wrench.
- To bleed the excess gases in the tubing, turn the oxygen and nitrous oxide regulator levers up, watch the balls rise and wait until the balls drop on flowmeter (Figure 18.9) and the tank gauges go down to zero. Then move oxygen and nitrous regulator levers back down.
- Turn the HVE off.
- Remove the nasal hood from the machine for sterilization.
- Unplug the scavenger system.
- Turn the unit off (button reads "PUSH OFF").
- Document (see Section Charting Template).

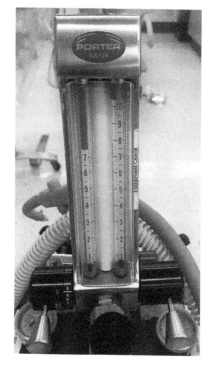

Figure 18.9 Flowmeter after bleeding the excess gases in the tubing.

Postoperative Instructions

- The effects of the nitrous oxide will have worn off by the time we remove your mask.
- You are free to go back to whatever plans you had for the rest of the day.
- You are able to drive after this.
- If your child received nitrous sedation today, it is a good idea to hold your child's hand at first.

Nitrous Oxide and Oxygen Sedation

Charting Template

NITROUS OXIDE/OXYGEN SEDATION

Indication(s) for nitrous oxide/oxygen:_____ e.g. dental phobia

Verbal and written informed consent obtained

Preoperative vitals:

    Blood pressure:_____

    Pulse:_____

    Respirations:_____

Postoperative vitals:

    Blood pressure:_____

    Pulse:_____

    Respirations:_____

    Tidal volume (l/min):_____

    Peak % nitrous oxide (%):_____

[*To calculate: nitrous oxide (liters) divided by tidal volume (liters) = % nitrous oxide*]

Length of sedation (minutes):_____

Length of postoperative 100% oxygen (minutes):_____

Recovery (observations): _____

[*Example: Patient responded very well, fully recovered and reported normalcy prior to dismissal*]

Adverse reactions/comments: _____

Dental procedure note:_____

Clinical Pearls

Troubleshooting

- If there are signs or symptoms of oversedation or inappropriate sedation, stop administering the nitrous oxide and administer 100% oxygen.
- If there are signs of diffusion hypoxia after the nasal hood is removed at the end of treatment, administer 100% oxygen for more time.
- If the patient vomits, turn the patient on their right side (left hip up) to prevent material entering the left bronchus.

Tips

- To prevent nausea in prolonged procedures, administer 100% oxygen every 45 minutes [1].
- Do not assume a patient's tidal volume will remain unchanged at different appointments. Factors that contribute to changes include the amount of food, mental or emotional state, amount of sleep, and increased tolerance with repeated administrations [1].
- The highest ratio of nitrous oxide recommended for safe administration is 50% nitrous oxide with 50% oxygen. Do not go beyond 50% nitrous oxide [1]. Studies have reported negative outcomes when nitrous oxide is used above 50%, and there are concerns with aspiration and loss of pharyngeal–laryngeal reflexes [2].

Miscellaneous

- Never leave the patient unaccompanied while under nitrous oxide/oxygen sedation [1].
- Occupational exposure:
  - Occupational exposure to nitrous is potentially toxic.
  - It is especially risky when a female dentist or dental staff members are pregnant and exposed to trace levels of nitrous oxide for more than three hours per week, and when scavenging equipment is not used. Studies have shown decreased fertility and increased rates of spontaneous abortion [4].
  - Minimize occupational exposure by testing the equipment, checking for leaks, minimizing the amount the patient is talking (and ensure the patient is breathing in and out of their nose and not their mouth [2]), and investigate air-monitoring devices (contact dental supply rep) [1].
- Medicolegal considerations:
  - Check with your state dental board if you are required to post a "Notice to Patients" sign on the wall warning of the risks of exposure to nitrous oxide sedation causing birth defects.
  - Always have a witness present to avoid any accusations from the patient.

Real-Life Questions and Comments Answered

Student Questions

- "I haven't done nitrous in a long time, can you run me through the steps?"
  - There is more to know than just the nitrous sedation steps for safe administration. Read this chapter.
- "My patient said he has a cold but he wants to get the procedure done today with nitrous. Is that OK?"
  - The patient must be able to breathe through their nose. Can your patient do this? If not, we will have to complete the procedure without nitrous or reschedule.
- "What do I do if my patient says his head hurts after the nitrous?"
  - Sounds like diffusion hypoxia. Did you administer 100% oxygen for five minutes after administering nitrous oxide? Let's continue oxygenating for another five minutes making sure the patient is breathing *only* through their nose and we will check in after five minutes to see how he feels.

Nitrous Oxide and Oxygen Sedation

Dental Assistant Comment

- "Hey doc, I'll get the kid started on the nitrous."
  - Check with your state dental board regarding permitted duties for dental assistants. Dental assistants may require formal training and certification in order to monitor or administer nitrous oxide.

Patients' Health Concerns

- "Is this safe for my child?"
  - The AAPD recognizes nitrous oxide/oxygen inhalation as a safe and effective technique to reduce anxiety and produce analgesia. There are no known allergies to nitrous oxide [1]. There have been no recorded fatalities or serious illness at the concentrations we use. Your child will still respond normally to verbal commands and have no loss of protective reflexes (be able to swallow/talk/cough). There is no loss of consciousness. This technique will simply help your child to relax and tolerate the dental procedure [2]. The most common adverse effect is nausea which is rare [3].
- "I heard someone's mouth caught on fire using nitrous."
  - Yes, there was a report in the media about a case in which there was a one to two-second fire in a patient's mouth. Fires require three ingredients, known as the fire triangle: oxygen, fuel, and heat. When nitrous oxide/oxygen sedation is administered, we provide oxygen at a high concentration. Fuel is anything that can be caught on fire such as gauze, cotton rolls, facial hair, grease, petroleum jelly. In this case the source of heat was a spark from the bur. We will not be causing any sparks in the mouth while administering nitrous oxide/oxygen. Sparks can happen when adjusting or sectioning ceramic and metal crowns and bridges, not when drilling on tooth structure [7].
    - o Once a fire has started:
      - Smother the air supply (oxygen). Close patient's mouth or cover mouth with hand.
      - Turn off the oxygen.
      - Cool materials with copious amounts of water.
      - Remove the source of fuel (anything that can catch on fire such as gauze, throat pack, cotton rolls, hair, nasal hood, rubber dam, bib, headrest covers) [8].
    - o Minimizing risk: try to avoid adjusting or sectioning crown and bridges intraorally when administering nitrous sedation. If unavoidable, use copious amounts of water when drilling and use moist throat packs (fuel). If necessary, when drilling or adjusting crowns or sectioning bridges, do this before or after administering nitrous oxide/oxygen sedation to avoid any sparks. Avoid using electrosurgery and lasers with nitrous oxide/oxygen sedation (heat) [8].
- "I may be pregnant. Is this safe?"
  - Thank you for sharing this with me. Our goal is to provide you with care that is safe for you and your baby. Sounds like you may be in your first trimester. It is safer to provide nitrous in the second and third trimester than the first trimester, and for a maximum of 30 minutes. The risk comes with repeated and prolonged exposures. The FDA has not assigned a pregnancy

risk category, as these studies would be unethical. I have to consult with your prenatal care provider before offering you nitrous oxide sedation [4].

Patients' Queries

- "I am extremely anxious about this appointment today."
  - What makes you anxious about today's appointment? Something we can offer you is nitrous oxide/oxygen sedation, also known as "laughing gas." Have you ever had this administered to you?
- "Can I get laughing gas today?"
  - We do offer laughing gas at our office. Just a few questions before we start:
    - ○ Have you recently eaten a large meal?
    - ○ Are you wearing contact lenses?
    - ○ Have you taken any medications or drugs in the last 72 hours? If so specify.
    - ○ Do you have debilitating cardiac or cerebrovascular disease?
    - ○ Are you able to breathe through your nose today? Nasal obstruction or deviation?
    - ○ COPD?
    - ○ Pneumothorax?
    - ○ Any earaches or surgery?
    - ○ Pregnant? Which trimester?
    - ○ Neutropenia?
    - ○ Claustrophobic?
    - ○ In recovery from alcoholism?
    - ○ Does the feeling of loss of control worry you?
    - ○ For more, see Section Contraindications.
- "What is nitrous oxide and oxygen sedation?"
  - See Section Introduction.
- "What will I feel?"
  - Everyone responds differently, but most feel relaxed, warm and comfortable [1]. Your arms and legs may feel tingly, you may feel lighter, and noises may sound more distant.
- "Can I drive home after this?"
  - Yes, nitrous oxide is excreted quickly from the lungs (both a rapid onset and recovery) within two to three minutes. The effects of the nitrous oxide will have worn off by the time we remove your mask. We will make sure you feel alert and back to normal before you leave.
- "I took some valium before this."
  - Nitrous oxide/oxygen sedation is a very safe way of achieving minimal or light to moderate sedation. If you have taken sedative drugs, such as Valium, it has an additive effect leading to deeper sedation. It is difficult to predict and control how you will respond to the nitrous oxide/oxygen sedation. For this reason, we do not recommend using the nitrous oxide and oxygen sedation today (unless trained in oral conscious sedation). Also, since you took Valium, do you have someone you know that will be driving you home after this appointment?
- "How is this different from IV sedation or general anesthesia?" (Table 18.2)

Nitrous Oxide and Oxygen Sedation

Table 18.2 Forms of sedation.

Form of sedation	Description	Driver needed?	Requires fasting?
Nitrous oxide and oxygen sedation	Known as laughing gas, when used alone is a very safe way of achieving minimal or light moderate sedation. The patient is able to respond normally to tactile stimulation and verbal commands and maintain an airway. Ventilatory and cardiovascular functions are unaffected	No	No
Oral sedation	A form of minimal or moderate sedation in which a medication is prescribed with a calming effect to reduce anxiety	Yes	Yes
Oral conscious sedation	A combination of nitrous oxide/oxygen sedation and oral sedation. The patient requires a driver to and from the appointment	Yes	Yes
IV sedation	Also known as "twilight sedation," a form of drug-induced sedation administered intravenously. The patient may be minimally, moderately, or deeply sedated but will not lose consciousness. If deeply sedated the patient may require assistance in breathing [9]	Yes	Yes
General anesthesia	Drug-induced loss of consciousness; patients often require assistance in maintaining breathing [10]	Yes	Yes

Patient Comment

- "My kid is fine. He doesn't need that gas."
  - "Billy does seem fairly calm right now. But as soon as some unfamiliar noises and sensations occur, he may become anxious. We would like to help Billy to remain calm and have a good visit today. The nitrous oxide helps him relax. He'll be breathing more oxygen [50–100% oxygen while ambient air is 21% oxygen] than you and I are right now. We'll get the work done faster. Does this information help you with your decision about the air? Do you have any other concerns?" [11]

References

1 Bowen, D.M. (1991, revised 2005). Aiding in the administration of Nitrous Oxide–Oxygen analgesia. http://www.yumpu.com/en/document/read/11506943/aiding-in-the-administration-of-nitrous-oxide-oxygen- (accessed 11 February 2020).

2 American Academy of Pediatric Dentistry (2018). Use of nitrous oxide for pediatric dental patients. http://www.aapd.org/research/oral-health-policies--recommendations/use-of-nitrous-oxide-for-pediatric-dental-patients (accessed 11 February 2020).

3 Casamassimo, P.S., Fields, H.W., McTigue, D.J., and Nowak, A.J. (2013). *Pediatric Dentistry: Infancy through Adolescence*, 5e. St. Louis, MO: Elsevier.

4 Little, J.W., Falace, D.A., Miller, G.S., and Rhodus, N.L. (2013). *Little and Falace's Dental*

Management of the Medically Compromised Patient, 8e. St. Louis, MO: Elsevier Mosby.

5 Skouteris, C.A. (ed.) (2018). *Dental Management of the Pregnant Patient*. Hoboken, NJ: Wiley Blackwell.

6 O'Neil, M. (2015). *The ADA Practical Guide to Substance Use Disorders and Safe Prescribing*. Hoboken, NJ: Wiley Blackwell.

7 Dentistry Today (2020). Only you can prevent oral fires. http://www.dentistrytoday.com/news/todays-dental-news/item/5891-only-you-can-prevent-oral-fires (accessed 4 February 2020).

8 Weaver, J.M. (2012). Prevention of fire in the dental chair. *Anesth. Prog.* 59 (3): 105–106.

9 American Society of Anesthesiologists (2020). Types of anesthesia: IV/monitored sedation. https://www.asahq.org/whensecondscount/anesthesia-101/types-of-anesthesia/ivmonitored-sedation (accessed 11 February 2020).

10 American Society of Anesthesiologists (2019). Continuum of depth of sedation: definition of general anesthesia and levels of sedation/analgesia. https://www.asahq.org/standards-and-guidelines/continuum-of-depth-of-sedation-definition-of-general-anesthesia-and-levels-of-sedationanalgesia (accessed 11 February 2020).

11 Wright, R. (1997). *Tough Questions, Great Answers: Responding to Patient Concerns about Today's Dentistry*. Chicago: Quintessence Publishing.

Nitrous Oxide and Oxygen Sedation

Appendix A

International Association of Dental Traumatology Guidelines

Chapter Outline

- Fractures and Luxations of Permanent Teeth
- Avulsion of Permanent Teeth
- Injuries in the Primary Dentition

Fractures and Luxations of Permanent Teeth [1]

See Tables A.1–A.13. For more detailed information refer to the reference.

Clinical Dentistry Daily Reference Guide, First Edition. William A. Jacobson.
© 2022 John Wiley & Sons, Inc. Published 2022 by John Wiley & Sons, Inc.

Table A.1 Permanent teeth: treatment guidelines for enamel infractions.

Enamel infraction	Clinical findings	Imaging, radiographic assessment, and findings	Treatment	Follow-up	Favorable outcomes	Unfavorable outcomes

An incomplete fracture (crack or crazing) of the enamel, without loss of tooth structure	• No sensitivity to percussion or palpation
	• Evaluate the tooth for a possible associated luxation injury or root fracture, especially if tenderness is observed
	• Normal mobility
	• Pulp sensibility tests usually positive
		• No radiographic abnormalities
		• Recommended radiographs:
		  - One parallel periapical radiograph
		  - Additional radiographs are indicated if signs or symptoms of other potential injuries are present
			• In case of severe infractions, etching and sealing with bonding resin should be considered to prevent discoloration and bacterial contamination of the infractions.
			• Otherwise, no treatment is necessary
				• No follow-up is needed if it is certain that the tooth suffered an infraction injury only
				• If there is an associated injury such as a luxation injury, that injury-specific follow-up regimen prevails
					• Asymptomatic
					• Positive response to pulp sensibility testing
					• Continued root developments immature teeth
						• Symptomatic
						• Pulp necrosis and infection
						• Apical periodontitis
						• Lack of further root developments immature teeth

Table A.2 Permanent teeth: treatment guidelines for uncomplicated crown fractures involving enamel only.

Uncomplicated crown fracture (enamel-only fracture)	Clinical findings	Imaging, radiographic assessment, and findings	Treatment	Follow-up	Favorable outcomes	Unfavorable outcomes
  A coronal fracture involving enamel only, with loss of tooth structure	• Loss of enamel • No visible sign of exposed dentin • Evaluate the tooth for a possible associated luxation injury or root fracture, especially if tenderness is present • Normal mobility • Pulp sensibility tests usually positive	• Enamel loss is visible • Missing fragments should be accounted for: – If fragment is missing and there are soft tissue injuries, radiographs of the lip and/or cheek are indicated to search for tooth fragments and/or foreign materials • Recommended radiographs: – One parallel periapical radiograph – Additional radiographs are indicated if signs or symptoms of other potential injuries are present	• If the tooth fragment is available, it can be bonded back on to the tooth • Alternatively, depending on the extent and location of the fracture, the tooth edges can be smoothed, or a composite resin restoration placed	Clinical and radiographic evaluations are necessary: • after 6–8 weeks • after 1 year • If there is an associated luxation or root fracture, or the suspicion of an associated luxation injury the luxation follow-up regimen prevails and should be used. Longer follow ups will be needed	• Asymptomatic • Positive response to pulp sensibility testing • Good quality restoration • Continued root development in immature teeth	• Symptomatic • Pulp necrosis and infection • Apical periodontitis • Loss of restoration • Breakdown of the restoration • Lack of further root development in immature teeth

Table A.3 Permanent teeth: treatment guidelines for uncomplicated crown fractures involving enamel and dentin.

Uncomplicated crown fracture (enamel–dentin fracture)	Clinical findings	Imaging, radiographic assessment, and findings	Treatment	Follow-up	Favorable outcomes	Unfavorable outcomes
A fracture confined to enamel and dentin without pulp exposure	• Normal mobility • Pulp sensibility tests usually positive • No sensitivity to percussion or palpation • Evaluate the tooth for a possible associated luxation injury or root fracture, especially if tenderness is present	• Enamel–dentin loss is visible. • Missing fragments should be accounted for: – If fragment is missing and there are soft tissue injuries, radiographs of the lip and/or cheek are indicated to search for tooth fragments and/or foreign materials • Recommended radiographs: – One parallel periapical radiograph – Additional radiographs are indicated if signs or symptoms of other potential injuries are present	• If the tooth fragment is available and intact, it can be bonded back on to the tooth. The fragment should be rehydrated by soaking in water or saline for 20 min before bonding • Cover the exposed dentin with glass-ionomer or use a bonding agent and composite resin • If the exposed dentin is within 0.5 mm of the pulp (pink but no bleeding), place a calcium hydroxide lining and cover with a material such as glass-ionomer	Clinical and radiographic evaluations are necessary: • after 6–8 weeks • after 1 year • If there is an associated luxation, root fracture or the suspicion of an associated luxation injury, the luxation follow-up regimen prevails and should be used. Longer follow ups will be needed	• Asymptomatic • Positive response to pulp sensibility testing • Good quality restoration • Continued root development in immature teeth	• Symptomatic • Pulp necrosis and infection • Apical periodontitis. • Lack of further root development in immature teeth • Loss of restoration • Breakdown of the restoration

Table A.4 Permanent teeth: treatment guidelines for complicated crown fractures.

Complicated crown fracture (enamel–dentin fracture with pulp exposure)	Clinical findings	Imaging, radiographic assessment, and findings	Treatment	Follow-up	Favorable outcomes	Unfavorable outcomes

A fracture confined to enamel and dentin with pulp exposure	• Normal mobility
	• No sensitivity to percussion or palpation.
	• Evaluate the tooth for a possible associated luxation injury or root fracture, especially if tenderness is present
	• Exposed pulp is sensitive to stimuli (e.g, air, cold, sweets)
		• Enamel–dentin loss is visible
		• Missing fragments should be accounted for:
		  – If fragment is missing and there are soft tissue injuries, radiographs of the lip and/or cheek are indicated to search for tooth fragments and/or foreign debris
		• Recommended radiographs:
		  – One parallel periapical radiograph
		  – Additional radiographs are indicated if signs or symptoms of other potential injuries are present
			• In patients where teeth have immature roots and open apices, it is very important to preserve the pulp. Partial pulpotomy or pulp capping are recommended in order to promote further root development
			• Conservative pulp treatment (e.g., partial pulpotomy) is also the preferred treatment in teeth with completed root development
			• Non-setting calcium hydroxide or non-staining calcium silicate cements are suitable materials to be placed on the pulp wound
			• If a post is required for crown retention in a mature tooth with complete root formation, root canal treatment is the preferred treatment
			• If the tooth fragment is available, it can be bonded back on to the tooth after rehydration and the exposed pulp is treated
			• In the absence of an intact crown fragment for bonding, cover the exposed dentin with glass-ionomer or use a bonding agent and composite resin
				Clinical and radiographic evaluations are necessary:
				• after 6–8 weeks
				• after 3 months
				• after 6 months
				• after 1 year
				• If there is an associated luxation, root fracture or the suspicion of an associated luxation injury, the luxation follow-up regimen prevails and should be used. Longer follow ups will be needed
					• Asymptomatic
					• Positive response to pulp sensibility testing
					• Good quality restoration
					• Continued root development in immature teeth
						• Symptomatic
						• Discoloration
						• Pulp necrosis and infection
						• Apical periodontitis
						• Lack of further root development in immature teeth
						• Loss of restoration
						• Breakdown of the restoration

Table A.5 Permanent teeth: treatment guidelines for uncomplicated crown–root fractures.

Uncomplicated crown–root fracture (crown–root fracture without pulp exposure)	Clinical findings	Imaging, radiographic assessment, and findings	Treatment	Follow-up	Favorable outcomes	Unfavorable outcomes
A fracture involving enamel, dentin and cementum (Note: Crown–root fractures typically extend below the gingival margin)	• Pulp sensibility tests usually positive • Tender to percussion. • Coronal, or mesial or distal, fragment is usually present and mobile • The extent of the fracture (sub- or supra-alveolar) should be evaluated	• Apical extension of fracture usually not visible • Missing fragments should be accounted for: – If fragment is missing and there are soft tissue injuries, radiographs of the lip and/or cheek are indicated to search for tooth fragments or foreign debris • Recommended radiographs: – One parallel periapical radiograph – Two additional radiographs of the tooth taken with different vertical and/or horizontal angulations – Occlusal radiograph • CBCT can be considered for better visualization of the fracture path, its extent, and its relationship to the marginal bone; also, useful to evaluate the crown–root ratio and to help determine treatment options	• Until a treatment plan is finalized, temporary stabilization of the loose fragment to the adjacent tooth/teeth or to the non-mobile fragment should be attempted • If the pulp is not exposed, removal of the coronal or mobile fragment and subsequent restoration should be considered • Cover the exposed dentin with glass-ionomer or use a bonding agent and composite resin Future Treatment Options: • *The treatment plan is dependent, in part, on the patient's age and anticipated cooperation. Options include:* • Orthodontic extrusion of the apical or non-mobile fragment, followed by restoration (may also need periodontal re-contouring surgery after extrusion) • Surgical extrusion • Root canal treatment and restoration if the pulp becomes necrotic and infected • Root submergence • Intentional replantation with or without rotation of the root • Extraction • Autotransplantation	Clinical and radiographic evaluations are necessary: • after 1 week • after 6–8 weeks • after 3 months • after 6 months • after 1 year • then yearly for at least 5 years	• Asymptomatic • Positive response to pulp sensibility testing • Continued root development in immature teeth • Good quality restoration	• Symptomatic • Discoloration • Pulp necrosis and infection • Apical periodontitis • Lack of further root development in immature teeth • Loss of restoration • Breakdown of the restoration • Marginal bone loss and periodontal inflammation

Table A.6 Permanent teeth: treatment guidelines for complicated crown–root fractures.

Complicated crown–root fracture (crown–root fracture with pulp exposure)	Clinical findings	Imaging, radiographic assessment, and findings	Treatment	Follow-up	Favorable outcomes	Unfavorable outcomes
A fracture involving enamel, dentin, cementum and the pulp (Note: Crown–root fractures typically extend below the gingival margin)	• Pulp sensibility tests usually positive • Tender to percussion. • Coronal, or mesial or distal, fragment is usually present and mobile • The extent of the fracture (sub- or supra-alveolar) should be evaluated	• Apical extension of fracture usually not visible • Missing fragments should be accounted for: – If fragment is missing and there are soft tissue injuries, radiographs of the lip and/or cheek are indicated to search for tooth fragments or foreign debris • Recommended radiographs: – One parallel periapical radiograph – Two additional radiographs of the tooth taken with different vertical and/or horizontal angulations – Occlusal radiograph – CBCTcan be considered for better visualization of the fracture path, its extent, and its relationship to the marginal bone; also useful to evaluate the crown–root ratio and to help determine treatment options	• Until a treatment plan is finalized, temporary stabilization of the loose fragment to the adjacent tooth/teeth or to the non-mobile fragment should be attempted • *In immature teeth with incomplete root formation, it is advantageous to preserve the pulp by performing a partial pulpotomy. Options* include: – Non-setting calcium hydroxide or non-staining calcium silicate cements are suitable materials to be placed on the pulp wound • *In mature teeth with complete root formation,* removal of the pulp is usually indicated – Cover the exposed dentin with glass-ionomer or use a bonding agent and composite resin Future Treatment Options: • *The treatment plan is dependent, in part, on the patient's age and anticipated cooperation. Options include:* • Completion of root canal treatment and restoration • Orthodontic extrusion of the apical segment (may also need periodontal re-contouring surgery after extrusion) • Surgical extrusion • Root submergence • Intentional replantation with or without rotation of the root • Extraction • Autotransplantation	Clinical and radiographic evaluations are necessary: • after 1 week • after 6–8 weeks • after 3 months • after 6 moths • after 1 year • then yearly for at least 5 years	• Asymptomatic • Continued root development in immature teeth • Good quality restoration	• Symptomatic • Pulp necrosis and infection • Apical periodontitis • Lack of further root development in immature teeth • Loss of restoration • Breakdown of the restoration • Marginal bone loss and periodontal inflammation

In immature teeth with incomplete root formation, it is advantageous to preserve the pulp by performing a partial pulpotomy. Rubber dam isolation is challenging but should be tried.

Table A.7 Permanent teeth: treatment guidelines for root fractures.

Root fracture	Clinical findings	Imaging, radiographic assessment, and findings	Treatment	Follow-up	Favorable outcomes	Unfavorable outcomes

A fracture of the root involving dentin, pulp and cementum. The fracture may be horizontal, oblique or a combination of both.	• The coronal segment may be mobile and may be displaced
	• The tooth may be tender to percussion
	• Bleeding from the gingival sulcus may be seen
	• Pulp sensibility testing may be negative initially, indicating transient or permanent neural damage
		• The fracture may be located at any level of the root
		• Recommended radiographs:
		  – One parallel periapical radiograph
		  – Two additional radiographs of the tooth taken with different vertical and/or horizontal angulations
		  – Occlusal radiograph
		• Root fractures may be undetected without additional imaging
		• In cases where the above radiographs provide insufficient information for treatment planning, CBCT can be considered to determine the location, extent and direction of the fracture
			• If displaced, the coronal fragment should be repositioned as soon as possible.
			• Check repositioning radiographically
			• Stabilize the mobile coronal segment with a passive and flexible splint for 4 weeks. If the fracture is located cervically, stabilization for a longer period of time (up to 4 months) may be needed
			• Cervical fractures have the potential to heal. Thus, the coronal fragment, especially if not mobile, should not be removed at the emergency visit
			• No endodontic treatment should be started at the emergency visit
			• It is advisable to monitor healing of the fracture for at least one year. Pulp status should also be monitored
			• Pulp necrosis and infection may develop later. It usually occurs in the coronal fragment only. Hence, endodontic treatment of the coronal segment only will be indicated. As root fracture lines are frequently oblique, determination of root canal length may be challenging. An apexification approach may be needed. The apical segment rarely undergoes pathological changes that require treatment
			• In mature teeth where the cervical fracture line is located above the alveolar crest and the coronal fragment is very mobile, removal of the coronal fragment, followed by root canal treatment and restoration with a post-retained crown will likely be required. Additional procedures such as orthodontic extrusion of the apical segment, crown lengthening surgery, surgical extrusion or even extraction may be required as future treatment options (similar to those for crown–root fractures outlined above).
				Clinical and radiographic evaluations are necessary:
				• after 4 weeks S+
				• after 6-8 weeks
				• after 4 months S++
				• after 6 months
				• after 1 year
				• then yearly for at least 5 years
					• Positive response to pulp sensibility testing; however, a false negative response is possible for several months. Endodontic treatment should not be started solely on the basis of no response to pulp sensibility testing
					• Signs of repair between the fractured segments
					• Normal or slightly more than physiological mobility of the coronal fragment
						• Symptomatic
						• Extrusion and/or excessive mobility of the coronal segment
						• Radiolucency at the fracture line
						• Pulp necrosis and infection with inflammation in the fracture line

Note: S+, splint removal (for mid-root and apical third fractures); S++, splint removal (for cervical third fractures).

Table A.8 Permanent teeth: treatment guidelines for alveolar fractures.

Alveolar fracture	Clinical findings	Imaging, radiographic assessment, and findings	Treatment	Follow-Up	Favorable outcomes	Unfavorable outcomes

The fracture involves the alveolar bone and may extend to adjacent bones.	• The alveolar fracture is complete and extends all the way from the buccal to the palatal bone in the maxilla and from the buccal to the lingual bony surface in the mandible
	
	• Segment mobility and displacement with several teeth moving together are common findings
	
	• Occlusal disturbances due to displacement and misalignment of the fractured alveolar segment are often seen
	
	• Teeth in the fractured segment may not respond to pulp sensibility testing
		• Fracture lines may be located at any level, from the marginal bone to the root apex
		
		• Recommended radiographs:
		  – One parallel periapical radiograph
		  – Two additional radiographs of the tooth taken with different vertical and/or horizontal angulations
		  – Occlusal radiograph
		
		• In cases where the above radiographs provide insufficient information for treatment planning, a panoramic radiograph and/ or CBCT can be considered to determine the location, extent and direction of the fracture
			• Reposition any displaced segment
			
			• Stabilize the segment by splinting the teeth with a passive and flexible splint for4 weeks
			
			• Suture gingival lacerations if present
			
			• Root canal treatment is contraindicated at the emergency visit
			
			• Monitor the pulp condition of all teeth involved, both initially and at follow ups, to determine if or when endodontic treatment becomes necessary
				Clinical and radiographic evaluations are necessary:
				• after 4 weeks S$^+$
				• after 6-8 weeks
				• after 4 months
				• after 6 months
				• after 1 year
				• then yearly for at least 5 years
				
				Bone and soft tissue healing must also be monitored
					• Positive response to pulp sensibility testing (a false negative response is possible for several months)
					
					• No signs of pulp necrosis and infection
					
					• Soft tissue healing
					
					• Radiographic signs of bone repair
					
					Slight tenderness of the bone to palpation may remain at the fracture line and/or on mastication for several months
						• Symptomatic
						
						• Pulp necrosis and infection
						
						• Apical periodontitis
						
						• Inadequate soft tissue healing
						
						• Non-healing of the bone fracture
						
						• External inflammatory (infection-related) resorption

Note: S$^+$, splint removal.

Table A.9 Permanent teeth: treatment guidelines for concussion injuries of the teeth.

Concussion	Clinical findings	Imaging, radiographic assessment, and findings	Treatment	Follow-up	Favorable outcome	Unfavorable outcome
	• Normal mobility • The tooth is tender to percussion and touch • The tooth will likely respond to pulp sensibility testing	• No radiographic abnormalities • Recommended radiographs: – One parallel periapical radiograph – Additional radiographs are indicated if signs or symptoms of other potential injuries are present	• No treatment is needed. • Monitor pulp condition for at least one year, but preferably longer	Clinical and radiographic evaluations are necessary: • after 4 weeks • after 1 year	• Asymptomatic • Positive response to pulp sensibility testing; however, a false negative response is possible for several months. Endodontic treatment should not be started solely on the basis of no response to pulp sensibility testing • Continued root development in immature teeth • Intact lamina dura	• Symptomatic • Pulp necrosis and infection • Apical periodontitis • No further root development in immature teeth

Table A.10 Permanent teeth: treatment guidelines for subluxation injuries of teeth.

Subluxation	Clinical findings	Imaging, radiographic assessment, and findings	Treatment	Follow-up	Favorable Outcome	Unfavorable outcome
An injury to the tooth-supporting structures with abnormal loosening, but without displacement of the tooth	• The tooth is tender to touch or light tapping • Tooth has increased mobility but is not displaced • Bleeding from the gingival crevice may be present • The tooth may not respond to pulp sensibility testing initially indicating transient pulp damage	• Radiographic appearance is usually normal • Recommended radiographs: – One parallel periapical radiograph – Two additional radiographs of the tooth taken with different vertical and/or horizontal angulations – Occlusal radiograph	• Normally no treatment is needed • A passive and flexible splint to stabilize the tooth for up to 2 weeks may be used but only if there is excessive mobility or tenderness when biting on the tooth • Monitor the pulp condition for at least one year, but preferably longer	Clinical and radiographic evaluations are necessary: • after 2 weeks S$^+$ • after 12 weeks • after 6 months • after 1 year	• Asymptomatic • Positive response to pulp sensibility testing; however, a false negative response is possible for several months. Endodontic treatment should not be started solely on the basis of no response to pulp sensibility testing • Continued root development in immature teeth • Intact lamina dura	• Symptomatic • Pulp necrosis and infection • Apical periodontitis • No further root development in immature teeth • External inflammatory (infection-related) resorption – if this type of resorption develops, root canal treatment should be initiated immediately, with the use of calcium hydroxide as an intra-canal medicament. Alternatively, corticosteroid/antibiotic medicament can be used initially, which is then followed by calcium hydroxide

Note: S$^+$, splint removal.

Table A.11 Permanent teeth: treatment guidelines for extrusive luxation injuries of the teeth.

Extrusive luxation	Clinical findings	Imaging, radiographic assessment, and findings	Treatment	Follow-up	Favorable outcome	Unfavorable outcome

Displacement of the tooth out of its socket in an incisal/axial direction	• The tooth appears elongated
	• The tooth has increased mobility
	• The tooth will appear elongated incisally
	• Likely to have no response to pulp sensibility tests
		• Increased periodontal ligament space both apically and laterally
		• Tooth will not be seated in its socket and will appear elongated incisally
		• Recommended radiographs:
		  One parallel periapical radiograph
		  Two additional radiographs of the tooth taken with different vertical and/or horizontal angulations
		  Occlusal radiograph
			• Reposition the tooth by gently pushing It back into the tooth socket under local anesthesia
			• Stabilize the tooth for 2 weeks using a passive and flexible splint. If breakdown/fracture of the marginal bone, splint for an additional 4 weeks
			• Monitor the pulp condition with pulp sensibility tests
			• If the pulp becomes necrotic and infected, endodontic treatment appropriate to the tooth's stage of root development is indicated
				Clinical and radiographic evaluations are necessary:
				• after 2 weeks S$^+$
				• after 4 weeks
				• after 8 weeks
				• after 12 weeks
				• after 6 months
				• after 1 year
				• then yearly for at least 5 years
				• Patients (and parents, where relevant) should be informed to watch for any unfavorable outcomes and the need to return to clinic if they observe any
				• Where unfavorable outcomes are identified, treatment is often required. This is outside the scope of these guidelines. Referral to a dentist with the relevant expertise, training and experience is advised
					• Asymptomatic
					• Clinical and radiographic signs of normal or healed periodontium.
					• Positive response to pulp sensibility testing; however, a false negative response is possible for several months. Endodontic treatment should not be started solely on the basis of no response to pulp sensibility testing
					• No marginal bone loss
					• Continued root development in immature teeth
						• Symptomatic
						• Pulp necrosis and infection
						• Apical periodontitis
						• Breakdown of marginal bone
						• External inflammatory (infection-related) resorption – if this type of resorption develops, root canal treatment should be initiated immediately, with the use of calcium hydroxide as an intra-canal medicament. Alternatively, corticosteroid/antibiotic medicament can be used initially, which is then followed by calcium hydroxide

Note: S$^+$, splint removal.

Lateral luxation	Clinical findings	Imaging, radiographic assessment, and findings	Treatment	Follow-up	Favorable outcome	Unfavorable outcome
Displacement of the tooth in any lateral direction, usually associated with a fracture or compression of the alveolar socket wall or facial cortical bone	• The tooth is displaced, usually in a palatal/lingual or labial direction • There is usually an associated fracture of the alveolar bone • The tooth is frequently immobile as the apex of the root is "locked" in by the bone fracture • Percussion will give a high metallic (ankylotic) sound • Likely to have no response to pulp sensibility tests	• A widened periodontal ligament space which is best seen on radiographs taken with horizontal angle shifts or occlusal exposures • Recommended radiographs: – One parallel periapical radiograph – Two additional radiographs of the tooth taken with different vertical and/or horizontal angulations – Occlusal radiograph	• Reposition the tooth digitally by disengaging it from its locked position and gently reposition it into its original location under local anesthesia. – Method: Palpate the gingiva to feel the apex of the tooth. Use one finger to push downwards over the apical end of the tooth, then use another finger or thumb to push the tooth back into its socket • Stabilize the tooth for 4 weeks using a passive and flexible splint. If breakdown/fracture of the marginal bone or alveolar socket wall, additional splinting may be required • Monitor the pulp condition with pulp sensibility tests at the follow-up appointments • At about 2 weeks post-injury, make an endodontic evaluation: • Teeth with incomplete root formation: – Spontaneous revascularization may occur. If the pulp becomes necrotic and there are signs of inflammatory (infection-related) external root resorption, root canal treatment should be started as soon as possible. – Endodontic procedures suitable for immature teeth should be used • Teeth with complete root formation: – The pulp will likely become necrotic. Root canal treatment should be started, using a corticosteroid/antibiotic or calcium hydroxide as an intra-canal medicament to prevent the development of inflammatory (infection-related) external resorption	Clinical and radiographic evaluations are necessary: • after 2 weeks • after 4 weeks S+ • after 8 weeks • after 12 weeks • after 6 months • after 1 year • then yearly for at least 5 years • Patients (and parents, where relevant) should be informed to watch for any unfavorable outcomes and the need to return to clinic if they observe any • Where unfavorable outcomes are identified, treatment is often required. This is outside the scope of these guidelines. Referral to a dentist with the relevant expertise, training and experience is advised	• Asymptomatic • Clinical and radiographic signs of normal or healed periodontium • Positive response to pulp sensibility testing; however, a false negative response is possible for several months. Endodontic treatment should not be started solely on the basis of no response to pulp sensibility testing • Marginal bone height corresponds to that seen radiographically after repositioning • Continued root developments immature teeth	• Symptomatic • Breakdown of marginal bone • Pulp necrosis and infection • Apical periodontitis • Ankylosis • External replacement resorption • External inflammatory (infection-related) resorption • External inflammatory (infection-related) resorption – if this type of resorption develops, root canal treatment should be initiated immediately, with the use of calcium hydroxide as an intra-canal medicament. Alternatively, corticosteroid/antibiotic medicament can be used initially, which is then followed by calcium hydroxide

Note: S+, splint removal.

Table A.13 Permanent teeth: treatment guidelines for intrusive luxation injuries of the teeth.

Intrusive luxation	Clinical findings	Imaging, radiographic assessment, and findings	Treatment	Follow-up	Favorable outcome	Unfavorable

Displacement of the tooth in an apical direction into the alveolar bone	• The tooth is displaced axially into the alveolar bone
	• The tooth is immobile
	• Percussion will give a high metallic (ankylotic) sound
	• Likely to have no response to pulp sensibility tests
		• The periodontal ligament space may not be visible for all or part of the root (especially apically)
		• The cemento-enamel junction is located more apically in the intruded tooth than in adjacent non-injured teeth
		• Recommended radiographs:
		  – One parallel periapical radiograph
		  – Two additional radiographs of the tooth taken with different vertical and/or horizontal angulations
		  Occlusal radiograph
			Teeth with incomplete root formation (immature teeth):
			• Allow re-eruption without intervention (spontaneous repositioning) for all intruded teeth independent of the degree of intrusion
			• If no re-eruption within 4 weeks, initiate orthodontic repositioning
			• Monitor the pulp condition
			• In teeth with incomplete root formation spontaneous pulp revascularization may occur. However, if it is noted that the pulp becomes necrotic and infected or that there are signs of inflammatory (infection-related) external resorption at follow-up appointments, root canal treatment is indicated and should be started as soon as possible when the position of the tooth allows. Endodontic procedures suitable for immature teeth should be used.
			• Parents must be informed about the necessity of follow-up visits
			Teeth with complete root formation (mature teeth):
			• Allow re-eruption without intervention if the tooth is intruded less than 3 mm. If no re-eruption within 8 weeks, reposition surgically and splint for 4 weeks with a passive and flexible splint Alternatively, reposition orthodontically before ankylosis develops
			• If the tooth is intruded 3–7 mm, reposition surgically (preferably) or orthodontically
			• If the tooth is intruded beyond 7mm, reposition surgically
			• In teeth with complete root formation, the pulp almost always becomes necrotic. Root canal treatment should be started at 2 weeks or as soon as the position of the tooth allows, using a corticosteroid/antibiotic or calcium hydroxide as an intra-canal medication. The purpose of this treatment is to prevent the development of inflammatory (infection-related) external resorption
				Clinical and radiographic evaluations are necessary:
				• after 2 weeks
				• after 4 weeks S⁺
				• after 8 weeks
				• after 12 weeks
				• after 6 months
				• after 1 year
				• then yearly for at least 5 years
				• Patients (and parents, where relevant) should be informed to watch for any unfavorable outcomes and the need to return to clinic if they observe any
				• Where unfavorable outcomes are identified, treatment is often required. This is outside the scope of these guidelines. Referral to a dentist with the relevant expertise, training and experience is advised
					• Asymptomatic
					• Tooth in place or is re-erupting
					• Intact lamina dura
					• Positive response to pulp sensibility testing; however, a false negative response is possible for several months. Endodontic treatment should not be started solely on the basis of no response to pulp sensibility testing
					• No signs of root resorption
					• Continued root development in immature teeth
						• Symptomatic
						• Tooth locked in place/ ankylotic tone to percussion
						• Pulp necrosis and infection
						• Apical periodontitis
						• Ankylosis
						• External replacement resorption
						• External inflammatory (infection-related) resorption – if this type of resorption develops, root canal treatment should be initiated immediately, with the use of calcium hydroxide as an intra-canal medicament. Alternatively, corticosteroid/antibiotic medicament can be used initially, which is then followed by calcium hydroxide

Note: S⁺, splint removal.

Avulsion of Permanent Teeth (Adapted from Fouad et al. [2])

- **General points for the patient**
  - Verify the tooth is a permanent tooth (primary teeth should not be replanted).
  - Pick up the tooth by the crown (avoid touching the root).
  - If the tooth is dirty, rinse with milk, saline, or the patient's saliva.
  - Place it back immediately into the socket.
  - The patient should bite on gauze, handkerchief or napkin to hold it in place.
  - If unable to replant the tooth, place the tooth in a storage medium within a few minutes. Storage mediums, in descending order of preference, include milk, Hanks' balanced salt solution (HBSS), saliva, saline, and water.
  - See the dentist immediately.
- **Tooth has been replanted immediately** (or within a very short time, about 15 minutes, at the place of the accident)
  - Clean the area with water, saline, or chlorhexidine.
  - Verify the correct position of the replanted tooth both clinically and radiographically.
  - Leave the tooth in the jaw (except where the tooth is malpositioned, in which case it needs to be corrected using slight digital pressure).
  - Administer local anesthesia, if necessary, and preferably with no vasoconstrictor.
  - If the tooth or teeth were replanted in the wrong socket or rotated, consider repositioning the tooth/teeth into the proper location for up to 48 hours after the trauma.
  - Stabilize the tooth for two weeks using a passive flexible wire of a diameter up to 0.016 inch (0.4 mm). Short immature teeth may require a longer splinting time. Keep the composite away from the gingival tissues and proximal areas. Alternatively, nylon fishing line (0.13–0.25 mm) can be used to create a flexible splint, using composite to bond it to teeth. In cases of associated alveolar or jawbone fracture, a more rigid splint is indicated and should be left in place for four weeks.
  - Suture gingival lacerations, if present.
- **Tooth has been kept in a storage medium (total extraoral dry time <60 minutes *or* total extraoral dry time >60 minutes regardless of tooth having been stored in a medium or not)**
  - If there is visible contamination, rinse the root surface with a stream of saline or osmolality-balanced media to remove gross debris.
  - Place or leave the tooth in a storage medium while taking a history, examining the patient clinically and radiographically, and preparing the patient for replantation.
  - Administer local anesthesia, if necessary, and preferably with no vasoconstrictor.
  - Irrigate the socket with sterile saline. Examine the alveolar socket; if there is a fracture of the socket wall, reposition the fractured fragment into its original position with a suitable instrument. Remove the coagulum with a saline stream.
  - Replant the tooth slowly with slight digital pressure (avoid excessive force).
  - Verify the correct position of the replanted tooth both clinically and radiographically.
  - Stabilize the tooth for two weeks using a passive flexible wire of a diameter up to 0.016 inch (0.4 mm). Short immature teeth may require a longer splinting time. Keep the composite away from the gingival tissues and proximal areas. Alternatively, nylon fishing line (0.13–0.25 mm) can be used to create a flexible splint, using composite to bond it to teeth. In cases of associated alveolar or jawbone fracture, a more rigid splint is indicated and should be left in place for four weeks.
  - Suture gingival lacerations, if present.

- **Endodontic treatment**
  - Teeth with a closed apex:
    - Initiate root canal treatment within two weeks after replantation. (Place rubber dam clamp on neighboring teeth to avoid further trauma.)
    - Administer systemic antibiotics.
    - Check tetanus status (refer patient to physician to evaluate need for tetanus booster).
  - Teeth with an open apex:
    - Revascularization of the pulp space, which can lead to further root development, is the goal. Risk of external infection-related root resorption should be weighed against the chances of revascularization. Such resorption is very rapid in children. If spontaneous revascularization does not occur, apexification, pulp revitalization/revascularization, or root canal treatment should be initiated as soon as pulp necrosis and infection is identified.
    - Administer systemic antibiotics.
    - Check tetanus status (refer patient to physician to evaluate need for tetanus booster).
- **Provide postoperative instructions**
  - Avoid participation in contact sports.
  - Maintain a soft diet for up to two weeks.
  - Brush teeth with soft toothbrush after each meal.
  - Use chlorhexidine (0.12%) mouthrinse twice a day for two weeks.
- **Clinical and radiographic follow-up**
  - Teeth with a closed apex:
    - Two weeks (when splint is removed)
    - Four weeks
    - Three months
    - Six months
    - One year
    - Yearly for at least five years.
  - Teeth with an open apex:
    - Two weeks (when splint is removed)
    - One month
    - Two months
    - Three months
    - Six months
    - One year
    - Yearly for at least five years.

Injuries in the Primary Dentition [3]

See Tables A.14–A.25. For more detailed information refer to the reference.

Table A.14 Treatment guidelines for primary teeth: enamel fractures.

Enamel fracture	Radiographic recommendations	Treatment	Follow-up	Favorable and unfavorable outcomes include some, but not necessarily all, of the following	
				Favorable outcomes	**Unfavorable outcomes**
Clinical findings: Fracture involves enamel only	• No radiographs recommended	• Smooth any sharp edges. • Parent/patient education: Exercise care when eating not to further traumatize the injured tooth while encouraging a return to normal function as soon as possible. Encourage gingival healing and prevent plaque accumulation by parents cleaning the affected area with a soft brush or cotton swab combined with an alcohol-free 0.1 to 0.2% chlorhexidine gluconate mouth rinse applied topically twice a day for 1 week	• No clinical or radiographic follow-up recommended	• Asymptomatic • Pulp healing with: – Normal color of the remaining crown No signs of pulp necrosis and infection Continued root development in immature teeth	• Symptomatic • Crown discoloration • Signs of pulp necrosis and infection, such as: Sinus tract, gingival swelling, abscess, or increased mobility Persistent dark gray discoloration with one or more other signs of infection Radiographic signs of pulp necrosis and infection • No further root development of immature teeth

Table A.15 Treatment guidelines for primary teeth: enamel–dentin fractures (with no pulp exposure).

Enamel–dentin fracture (with no pulp exposure)	Radiographic recommendations	Treatment	Follow-up	Favorable and unfavorable outcomes include some, but not necessarily all, of the following	
				Favorable outcome	Unfavorable outcome
Clinical findings: Fracture involves enamel and dentin. The pulp is not exposed • The location of missing tooth fragments should be explored during the trauma history and examination, especially when the accident was not witnessed by an adult or there was a loss of consciousness • Note: While fragments are most often lost out of the mouth, there is a risk that they can be embedded in the soft tissues, ingested, or aspirated	• Baseline radiograph optional • Take a radiograph of the soft tissues if the fractured fragment is suspected to be embedded in the lips, cheeks, or tongue	• Cover all exposed dentin with glass ionomer or composite • Lost tooth structure can be restored using composite immediately or at a later appointment • Parent/patient education: – Exercise care when eating not to further traumatize the injured tooth while encouraging a return to normal function as soon as possible – Encourage gingival healing and prevent plaque accumulation by parents cleaning the affected area with a soft brush or cotton swab combined with an alcohol-free 0.1–0.2% chlorhexidine gluconate mouth rinse applied topically twice a day for 1 week	• Clinical examination after 6–8 weeks • Radiographic follow-up indicated only when clinical findings are suggestive of pathosis (e.g., signs of pulp necrosis and infection) • Parents should watch for any unfavorable outcomes. If seen, the child needs to return to the clinic as soon as possible. When unfavorable outcomes are identified, treatment is often required • The follow-up treatment, which frequently requires the expertise of a child-oriented team, is outside the scope of these guidelines	• Asymptomatic • Pulp healing with: – Normal color of the remaining crown – No signs of pulp necrosis and infection – Continued root development in immature teeth	• Symptomatic • Crown discoloration • Signs of pulp necrosis and infection, such as: – Sinus tract, gingival swelling, abscess, or increased mobility – Persistent dark gray discoloration with one or more other signs of root canal infection – Radiographic signs of pulp necrosis and infection • No further root development of immature teeth

Table A.16 Treatment guidelines for primary teeth: complicated crown fractures (with pulp exposure).

Complicated crown fracture (i.e., with exposed pulp)	Radiographic recommendations	Treatment	Follow-up	Favorable and unfavorable outcomes include some, but not necessarily all, of the following	
				Favorable outcome	**Unfavorable outcome**

Clinical findings: Fracture involves enamel and dentin plus the pulp is exposed.

- The location of missing tooth fragments should be explored during the trauma history and examination, especially when the accident was not witnessed by an adult or there was a loss of consciousness

- Note: While fragments are most often lost out of the mouth, there is a risk that they can be embedded in the soft tissues, ingested, or aspirated

Radiographic recommendations

- A periapical radiograph (using a size 0 sensor/film and the paralleling technique) or an occlusal radiograph (with a size 2 sensor/film) should be taken at the time of initial presentation for diagnostic purposes and to establish a baseline

- Take a radiograph of the soft tissues if the fractured fragment is suspected to be embedded in the lips, cheeks, or tongue

Treatment

- Preserve the pulp by partial pulpotomy. Local anesthesia will be required. A non-setting calcium hydroxide paste should be applied over the pulp and cover this with a glass ionomer cement and then a composite resin. Cervical pulpotomy is indicated for teeth with large pulp exposures. The evidence for using other biomaterials such as nonstaining calcium silicate-based cements is emerging. Clinicians should focus on appropriate case selection rather than the material used

- Treatment depends on the child's maturity and ability to tolerate procedures. Therefore, discuss different treatment options (including pulpotomy) with the parents. Each option is invasive and has the potential to cause longterm dental anxiety. Treatment is best performed by a child-oriented team with experience and expertise in the management of pediatric dental injuries. Often no treatment may be the most appropriate option in the emergency situation, but only when there is the potential for rapid referral (within several days) to the child-oriented team

- Parent/patient education:
  - Exercise care when eating not to further traumatize the injured tooth while encouraging a return to normal function as soon as possible.
  - To encourage gingival healing and prevent plaque accumulation, parents should clean the affected area with a soft brush or cotton swab combined with an alcohol-free 0.1–0.2% chlorhexidine gluconate mouth rinse applied topically twice a day for 1 week

Follow-up

- Clinical examination after:
  - 1 week
  - 6–8 weeks
  - 1 year

- Radiographic follow-up at 1 year following pulpotomy or root canal treatment. Other radiographs are only indicated where clinical findings are suggestive of pathosis (e.g., an unfavorable outcome)

- Parents should watch for any unfavorable outcomes. If seen, the child needs to return to the clinic as soon as possible. Where unfavorable outcomes are identified, treatment is often required.

- The follow-up treatment, which frequently requires the expertise of a childoriented team, is outside the scope of these guidelines

Favorable outcome

- Asymptomatic
- Pulp healing with:
  - Normal color of the remaining crown
  - No signs of pulp necrosis and infection
  - Continued root development in immature teeth

Unfavorable outcome

- Symptomatic
- Crown discoloration
- Signs of pulp necrosis and infection, such as:
  - Sinus tract, gingival swelling, abscess, or increased mobility
  - Persistent dark gray discoloration with one or more signs of root canal infection
  - Radiographic signs of pulp necrosis and infection
- No further root development of immature teeth

Table A.17 Treatment guidelines for primary teeth: crown–root fractures.

Crown-root fracture	Radiographic recommendations	Treatment	Follow-up	Favorable and unfavorable outcomes include some, but not necessarily all, of the following	
				Favorable outcome	**Unfavorable outcome**

Clinical findings: Fracture involves enamel, dentin, and root; the pulp may or may not be exposed (i.e., complicated or uncomplicated)
 	
• Additional findings may include loose, but still attached, fragments of tooth
	• A periapical radiograph (using a size 0 sensor/film and the paralleling technique) or an occlusal radiograph (with a size 2 sensor/film) should be taken at the time of initial presentation for diagnostic purposes and to establish a baseline	• Often no treatment may be the most appropriate option in the emergency situation, but only when there is the potential for rapid referral (within several days) to a child-oriented team
		• If treatment is considered at the emergency appointment, local anesthesia will be required
		• Remove the loose fragment and determine if the crown can be restored
		• Option A:
		  – If restorable and no pulp exposed, cover the exposed dentin with glass ionomer
		  – If restorable and the pulp is exposed, perform a pulpotomy (see crown fracture with exposed pulp) or root canal treatment, depending on the stage of root development and the level of the fracture.
		• Option B:
		  – If unrestorable, extract all loose fragments taking care not to damage the permanent successor tooth and leave any firm root fragment in situ, or extract the entire tooth
		• Treatment depends on the child's maturity and ability to tolerate the procedure. Therefore, discuss treatment options (including extraction) with the parents. Each option is invasive and has the potential to cause long-term dental anxiety. Treatment is best performed by a child-oriented team with experience and expertise in the management of pediatric dental injuries
		• Parent/patient education:
		  – Exercise care when eating not to further traumatize the injured tooth while encouraging a return to normal function as soon as possible
		  – To encourage gingival healing and prevent plaque accumulation, parents should clean the affected area with an soft brush or cotton swab combined with an alcohol-free 0.1–0.2% chlorhexidine gluconate mouth rinse applied topically twice a day for 1 week
			• Where tooth is retained, clinical examination after:
			  – 1 week
			  – 6–8 weeks
			  – 1 year
			• Radiographic follow-up after 1 year following pulpotomy or root canal treatment. Other radiographs only indicated where clinical findings are suggestive of pathosis (e.g., an unfavorable outcome)
			• Parents should watch for any unfavorable outcomes. If seen, the child needs to return to the clinic as soon as possible. Where unfavorable outcomes are identified, treatment is often required
			• The follow-up treatment, which frequently requires the expertise of a child-oriented team, is outside the scope of these guidelines
				• Asymptomatic
				• Pulp healing with:
				  – Normal color of the remaining crown
				• No signs of pulp necrosis and infection
				• Continued root development in immature teeth
					• Symptomatic
					• Crown discoloration
					• Signs of pulp necrosis and infection, such as:
					  – Sinus tract, gingival swelling, abscess, or increased mobility
					  – Persistent dark gray discoloration with one or more signs of root canal infection
					• Radiographic signs of pulp necrosis and infection
					• No further root development of immature teeth

Table A.18 Treatment guidelines for primary teeth: root fractures.

Root fracture	Radiographic recommendations and findings	Treatment	Follow-up	Favorable and unfavorable outcomes include some, but not necessarily all, of the following	
				Favorable outcome	Unfavorable outcome
Clinical findings: Depends on the location of fracture • The coronal fragment may be mobile and may be displaced • Occlusal interference may be present	• A periapical (size 0 sensor/film, paralleling technique) or occlusal radiograph (size 2 sensor/film) should be taken at the time of initial presentation for diagnostic purposes and to establish a baseline • The fracture is usually located mid-root or in the apical third	• If the coronal fragment is not displaced, no treatment is required • If the coronal fragment is displaced and is not excessively mobile, leave the coronal fragment to spontaneously reposition even if there is some occlusal interference • If the coronal fragment is displaced, excessively mobile and interfering with occlusion, two options are available, both of which require local anesthesia • **Option A:** Extract only the loose coronal fragment. The apical fragment should be left in place to be resorbed • **Option B:** Gently reposition the loose coronal fragment. If the fragment is unstable in its new position, stabilize the fragment with a flexible splint attached to the adjacent uninjured teeth. Leave the splint in place for 4 weeks • The treatment depends on the child's maturity and ability to tolerate the procedure. Therefore, discuss treatment options with the parents. Each option is invasive and has the potential to cause long-term dental anxiety. Treatment is best performed by a child-oriented team with experience and expertise in the management of pediatric dental injuries. Often no treatment may be the most appropriate option in the emergency scenario, but only when there is the potential for rapid referral (within several days) to the child-oriented team • Parent/patient education: - Exercise care when eating not to further traumatize the injured tooth while encouraging a return to normal function as soon as possible - To encourage gingival healing and prevent plaque accumulation, parents should clean the affected area with a soft brush or cotton swab combined with an alcohol-free 0.1–0.2% chlorhexidine gluconate mouth rinse applied topically twice a day for 1 week	• Where no displacement of coronal fragment, clinical examination after: - 1 week - 6–8 weeks - 1 year and where there are clinical concerns that an unfavorable outcome is likely. - Then continue clinical follow-up each year until eruption of permanent teeth • If coronal fragment has been repositioned and splinted, clinical examination after: - 1 week - 4 weeks for splint removal - 8 weeks - 1 year • If coronal fragment has been extracted, clinical examination after 1 year • Where there are concerns that an unfavorable outcome is likely, then continue clinical follow-up each year until eruption of permanent teeth • Radiographic follow-up only indicated where clinical findings are suggestive of pathosis (e.g., an unfavorable outcome) • Parents should be informed to watch for any unfavorable outcomes and the need to return to the clinic as soon as possible. Where unfavorable outcomes are identified, treatment is often required. The follow-up treatment, which frequently requires the expertise of a child-oriented team, is outside the scope of these guidelines	• Asymptomatic • Pulp healing with: - Normal color of the crown or transient red/gray or yellow discoloration and pulp canal obliteration - No signs of pulp necrosis and infection - Continued root development in immature teeth • Realignment of the root-fractured tooth • No mobility • Resorption of the apical fragment	• Symptomatic • Signs of pulp necrosis and infection, such as: - Sinus tract, gingival swelling, abscess, or increased mobility - Persistent dark gray discoloration with one or more signs of root canal infection - Radiographic signs of pulp necrosis and infection - Radiographic signs of infection-related (inflammatory) resorption • No further root development of immature teeth • No improvement in the position of the root-fractured tooth

Table A.19 Treatment guidelines for primary teeth: alveolar fractures.

Alveolar fracture	Radiographic recommendations and findings	Treatment	Follow-up	Favorable and unfavorable outcomes include some, but not necessarily all, of the following	
				Favorable outcome	Unfavorable outcome
Clinical findings: The fracture involves the alveolar bone (labial and palatal/lingual) and may extend to the adjacent bone • Mobility and dislocation of the segment with several teeth moving together are common findings • Occlusal interference is usually present	• A periapical (size 0 sensor/film, paralleling technique) or occlusal radiograph (size 2 sensor/film) should be taken at the time of initial presentation for diagnostic purposes and to establish a baseline • A lateral radiograph may give information about the relationship between the maxillary and mandibular dentitions and if the segment is displaced in a labial direction • Fracture lines may be located at any level, from the marginal bone to the root apex or beyond, and they may involve the primary teeth and/or their permanent successors • Further imaging may be needed to visualize the extent of the fracture(s) but only where it is likely to change the treatment provided.	• Reposition (under local anesthesia) any displaced segment which is mobile and/or causing occlusal interference • Stabilize with a flexible splint to the adjacent uninjured teeth for 4 weeks • Treatment should be performed by a child-oriented team with experience and expertise in the management of pediatric dental injuries • Parent/patient education: – Exercise care when eating not to further traumatize the injured teeth while encouraging a return to normal function as soon as possible – To encourage gingival healing and prevent plaque accumulation, parents should clean the affected area with a soft brush or cotton swab combined with an alcohol-free 0.1–0.2% chlorhexidine gluconate mouth rinse applied topically twice a day for 1 week	• Clinical examination after: – 1 week – 4 weeks for splint removal – 8 weeks – 1 year – Further follow-up at 6 years of age is indicated to monitor eruption of the permanent teeth • Radiographic follow-up at 4 weeks and 1 year to assess impact on the primary tooth and the permanent tooth germs in the line of the alveolar fracture. This radiograph may indicate a more frequent follow-up regimen is needed. Other radiographs are indicated only where clinical findings are suggestive of pathosis (e.g., an unfavorable outcome) • If the fracture line is located at the level of the primary root apex, an abscess can develop. A periapical radiolucency can be seen on the radiograph • Parents should be informed to watch for any unfavorable outcomes and the need to return to the clinic as soon as possible. Where unfavorable outcomes are identified, treatment is often required • The follow-up treatment, which frequently requires the expertise of a child-oriented team, is outside the scope of these guidelines	• Asymptomatic • Pulp healing with: – Normal crown color or transient red/gray or yellow discoloration and pulp canal obliteration – No signs of pulp necrosis and infection – Continued root development in immature teeth • Periodontal healing • Realignment of the alveolar segment with the original occlusion restored • No disturbance to the development and/or eruption of the permanent successor	• Symptomatic • Signs of pulp necrosis and infection, such as: – Sinus tract, gingival swelling, abscess, or increased mobility – Persistent dark gray discoloration plus one or more signs of root canal infection – Radiographic signs of pulp necrosis and infection including infection-related (inflammatory) resorption • No further root development in immature teeth • Limited or no improvement in the position of the displaced segment and the original occlusion is not re-established • Negative impact on the development and/or eruption of the permanent successor

Table A.20 Treatment guidelines for primary teeth: concussion.

Concussion	Radiographic recommendations	Treatment	Follow-up	Favorable and unfavorable outcomes include some, but not necessarily all, of the following	
				Favorable outcome	Unfavorable outcome
Clinical findings: The tooth is tender to touch but it has not been displaced • It has normal mobility and no sulcular bleeding	• No baseline radiograph recommended	• No treatment is needed. • Observation • Parent/patient education: – Exercise care when eating not to further traumatize the injured tooth while encouraging a return to normal function as soon as possible – To encourage gingival healing and prevent plaque accumulation, parents should clean the affected area with a soft brush or cotton swab combined with an alcoholfree 0.1–0.2% mouth rinse chlorhexidine gluconate applied topically twice a day for 1 week	• Clinical examination after: – 1 week – 6–8 weeks • Radiographic follow-up only indicated where clinical findings are suggestive of pathosis (eg, an unfavorable outcome) • Parents should be informed to watch for any unfavorable outcomes and the need to return to the clinic as soon as possible. Where unfavorable outcomes are identified, treatment is often required • The follow-up treatment, which frequently requires the expertise of a child-oriented team, is outside the scope of these guidelines	• Asymptomatic • Pulp healing with: – Normal color of the crown or transient red/gray or yellow discoloration and pulp canal obliteration – No signs of pulp necrosis and infection • Continued root development in immature teeth • No disturbance to the development and/or eruption of the permanent successor	• Symptomatic • Signs of pulp necrosis and infection, such as: – Sinus tract, gingival swelling, abscess, or increased mobility – Persistent dark gray discoloration plus one or more other signs of root canal infection • Radiographic signs of pulp necrosis and infection • No further root development of immature teeth • Negative impact on the development and/or eruption of the permanent successor

Table A.21 Treatment guidelines for primary teeth: subluxation.

Subluxation	Radiographic recommendations and findings	Treatment	Follow-up	Favorable and unfavorable outcomes include some, but not necessarily all, of the following	
				Favorable outcome	Unfavorable outcome
Clinical findings: The tooth is tender to touch and it has increased mobility, but it has not been displaced • Bleeding from gingival crevice may be noted	• A periapical (size 0 sensor/ film, paralleling technique) or occlusal radiograph (size 2 sensor/film) should be taken at the time of initial presentation for diagnostic purposes and to establish a baseline • Normal to slightly widened periodontal ligament space will be visible	• No treatment is needed. • Observation • Parent/patient education: – Exercise care when eating not to further traumatize the injured teeth while encouraging a return to normal function as soon as possible – To encourage gingival healing. Parents should clean the affected area with a soft brush or cotton swab combined with an alcoholfree 0.1%–0.2% chlorhexidine gluconate mouth rinse applied topically twice a day for 1 week	• Clinical examination after: – 1 week – 6–8 weeks • Where there are concerns that an unfavorable outcome is likely, then continue clinical follow up each year until eruption of the permanent teeth • Radiographic follow-up only indicated where clinical findings are suggestive of pathosis (e.g., an unfavorable outcome) • Parents should be informed to watch for any unfavorable outcomes and the need to return to the clinic as soon as possible. Where unfavorable outcomes are identified, treatment is often required • The follow-up treatment, which frequently requires the expertise of a child-oriented team, is outside the scope of these guidelines	• Asymptomatic • Pulp healing with: – Normal color of the crown or transient red/gray or yellow discoloration and pulp canal obliteration – No signs of pulp necrosis and infection • Continued root development in immature teeth • No disturbance to the development and/or eruption of the permanent successor	• Symptomatic • Signs of pulp necrosis and infection, such as: – Sinus tract, gingival swelling, abscess, or increased mobility – Persistent dark gray discoloration plus one or more signs of root canal infection • Radiographic signs of pulp necrosis and infection • No further root development of immature teeth • Negative impact on the development and/or eruption of the permanent successor

Table A.22 Treatment guidelines for primary teeth: extrusive luxation.

Extrusive luxation	Radiographic recommendations and findings	Treatment	Follow-up	Favorable and unfavorable outcomes include some, but not necessarily all, of the following:	
				Favorable outcome	Unfavorable outcome
Clinical findings: Partial displacement of the tooth out of its socket • The tooth appears elongated and can be excessively mobile. • Occlusal interference may be present	• A periapical (size 0 sensor/film, paralleling technique) or occlusal radiograph (size 2 sensor/film) should be taken at the time of initial presentation for diagnostic purposes and to establish a baseline • Slight increase to substantially widened periodontal ligament space apically	• Treatment decisions are based on the degree of displacement, mobility, interference with the occlusion, root formation, and the ability of the child to tolerate the emergency situation • If the tooth is not interfering with the occlusion—let the tooth spontaneously reposition itself • If the tooth is excessively mobile or extruded > 3 mm, then extract under local anesthesia • Treatment should be performed by a child-oriented team with experience and expertise in the management of pediatric dental injuries. Extractions have the potential to cause long-term dental anxiety • Parent/patient education: • Exercise care when eating not to further traumatize the injured tooth while encouraging a return to normal function as soon as possible. • To encourage gingival healing and prevent plaque accumulation, parents should clean the affected area with a soft brush or cotton swab combined with an alcohol-free 0.1–0.2% chlorhexidine gluconate mouth rinse applied topically twice a day for 1 week	• Clinical examination after: • 1 week • 6–8 weeks • 1 year • Where there are concerns that an unfavorable outcome is likely, then continue clinical follow-up each year until eruption of the permanent teeth • Radiographic follow-up only indicated where clinical findings are suggestive of pathosis (eg, an unfavorable outcome) • Parents should be informed to watch for any unfavorable outcomes and the need to return to the clinic as soon as possible. Where unfavorable outcomes are identified, treatment is often required • The follow-up treatment, which frequently requires the expertise of a child-oriented team, is outside the scope of these guidelines	• Asymptomatic • Pulp healing with: • Normal color of the crown or transient red/gray or yellow discoloration and pulp canal obliteration • No signs of pulp necrosis and infection • Continued root development in immature teeth • Realignment of the extruded tooth • No interference with the occlusion • No disturbance to the development and/or eruption of the permanent successor	• Symptomatic • Signs of pulp necrosis and infection, such as: • Sinus tract, gingival swelling, abscess, or increased mobility • Persistent dark gray discoloration plus one or more signs of root canal infection • Radiographic signs of pulp necrosis and infection • No further root development of immature teeth • No improvement in the position of the extruded tooth • Negative impact on the development and/or eruption of the permanent successor

Table A.23 Treatment guidelines for primary teeth: lateral luxation.

Lateral luxation	Radiographic recommendations and findings	Treatment	Follow-up	Favorable and unfavorable outcomes include some, but not necessarily all, of the following	
				Favorable outcome	Unfavorable outcome
Clinical findings: The tooth is displaced, usually in a palatal/lingual or labial direction • The tooth will be immobile • Occlusal interference may be present	• A periapical (size 0 sensor/film, paralleling technique) or occlusal radiograph (size 2 sensor/film) should be taken at the time of initial presentation for diagnostic purposes and to establish a baseline • Increased periodontal ligament space apically (most clearly seen on an occlusal radiograph, especially if tooth is displaced labially)	• If there is minimal or no occlusal interference, the tooth should be allowed to spontaneously reposition itself • Spontaneous repositioning usually occurs within 6 months • In situations of severe displacement, two options are available, both of which require local anesthesia: **Option A:** • Extraction when there is a risk of ingestion or aspiration of the tooth **Option B:** • Gently reposition the tooth • If unstable in its new position, splint for 4 weeks using a flexible splint attached to the adjacent uninjured teeth • Treatment should be performed by a child-oriented team with experience and expertise in the management of pediatric dental injuries. Extractions have the potential to cause long-term dental anxiety Parent/patient education: • Exercise care when eating not to further traumatize the injured teeth while encouraging a return to normal function as soon as possible • To encourage gingival healing and prevent plaque accumulation, parents should clean the affected area with a soft brush or cotton swab combined with an alcoholfree chlorhexidine gluconate 0.1%– 0.2% mouth rinse applied topically twice a day for 1 week	• Clinical examination after: • 1 week • 6–8 weeks • 6 months • 1 year • If repositioned and splinted, review after: • 1 week • 4 weeks for splint removal • 8 weeks • 6 months • 1 year • Where there are concerns that an unfavorable outcome is likely, then continue clinical follow-up each year until eruption of the permanent teeth • Radiographic follow-up only indicated where clinical findings are suggestive of pathosis (e.g., an unfavorable outcome) • Parents should be informed to watch for any unfavorable outcomes and the need to return to the clinic as soon as possible. Where unfavorable outcomes are identified, treatment is often required • The follow-up treatment, which frequently requires the expertise of a child-oriented team, is outside the scope of these guidelines	• Asymptomatic • Pulp healing with: • Normal color of the crown or transient red/gray or yellow discoloration and pulp canal obliteration • No signs of pulp necrosis and infection • Continued root development in immature teeth • Periodontal healing • Realignment of the laterally luxated tooth • Normal occlusion • No disturbance to the development and/or eruption of the permanent successor	• Symptomatic • Signs of pulp necrosis and infection, such as: • Sinus tract, gingival swelling, abscess, or increased mobility • Persistent dark gray discoloration plus one or more signs of root canal infection • Radiographic signs of pulp necrosis and infection • Ankylosis • No further root development of immature teeth • No improvement in position of the laterally luxated tooth • Negative impact on the development and/ or eruption of the permanent successor

Table A.24 Treatment guidelines for primary teeth: intrusive luxation.

Intrusive luxation	Radiographic recommendations and findings	Treatment	Follow-up	Favorable and unfavorable outcomes include some, but not necessarily all, of the following	
				Favorable outcome	Unfavorable outcome
Clinical findings: The tooth is usually displaced through the labial bone plate, or it can impinge on the permanent tooth bud • The tooth has almost completely disappeared into the socket and can be palpated labially	• A periapical (size 0 sensor/ film, paralleling technique) or occlusal radiograph (size 2 sensor/film) should be taken at the time of initial presentation for diagnostic purposes and to establish a baseline • When the apex is displaced toward or through the labial bone plate, the apical tip can be seen and the image of the tooth will appear shorter (foreshortened) than the contralateral tooth • When the apex is displaced toward the permanent tooth germ, the apical tip cannot be visualized and the image of the tooth will appear elongated	• The tooth should be allowed to spontaneously reposition itself, irrespective of the direction of displacement • Spontaneous improvement in the position of the intruded tooth usually occurs within 6 months • In some cases, it can take up to 1 year • A rapid referral (within a couple of days) to a child-oriented team that has experience and expertise in the management of pediatric dental injuries should be arranged • Parent/patient education: – Exercise care with eating not to further traumatize the injured tooth while encouraging a return to normal function as soon as possible – To encourage gingival healing and prevent plaque accumulation, parents should clean the affected area with a soft brush or cotton swab combined with an alcoholfree 0.1–0.2% chlorhexidine gluconate mouth rinse applied topically twice a day for 1 week	• Clinical examination after: – 1 week – 6–8 weeks – 6 months – 1 year – Further follow-up at 6 years of age is indicated for severe intrusion to monitor eruption of the permanent tooth • Radiographic follow-up only indicated where clinical findings are suggestive of pathosis (eg, an unfavorable outcome) • Parents should be informed to watch for any unfavorable outcomes and the need to return to the clinic as soon as possible. Where unfavorable outcomes are identified, treatment is often required • The follow-up treatment, which frequently requires the expertise of a child-oriented team, is outside the scope of these guidelines	• Asymptomatic • Pulp healing with: – Normal color of the crown or transient red/gray or yellow discoloration and pulp canal obliteration – No signs of pulp necrosis and infection • Continued root development in immature teeth • Periodontal healing • Re-eruption/ realignment of the intruded tooth • No disturbance to the development and/ or eruption of the permanent successor	• Symptomatic • Signs of pulp necrosis and infection, such as: – Sinus tract, gingival swelling, abscess, or increased mobility – Persistent dark gray discoloration with one or more signs of infection • Radiographic signs of pulp necrosis and infection • No further root development of immature teeth • Ankylosis • Negative impact on the development and/ or eruption of the permanent successor

Table A.25 Treatment guidelines for primary teeth: avulsion.

Avulsion	Radiographic recommendations and findings	Treatment	Follow-up	Favorable and unfavorable outcomes include some, but not necessarily all, of the following	
				Favorable outcome	**Unfavorable outcome**
Clinical findings: The tooth is completely out of the socket	• A periapical (size 0 sensor/ film, paralleling technique) or occlusal radiograph (size 2 sensor/film) is essential where the primary tooth is not brought into the clinic to ensure that the missing tooth has not been intruded	• Avulsed primary teeth should not be replanted	• Clinical examination after:	• No signs of disturbance to development and/or eruption of the permanent successor	• Negative impact on the development and/or eruption of the permanent successor
• The location of the missing tooth should be explored during the trauma history and examination, especially when the accident was not witnessed by an adult or there was a loss of consciousness.		• Parent/patient education:	– 6–8 weeks		
		Exercise care when eating not to further traumatize the injured soft tissues	Further follow-up at 6 years of age is indicated to monitor eruption of the permanent tooth		
• While avulsed teeth are most often lost out of the mouth, there is a risk that they can be embedded in soft tissues of the lip, cheek, or tongue, pushed into the nose, ingested or aspirated.	• The radiograph will also provide a baseline for assessment of the developing permanent tooth and to determine whether it has been displaced	To encourage gingival healing and prevent plaque accumulation, parents should clean the affected area with a soft brush or cotton swab combined with an alcohol-free 0.1–0.2% chlorhexidine gluconate mouth rinse applied topically twice a day for 1 week	• Radiographic follow-up only indicated where clinical findings are suggestive of pathosis (e.g., an unfavorable outcome)		
• If the avulsed tooth is not found, the child should be referred for medical evaluation to an emergency room for further examination, especially where there are respiratory symptoms			• Parents should be informed to watch for any unfavorable outcomes and the need to return to the clinic as soon as possible. Where unfavorable outcomes are identified, treatment is often required		
			• The follow-up treatment, which frequently requires the expertise of a child-oriented team, is outside the scope of these guidelines		

References

1 Bourguignon, C., Cohenca, N., and Lauridesn, E. (2020). International Association of Dental Traumatology guidelines for the management of traumatic dental injuries: 1. Fractures and luxations. *Dent. Traumatol.* 36 (4): 314–330. https://doi.org/10.1111/edt.12578.

2 Fouad, A., Abbott, P., Tsilingaridis, G. et al. (2020). International Association of Dental Traumatology guidelines for the management of traumatic dental injuries: 2. Avulsion of permanent teeth. *Dent. Traumatol* 36 (4): 331–342. https://doi.org/10.1111/edt.12573.

3 Day, P., Flores, M., O'Connell, A. et al. (2020). International Association of Dental Traumatology guidelines for the management of traumatic dental injuries: 3. Injuries in the primary dentition. *Dent. Traumatol.* 36 (4): 343–359. https://doi.org/10.1111/edt.12576.

Appendix B

Basic Life Support

Chapter Outline

- Relevance
- Radiographic Exam
- American Heart Assocation CPR Techniques for the BLS Provider
- Recipe for Life
- Team Dynamics
- Additional Notes
- Prognosis
- Dental-Related Tips
- Miscellaneous

Relevance

Licensed dentists are required to maintain an *active* Basic Life Support (BLS) certificate, which involves recertifying every two years. An understanding of BLS is necessary for responding to someone experiencing cardiac arrest, respiratory distress, or an obstructed airway.

Radiographic Exam

If a patient swallows or aspirates a foreign object while in the dental chair and it cannot be retrieved, immediately refer the patient to a hospital to have an abdominal and chest X-ray. The radiologist or physician will interpret the findings to determine if intervention is required.

Clinical Dentistry Daily Reference Guide, First Edition. William A. Jacobson.
© 2022 John Wiley & Sons, Inc. Published 2022 by John Wiley & Sons, Inc.

American Heart Association CPR Techniques for the BLS Provider

Summary

Action	Adult and adolescents	Child (one year to puberty)	Infant (under one year of age)
Scene safety	Make sure the environment is safe for the rescuer		
Determine unresponsiveness/ cardiac arrest	Check for responsiveness Scan for normal breathing or gasping (gasping is not normal breathing) No definite pulse felt within 10 seconds (pediatric ≤60 bpm)		
You activate EMS	If alone call emergency number; otherwise send someone to call emergency number	Yell for help. Stay and perform two minutes of CPR before you leave and call emergency number	
Hand placement	Two hands on the lower half of the breastbone (sternum)	Two hands or one hand on the lower half of the breastbone (sternum)	Two to three fingers, center of the chest, just below the nipple line
Compression depth	2 inches (5 cm)	2 inches (5 cm)	1.5 inches (3.8 cm)
Compression rate	100–120 compressions per minute		
Airway breathing	Head tilt/chin lift (suspected trauma, use jaw thrust) Two effective breaths; each one second (just enough to see the chest rise)		
Compression/ ventilation ratio	30 : 2 (one or two rescuers)	30 : 2 (single rescuer) 15 : 2 (two rescuers)	30 : 2 (single rescuer) 15 : 2 (two rescuers)
Compression/ ventilation ratio with advanced airway	Continuous compressions at rate of 100–120/min Give one breath every six seconds (10 breaths/min)		
Chest recoil/ minimize interruptions	Allow full recoil of chest after each compression. Do not lean on chest Limit interruptions in chest compressions to less than 10 seconds		

Source: Courtesy of Heartbeat CPR Educators.

Defibrillation

AED	Adult	Child (under eight years of age)	Infant
1. Turn on and follow directions 2. Pads on chest 3. Clear to analyze 4. Push shock button if advised 5. Resume CPR	● Use adult pads ● Do not use child pads/child system on victims eight years or older	● Use AED as soon as available for sudden collapse ● Use child pads (if not available use adult pads)	● A manual defibrillator is preferred ● (If not available) an AED with pediatric attenuation is desirable

Rescue Breathing for the BLS Provider

Adult	Child	Infant
One breath every 5–6 seconds	One breath every 3–5 seconds	One breath every 3–5 seconds

Obstructed Airway for the BLS Provider

Adult	Child	Infant
Responsive victim (conscious)		
Standing abdominal thrust (Heimlich maneuver)		Five back slaps, five chest thrusts
Unresponsive victim (unconscious)		
Activate EMS (if alone, call after two minutes)		
Start CPR, beginning with chest compressions		
Open airway		
Look for object before attempting breaths		
Do not blind finger sweep any victim		

Recipe for Life

- Make sure scene is safe.
- Check for responsiveness.
- Check for normal breathing.
- Check for the carotid pulse (adult and child) or brachial pulse (infant).
  - Breathing and pulse check can be performed simultaneously in less than 10 seconds.
- Activate EMS, call emergency number.
- C: Compress (circulate blood).
- A: Airways: open (head tilt/chin lift).
- B: Breath (ventilate, two full breaths).
- D: Defibrillate.

Team Dynamics

- Successful resuscitation teams:
  - Clear roles and responsibilities: know positions and tasks
  - Know your limitations – boundaries
  - Constructive intervention
- What to communicate:
  - Knowledge sharing
  - Summarizing and reevaluation
- How to communicate:
  - Closed loop communication
  - Clear messages
  - Mutual respect
- Debriefing [1]

Additional Notes

- **Age assessment**
  - Since age is a factor with specific BLS recommendations, it must be defined.
  - Adults: adolescents and older.
  - Children: one year of age to puberty.
  - Infants: less than one year of age [2].
- **Assessment/calling for help**
  - If the victim collapses or is seen collapsed, tap the victim's shoulder and shout "Are you OK?" (If an infant, tap the heel of the foot.)

- ○ Check for responsiveness:
  - ◾ Scan for normal breathing.
  - ◾ Check the pulse (palpate the carotid artery on adults/children; palpate the brachial artery on an infant).
  - ○ If alone call EMS and get the AED. If someone is nearby, shout "Call EMS and retrieve the AED."
- **Abnormal breathing**
  - – Abnormal breathing includes gasping, which may sound like a snort, a snore, a groan, forceful or weak breathing. These are signs of cardiac arrest.
- **Abnormal breathing with a pulse**
  - – If patient has no normal breathing but has a definite pulse, provide rescue breathing of one breath every five to six seconds and after two minutes call EMS. Continue with rescue breathing and checking pulse every two minutes; if no pulse, then begin CPR.
- **EMS**: the trained medical professionals who respond to the emergency call and treat and transport patient to nearby hospitals.
- **Communication**
  - – Closed loop communication: for example, rescuer 1 says "Call EMS and get the AED"; rescuer 2 says "I'm calling EMS and getting the AED."
  - – Constructive intervention: instead of taking over the other rescuer's role, communicate to the rescuer, for example "Compress at a faster rate of 100–120 compressions per minute."
- **Compressions**
  - – Give compression on adults between the nipples.
  - – 100–120 compressions per minute is about twocompressions per second – this is fast.
  - – Lock arms and shoulders so they are stiff during compressions.
- **Ventilation**
  - – Head tilt/chin lift lifts the tongue allowing for a more open airway.
  - – For mouth-to-mouth breathing, pinch the victim's nose closed, seal your lips around the victim's mouth creating an airtight seal and take regular breaths (not deep) and watch for the chest to rise. If chest does not rise repeat the head tilt/chin position and repeat.
  - – If breaths are too rapid or too forceful can cause gastric inflation, which can lead to vomiting, aspiration and pneumonia.
  - – If not comfortable giving mouth-to-mouth, continue giving compressions until further help arrives
  - – Pocket masks are useful as they often have a one-way valve to prevent exhaled air, blood or bodily fluids entering the rescuer's mouth. Make sure the seal is airtight with the mask device, or the ventilation will be ineffective [2].
- **Victim assessment**
  - – Reassess every two minutes: check pulse and breathing and count to five.
  - – Count out loud when checking pulse, checking breathing, when doing compressions, and when giving ventilation. This helps you stay focused as a rescuer and communicates with others around you.
- **Automated external defibrillator (AED)**
  - – The AED is a lightweight, portable, simple-to-operate device that can both identify an abnormal heart rhythm and provide a shock to the victim to restore the normal cardiac rhythm. Arrhythmias, or abnormal heartbeats, prevent the heart from filling and pumping adequate amounts of blood to the tissues and organs of the body. Two life-threatening arrhythmias include:
    - ○ Pulseless ventricular tachycardia: the ventricles, or lower chambers of the heart, contract at such a rapid pace that the blood is not pumped throughout the body. No pulse is detected.

- Ventricular fibrillation: the heart muscles quiver in an unsynchronized way and the heart does not pump blood properly to the body. No pulse is detected.
- How to operate the AED
  - Turn on the AED (some models power on automatically when opening the case).
  - Follow the directions.
  - Attach two electrode pads to the bare chest.
    - Pad size selection:
      a Use adult and child-sized pads appropriately.
      b If only adult-sized pads, these can be used on a child or an infant.
      c If only child-sized pads available, the shock dose will likely be too low for an adult.
  - Pad placement:
    - Remove shirt and bra if present. If bra is kept on chest, patient may experience burns.
    - Special scenarios:
      a) If the chest is hairy, either shave the hair with a razor or press firmly with the pad, rip off and apply a new pad.
      b) If the chest is wet, dry the chest or remove victim from water and dry the chest.
      c) If a transdermal medication patch is present, remove the patch with gloves on, and then attach pads.
      d) If an implanted defibrillator or pacemaker is present, it is not a contraindication. Simply avoid placing the pads over the implanted device as the shock will be less effective.
  - Position of AED electrode pads (as illustrated on the pads):
    - Adults: place one pad below the right collarbone and the other pad to the left of the left nipple a few inches below the left armpit (form a "heart sandwich" [3]).
    - Children and infants: may be placed on the chest and back.
- Shout "clear" for the AED to analyze the rhythm (verify no one is touching the victim).
- If the AED advises a shock, shout "Everybody clear" and verify no one is touching the victim.
  - Press the shock button.
  - The victim's muscles will contract.
  - Immediately resume CPR starting with compressions.
- If the AED does not advise a shock, immediately resume CPR starting with compressions [2]

- **Foreign-body airway obstruction**
  - Adults and adolescents:
    - If the victim appears to be choking and able to forcibly cough, say "Continue coughing."
    - If patient shows no or diminished air exchange, is unable to cough, is wheezing, shows cyanosis (turning blue), is unable to speak, or showing the universal choking symbol:
      - Stand behind victim.
      - Wrap your arms around the middle abdomen below the breastbone and above the belly button.
      - Place one hand into a fist and cover it with your other hand.
      - Thrust upward with quick repeated motions (abdominal thrusts known as the Heimlich maneuver) until the victim expels the object or becomes unresponsive. If unresponsive begin CPR.
  - Infants
    - Five back slaps followed by five chest thrusts and repeat until the object is expelled or the victim becomes unresponsive. If unresponsive begin CPR.
  - If pregnant or obese victim: perform chest thrusts instead of abdominal thrusts [2].

Prognosis

- "Sudden cardiac arrest is a leading cause of death" [2].
- "Death occurs in minutes if the victim does not receive immediate lifesaving treatment" [2].
- "Rapid defibrillation in combination with high-quality CPR can double or triple the chances of survival" [2].

Dental-Related Tips

- When removing an amalgam restoration, isolate with a rubber dam or isolation system (e.g. DryShield, Isovac) to prevent large pieces of amalgam being swallowed or aspirated (leading to airway obstruction).
- When recementing a poorly retentive crown or designing a partial denture, consider if it could lead to an airway obstruction.
- Be careful when trying in a posterior crown. Saliva makes the crown slippery. Have the patient turn their head to the side so that if the crown slips out of your hand it will land on their cheek, as opposed to going down the patient's throat.
- Always place a throat pack (gauze) when doing extractions or sectioning a bridge/crown to prevent foreign objects from being swallowed/aspirated.
  - Caution with the gauze throat pack. If the patient has to cough, they will inhale deeply first and the gauze could become aspirated!
- With medical emergencies it is important to interpret the signs and symptoms as the diagnosis dictates the treatment. One good book to have in your office is:
  - Meiller, T.F., Wynn, R.L., McMullin, A.M., et al. (2016). *Dental Office Medical Emergencies: A Manual of Office Response Protocols*, 6th edn. Hudson, OH: Lexicomp.

Miscellaneous

- Cardiac arrest versus heart attack
  - Cardiac arrest: occurs when the heart has an abnormal rhythm and cannot pump blood to the organs. Within seconds the person becomes unresponsive and is not breathing normally and has no pulse.
  - Heart attack: occurs when there is a blockage of blood flow to the heart muscle causing the muscle to die. Signs include severe discomfort in the chest, pain in the jaw, arms, back or neck, shortness of breath, cold sweats, nausea/vomiting [2]. For heart attack treatment refer to *Dental Office Medical Emergencies: A Manual of Office Response Protocols*.
- CPR versus BLS
  - The main difference is in the curriculum. BLS in general is more advanced training than CPR training and required for those working in healthcare. CPR training is more suited for other professionals such as teachers, coaches, and daycare workers [4].

References

1 HeartBeat CPR Educators (2017). American Heart Association Cardiopulmonary Resuscitation (CPR) Techniques for the Basic Life Support (BLS) provider. www.heartbeatcpr.com (accessed 14 February 2020).

2 American Heart Association. (2016). *Basic Life Support: Provider Manual*. Dallas, TX: AHA.

3 BLS recertification course (2020). www.acls.com (accessed 14 February 2020).

4 National CPR Foundation (2018). BLS vs. CPR: what's the difference? http://www.nationalcprfoundation.com/bls-cpr-differences (accessed 12 February 2020).

Appendix C

Evidence-based Dentistry Pyramid

Relevance

As a dentist you are inundated with dental journal articles, advertisements, sales reps trying to sell you their latest dental products, and patients' questions or claims about topics they've researched online. It will be up to you to decipher the strength of the studies supporting these claims.

Evidence-based dentistry is a "patient-centered approach to treatment decisions, which provides personalized dental care based on the most current scientific knowledge" [1]. The evidence pyramid (Figure C.1) is a visual representation of study designs organized by strength of evidence as one aid to guide you with your analysis of the research.

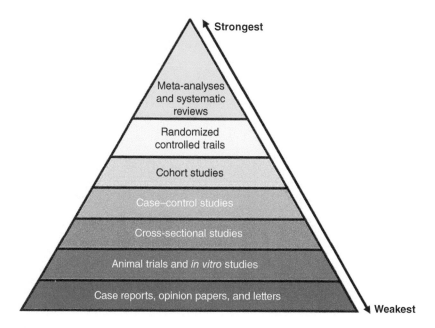

Figure C.1 Hierarchy of scientific evidence [2]. *Source:* The Logic Of Science, Hierarchy of Evidence. Public domain. Licensed under CC BY-SA 4.0.

Clinical Dentistry Daily Reference Guide, First Edition. William A. Jacobson.
© 2022 John Wiley & Sons, Inc. Published 2022 by John Wiley & Sons, Inc.

References

1 American Dental Association (2021). About EBD. https://ebd.ada.org/en/about (accessed 21 March 2021).

2 The University of Alabama at Birmingham (2021). Evidence-based dentistry: determining strength of evidence. https://guides.library.uab.edu/ebd/evidencestrength (accessed 16 March 2021).

Appendix D

Ergonomics for the Dentist, Patient, and Dental Assistant

Dentist

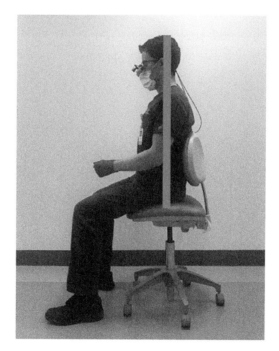

Figure D.1   Sit in a neutral position aligning the ears to shoulders to hips [1].

Clinical Dentistry Daily Reference Guide, First Edition. William A. Jacobson.
© 2022 John Wiley & Sons, Inc. Published 2022 by John Wiley & Sons, Inc.

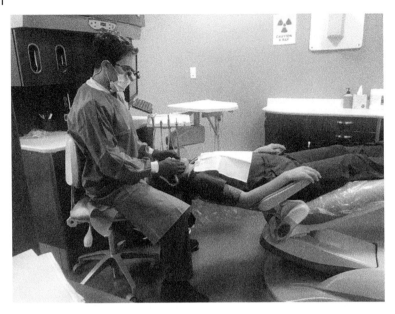

Figure D.2 With your shoulders relaxed, position patient's mouth so it is below your elbow [1].

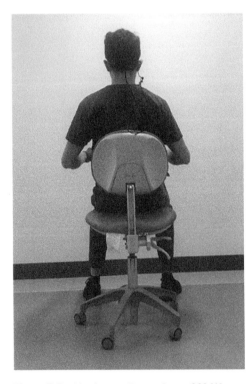

Figure D.3 Maximum elbow raise to 20° [1].

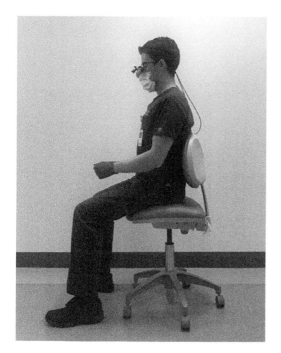

Figure D.4 Maximum head tilt to 20°. Instead of lowering your head more, look down with your eyes [1].

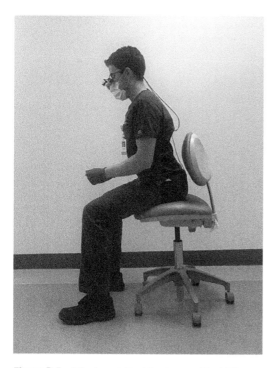

Figure D.5 Hinging at the hips is permitted [1].

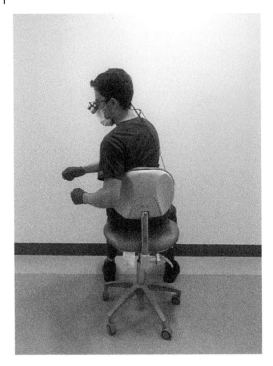

Figure D.6   Avoid twisting when working or to grab instruments. Instead swivel in the chair [1].

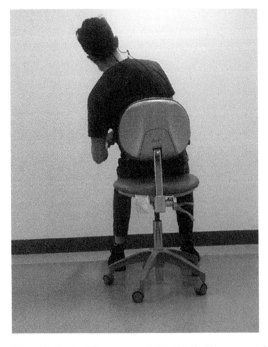

Figure D.7   Avoid uneven weight distribution on one hip [1].

Patient

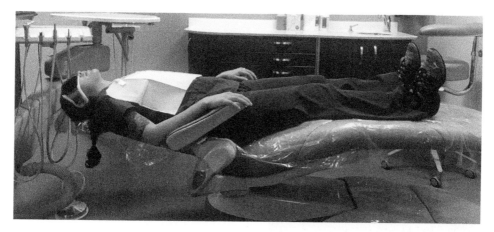

Figure D.8   When working on the maxillary arch the patient should be supine with their chin up.

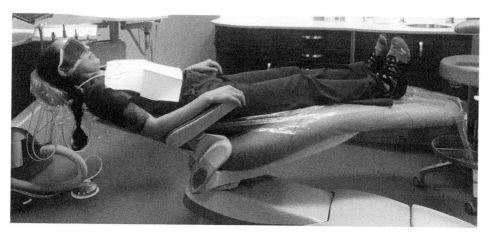

Figure D.9   When working on the mandibular arch the patient should be semi-supine (15–20°) with their chin down.

Dental Assistant

Picture the patient's face being a clock. When working with a right-handed dentist sitting at 9–12 o'clock, the assistant will sit at 2–4 o'clock. When working with a left-handed dentist sitting at 12–3 o'clock, the assistant will sit at 8–10 o'clock. If the dentist is standing for a procedure (typically with oral surgery), the assistant will also stand.

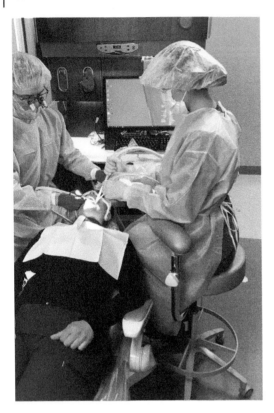

Figure D.10 The height of the assistant's chair must be higher than that of the dentist's chair (6 inches [15 cm] above the dentist's eye level [1]) with the assistant's feet on the footrest. The elbows should rest on the arm rest. The assistant should not lean their body weight or stomach on the arm rest or the chair can fall over onto the patient.

Reference

1 Gehrig, J.S., Sroda, R., and Saccuzzo, D. (2016). *Fundamentals of Periodontal Instrumentation*, 8e. Burlington, MA: Jones and Bartlett Learning.

Appendix E

"CAMBRA" CAries Management By Risk Assessment*

Chapter Outline

- Background
- Low Risk
- Moderate Risk
- High Risk
- Extreme Risk

Background

- Based on studies conducted at University of California San Francisco (USCF).
- CAMBRA is an evidence-based approach to preventing, reversing, and treating dental caries.
- In order to reduce the caries risk level, it requires minimally invasive restorative work, chemical therapy, and behavioral change.
- One major takeaway from the CAMBRA studies is that simply placing restorations (also known as "drilling and filling") did not lower the caries risk level of an individual.
- CAMBRA intervention studies showed a significant reduction in the caries risk level and caries disease indicators (i.e. new caries lesions) in thousands of patients.

Low Risk

- The results of your exam indicate that you are at **low risk** for development of new cavities in the future.
    - Keep doing what you are doing and make sure to:
        - Use an over-the-counter fluoride toothpaste (1000–1450 ppm F) twice daily.
        - Floss before brushing at night.
        - Visit the dentist for follow-up visits every 12 months.

Moderate Risk

- The results of your exam indicate that you are at **moderate risk** for development of new cavities in the future.
    - To reduce the risk, please do the following:
        - Option 1:
            - Brush twice a day with over-the-counter fluoride toothpaste.

Clinical Dentistry Daily Reference Guide, First Edition. William A. Jacobson.
© 2022 John Wiley & Sons, Inc. Published 2022 by John Wiley & Sons, Inc.

a) Brush after breakfast, and at night floss before brushing.
- Rinse with a 0.05% sodium fluoride mouthrinse before going to sleep.
  - Option 2:
    - Brush twice a day with prescription-strength toothpaste (Clinpro 5000 or Prevident 5000) instead of your regular toothpaste. After brushing spit, don't rinse with water. Do not eat or drink for 30 minutes after.
      b) Brush teeth after breakfast, and at night floss before brushing.
    - Reduce the number of between-meal carbohydrate-rich snacks.
    - Visit the dentist for follow-up visits every six months.

High Risk

- The results of your exam indicate that you are at **high risk** for development of new cavities in the future.
  - To reduce the risk, please do the following:
    - Visit the dentist for fluoride varnish application every four to six months.
    - Brush twice a day with prescription-strength toothpaste (Clinpro 5000 or Prevident 5000) instead of your regular toothpaste. After brushing spit, don't rinse with water. Do not eat or drink for 30 minutes after.
      - Brush teeth after breakfast. Before bed, floss your teeth before brushing.
    - 0.12% Chlorhexidine gluconate mouthrinse: swish one tablespoon (15 mL) for one minute and expectorate (spit) after breakfast and before bed after brushing.
      - Use this rinse twice a day for one week (seven days) per month. You could do this the first.
      - This should be one hour apart from the fluoride toothbrushing.
      - To be continued for a least a year until the disease is controlled and the risk level is lowered.
    - Reduce the number of between-meal carbohydrate-rich snacks
    - Visit the dentist for fluoride varnish application every four to six months.
    - Visit the dentist for follow-up visits every four to six months.

Extreme Risk

- The results of your exam indicate that you are at **extreme risk** for development of new cavities in the future.
  - To reduce the risk, please do the following:
    - Visit the dentist for fluoride varnish application every four to six months.
    - Brush twice a day with prescription-strength toothpaste (Clinpro 5000 or Prevident 5000) instead of your regular toothpaste. After brushing spit, don't rinse with water. Do not eat or drink for 30 minutes after.
      - Brush teeth after breakfast. Before bed, floss your teeth before brushing.
    - 0.12% Chlorhexidine gluconate mouthrinse: swish one tablespoon (15 mL) for one minute and expectorate (spit) after breakfast and before bed after brushing.
      - Use this rinse twice a day for one week (seven days) per month. You could do this the first.
      - This should be one hour apart from the fluoride toothbrushing.
      - To be continued for a least a year until the disease is controlled and the risk level is lowered.

- ○ Rinse as often as desired throughout the day with a baking soda solution to control the pH level in the mouth.
  - ▪ Must be made fresh daily.
  - ▪ Two teaspoons of baking soda in 8 ounces (250 ml) of water.
- ○ Reduce the number of between-meal carbohydrate-rich snacks.
- ○ Visit the dentist for fluoride varnish application every four to six months.
- ○ Visit the dentist for follow-up visits every three to four months.
  - ▪ *If risk is not being lowered, you may require a custom fluoride tray fabricated at the dentist with a prescription 5000 ppm fluoride gel to be used for five minutes daily.*

Index